To Lisa, Margaret, and David Babikian for their unwavering love and support.
They are the source of my inspiration.

To my loving and understanding wife, Phyllis Cook Wechsler

With all my love to my wife, Jeannie Higashida, M.D.

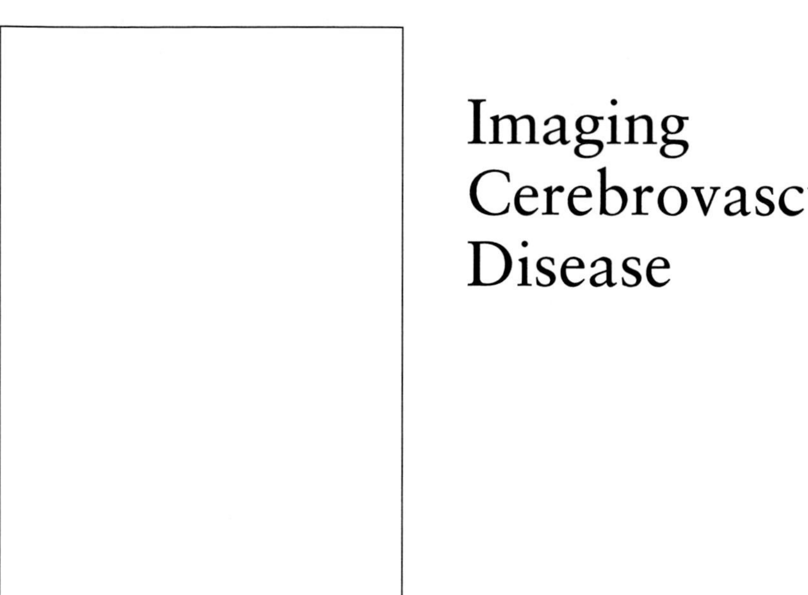

Imaging Cerebrovascular Disease

Imaging Cerebrovascular Disease

Edited by

Viken L. Babikian, M.D.

Professor of Neurology, Boston University School of Medicine; Stroke Service, Boston Medical Center and Boston Veterans Administration Medical Center

Lawrence R. Wechsler, M.D.

Professor of Neurology, University of Pittsburgh School of Medicine; Director, University of Pittsburgh Medical Center Stroke Institute

Randall T. Higashida, M.D.

Clinical Professor of Radiology, Neurological Surgery, Neurology, and Anesthesiology, Director, Division of Interventional Neurovascular Radiology, University of California, San Francisco, Medical Center

With 38 Contributing Authors

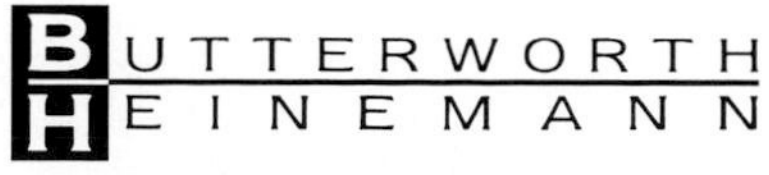

An imprint of Elsevier Science

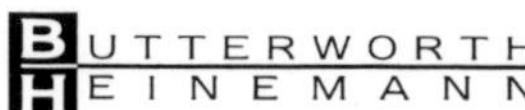

An imprint of Elsevier Science

The Curtis Center
Independence Square West
Philadelphia, PA 19106

Imaging Cerebrovascular Disease 0-7506-7302-8

Notice

Neurology is an ever-changing field. Standard safety precautions must be followed, but as new research and clinical experience broaden our knowledge, changes in treatment and drug therapy may become necessary or appropriate. Readers are advised to check the most current product information provided by the manufacturer of each drug to be administered to verify the recommended dose, the method and duration of administration, and contraindications. It is the responsibility of the treating physician, relying on experience and knowledge of the patient, to determine dosages and the best treatment for each individual patient. Neither the Publisher nor the author assume any liability for any injury and/or damage to persons or property arising from this publication.

The Publisher

Library of Congress Cataloging-in-Publication Data

Imaging cerebrovascular disease / [edited by] Viken L. Babikian, Lawrence R. Wechsler, and Randall T. Higashida.— 1st ed.
p. ; cm.
Includes bibliographical references and index.
ISBN 0-7506-7302-8
1. Cerebrovascular system—Imaging. 2. Diagnostic imaging. I. Babikian, Viken L. II. Wechsler, Lawrence R. III. Higashida, Randall T.
[DNLM: 1. Cerebrovascular Diseases—diagnosis. 2. Diagnostic Imaging—methods. WG 141 I307 2003]
RC683.5.I42 I427 2003
616.1'0754—dc21

2002071226

Publisher: Susan F. Pioli
Editorial Assistant: Joan Ryan

SSC/DN

Printed in China

9 8 7 6 5 4 3 2 1

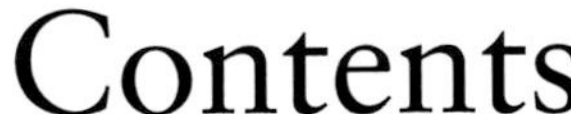

Contents

Contributing Authors

Nafi Aygun, M.D.
Staff, Department of Radiology, Section of Neuroradiology, The Cleveland Clinic Foundation

Viken L. Babikian, M.D.
Professor of Neurology, Boston University School of Medicine; Stroke Service, Boston Medical Center and Boston Veterans Administration Medical Center

Jean-Claude Baron, M.D.
Professor of Stroke Medicine, Department of Neurology, University of Cambridge, Cambridge, United Kingdom; Honorary Consultant in Neurology, Addenbrooke's Hospital, Cambridge

John D. Barr, M.D.
Chief, Interventional Neuroradiology, Department of Neuroradiology, Baptist Memorial Hospital, Memphis, Tennessee

Robert J. Bert, M.D.
Assistant Professor of Radiology, Tufts University School of Medicine; Neuroradiologist, Tufts-New England Medical Center, Boston

William G. Bradley, Jr., M.D., Ph.D., F.A.C.R.
Professor and Chairman, Department of Radiology, University of California, San Diego, School of Medicine

Bohdan W. Chopko, M.D., Ph.D.
Assistant Professor, Department of Neurobiology, Northeastern Ohio Universities College of Medicine, Rootstown; Chief, Endovascular Surgery, Surgical Neurology of North Central Ohio, Mansfield

DeWitte T. Cross III, M.D.
Associate Professor of Radiology, Mallinckrodt Institute of Radiology, Washington University School of Medicine, St. Louis; Director of Interventional Neuroradiology, Barnes-Jewish Hospital, St. Louis

William P. Dillon, M.D.
Professor of Radiology, Neurology, and Neurosurgery, Chief, Section of Neurology, University of California, San Francisco, School of Medicine

Christopher F. Dowd, M.D.
Associate Clinical Professor of Radiology, Neurological Surgery, Neurology, Anesthesiology, and Perioperative Care, The Neurovascular Medical Group, University of California, San Francisco, Medical Center

Marc Fisher, M.D.
Professor and Vice Chairman, Department of Neurology, University of Massachusetts Medical School, Worcester; Director of Stroke Services, University of Massachusetts Memorial Health Care, Worcester

Alejandro M. Forteza, M.D.
Associate Professor of Neurology, University of Miami School of Medicine; Director, Stroke Service, Department of Neurology, Jackson Memorial Hospital, Miami

Daryl R. Gress, M.D.
Associate Professor of Clinical Neurology and Neurosurgery, Department of Neurology, University of California, San Francisco, School of Medicine; Director, Neurovascular Service, Department of Neurology, University of California, San Francisco, Medical Center

Van Halbach, M.D.
Clinical Professor of Radiology, Neurological Surgery, Neurology, and Anesthesiology, University of California, San Francisco, Medical Center

Randall T. Higashida, M.D.
Clinical Professor of Radiology, Neurological Surgery, Neurology, and Anesthesiology, Director, Division of Interventional Neurovascular Radiology, University of California, San Francisco, Medical Center

David T. Jeck, M.D.
Interventional Neuroradiologist, Radiology Limited, Tucson, Arizona

Tudor G. Jovin, M.D.
Assistant Professor of Neurology, University of Pittsburgh School of Medicine; University of Pittsburgh Medical Center Stroke Institute, Presbyterian University Hospital

Manfred Kaps, M.D., Ph.D.
Chairman of Neurology, Justus-Liebig-University Giessen, Giessen, Germany

Sebastian Koch, M.D.
Assistant Professor of Neurology, University of Miami School of Medicine; Stroke Service, Department of Neurology, Jackson Memorial Hospital, Miami

Walter J. Koroshetz, M.D.
Associate Professor, Department of Neurology, Harvard Medical School, Boston; Vice Chair, Department of Neurology, Massachusetts General Hospital, Boston

Jaroslaw Krejza, M.D., Ph.D.
Associate Professor of Radiology, Bialystok University School of Medicine, Bialystok, Poland; Director, Cerebrovascular Laboratory, University Hospital of Bialystok Medical Academy, Bialystok

Theodore J. Lee, M.D.
Resident Physician, Department of Radiology, University of California, San Francisco, School of Medicine

Elad I. Levy, M.D.
Endovascular Fellow, Department of Neurosurgery, University at Buffalo School of Medicine and Biomedical Sciences, Buffalo, New York

José C. Masdeu, M.D., Ph.D.
Professor and Director, Department of the Neurological Sciences, University of Navarre Medical School, Pamplona, Spain; Director, Neuroscience Center, University Hospital, Pamplona

Peter J. Mitchell, M.B., F.R.A.N.Z.C.R.
Director of Neurointerventional Radiology, Department of Radiology, The University of Melbourne, The Royal Melbourne Hospital, Melbourne, Victoria, Australia

Gary M. Nesbit, M.D.
Associate Professor, Division of Neuroradiology, Oregon Health Sciences University School of Medicine; Dotter Interventional Institute, Portland

Walter D. Obrist, Ph.D.
Professor Emeritus of Neurological Surgery, University of Pittsburgh School of Medicine

John Perl II, M.D.
Director, Endovascular Neurosurgery, Departments of Neuroradiology and Neurosurgery, The Cleveland Clinic Foundation

Heidi C. Roberts, M.D.
Associate Professor of Radiology, Department of Medical Imaging, University of Toronto Faculty of Medicine

Timothy P. L. Roberts, Ph.D.
Associate Professor, Director of Research and Vice-Chair, Canada Research Chair in Imaging Research; Department of Medical Imaging, University of Toronto Faculty of Medicine

Vineeta Singh, M.D.
Assistant Clinical Professor, Department of Neurology, Division of Neurovascular and Neurocritical Care, University of California, San Francisco, School of Medicine

Michael A. Sloan, M.D.
Associate Professor of Neurological Sciences and Neurosurgery, Rush Medical College; Director, Inpatient Stroke Service, Director, Cerebrovascular Ultrasonography Laboratory, Rush Presbyterian St. Luke's Medical Center

Erwin P. Stolz, M.D.
Attending Physician, Department of Neurology, Justus-Liebig-University Giessen, Giessen, Germany

Robert W. Tarr, M.D.
Associate Professor of Radiology, Neurology, and Neurosurgery, Case Western Reserve Medical School, Cleveland, Ohio; Director of Interventional Neuroradiology, University Hospitals of Cleveland

David E. Thaler, M.D.
Assistant Professor of Neurology, Tufts University School of Medicine; Co-Director, Tufts Comprehensive Stroke Center at New England Medical Center

Tjhi Wen Tjauw, M.D.
Assistant Professor, Department of Diagnostic Radiology, Oregon Health Sciences University School of Medicine, Portland; Neuroradiologist, Department of Diagnostic Radiology, Oregon Health Sciences University School of Medicine

Lawrence R. Wechsler, M.D.
Professor of Neurology, University of Pittsburgh School of Medicine; Director, University of Pittsburgh Medical Center Stroke Institute

Howard Yonas, M.D.
Peter J. Jannetta Professor and Vice Chairman of Academic Affairs, Department of Neurological Surgery, University of Pittsburgh School of Medicine; Chief of Cerebrovascular Surgery, Department of Neurological Surgery, Co-Director of University of Pittsburgh Medical Center Stroke Institute, Presbyterian University Hospital

Preface

A detailed history and examination are the main techniques on which clinicians have traditionally relied to make a diagnosis of stroke and prescribe appropriate treatment. Although they remain the cornerstones of clinical medicine, advances over the past two decades in imaging the brain and its vasculature and new neurointerventional technologies have reshaped the basic understanding of cerebrovascular disease processes. They have also substantially improved both the diagnostic and therapeutic landscapes. It is virtually impossible today to provide care to patients with acute stroke or chronic cerebrovascular disease without some diagnostic testing, and it is not uncommon for the neuroimaging test to force a rethinking of the initial clinical impression.

Imaging Cerebrovascular Disease stems from this background. It aims at integrating the clinical and radiologic features of cerebrovascular diseases, and it addresses both the diagnostic and therapeutic aspects of disease management. What are the basic anatomic and physiologic disease processes, and how is neuroimaging technology helping in their understanding? How is this understanding translating into patient care today? Where is the future of these diagnostic and therapeutic techniques headed? These are questions the authors have asked themselves, and this book is designed to provide at least some answers.

The management of patients with acute or chronic cerebrovascular diseases increasingly requires the coordination of the efforts of physicians from different specialties. To improve the quality of care for stroke patients, interdepartmental boundaries were crossed, and an integrated team approach was introduced at major medical centers during the early 1990s. *Imaging Cerebrovascular Disease* was written with the "Stroke Team" in mind. It represents the combined efforts of radiology, neurology, neurosurgery, and intensive care specialists who recognize that it is no longer sufficient for a specialist to master only the knowledge base of his or her own area of expertise. Improved patient care necessitates a broader and more detailed understanding of the problems faced by patients with cerebrovascular disease. We hope *Imaging Cerebrovascular Disease* facilitates this understanding.

Viken L. Babikian, M.D.
Lawrence R. Wechsler, M.D.
Randall T. Higashida, M.D.

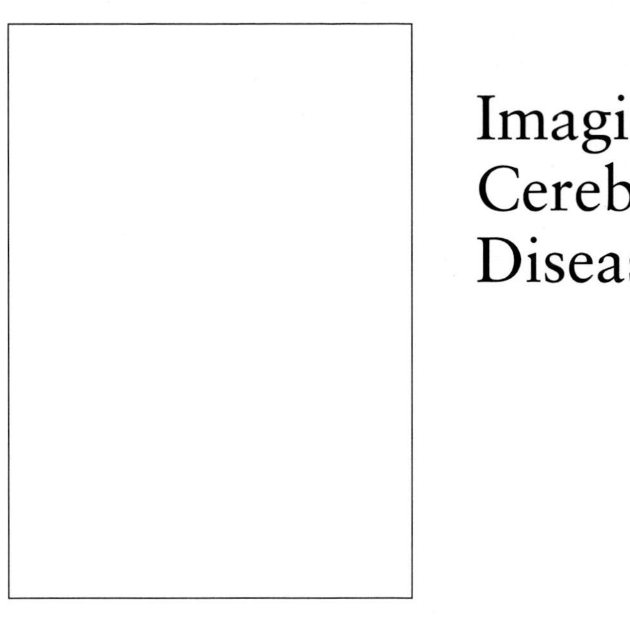

Imaging Cerebrovascular Disease

Section

I

Cerebral Vascular Imaging

CHAPTER

1

Ultrasound Imaging of Cerebrovascular Disease

Alejandro M. Forteza, Jaroslaw Krejza, Sebastian Koch, and Viken L. Babikian

Introduced to clinical use as echoencephalography[1] in the early 1950s, ultrasonic imaging of the brain has evolved considerably since, and a variety of techniques are used today to study the cerebral vasculature and blood flow. Ultrasonic imaging is considered an integral part of the evaluation of patients with cerebrovascular disease because it is noninvasive, relatively inexpensive, and readily accessible. This chapter summarizes the state of the art regarding the clinical applications of ultrasound imaging for cerebrovascular disease.

SOME PHYSICAL PRINCIPLES OF ULTRASONOGRAPHY

A comprehensive review of the physical principles that form the basis of medical ultrasonography is beyond the scope of this chapter. In the following paragraphs, a brief definition of terms is presented.

Interactions of Ultrasound with Tissue

Ultrasonic waves entering human tissue are transmitted, absorbed, reflected, and scattered (Figure 1-1).[2,3] The transmission properties of a tissue depend on its density and elasticity. Density and speed of propagation of ultrasound waves determine a tissue's acoustic impedance. In homogeneous tissues, sound waves propagate until all their energy is dissipated and has been converted to heat. In nonhomogeneous tissues, when ultrasound waves strike a medium with a different acoustic impedance, reflection, scattering, transmission, or a combination of these processes occurs. The larger the difference in acoustic impedance between tissues is, the more ultrasound waves are reflected. Reflection further depends on the angle of insonation, and stronger echoes are received when the angle of insonation is zero. Reflected waves return to the transducer as echoes, and the corresponding signals are processed to create images of the tissue of interest. Strongly reflective interfaces such as bone or air prevent imaging of weaker echoes from deeper tissue and cast an acoustic shadow behind them. This prevents imaging of distal structures. Tissues that strongly reflect ultrasound are called *hyperechoic*, whereas poorly reflective tissues are described as *hypoechoic*. Fluids, which do not reflect ultrasound, are called *anechoic* or *sonolucent*.

Echo Display Modes

Structures imaged by B-mode, or brightness mode, imaging are displayed proportionally to the intensity of returning echoes.[2,3] An ultrasonic beam scanning through a tissue plane produces a two-dimensional gray-scale image. In routine clinical practice, the beam is swept quickly through the field of view, and the image is continuously renewed, allowing a real-time visualization of the underlying tissue anatomy. In M-mode imaging, a vertical time-base trace driven from left to right across the display is simultaneously generated.[2] The echoes converted to bright spots are displayed and swept across the screen over time. They are spaced vertically as the depth of ultrasound penetration increases. The M-mode method is used to evaluate the motion of well-defined surfaces such as blood vessel walls.[4,5]

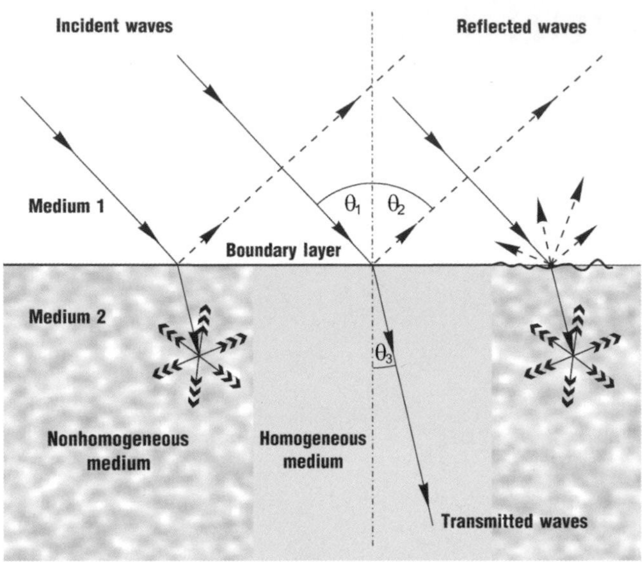

FIGURE 1-1. Interactions of ultrasound with tissues. The interface of medium 1 and medium 2 is regular, and incident ultrasound waves are reflected and transmitted. An irregular interface surface additionally causes scattering of the ultrasound beam, as seen on the right of the figure. (θ_1 = insonation angle; θ_2 = reflection angle; θ_3 = refraction angle.)

Doppler Display Modes and Blood Velocity Measurements

The difference in frequency between emitted and returning ultrasonic echoes is the Doppler frequency shift.[2] The magnitude of the shift depends on the ultrasound transmission velocity in the insonated tissue (*C*), the relative velocities of the reflector (blood, *V*), and the frequency of the source (*Fo*). The observed frequency shift (ΔF) is $\Delta F = 2VFo/C$.[2,4] The shift is measured only for that component of motion occurring along the axis of the ultrasound beam. Therefore, absolute velocity measurements require that a correction be made for the angle (θ) between the vessel and the beam as follows: $V = \Delta FC/(2Fo \cos \theta)$. In routine clinical practice, Doppler modes are used to measure flow velocity (Figure 1-2). The frequency shift is proportional to the velocity of moving blood.

Continuous-Wave Doppler

The simplest Doppler ultrasound instrument has two identical piezoelectric crystal transducers. One crystal continuously emits toward the region of interest, and the other continuously receives reflected echoes. Flow toward the transducer produces an increase in the received frequency, whereas flow away from the transducer causes a drop. Continuous Doppler systems can measure a wide range of velocities without a limit. However, they do not provide any information about the

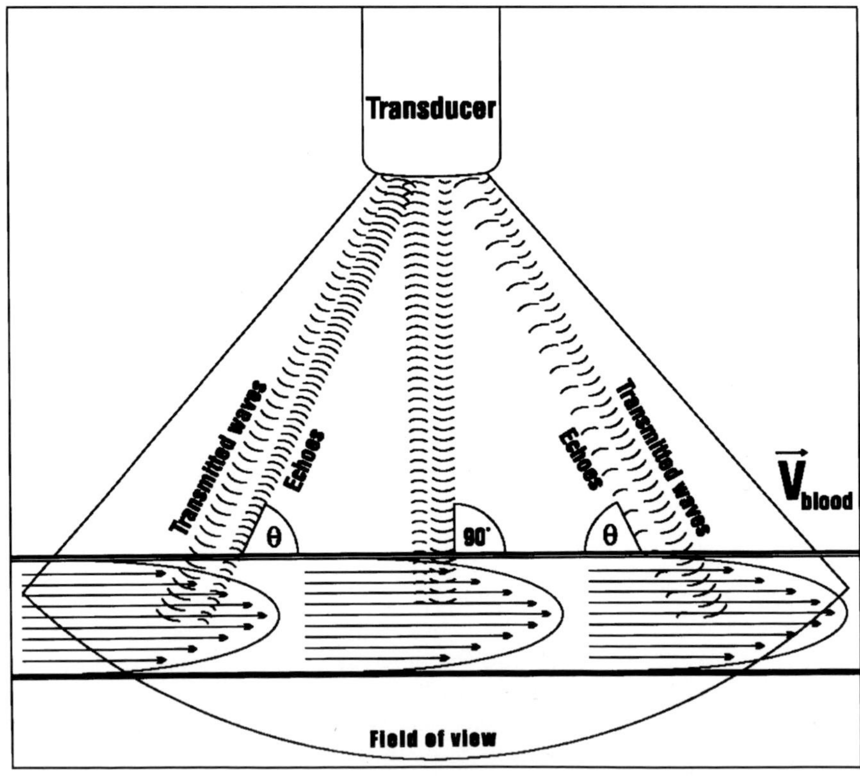

FIGURE 1-2. Doppler effect. As blood flows toward the transducer, returning echoes have a shortened wavelength. The opposite occurs as blood flows away from the transducer. The angle of insonation is θ. (V = blood flow velocity.)

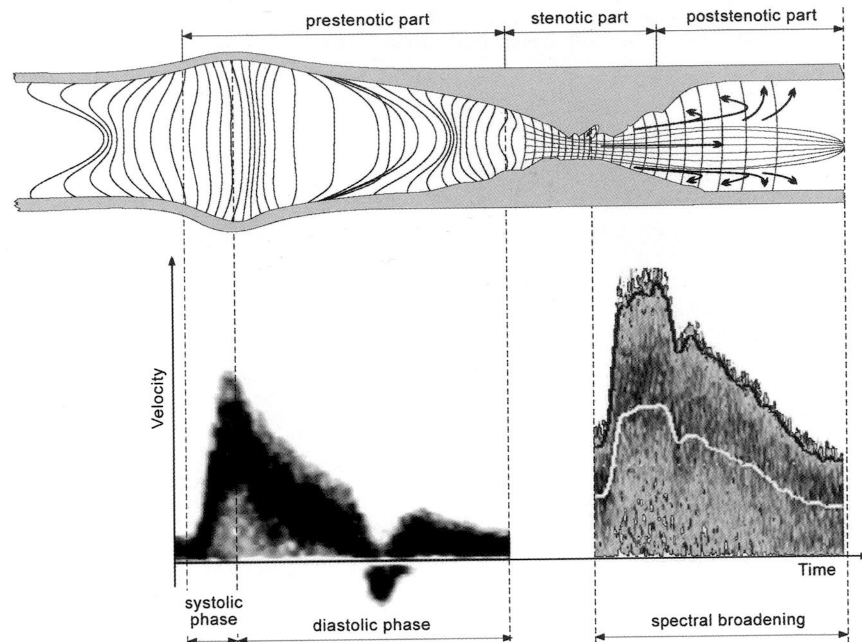

FIGURE 1-3. Effect of arterial stenosis on laminar blood flow. In the prestenotic segment, the spectral image shows a laminar flow pattern. In the poststenotic segment, the peak systolic and end-diastolic velocities are increased, and spectral broadening is present.

depth of the reflecting tissue because any moving object in the beam's pathway reflects echoes.

Pulsed-Wave Doppler

The depth or position insensitivity of continuous-wave Doppler is overcome to a large extent by using pulsed-wave Doppler. In this technique, a single transducer generates ultrasound pulses and detects returning echoes. Assuming that the speed of transmission of ultrasound in human tissues is a constant, the time delay between the emitted pulse and the returning echo enables the sampled structure's depth to be determined. However, anatomy is not displayed, and the pulse's duration and repetition frequency impose limits on the maximum velocity that can be measured. This technique is used for conventional transcranial Doppler ultrasound (TCD).

Duplex Doppler

Duplex imaging combines pulsed-wave Doppler with two-dimensional, real-time, gray-scale imaging. The gray-scale image of a selected vessel is displayed, allowing precise placement of the Doppler sample volume in the vessel to measure flow velocity throughout the cardiac cycle. Optimal angle correction for velocity calculations can be performed, as the course of the vessel in relation to the ultrasound beam is visually depicted.

Color-Flow Doppler

Color duplex is the most commonly used technology today for extracranial carotid imaging. It is also used for transcranial color Doppler ultrasonography (TCCD). Color is superimposed on a conventional gray-scale image to enhance the image of the Doppler frequency shift. Red indicates flow toward the transducer, whereas blue represents flow away from the transducer. High flow velocities are depicted with increasing brightness. As a result, the presence of flow, its direction, and hemodynamic disturbances can be quickly assessed.

Power Doppler

Power Doppler ultrasonography emphasizes the display of amplitude information rather than velocity. The color map in color Doppler ultrasonography displays the integrated power of the Doppler signal, which is related to the number of red blood cells that produce the Doppler shift. Advantages of power Doppler include independence from the angle of insonation, absence of aliasing, and the ability to detect very low flows.

Normal and Abnormal Flow Patterns

In healthy individuals, arterial flow is pulsatile and laminar.[6] The development of focal stenoses causes the laminar flow pattern in diastole to undergo early disruptions (Figure 1-3). Additionally, the presence of turbulence at, and distal to, the stenosed area causes an increase in the range of flow velocities, a phenomenon known as *spectral broadening*.[2] As the degree of stenosis progresses, flow velocities—particularly the peak systolic velocity—increase at the point of maximum narrowing. In very severe stenosis, marked reductions in the residual

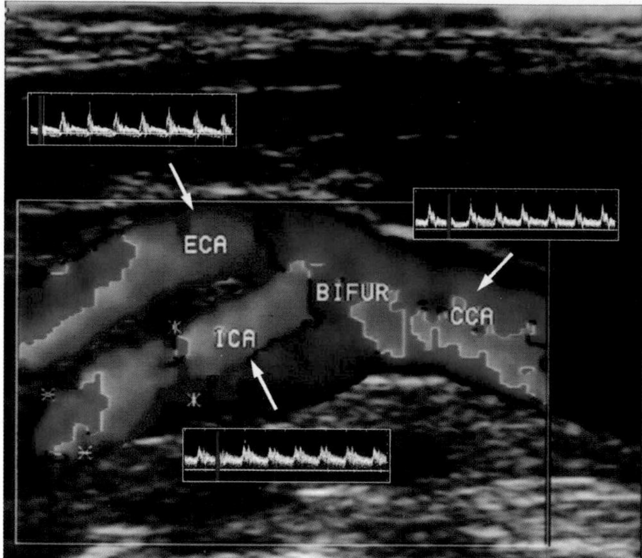

FIGURE 1-4. Common carotid artery (CCA) bifurcation (BIFUR). The Doppler waveforms depict the characteristic flow patterns of the internal carotid artery (ICA), external carotid artery (ECA), and CCA. A low-resistance flow pattern is seen in the ICA, a relatively elevated resistance flow pattern is seen in the ECA, and an intermediate resistance flow pattern is seen in the CCA. These patterns aid in the ultrasonographic identification of the vessels.

lumen cause flow velocities to fall, ultimately leading to flow cessation with complete lumen obliteration. Doppler insonation proximal to an occluded vessel assumes a stump flow pattern.

Impedance Indices

The downstream cerebrovascular impedance can be estimated with the pulsatility and resistance indices,[7,8] which can be calculated from the Doppler velocity waveform (Figure 1-4). Flow, in the external carotid artery, supplying high-resistance arterial beds, is characterized by high-impedance indices. Internal carotid artery (ICA) and intracranial artery waveforms have relatively low-impedance indices because they supply the low-resistance vascular bed of the brain.

Transducers

Piezoelectric crystals arranged geometrically into an array inside the transducer produce the ultrasound beam. A linear array produces a rectangular field of view, which is most useful in carotid imaging. A phased array is used for TCD and produces a wedge-shaped field of view. The frequencies generally used for neurosonology range from 1.0 to 3.5 MHz for transcranial imaging and 7.5 to 16.0 MHz for carotid imaging.

DUPLEX IMAGING OF EXTRACRANIAL ARTERIES

Vascular Pathology as Seen by Ultrasound

Atherosclerosis is a dynamic process. The earliest atherosclerotic changes include intimal thickening secondary to lipid deposits and lipid-laden macrophage infiltration of the arterial wall.[9,10] These events are displayed on B-mode ultrasonography as a thickening of the intima and media. As the process advances, atheromatous plaques begin to protrude into the arterial lumen. Initially, these plaques are covered with a fibrous cap that gives them mechanical stability.[9] Fibrous plaques are rarely associated with neurologic symptoms.[11,12] On ultrasound, they appear smooth, isoechoic, and homogenous (Figure 1-5A). During subsequent stages, increasing amounts of extracellular lipids and cholesterol esthers are deposited, calcification occurs, and intraplaque hemorrhages develop,[9] giving the plaque a heterogeneous appearance on ultrasonographic examination. When the mechanical support of the plaque surface erodes, embolization of plaque contents may occur. In addition, plaque surface ulcers may develop and serve as foci for thrombus formation. These plaques appear heterogeneous with variable echodensities, calcific shadows, and surface irregularities[11,12] (see Figure 1-5B).

Morphologic and physiologic features readily assessed with ultrasonography and associated with an increased risk of cerebral infarction include intraplaque echolucency, surface ulceration, and, most important, degree of stenosis.

Plaque Echolucency and Surface Ulceration

Chemical composition and some morphologic features are related to plaque stability and emboligenic potential. Pathologic studies of carotid endarterectomy specimens obtained from symptomatic patients reveal an increase in intraplaque hemorrhage and in the relative proportion of lipids.[13–15] These areas appear echolucent on ultrasonographic examination[16,17] (see Figure 1-5C), and a classification of the severity of echolucency has been proposed.[18] Prospective studies have confirmed the increased stroke risk associated with carotid plaque echolucency.[19–22] A surface alteration such as ulceration is thought to serve as a nidus for the generation of mural platelet-fibrin thromboemboli.[23] The notion is further supported by pathologic studies[24] and by large clinical trials. In the North American Symptomatic Carotid Endarterectomy Trial (NASCET), even when severe stenosis was present, plaque ulceration almost doubled the risk of stroke in medically treated patients.[25] When compared to endarterectomy specimens, the B-mode ultrasonographic and angiographic detection of ulceration has been poor,[26–28] thus limiting the clinical usefulness of

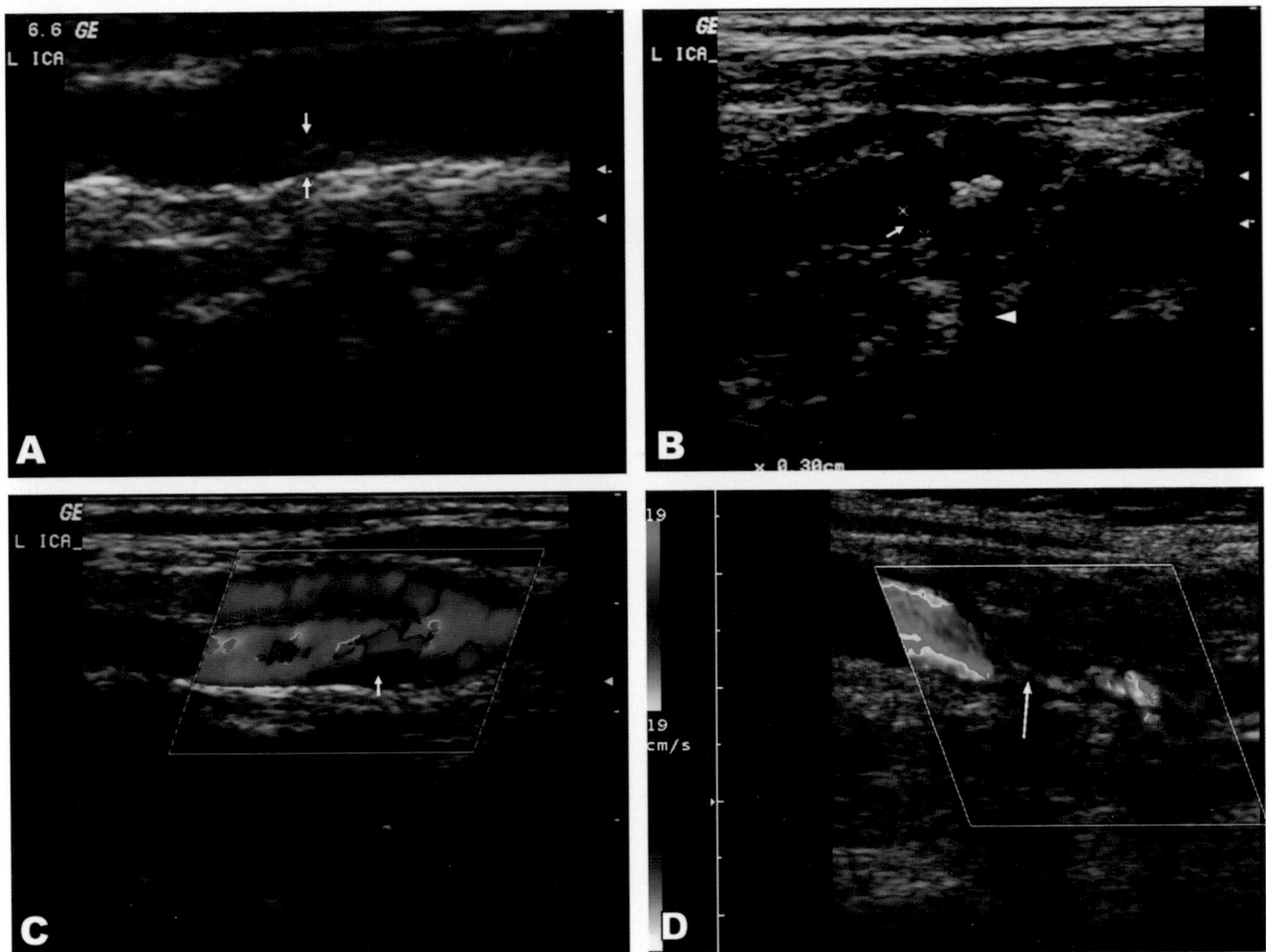

FIGURE 1-5. Atherosclerotic plaques. **A.** Homogenous, soft, and fibrous plaque (*arrows*) at the internal carotid artery (ICA) origin. **B.** Heterogeneous, complex plaque. Hypoechoic area (*arrow*) and an acoustic shadow (*arrowhead*) caused by calcification. **C.** Echolucent plaque (*arrow*) at the origin of the ICA. **D.** High-grade ICA stenosis causing aliasing (*arrow*) on color Doppler.

the observation. Color duplex testing has improved the clinician's diagnostic capability. It has an accuracy of 94% when compared to surgical findings.[29,30]

Degree of Stenosis

The NASCET, the European Carotid Surgery Trial (ECST), and the Asymptomatic Carotid Artery Surgery (ACAS) trial demonstrated the benefit of endarterectomy in symptomatic and asymptomatic patients with moderate and severe carotid stenosis.[31–34] In the NASCET, however, endarterectomy was only marginally beneficial if the degree of stenosis was between 50% and 70%,[33] underscoring the importance of accurately measuring the severity of stenosis. Ultrasonography must, therefore, be able to distinguish between a carotid stenosis of 50–70% in symptomatic patients and to identify a 60% diameter stenosis in asymptomatic patients.

Catheter angiography, the diagnostic gold standard for the evaluation of the cerebral vasculature, carries a small but non-negligible risk of cerebral ischemia.[35] Noninvasive evaluation of the extracranial ICA with color duplex ultrasonography and magnetic resonance angiography (MRA) is increasingly regarded as a replacement, but its role is not undisputed.[36] In a recent study comparing duplex ultrasonography to catheter angiography, duplex ultrasonography misclassified 28% of patients considered candidates for carotid endarterectomy.[37] Other studies suggest that this classification can be performed accurately if high standards of ultrasonography are maintained.[38,39]

Various diagnostic criteria have been proposed for determining the percentage of stenosis. These include peak systolic velocity (PSV), end-diastolic velocity (EDV), and the ratio of PSVs in the ICA to the mid–common carotid artery (CCA) (ICA:CCA PSV

TABLE 1-1. Normal Reference Values for Blood Flow Velocities (in cm/sec) in the Carotid and Vertebral Arteries in Different Age Groups*

Blood flow velocity	*All (n = 182)*	*20–40 Yrs (n = 71)*	*41–60 Yrs (n = 64)*	*>60 Yrs (n = 47)*
Common carotid artery				
Peak systolic	80 (34–126)	96 (55–135)	75 (39–110)	61 (29–93)
End diastolic	21 (9–33)	23 (12–34)	21 (10–31)	16 (6–26)
Internal carotid artery				
Peak systolic	61 (27–94)	65 (40–92)	61 (24–97)	51 (21–81)
End diastolic	24 (9–39)	27 (15–38)	25 (9–50)	18 (7–30)
Vertebral artery				
Peak systolic	48 (26–69)	49 (29–69)	48 (23–73)	45 (26–63)
End diastolic	16 (10–23)	17 (11–23)	17 (10–27)	14 (8–20)

*Range of velocities (calculated as mean ± 2 standard deviations) is given in parentheses. Data from 182 healthy volunteers.
Source: Neurovascular Laboratory, Bialystok Medical Academy, Poland.

ratio). The PSV has traditionally been believed to provide the closest angiographic correlation and is easily obtained[40–43]; however, many laboratories rely also on the EDV or the ICA:CCA PSV ratio for improved diagnostic accuracy and to correct for factors that may alter the carotid blood flow. Such factors include low cardiac output, valvular disease, acute elevations in blood pressure, anemia, and abnormal collateral flow.[44,45] Any of these conditions may lead to flow alterations across a carotid plaque and may lead to either over- or underestimation of the true degree of stenosis.[46] In these instances, the ICA:CCA PSV ratio often helps in correcting hemodynamic disturbances, but it has limitations.[47] The diagnostic impression is further confirmed by B-mode and color flow imaging, which allow visual inspection of the degree of stenosis caused by the plaque (see Figure 1-5D). A quantitative cross-sectional analysis of plaque stenosis derived from color flow images was recently proposed, and it further increases diagnostic accuracy.[48]

Reference Values

A wide range of criteria has been proposed to identify the clinically relevant degrees of ICA stenosis. They are summarized in Tables 1-1 through 1-4. The diagnostic accuracy of duplex ultrasonography ranges between 85% and 95% and varies among laboratories. A survey of diagnostic criteria used by vascular laboratories in Great Britain showed that at least nine different diagnostic parameters are currently used to measure the severity of stenosis.[60] These differences among laboratories illustrate the fact that ultrasound testing is equipment and operator dependent, and they emphasize the necessity for each laboratory to develop its own diagnostic criteria based on angiographic correlations.[61,62]

Clinical Utility of Carotid Duplex

Characterization of plaque morphology and determination of degree of vessel stenosis are the most common clinical applications of carotid ultrasonography, and they are reviewed in the preceding paragraphs. In the day-to-day practice of stroke medicine, carotid ultrasound is also used in the following areas.

Progression of Atherosclerotic Plaques

Longitudinally monitored internal carotid artery plaques progress in approximately 30–60% of untreated patients and regress in approximately 20%.[63–65] A wide degree of variability exists in the rate of disease progression among individuals. Progression is associated with an increased risk of stroke,[63–65] and color duplex imaging allows accurate noninvasive follow-up of this process.[66] Noninvasive monitoring is particularly useful in asymptomatic patients, but its value on stroke prevention remains to be seen.[67]

Criteria regarding the frequency of follow-up testing have not been established. Based on their collective experience, the authors recommend yearly color duplex ultrasound testing for patients with asymptomatic stenosis in the 50–70% range and repeat imaging every 6 months for higher degrees of stenosis. The finding of complicated plaque features on B-mode imaging should prompt more frequent testing, whereas lack of progression may be sufficient reason to retest at longer intervals.

Monitoring after Revascularization Procedures

Although the practice of serial follow-up examinations after endarterectomy is intuitively appealing, the value of routine postoperative surveillance is uncertain. The incidence of restenosis (defined as a reduction in diameter of

TABLE 1-2. Diagnostic Parameters for Internal Carotid Artery Stenosis of 70% or More

Authors (yr)	*Diagnostic criteria**	*Sensitivity (%)*	*Specificity (%)*	*Accuracy (%)*
Hunink[42] (1993)	PSV >230	80	90	Not reported
Moneta[49] (1993)	PSV >325	83	100	88
	ICA:CCA PSV ratio >4	91	87	88
Faught[50] (1994)	EDV >100	77	85	80
	PSV >210	89	94	93
	PSV >130 and EDV >100	81	98	95
Neale[51] (1994)	PSV >270	96	86	88
	EDV >110	91	93	93
	PSV >270 and EDV >110	96	91	93
Carpenter[52] (1996)	EDV >70	92	60	77
	ICA:CCA EDV ratio >3.3	100	65	79
	PSV >210	94	77	83
	ICA:CCA PSV ratio >3	91	78	83
Hood[53] (1996)	PSV >130 and EDV >100	87	97	95
Huston[54] (2000)	PSV >230	86	90	89
	EDV >70	82	89	87
	ICA:CCA PSV ratio >3.2	87	90	89

CCA = common carotid artery; EDV = end-diastolic velocity; ICA = internal carotid artery; PSV = peak systolic velocity.
*All velocities in cm/sec.

more than 50%) varies between 2% and 20% at 2–3 years after surgery,[68,69] but the incidence of recurrent symptoms is low.[70,71] Restenosis within 2 years of surgery is usually secondary to intimal hyperplasia and carries a benign prognosis because the risk of distal embolism is low and lesions often regress.[71,72] Late restenosis is most likely secondary to recurrent atherosclerosis, and the associated risk of ipsilateral hemispheric or retinal symptoms may not be different from that of the original primary lesion.[72] In a small percentage of cases, postoperative testing shows evidence of thrombus formation at the endarterectomy site, intimal flaps, and occlusion.

Intracarotid and intravertebral stent placement is being performed with increasing frequency. Repeat testing after stent placement usually reveals an improvement of the intraluminal hemodynamic pattern. It is unclear, though, whether the diagnostic criteria presented in Tables 1-2 through 1-4 are applicable in the detection and monitoring of stent stenosis (Figure 1-6).

Intima-Media Thickness

High-resolution gray-scale imaging is currently the only imaging technique that allows assessment of the intima-

TABLE 1-3. Diagnostic Parameters for Internal Carotid Artery Stenosis of 60% or More

Authors (yr)	*Diagnostic criteria**	*Sensitivity (%)*	*Specificity (%)*	*Accuracy (%)*
Moneta[49] (1995)	PSV >260 and EDV >70	84	94	90
Carpenter[55] (1995)	ICA:CCA PSV ratio >2	97	73	76
	EDV >40	97	52	86
	ICA:CCA EDV ratio >2.4	100	80	88
	PSV >170	98	87	92
Jackson[56] (1998)	PSV >245 and EDV >65	89	92	Not reported

CCA = common carotid artery; EDV = end-diastolic velocity; ICA = internal carotid artery; PSV = peak systolic velocity.
*All velocities in cm/sec.

TABLE 1-4. Diagnostic Parameters for Internal Carotid Artery Stenosis of Fifty Percent or More

Authors (yr)	*Diagnostic criteria**	*Sensitivity (%)*	*Specificity (%)*	*Accuracy (%)*
Ballard[57] (1994)	PSV >120	79	84	82
Faught[50] (1994)	PSV >130	97	97	97
Paivansalo[58] (1996)	ICA:CCA PSV ratio >1.6	95	92	93
Wikelaar[59] (1999)	EDV >50	91	86	89
	PSV >150	98	84	92
	ICA:CCA PSV ratio >2	96	89	93
Huston[54] (2000)	ICA:CCA PSV ratio >1.6	93	83	88
	PSV >130	92	90	91

CCA = common carotid artery; EDV = end-diastolic velocity; ICA = internal carotid artery; PSV = peak systolic velocity.
*All velocities in cm/sec.

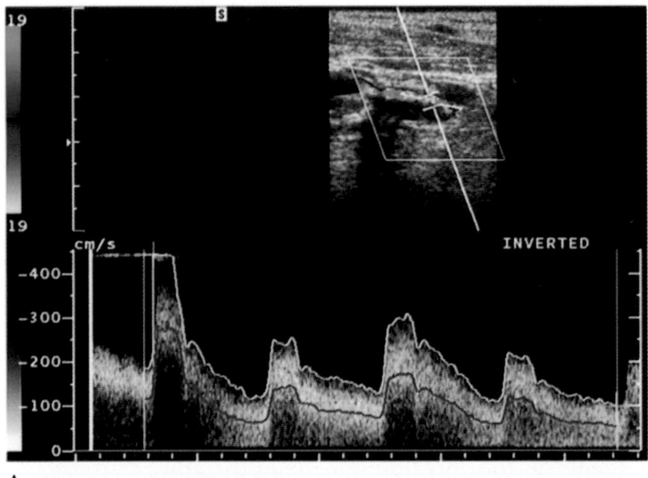

A

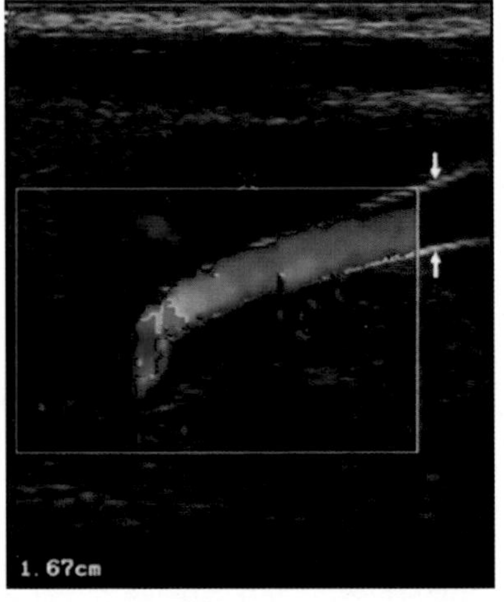

B

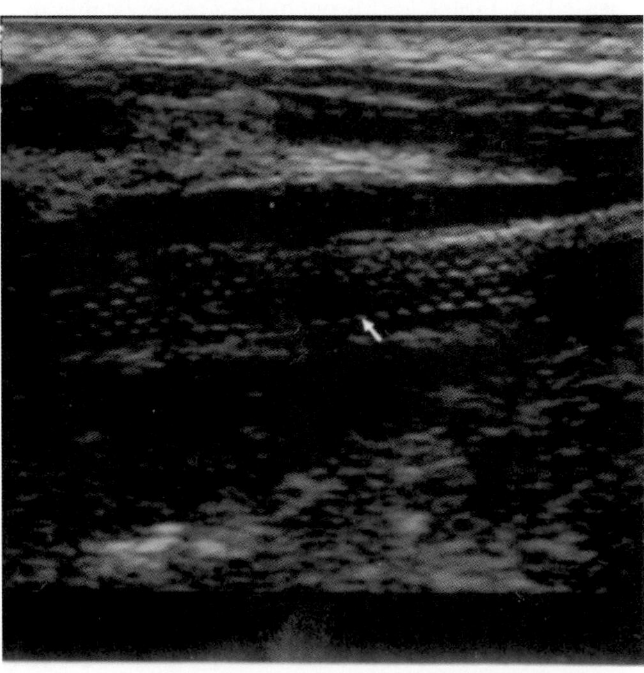

C

FIGURE 1-6. Stenting. **A.** High-grade symptomatic internal carotid artery origin stenosis with increased flow velocities. **B.** Stent (*arrows*) deployed successfully across the lesion. **C.** The mesh-like structure of the stent is well seen with B-mode imaging (*arrow*).

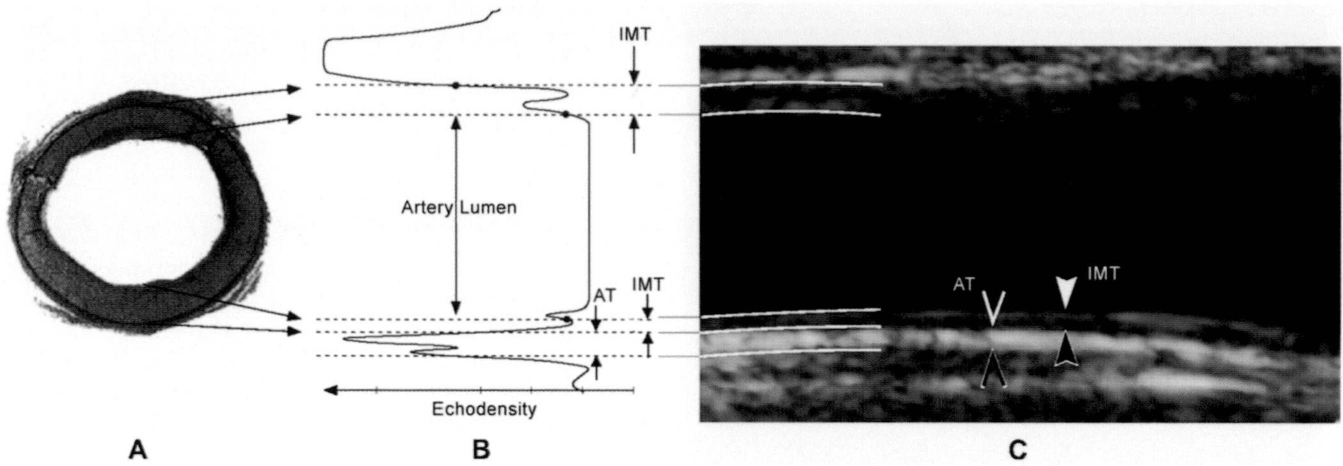

FIGURE 1-7. Histologic and ultrasonic correlation of intima-media thickness (IMT). **A.** The sets of two arrows at the top and bottom outline the IMT between the luminal border of the intima and the junction of the media and adventitia (AT). **B.** Graph depicting the echogenicity profiles of the AT, media, intima, and arterial lumen. **C.** The IMT and AT are respectively outlined by the closed and open arrowheads.

media thickness (IMT), a valuable marker for generalized atherosclerosis. Far-wall measurements of IMT are considered to be more accurate than near-wall measurements.[73] Measurements should be done at an arterial segment that allows easy reproducibility such as the one just distal to the carotid bifurcation.[74]

The normal IMT of carotid arteries in adults ranges between 0.5 and 1.0 mm (Figure 1-7).[74] Thickening exceeding 1.0 mm is associated with established cardiovascular risk factors.[75–78] Increased IMT of the CCA is associated with stroke, whereas increased thickness at the carotid bifurcation is associated with coronary artery disease.[79] Regression of the IMT indicates reduced cardiovascular morbidity and mortality.[80]

Arterial Dissection

The ultrasonographic features of dissection are less specific than those observed with angiography, and they usually reflect flow abnormalities seen in high-grade stenosis secondary to any etiology: high flow velocities, high resistance flow patterns, or complete absence of flow.[81,82] Despite the advantage of ultrasonography in displaying luminal irregularities, an intimal flap is infrequently seen,[83] possibly because the size of the flap lies beyond the resolution of ultrasound. Ultrasonography is helpful in monitoring the course of natural repair.[81,82]

Vertebral dissections follow a similar fate. Vertebral artery flow disturbances are nonspecific and show the same patterns as any stenotic lesion associated with intraluminal hemodynamic change. Such patterns include absence of a flow signal, bidirectional or dampened flow, and elevated flow velocities with associated turbulence.[84,85]

Pitfalls of Carotid Ultrasonography

Carotid Occlusion

Ultrasonographic diagnosis of a carotid occlusion remains unreliable, because a minimally patent arterial lumen with a trickle of flow can be missed. In the case of symptomatic atherosclerotic disease, such a differentiation is vital because endarterectomy is clearly indicated in a patent vessel but is generally not possible in the case of occlusion. Early reports suggested a diagnostic accuracy of 85% for carotid artery occlusion, but in more recent studies based on color duplex imaging, the accuracy was shown to exceed 96%.[86–88]

Difficulties arise from the presence of calcific plaque formation and the low-flow volume in near occlusions.[88] In addition, arterial tortuosity may cause angle artifacts, further compromising sensitivity. The angle independence of the power Doppler technique helps to overcome this, and its negative predictive value is 98%.[89] The use of ultrasound contrast further increases the ability of duplex imaging to differentiate a pseudo-occlusion from a true occlusion.[88] Diagnostic confusion may also arise when an external carotid artery branch overlies the ICA occlusion and is incorrectly identified as a patent residual lumen.[90] In some patients with ICA occlusion, the external carotid artery assumes a low-resistance pattern as it provides collateral flow to the brain. Tapping the fingers over the temporalis muscle and the identification of vascular branches may help differentiate the external carotid artery from the ICA.

ICA occlusion and high-grade stenosis also lead to diagnostic difficulties in determining the degree of stenosis on the contralateral side. Increased contralateral flow velocities may be secondary to collateral flow and lead

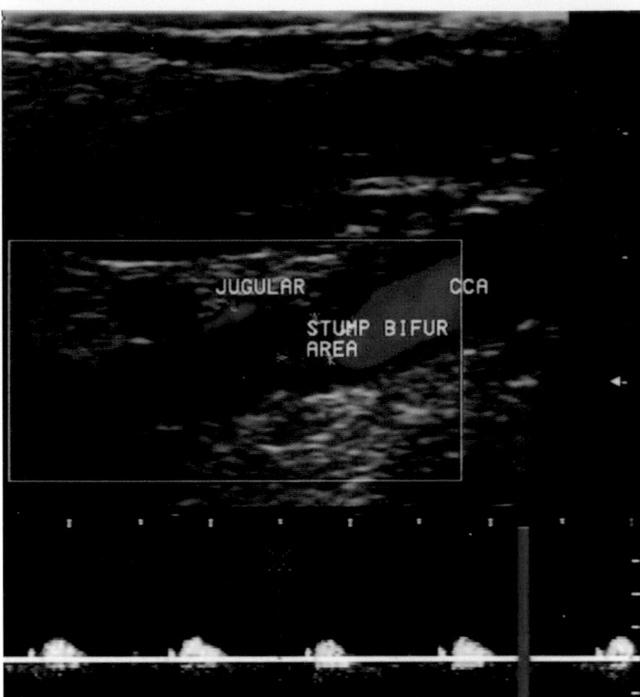

FIGURE 1-8. Suspected internal carotid artery occlusion. Color-flow Doppler fails to show flow in the internal carotid artery, and the spectral image (*bottom*) depicts a stump-flow pattern. (BIFUR = bifurcation; CCA = common carotid artery.)

the sonographer to overestimate the degree of true stenosis. In such cases, the use of PSV alone is insufficient and misleading. The overestimation is proportional to the degree of contralateral stenosis.[46] Increasing the number of diagnostic criteria in the setting of contralateral stenosis improves the diagnostic accuracy.[91] The ICA:CCA PSV ratio may accurately reflect the degree of stenosis in this setting (Figure 1-8).

Calcification

Heavily calcified plaques often cast an acoustic shadow that prevents duplex examination. Doppler velocities can then only be measured proximal and distal to the lesion, and elevated flow velocities at the level of the stenotic plaque can be missed. If the width of the acoustic shadow does not exceed 1 cm, it may be inferred from normal distal flow velocities that a high-grade lesion is not present.[92]

Tortuosity

With the aging process, the cervical carotid artery can develop loops or kinks. These may cause increases in flow velocity, suggesting a focal area of stenosis. Color duplex and power Doppler examinations are particularly helpful in these cases.

High Bifurcation

In patients with high CCA bifurcation, the mandible interferes with the ultrasonographic evaluation. A posterior approach, in these instances, allows a better evaluation of the artery.

Extracranial Vertebral Artery

Atherosclerotic plaques of the extracranial vertebral artery are usually localized at the artery's origin from the subclavian artery,[93] and they also tend to involve to the vertebrobasilar junction. In addition, the vertebral artery is susceptible to dissection at the V1 and V3 segments. Intraluminal flow characteristics can be readily assessed with extracranial ultrasound. However, velocities are usually measured only in the V2 intravertebral segment. Interrogation at this point allows determination of flow direction and pattern, but it gives only indirect evidence about proximal or distal stenotic lesions. Insonation of the vertebral artery origin is technically difficult due to its deep intrathoracic location, which does not always allow for optimal angle correction. Normal values range between 19 and 98 cm per second for PSV and 6 and 30 cm per second for EDV.[94,95] For the normal vertebral artery origin, a PSV of 69 cm per second and EDV of 16 cm per second have recently been reported.[83,96] When compared to the ICA and the middle cerebral artery, flow is slower in the vertebrobasilar trunk.

There are no established ultrasonographic criteria for vertebral artery stenosis. Hemodynamically significant vertebral artery disease can be inferred when a focal flow velocity increase of 50% or more is detected. The presence of a high-resistance pattern suggests high-grade distal stenosis.[97] However, because the resistance pattern is highly variable in the vertebral artery, it is an unreliable finding.[83] This is further confounded by the frequent presence of congenital variants in the vertebrobasilar circulation, including vertebral artery hypoplasia.[98] Flow in a hypoplastic vessel may be dampened, mimicking a high-resistance pattern with almost absent diastolic flow. This confuses the interpreter and affects the test's accuracy.[94] Experience with extracranial vertebral artery ultrasonography remains limited, and the technique is not used as often as for ICA disease (Figure 1-9).

The subclavian steal syndrome is usually a result of high-grade stenosis or occlusion of the proximal subclavian artery. As perfusion pressure and blood flow in the arm drop, the ipsilateral vertebral artery acts as a collateral vessel, channeling blood distal to the obstruction. Flow direction in the vertebral artery is reversed. The syndrome can be diagnosed with ultrasound with high sensitivity.[94,99,100]

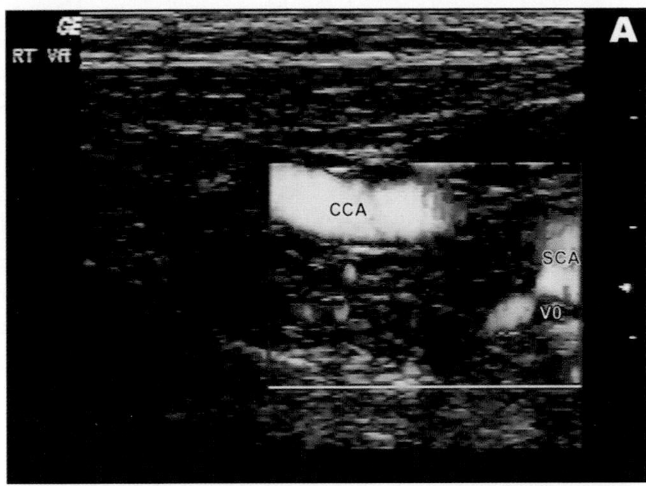

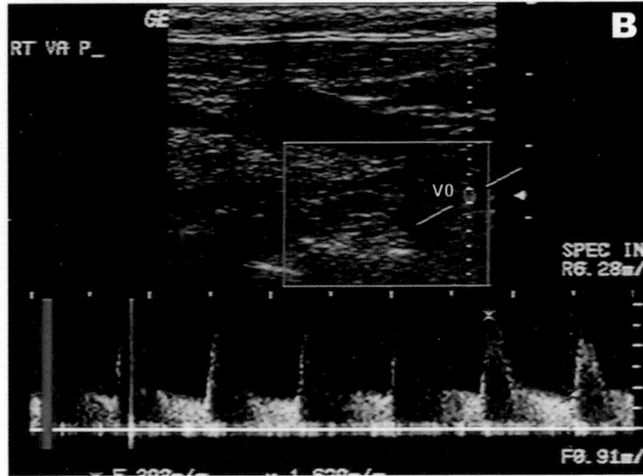

FIGURE 1-9. Vertebral artery origin stenosis. **A.** Power Doppler image. **B.** Color duplex and Doppler waveform (*bottom*). (CCA = common carotid artery; RT VA = right vertebral artery; SCA = subclavian artery; V0 = vertebral artery origin.)

TRANSCRANIAL ULTRASOUND IMAGING

Introduced to clinical use in the early 1980s by Aaslid et al.,[101] TCD imaging permits insonation of the basal brain arteries. TCD technology substantially evolved during the mid- to late 1990s, and TCCD is increasingly used today. Each of these technologies has specific advantages. TCD is based on pulsed-wave Doppler measurements of blood flow velocity. Its 2-MHz, relatively small transducers are easy to use, particularly when prolonged monitoring is performed. Experience with this technology is extensive, but the angle of insonation cannot be assessed, leading to an error in velocity measurements. TCCD combines two-dimensional, gray-scale, real-time imaging with pulsed-wave Doppler and color-coded display of velocity information. It is performed with phased-array, 1.0- to 3.5-MHz transducers that are slightly larger and less easy to manipulate than their TCD counterparts. In contrast to TCD, however, TCCD enables the sonographer to outline some intracranial parenchymal structures, to place the Doppler sample at a specific site of the insonated artery, and to visualize segments of the basal cerebral arteries in color. These advantages permit more rapid studies, provide more information, and improve the sonographer's confidence as well as the test's accuracy. TCCD equipment is substantially more expensive than TCD technology. Information derived from both technologies is used in this section of the chapter in which common clinical applications of transcranial ultrasonography are reviewed.

The technique of transcranial ultrasound insonation has been described elsewhere.[102] Both TCD and TCCD are noninvasive and enable bedside testing. Measurements are also highly reproducible.[103] Inadequate ultrasonic windows, present in 10–20% of patients, and limited accuracy constitute the major disadvantages that limit a more widespread use of the technology (Figures 1-10 and 1-11).

Reference Values

When compared to values obtained with conventional, blind TCD, flow velocities measured by TCCD are higher by approximately 10–30%.[104–107] TCCD measurements are considered more accurate because velocities are corrected for the angle of insonation. With conventional TCD, a small angle of insonation of less than 30 degrees is assumed,[108] but, in fact, the angle has been shown to vary widely in healthy controls[109] and may be even wider in patients with intracranial arterial stenosis. Therefore, TCD reference values cannot be used for TCCD measurements. Normal reference TCCD data for flow velocities have been published.[109] They are also presented in Table 1-5.

Velocity values are highest during the first decade of life and drop during the fifth and sixth decades.[106] Women tend to have higher velocity values up to the age of 60. This may be partially explained by the effect of hormonal fluctuations that affect the reactivity and tone of the cerebral microcirculation.[110,111] Other factors that affect flow velocities include intracranial pressure, hematocrit, fibrinogen, cardiac rhythm disorders, and several medications.

Acute Stroke

The "blind" administration of thrombolytic agents in acute stroke has been criticized because, in approximately 20–40% of cases, an arterial embolic occlusion is not present on early conventional contrast angiography. It has been argued that these patients are exposed to a

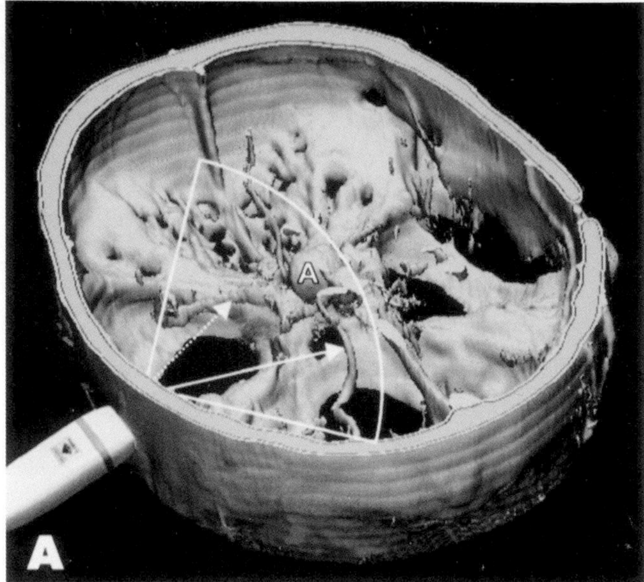

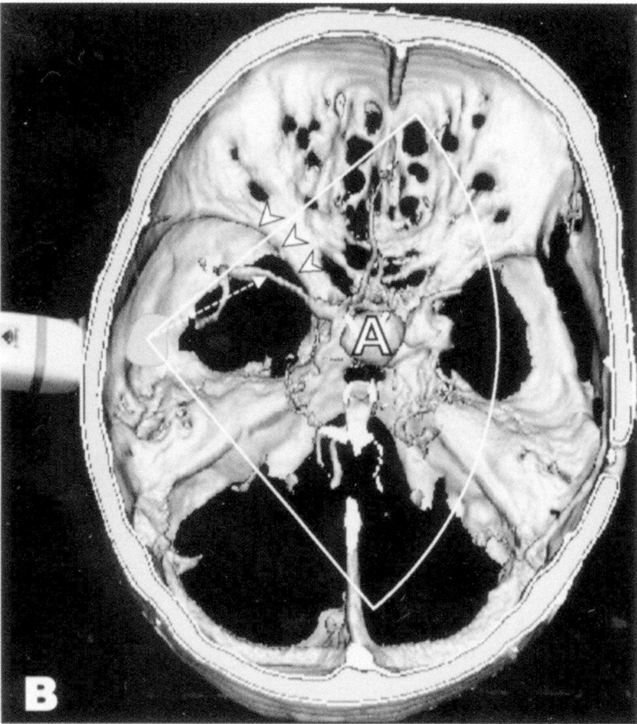

FIGURE 1-10. Three-dimensional computed tomographic reconstruction depicting the transcranial ultrasound field of view. **A.** An aneurysm (A). Transtemporal insonation enables imaging of the middle cerebral artery (*dashed arrow*) and, occasionally, the distal segment of the basilar artery (*solid arrow*). **B.** Origin and course of the middle cerebral artery (*dashed arrow*) and its spatial relationship with the sphenoid wing (*arrowheads*) are seen.

dangerous treatment with no potential for benefit. Early vascular imaging with MRA, computed tomography (CT) angiography, or transcranial ultrasound can be helpful in selecting patients most likely to benefit from this therapy.

TCD and TCCD have been used to monitor the effects of thrombolytic agents and to adjust medication dosage.[112] Intravenous tissue-type plasminogen activator is associated with partial or complete recanalization in 70% of patients. This result is achieved within 60 minutes of bolus administration in 75% of those who recanalize,[113] and the speed of recanalization correlates inversely with the onset of improvement.[113] Follow-up studies at 24 and 48 hours after treatment can determine the presence of recanalization or recurrent occlusion with acceptable accuracy, and they correlate with the clinical outcome.[114] TCD has also been used to monitor the effects of intra-arterial tissue-type plasminogen activator and intravenous streptokinase.[115]

As indicated in the introduction to this section, ultrasound monitoring is limited by technical shortcomings, such as the absence of adequate temporal bone windows. This limits its use in the emergency room, where acute stroke patients are usually seen. In addition, in more than 25% of cases, embolic occlusions involve middle, anterior, or posterior cerebral artery distal branches, segments that are beyond the reach of routine transcranial ultrasound imaging. The increased use of TCCD in this setting, with or without contrast agents, has improved the diagnostic utility of the technique.[116,117]

Can exposing a thrombus to low-frequency ultrasound facilitate thrombolysis? In laboratory animals and in patients with coronary artery disease, the answer is a tentative "yes."[118] Recent laboratory studies based on a low-intensity (<1 MHz) transducer[119] and some clinical investigations suggest that thrombolysis can also be enhanced with transcranial ultrasound in humans. Although these preliminary studies are promising, it is too early to determine whether they will translate into actual clinical applications.

Chronic Cerebrovascular Disease

Intracranial Arterial Stenosis

Intracranial atherosclerotic stenoses are the cause of stroke in approximately 5–10% of all patients, and lesions at the ICA siphon, middle cerebral artery M1 segment, vertebral artery V4 segment, and proximal to mid-basilar artery are particularly common. The prevalence of these lesions is higher in African-American and Asian populations. The mechanism(s) by which these lesions cause cerebral ischemia are not well understood, but some plaques can act as sources of distal microembolism.[120] Most are within the reach of transcranial ultrasound imaging. The corresponding main finding consists of increased peak systolic, end-diastolic, and mean velocities. Although this increase is proportional to the severity of arterial stenosis,[121] the relationship of velocity to artery diameter and flow is not a simple one.[122] Additional findings caused by turbulent or dis-

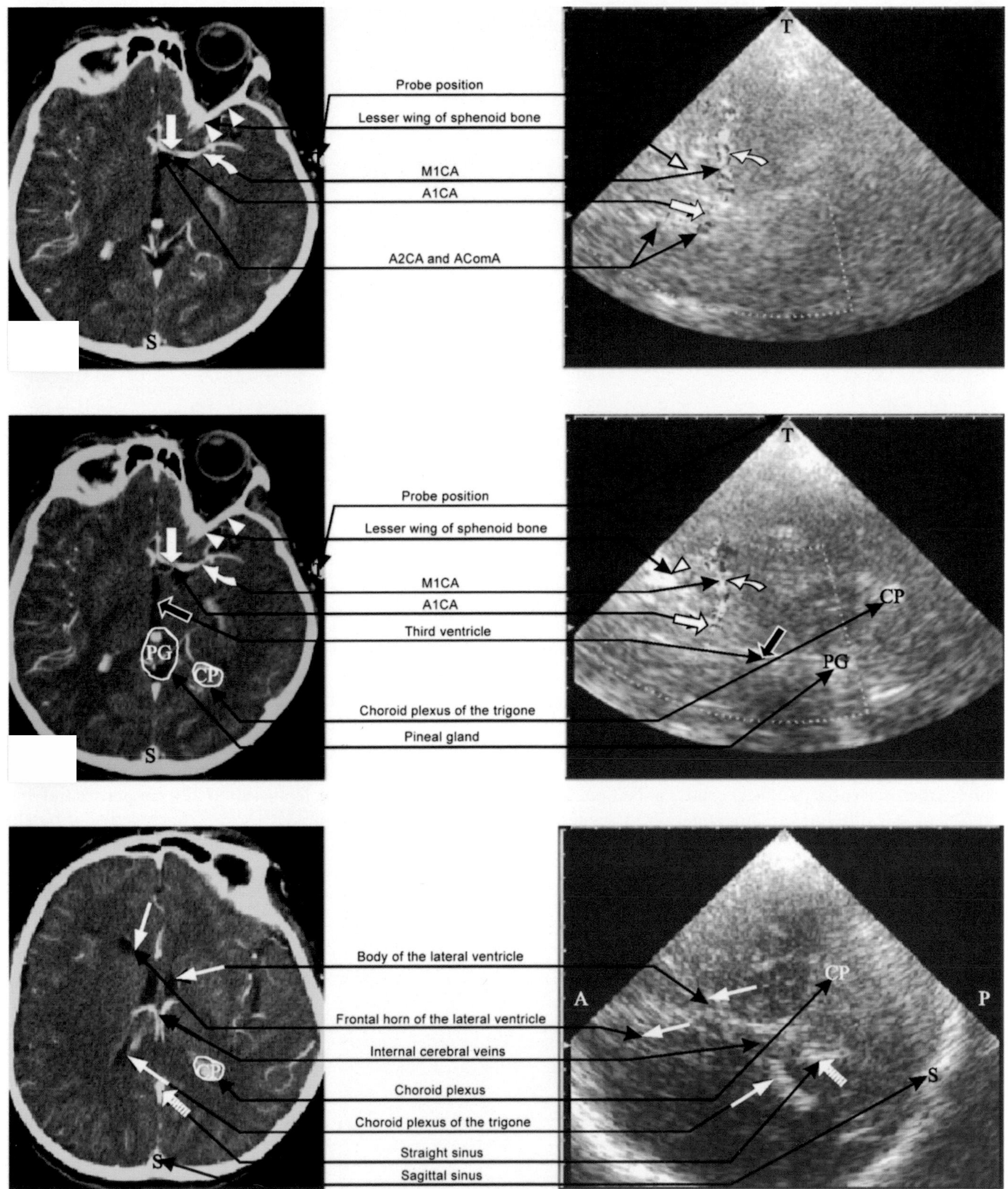

FIGURE 1-11. Transcranial color Doppler sonography and computed tomographic anatomic correlation. (A = anterior; A1CA = A1 segment of anterior cerebral artery; A2CA = A2 segment of anterior cerebral artery; AcomA = anterior communicating artery; CP = choroid plexus; M1CA = M1 segment of middle cerebral artery; P = posterior; PG = pineal gland; S = sinus; T = transducer.)

TABLE 1-5. Normal Reference Values for Blood Flow Velocities (cm/sec) in the Basal Cerebral Arteries in Different Age Groups*

Blood flow velocity	*N*	*All*	*20–40 Yrs*	*41–60 Yrs*	*>60 Yrs*
Anterior cerebral artery	313				
Peak systolic		79 (37–121)	82 (40–124)	80 (36–124)	72 (52–102)
Mean (TAMAX)		53 (33–83)	56 (42–84)	53 (37–85)	44 (22–66)
End diastolic		35 (13–57)	38 (16–60)	35 (13–57)	28 (12–44)
Middle cerebral artery	335				
Peak systolic		110 (54–166)	120 (64–176)	109 (65–175)	92 (58–126)
Mean (TAMAX)		73 (33–133)	81 (41–121)	73 (35–111)	59 (37–81)
End diastolic		49 (21–77)	55 (29–81)	49 (23–75)	37 (21–53)
Posterior cerebral artery	336				
Peak systolic		71 (39–103)	75 (43–107)	74 (40–108)	62 (38–86)
Mean (TAMAX)		49 (25–73)	52 (28–76)	51 (25–75)	40 (22–58)
End diastolic		33 (15–51)	36 (20–52)	34 (18–50)	26 (14–38)

TAMAX = time-averaged maximum velocity.
*Range of velocities (calculated as mean ± 2 standard deviations) is given in parentheses.
Source: Adapted from J Krejza, Z Mariak, J Walecki, et al. Transcranial color Doppler sonography of basal cerebral arteries in 182 healthy subjects: age and sex variability and normal reference values for blood parameters. AJR Am J Roentgenol 1999;172:213–218.

turbed flow include increased wall covibration, low-frequency, bidirectional signals during systole, and spectral broadening (Figure 1-12).[4]

There is no consensus in the literature today regarding specific criteria for the severity of stenosis. A threshold flow velocity corresponding to 50% stenosis, usually considered clinically relevant, has not been established for the main basal arteries. The investigators of the Stroke Outcomes and Neuroimaging of Intracranial Atherosclerosis (SONIA) study, a National Institutes of Health–funded investigation assessing the accuracy of TCD and MRA in patients with symptomatic intracranial stenosis, opted for a mean velocity of 100 cm per second for the middle cerebral artery, 90 cm per second for the internal carotid siphon and supraclinoid segment, and 80 cm per second for the distal vertebral and proximal basilar arteries as the minimal cutoff points to enroll patients in the study. These velocities are presumed to indicate a severity of stenosis of 50% in corresponding arteries. Higher peak systolic cutoff point velocities, ranging from 180 to 220 cm per second, have been proposed for TCCD.[123,124] Irrespective of baseline

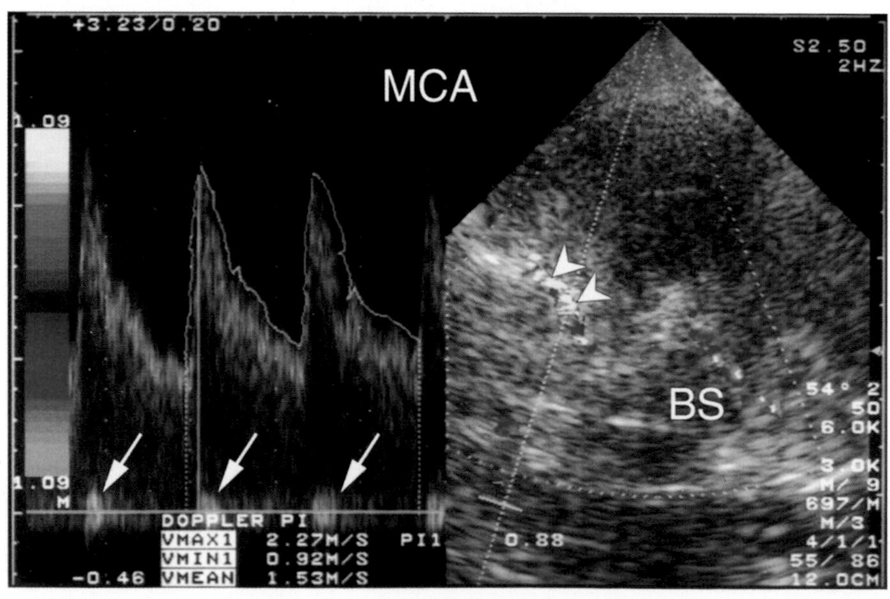

FIGURE 1-12. Middle cerebral artery (MCA) stenosis. Transcranial color Doppler ultrasound shows the MCA M1 segment (*right, arrowheads*). The peak systolic velocity of 227 cm per second (*left*) is not angle corrected. Spectral broadening and low-frequency bidirectional signals (*arrows*) are detected. (BS = brain stem.)

velocities, longitudinal monitoring enables the assessment of disease progression over time.[125]

The overall accuracy of TCD and TCCD in detecting intracranial stenoses has not been adequately established in well-designed and conclusive studies. Note should be made, however, that although contrast angiography is considered the gold standard for detecting these lesions, its accuracy has also been questioned. TCD has been studied more often than TCCD, and available data suggest that when compared to contrast angiography, TCD is approximately 80–90% sensitive in detecting stenotic lesions of the ICA siphon and middle cerebral artery M1 segment.[126] The specificity is in excess of 95%.[126] In expert hands, both the sensitivity and specificity of TCCD for the same arterial segments are more than 98%.[123,124] Both techniques are less accurate when evaluating lesions of the vertebral artery V4 segment and proximal basilar artery, with sensitivity and specificity respective values of 70% and 85% for TCD[127] and 70% and 98% for TCCD.[128,129] For these lesions, CT or MRA may be more useful, particularly in patients with acute distal basilar artery occlusion (Figure 1-13).[130]

Although TCD is less accurate in detecting arterial occlusions than stenoses, a recent investigation of acute stroke patients showed acceptable accuracy in detecting acute occlusions.[131] TCCD is more accurate than TCD in detecting occlusions. The color scale must be adjusted to the lowest possible limit to detect low velocity. Flow and color are undetectable in the occluded artery but may be seen in adjacent vessels. The occluded artery can frequently be identified in gray-scale images in relation to adjacent parenchymal and bony structures. The sensitivity and specificity of TCCD in the diagnosis of middle cerebral artery occlusion vary from 70% to 100%.[129,132] The administration of contrast agents substantially improves the test's diagnostic accuracy.[133] Transcranial ultrasonography is not useful in detecting occlusion of middle cerebral artery branches.[132]

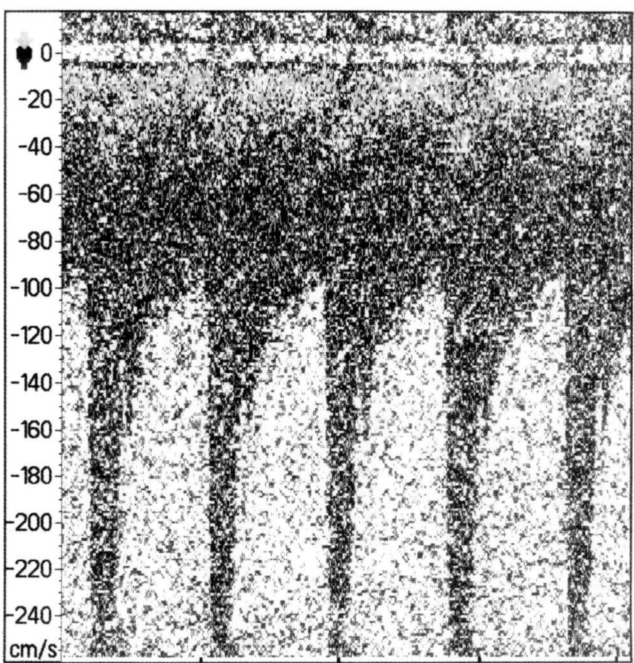

FIGURE 1-13. Basilar artery stenosis. Increased peak systolic (>240 cm per second) and end-diastolic (95 cm per second) flow velocities at a depth of insonation of 90 mm (occipital window) are consistent with severe proximal basilar artery stenosis.

Intracranial Hemodynamic Changes

Rapid changes in cerebral perfusion are notoriously difficult to image or monitor. The real-time capability of TCD can be quite useful in these settings.[134–136] In positional cerebral ischemia, flow velocities drop distal to the occluded artery after postural changes.[134] In cough syncope, a transient cerebral circulatory arrest coincides with the fainting episode.[135]

In addition to their local hemodynamic effects, extracranial ICA stenoses also affect flow in the middle and anterior cerebral arteries. Flow velocities in these arteries usually drop distal to ICA stenosis of more than 70%, and a comparison with the contralateral, unaffected side may be diagnostically useful. In addition, as the blood pressure distal to a severe stenosis drops, collateral flow channels become functional. In the anterior circulation, these channels include the ophthalmic artery, in which flow becomes retrograde, and the anterior and posterior communicating arteries. Collateral flow through the anterior communicating artery is usually a sign of well-preserved hemodynamic status, whereas flow limited only to the posterior communicating artery denotes poorly compensated perfusion.[137] Collateral channels are particularly well imaged with TCCD.[138,139]

The development of collateral flow is associated with changes in cerebral autoregulation and vasoreactivity. Changes in response to fluctuations in perfusion pressure or arterial carbon dioxide concentration are mediated through the dilatation or constriction of pial arterioles and, to a lesser degree, of large arteries at the base of the brain. Compensatory vasodilatation causes a fall of vascular impedance and of pulsatility index values. The acceleration time (i.e., the time of arrival of PSV) increases upstream in the artery.[140] Thus, in individuals with severe stenosis of the extracranial ICA, impaired distal vasoreactivity denotes a state of arteriolar and arterial dilatation (Figure 1-14). When detected in a subgroup of asymptomatic patients, it is associated with an increased risk of future ischemic events.[141] The brain CT characteristics of the corresponding lesions are those of "low-flow" infarcts.[142] Impaired vasoreactivity

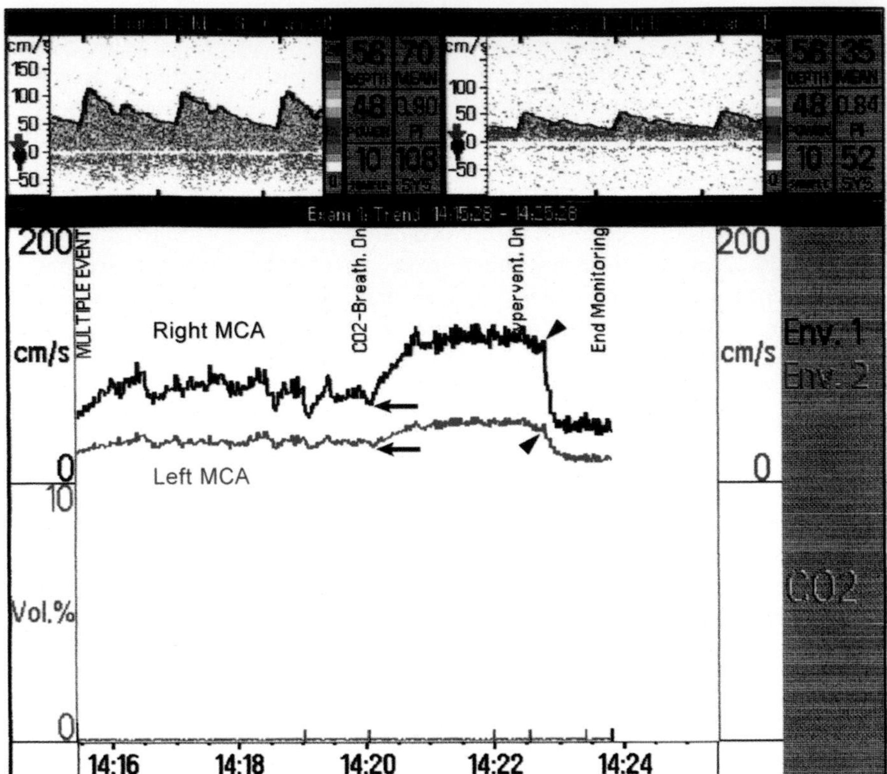

FIGURE 1-14. Vasomotor reactivity. The left internal carotid artery is occluded. At baseline, the right middle cerebral artery (MCA) waveform (*top left*) is normal, whereas the waveform of the left MCA is dampened (*top right*). After carbon dioxide inhalation (*bottom*), MCA flow velocities are increased on the right (*black line*) more than the left (*green line, arrows*). Furthermore, hyperventilation causes a rapid drop in the right MCA flow velocities (*arrowhead*), but the response is blunted on the left.

can also be seen in elderly hypertensive patients without extracranial arterial stenosis[143] and is considered a risk marker for lacunar brain infarction.[144]

Cerebral Vein Thrombosis

The straight sinus, basal cerebral veins, cavernous sinus, and superior and inferior sagittal sinuses can be insonated with TCD and TCCD. Normal PSVs usually range from 5 cm per second to 35 cm per second, varying from one sinus to the other. In sinus thrombosis, flow velocities may decrease,[145] or they may markedly increase to above 100 cm per second, most likely indicating increased collateral circulation.[146,147] Follow-up studies show gradual normalization after a period of months.[147] Venous flow velocities are also affected by intracranial pressure changes.[148] Experience with cerebral vein insonation remains limited.

Sickle Cell Disease

Neurologic complications, including seizures and strokes, occur in 5–10% of patients with sickle cell anemia, mostly in the pediatric age group.[149] An occlusive arteriopathy involves intracranial arteries with a particular predilection for distal ICAs and proximal middle cerebral arteries.

Anemia and young age contribute to the mild to moderate diffuse increase of flow velocities detected in most patients with sickle cell disease. The increase tends to be most pronounced at the level of the ICA bifurcation into middle and anterior cerebral arteries, and a time-averaged mean-maximum velocity of 200 cm per second in that arterial segment is strongly associated with an increased risk of ischemic stroke.[150] Blood transfusions reduce the risk of first stroke.[151] A 1997 Clinical Alert from the National Heart, Lung, and Blood Institute[152] recommends that children aged 2 to 16 years with sickle cell disease receive TCD screening. Those with normal studies should be restudied every 6 months (Figure 1-15).[152]

Vasospasm after Subarachnoid Hemorrhage

Cerebral vasospasm is frequently detected after aneurysmal or traumatic subarachnoid hemorrhage and significantly contributes to its morbidity and mortality by causing brain ischemia. Early diagnosis of vasospasm is of particular importance, because it allows the institution of aggressive medical therapy even before symptoms develop.[153] Balloon angioplasty and intra-arterial papaverine infusion are increasingly used to treat selected patients with severe vasospasm.[154] These therapeutic interventions, however, are based on the assumption that vasospasm can be reliably detected. Cerebral angiography, the gold standard diagnostic test,[155] cannot be repeated as often as clinically indicated because it is invasive and increases the risk of cerebral ischemia, especially in symptomatic patients with subarachnoid hemorrhage.

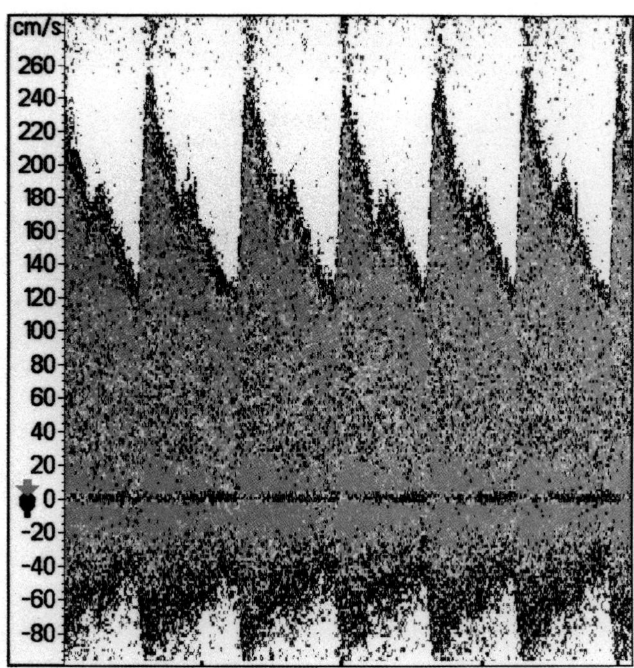

FIGURE 1-15. Sickle cell disease in a child. Moderately to severely increased flow velocities at a depth of insonation corresponding to the proximal middle cerebral artery are consistent with the vasculopathy seen in this condition.

TCD provides a means to detect vasospasm, before it becomes symptomatic, and may be used to monitor its evolution.[156–159] Patients who develop symptomatic cerebral ischemia generally demonstrate rapidly rising middle cerebral artery mean velocities to values exceeding 200 cm per second during the first week.[157] Although symptoms of vasospasm usually appear several days after the hemorrhage, increases in flow velocity often precede the onset of symptoms by hours or days.[156] Increased velocities can persist for more than 3 weeks after the onset of hemorrhage.

Several studies have focused on establishing a threshold velocity that reliably distinguishes between normal and vasospastic arteries. For the middle cerebral artery, the most commonly cited threshold is a mean velocity of 120 cm per second. The clinical relevance of the concept of threshold has been questioned by some investigators, who have emphasized that vasospasm is not an all-or-nothing phenomenon,[160–165] and it has been pointed out that during the 2-week period after hemorrhage, some degree of asymptomatic vasospasm can be detected by angiography in more than 50% of patients. The middle cerebral artery mean velocity value of 200 cm per second has the best positive predictive value (Table 1-6; Figure 1-16).[160,165]

TABLE 1-6. Sensitivity and Specificity of Transcranial Doppler Ultrasonography for Detection of Vasospasm Affecting the M1 Segment of the Middle Cerebral Artery*

Authors	*No. of arteries*	*No. of patients*	*Prevalence of spasm (%)*	*Mean velocity (cm/sec)*	*Sensitivity (%)*	*Specificity (%)*	*Positive predictive value (%)*	*Negative predictive value (%)*
Transcranial Doppler ultrasonography								
Aaslid[171]	76	38	8	120	100	95	60	100
Grolimund[172]	NA	93	15	120	100	89	61	100
Compton[167]	35	26	11	100	40	96	80	80
Lindegaard[169]	112	76	31	110	85	98	95	94
Sekhar[173]	NA	21	38	155	80	98	85	85
Lennihan[166]	66	41	11	120	86	86	43	98
Sloan[174]	52	34	48	120	88	86	84	89
Sloan[165]	131	NA	25	120	52	79	45	83
Burch[175]	87	49	44	120	39	94	83	66
Vora[160]	264	135	48	120	88	72	55	94
Vora[160]	264	135	48	160	46	90	61	83
Vora[160]	264	135	48	200	27	98	87	77
Proust[176]	40	20	18	122	83	94	NA	NA
Transcranial color Doppler ultrasonography								
Proust[176]	38	20	18	120	100	93	100	94

NA = not available.

*The specified measures of accuracy were calculated from data reported in the papers.

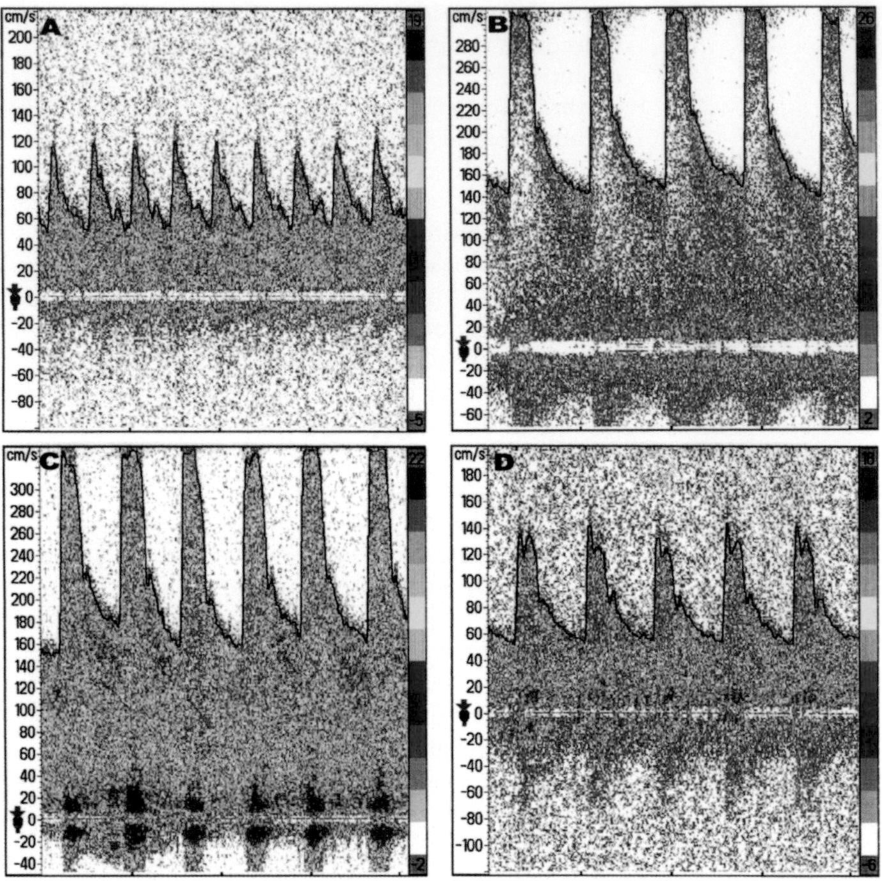

FIGURE 1-16. Middle cerebral artery vasospasm after subarachnoid hemorrhage. **A.** Baseline study 12 hours after hemorrhage. The peak systolic flow velocity is approximately 120 cm per second. **B.** Eighth day after hemorrhage and 1 day before neurologic deterioration. The peak systolic velocity is in excess of 300 cm per second. **C.** Tenth day after hemorrhage. Patient is lethargic and hemiparetic. The peak systolic velocity is now more than 320 cm per second. **D.** Flow velocities have returned to baseline values 18 days after the onset of hemorrhage.

Results regarding the accuracy of TCD in detecting vasospasm vary widely from one study to another (see Table 1-6). TCD has a sensitivity of 80–90% and a specificity exceeding 85% when detecting vasospasm of the middle cerebral artery M1 segment (see Table 1-6). Vertebral or basilar artery spasm is diagnosed with a 75% sensitivity and an 80% specificity. TCD is not reliable when assessing spasm of the anterior cerebral artery or the middle cerebral artery's distal segments.[165–167] Hyperperfusion, anemia, the angle of insonation, and increased intracranial pressure are some of the factors that affect the technique's accuracy, and additional Doppler parameters have been introduced to improve the latter. Among them are the Lindegaard ratio of middle cerebral artery to ipsilateral extracranial ICA velocity, and the pulsatility index.[168–170] Whether these parameters substantially enhance the predictive value of absolute velocities is not known.[160,161]

It is expected that the introduction of TCCD will substantially improve accuracy in the ultrasonic diagnosis of cerebral vasospasm. Although available data are scarce, they suggest a high sensitivity and specificity in detecting spasm of the middle cerebral artery M1 and the anterior cerebral artery A1 segments.[176,177] Large and medium-sized aneurysms of the circle of Willis can also be detected by TCCD,[178] and their visualization is improved by the administration of echo contrast agents.[179]

Increased intracranial pressure is common in subarachnoid hemorrhage, and it affects ultrasound findings. The earliest changes include increased pulsatility values associated with decreased diastolic velocities. With progressive increases of the intracranial pressure, the diastolic flow becomes retrograde, and the systolic flow starts to drop. Eventually, only small systolic peaks persist, or flow stops altogether, indicating cerebral circulatory arrest.[180]

Vascular Malformations

Arteriovenous malformations can be detected by transcranial ultrasound imaging. TCCD studies show a focal accumulation of vascular convolutions as a color mosaic with abnormal Doppler waveforms.[181–183] The hemodynamic abnormalities in feeding cerebral arteries and draining veins are detected by TCCD or TCD.[181,182] Typically, flow velocities in feeding vessels are high, ranging from 140 to 200 cm per second, and impedance indexes are low, indicating a drop in distal resistance.[181,184] Draining veins are enlarged, channeling pulsatile and arterialized blood.

The diagnostic accuracy of TCD and TCCD in detecting arteriovenous malformations is not known.

Large (>4 cm) and medium-sized (2–4 cm) radiologically proven malformations are regularly detected.[185] Because more than one-third of small (<2 cm) arteriovenous malformations can be missed,[185] transcranial ultrasonography is not considered as a reliable routine diagnostic tool in this setting. Nevertheless, it is useful in monitoring the effects of therapeutic procedures.[183,186,187]

Transcranial Doppler Microembolus Detection

Reflected echoes from red blood cells originate the normal TCD wave pattern. When aggregates of cells or platelets forming larger particles traverse the sample volume being interrogated, high-intensity transient signals, often called microembolic signals (MESs), appear in the spectral envelope.[188,189] Each signal's intensity and duration can be measured, and these characteristics depend on the physical properties of the embolic particle.[190] MESs are usually observed within the spectral envelope, whereas artifacts, which can resemble them, extend outside the envelope and are bidirectional.[191–195] In laboratory models, the size and composition of embolic particles can be estimated, with larger particles causing signals of longer duration and higher intensity.[196,197] Strongly echogenic gaseous materials elicit higher-intensity signals than those caused by fat or thrombus. In clinical practice, however, it is difficult to determine whether a given MES corresponds to a large platelet embolus or to a small atheroma due to a considerable overlap between MES characteristics.[196] Several techniques have been proposed to resolve these issues.[198–201]

Technical limitations present considerable difficulties. For example, using a higher decibel threshold improves reproducibility,[202] but it can decrease sensitivity. In an attempt to establish a general consensus among investigators, a committee of experts has defined MES characteristics.[203] Manual saving of suspicious signals by the recording operator and subsequent off-line analysis is the standard practice today, but it is cumbersome and time consuming. Automated systems for embolus detection have been developed.[192,204] Their accuracy remains limited. Although the optimal duration of insonation needed to achieve maximum sensitivity is unknown, most centers monitor for 30 minutes to 1 hour. Longer periods of insonation,[205] or repeat studies,[206] may be needed in some instances.

Acute Stroke and Stroke-Prone Patients

Acute stroke and stroke-prone patients have been evaluated extensively for the presence of microembolism,[207–244] and MES can be detected in approximately 15–30% of these subjects.[207–210] MESs are particularly common in symptomatic internal carotid atherosclerotic stenosis,[211–213] carotid dissection,[214–216] some cardiac conditions associated with embolism,[217–219] aortic arch atherosclerosis,[220] carotid occlusion,[221] and hypercoagulable disorders.[222] They are not usually detected when distal hypoperfusion is thought to be the cause of cerebral ischemia[225,226] or in patients with lacunar infarction.[230,232] The prevalence of MES varies among conditions, depending on the particular embolic source and its degree of activity or quiescence.

Multiple clinical studies have confirmed the high prevalence rate of MES shortly after transient ischemic attacks and acute stroke.[228–232] In this setting, the presence of MES indicates an increased risk for recurrent ischemia.[211] Interestingly, MES has also been observed to be an independent marker of future stroke risk in asymptomatic carotid stenosis.[233] Microemboli are also observed at the time of arterial recanalization after thrombolysis, allowing real-time, noninvasive monitoring of the very process intended to modify: arterial occlusion.[235]

Transcranial Doppler monitoring offers the possibility of titrating antithrombotic drug therapy using the presence of MES as a potential surrogate marker for disease activity.[216,236–238] Intravenous aspirin administration can markedly reduce the MES count,[236] but the effect of heparin remains unknown. During the immediate postoperative period after carotid endarterectomy, intravenous dextran-40 stops all microembolism, contributing to the improved perioperative morbidity.[239–242] Intravenously administered L-arginine also reduces microembolism.[243,244] Although promising, these findings have not yet translated into routine clinical applications.

Carotid Artery Disease

Artery-to-artery embolism is considered a common pathogenetic process causing cerebral and ocular ischemia in atherosclerotic ICA disease,[245] and, as indicated in the preceding paragraphs of this section, it has been extensively evaluated. MESs correlate with the degree of arterial stenosis, the presence of neurologic symptoms, plaque morphology, and the presence of ulceration.[202,203,213,246–248] Their presence constitutes a prognostic marker of future risk of brain ischemic events independently of the degree of stenosis.[233,249,250] Microembolism is transient in this context.[212,251–253]

Carotid Endarterectomy

Brain infarction is the most common major complication of carotid endarterectomy, occurring in 2–11% of patients.[254,255] Embolism and hypoperfusion during the procedure and embolism and hyperperfusion during the 24–48 hour period after it, are the main causes of perioperative stroke. These processes can be monitored by TCD.

The middle cerebral artery on the side of endarterectomy is the artery usually insonated. A predictable

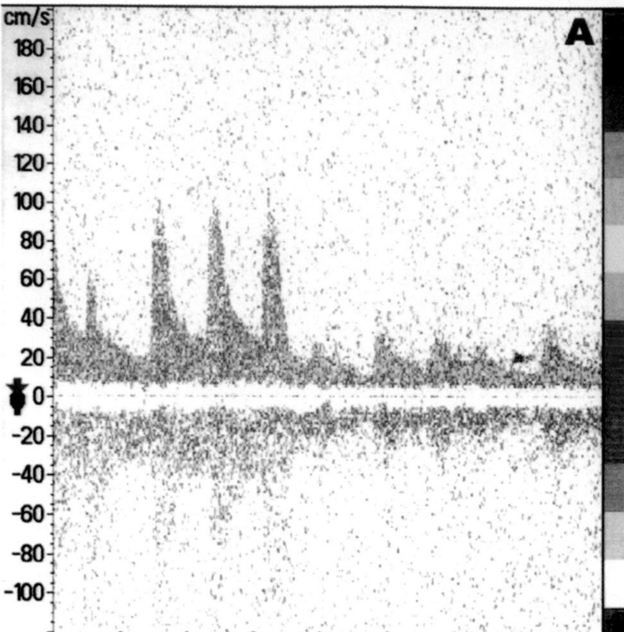

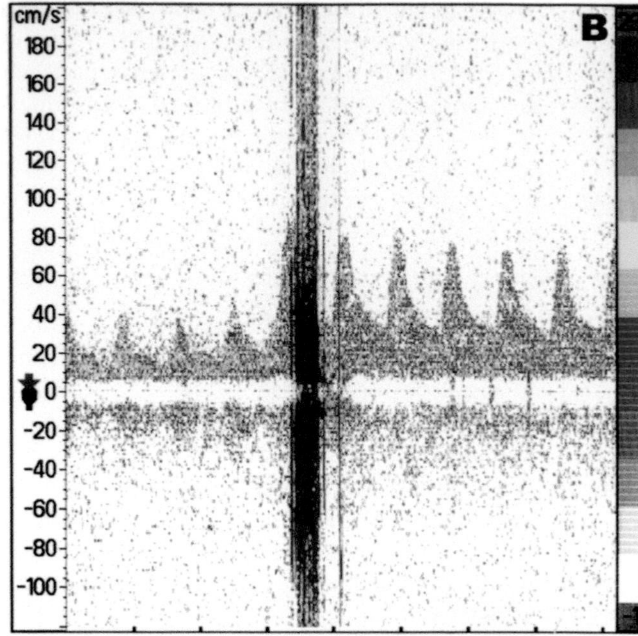

FIGURE 1-17. Carotid endarterectomy. **A.** At cross-clamping, flow velocities in the ipsilateral middle cerebral artery drop to 30 cm per second. **B.** At clamp release, the flow velocities rebound to approximately 90 cm per second, and a signal (*red*), suggestive of air embolism, is seen.

course of intracranial events occurs as the operation progresses. Velocities drop slightly with the administration of anesthetic agents but then stabilize until the time of cross-clamping—the true hemodynamic test of the operation. In most patients, flow velocities in the monitored middle cerebral artery drop to 60–90% of preclamp values at cross-clamping (Figure 1-17A); a more severe drop leading to a mean velocity of less than 15 cm per second is detected in 10–20% of cases.[256,257] These changes in flow velocity parallel changes in flow volume.[258] The 15 cm per second threshold has been associated with a regional cerebral blood flow of 9 ml/100 g tissue per minute and suppression of electroencephalographic activity, which leads to clinically evident brain ischemia if not corrected.[256,259,260] Slightly higher velocity and flow values are usually considered appropriate for shunting to provide a margin of safety. Thus, patients with moderate or severe flow velocity drops are considered candidates for shunting. The latter restores flow back to 50–120% of preclamp values. Some surgeons avoid shunting altogether and use, with good results, high-dose thiopental sodium anesthesia during this phase of the operation.[261] A moderate increase in velocities is not uncommon during the days after the operation. A persistent and severe increase is seen in patients who develop the hyperperfusion syndrome.

Embolism is considered the most common cause of perioperative brain infarction. Microembolic signals are detected by TCD throughout the course of surgery, and both particulate microemboli and air microbubbles occur. Microembolism is particularly prevalent at clamp release (see Figure 1-17B), but only signals detected during dissection, wound closure, and the immediate postoperative phase of surgery have been associated with brain infarction.[262–264] The latter is not always symptomatic, and some small subcortical infarcts can be demonstrated only by CT or magnetic resonance imaging studies.[263] The detection of microembolism is useful because it prompts the surgeon to change the operative technique during the dissection phase or to use antithrombotic agents during the immediate postoperative period.[239] Shunting is also associated with ipsilateral microembolism.

Several studies indicate that monitoring leads to a reduction in the perioperative stroke rate.[262,265] Despite these reports, some investigators have been reluctant to base intraoperative decisions solely on TCD findings.[266] Although available data suggest that TCD can provide useful intraoperative information to the surgeon, TCD criteria based on prospective and well-designed studies are lacking at this time. Published studies provide a useful frame of reference, however. A more than 70% drop in middle cerebral artery flow velocities at cross-clamping is considered an adequate criterion for shunting by some authors.[265,267] Other investigators are stricter and require a 90% or more drop in the PSV[262] or an 85% or more decrease in mean flow velocity[256] to shunt. The positive and negative predictive values of these thresholds have not been established. Published case reports also show that embolic perioperative brain infarcts are associated with a "massive"[267] increase of microembolism.[259,268,269] More

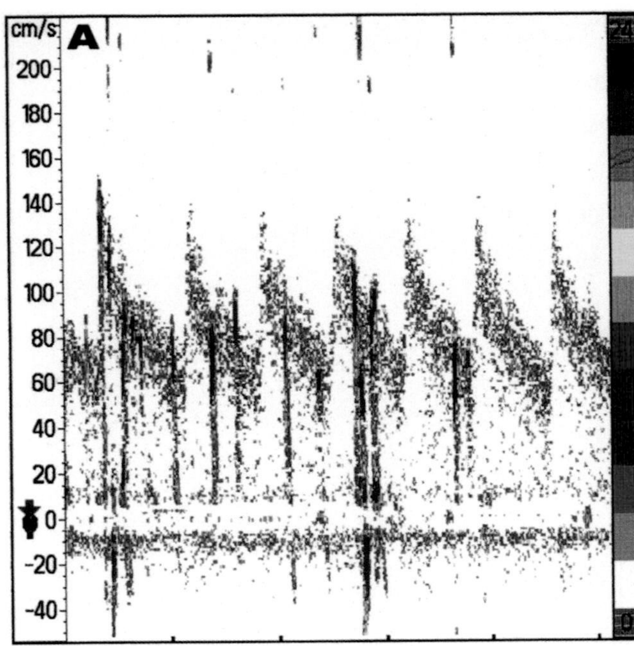

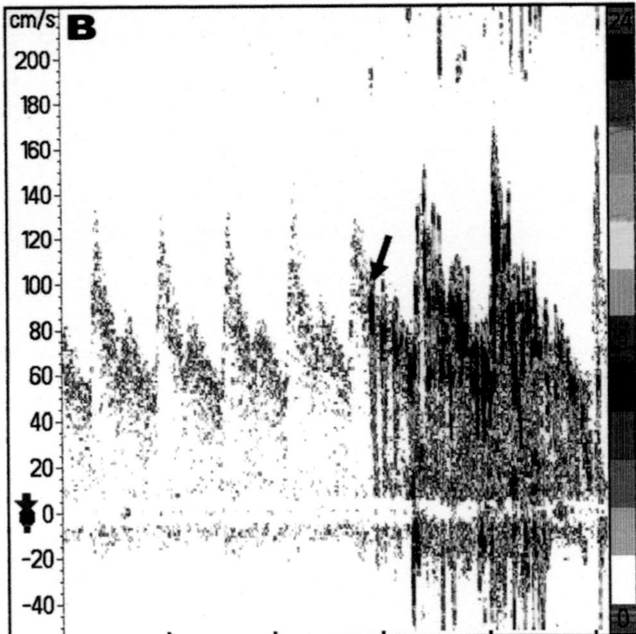

FIGURE 1-18. Patent foramen ovale. **A.** Microembolic signals appear in the middle cerebral artery less than 10 seconds after intravenous injection of an air-saline–agitated solution into a brachial subcutaneous vein. **B.** The injection was repeated during a Valsalva maneuver, which resulted in an increase of signals (*arrow*).

than 10 MESs during the dissection phase of the surgery[270] and more than 20 microemboli per hour during the immediate postoperative phase are associated with clinically or radiologically detected brain infarcts.[263,264]

Carotid Angioplasty and Stenting

MESs have also been observed during carotid angioplasty and stenting.[271] This high frequency of MESs is not associated with a chronic cognitive impairment.[272] TCD monitoring can help in assessing the efficacy of cerebral protection devices deployed during stenting.[273,274]

Cardiac Disease

MESs are detected in approximately one-third of patients with atrial fibrillation and stroke,[275–278] but they are not observed in asymptomatic patients with lone atrial fibrillation.[279] They are also observed in patients with prosthetic cardiac valves,[217,219] but in this setting, stroke symptoms do not seem to correlate with their number. Compared to signals detected in carotid disease, MES in patients with prosthetic heart valves have greater intensities, longer durations,[219,280,281] and some characteristics of gaseous emboli.[282] The phenomenon of "cavitation" secondary to the movement of prosthetic valves has been suggested as a cause of microbubble formation responsible for the MESs. This explains the resistance of MESs to antithrombotic therapy in this condition,[219,283–285] as well as their suppression with inhaled oxygen.[286] Several techniques have been introduced to differentiate gaseous and particulate microemboli.[200,280,286] MESs have also been described in patients with cardiomyopathy and with left ventricular assist devices.[217,218,238,287]

Paradoxical embolism through a patent foramen ovale is a relatively common cause of stroke, especially in young adults.[288,289] A right-to-left shunt can be diagnosed by TCD when MESs appear over both middle cerebral arteries within 10 seconds of the injection of agitated saline into a brachial vein (Figure 1-18). The administration of ultrasonic contrast agents and performance of the Valsalva maneuver can improve the test's sensitivity.[290,291] When compared to transesophageal echocardiography, the current gold standard, TCD has a sensitivity of 91–100% and a specificity between 65% and 93%.[290,292] TCD has also the advantage of being able to detect extracardiac shunts, such as pulmonary arteriovenous fistulas[293] that may be missed with echocardiography.

Cardiac Surgery

Brain injury during cardiac surgery usually presents clinically as encephalopathy or acute stroke,[294,295] and more than one-third of patients continue to have cognitive abnormalities 1 year after the operation.[296] Although hypoperfusion may be a cause of these complications,[297,298] brain embolism is often suspected. Persistent neuropsychological abnormalities are particularly common at 8 weeks after surgery in patients with high rates

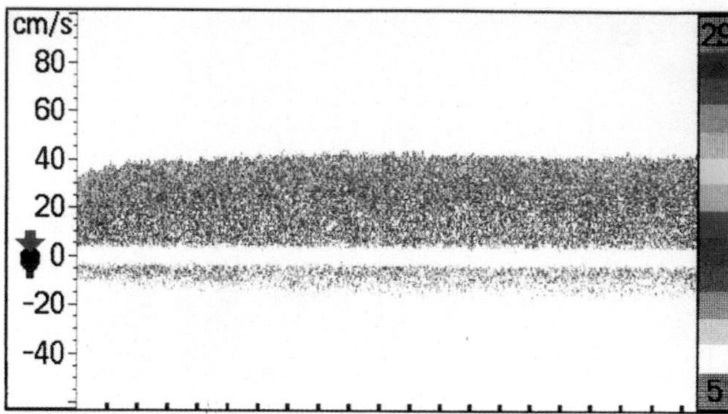

FIGURE 1-19. Coronary artery bypass graft surgery. Flow in the middle cerebral artery is nonpulsatile during cardiopulmonary bypass, and a microembolic signal is seen (*red*).

of brain microembolism during the procedure.[299] MESs are commonly observed during cardiac surgery,[300] and microembolism has been detected by funduscopic[301] and magnetic resonance imaging[302,303] examinations.

Both overt stroke and subtle cognitive dysfunctions have been correlated with the number of intraoperative MESs.[304] The composition of MESs during cardiopulmonary bypass has not been completely elucidated, but evidence of gaseous particles, atherosclerotic plaque components, platelet-fibrin aggregates, and lipid-laden or fatty particles exists.[305,306] The introduction of membrane rather than bubble oxygenators and in-line filtration markedly decreases the number of MESs during cardiopulmonary bypass.[307]

Just as in other invasive procedures, MESs do not appear at random during the course of cardiac surgery.[308,309] Clamping and unclamping of the aorta account for more than 60% of the total number of microemboli,[308–312] and it is recognized that the release of an aortic clamp placed over an atherosclerotic plaque is strongly related to the risk of cerebral embolism.[313,314] The number of MESs is especially high during cardiac ejection after the release of aortic cross-clamps and immediately after bypass. These signals correspond to atheromatous debris arising from the aorta. Better selection of the site of clamp placement by epiaortic ultrasound and the use of filters distal to the clamp may lead to a reduction in perioperative stroke.[315,316] Coronary artery bypass surgery performed off-pump decreases the number of microemboli when compared to the conventional on-pump bypass technique[317] (Figure 1-19).

Fat Embolism Syndrome

The fat embolism syndrome usually occurs in the setting of bone fractures and is characterized by neurologic and pulmonary dysfunction as well as skin petechiae. MESs can be detected in the brain arteries of patients with this syndrome (Figure 1-20). As trauma victims may also suf-

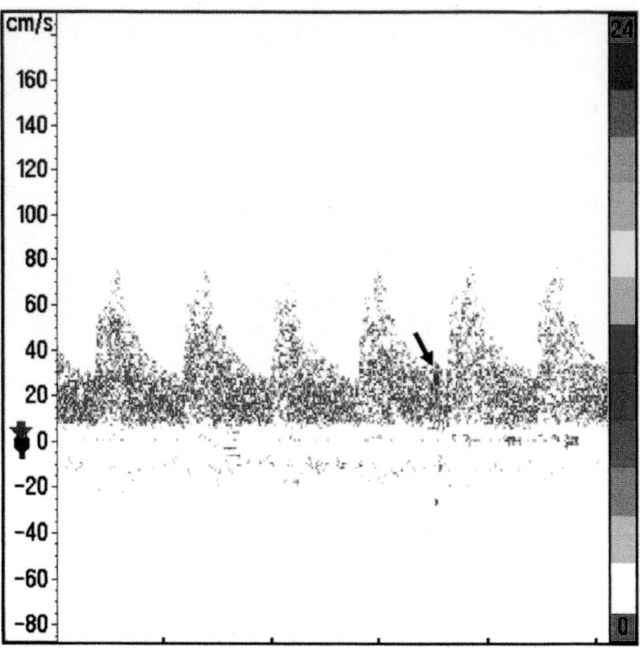

FIGURE 1-20. Fat embolism syndrome. Characteristic microembolic signal (*arrow*) in a patient with fat embolism.

fer concomitant head and chest injuries that can blur the clinical picture, the detection of MESs in several cerebral arteries, in this context, may point to the correct diagnosis.[223] MESs detected after fractures of the femur are associated with the development of neurologic symptoms. The simultaneous presence of a right-to-left cardiac shunt adversely affects the outcome.[318]

REFERENCES

1. White DN. The early development of neurosonology: I. Echoencephalography in adults. Ultrasound Med Biol 1992;18:115–165.

2. Nelson TR, Pretorius DH. The Doppler signal: where does it come from and what does it mean? AJR Am J Roentgenol 1991;151:439–447.

3. Taylor KJW, Burns PN, Wells PNT. Clinical Applications of Doppler Ultrasound. New York: Raven Press, 2001.

4. Hoeks APG, Reneman SR. Biophysical principles of vascular diagnosis. J Clin Ultrasound 1995; 23:71–79.

5. Juul R, Slordahl AS, Torp H, et al. Flow estimation using ultrasound imaging (color M-mode) and computer postprocessing. J Cereb Blood Flow Metab 1991;11:879–882.

6. McDonald DA. Blood Flow in Arteries. Baltimore: Williams & Wilkins, 1974.

7. Gosling RG, King DH. Arterial assessment by Doppler-shift ultrasound. Proc R Soc Med 1974;67: 447–449.

8. Pourcelot L. Applications cliniques de l'examen Doppler transcutane. Coloques de l'Inst Natl Sante Rech Med 1974;12:1376–1380.

9. Stary HC, Chandler AB, Dinsmore RE, et al. A definition of advanced types of atherosclerotic lesions and a histological classification of atherosclerosis. A report from the Committee on Vascular Lesions of the Council on Arteriosclerosis, American Heart Association. Circulation 1995;92:1355–1374.

10. Stary HC, Chandler AB, Glagou S, et al. A definition of initial, fatty streak and intermediate lesions of atherosclerosis. A report from the Committee on Vascular Lesions of the Council on Arteriosclerosis, American Heart Association. Arterioscler Thromb 1994;14:840–856.

11. Goes E, Janssens W, Maillet B. Tissue characterization of atheromatous plaques: correlation between ultrasound image and histological findings. J Clin Ultrasound 1990;18:611–617.

12. Hennerici M, Reifschneider G, Trockel U, Aulich A. Detection of early atherosclerotic lesions by duplex scanning of the carotid artery. J Clin Ultrasound 1984;12:455–464.

13. Lusby RJ, Ferrell LD, Ehrenfeld WK, et al. Carotid plaque hemorrhage: its role in production of cerebral ischemia. Arch Surg 1982;117:1479–1488.

14. Imparato AM, Riles TS, Gorstein F. The carotid bifurcation plaque: pathologic findings associated with cerebral ischemia. Stroke 1979;10:238–245.

15. Seeger J, Klingman N. The relationship between carotid plaque composition and neurological symptoms. J Surg Res 1987;43:78–85.

16. O'Donnell TF, Erdoes L, Mackey WC, et al. Correlation of B-mode ultrasound imaging and arteriography with pathological findings at carotid endarterectomy. Arch Surg 1985;120:443–449.

17. Bluth E, Kay D, Merritt C, et al. Sonographic characterization of carotid plaque: detection of hemorrhage. AJR Am J Roentgenol 1986;146:1061–1065.

18. Geroulakos G, Ramaswami G, Nicolaides A, et al. Characterization of symptomatic and asymptomatic carotid plaques using high-resolution real-time ultrasonography. Br J Surg 1993;80:1274–1277.

19. Mathiesen EB, Bonaa KH, Joakimsen O. Echolucent plaques are associated with high risk of ischemic cerebrovascular events in carotid stenosis: the Tromso Study. Circulation 2001;103:2171–2175.

20. O'Holleran LW, Kennelly MM, McClurken M, Johnson JM. Natural history of asymptomatic carotid plaque: five year follow-up study. Am J Surg 1987;154:659–662.

21. Sterpetti AV, Schultz RD, Feldhaus RJ, et al. Ultrasonographic features of carotid plaque and the risk of subsequent neurological deficits. Surgery 1988;104:652–660.

22. Polak JF, Shemanski L, O'Leary D, et al. Hypoechoic plaque at US of the carotid artery: an independent risk factor for incident stroke in adults aged 65 or older. Radiology 1998;208:649–654.

23. Gomez CR. Carotid plaque morphology and risk for stroke. Stroke 1990;21:148–151.

24. Imparato A, Riles T, Mintzer R, Baumann FG. The importance of hemorrhage in the relationship between gross morphological characteristics and cerebral symptoms in 376 carotid artery plaques. Ann Surg 1983;197:195–203.

25. Eliasziw M, Streifler J, Fox A, et al. Significance of plaque ulceration in symptomatic patients with high-grade carotid stenosis. North American Symptomatic Carotid Endarterectomy Trial. Stroke 1994;25: 304–308.

26. Wechsler LR. Ulcerations and carotid artery disease. Stroke 1988;19:650–653.

27. O'Leary DH, Holen J, Ricotta JJ, et al. Carotid bifurcation disease: prediction of ulceration with B-mode ultrasound. Radiology 1987;162:523–525.

28. Bluth EI, McVay LV 3rd, Merritt CR, Sullivan MA. The identification of ulcerative plaque with high resolution duplex carotid scanning. J Ultrasound Med 1988;7:73–76.

29. Furst H, Hartl WH, Jansen I, et al. Color-flow Doppler sonography in the identification of ulcerative plaques in patients with high-grade carotid artery stenosis. Am J Neuroradiol 1992;13:1581–1587.

30. Steinke W, Hennerici M, Rautenberg W, Mohr JP. Symptomatic and asymptomatic high-grade carotid stenoses in Doppler color-flow imaging. Neurology 1992;42:131–138.

31. European Carotid Surgery Trialists' Collaborative Group. MRC European Carotid Surgery Trial: interim results for symptomatic patients with severe [70-99%] or with mild [0-29%] carotid stenosis. Lancet 1991;337:1235–1243.

32. North American Symptomatic Carotid Endarterectomy Trial Collaborators. Beneficial effect of carotid endarterectomy in symptomatic patients with high-grade stenosis. N Engl J Med 1991;325:445–453.

33. Barnett HJM, Taylor DW, Eliasziw M. North American Symptomatic Carotid Endarterectomy Trial Collaborators. Benefits of carotid endarterectomy in patients with symptomatic moderate or severe stenosis. N Engl J Med 1998;339:1415–1425.

34. Executive Committee for the Asymptomatic Carotid Atherosclerosis Study. Endarterectomy for asymptomatic carotid artery stenosis. JAMA 1995;273: 1421–1428.

35. Earnest F 4th, Forbes G, Sandok BA, et al. Complications of cerebral angiography: prospective assessment of risk. AJR Am J Roentgenol 1984;142: 247–253.

36. New G, Roubin GS, Oetgen ME, et al. Validity of duplex ultrasound as a diagnostic modality for inter-

nal carotid artery disease. Catheter Cardiovasc Interv 2001;52:9–15.

37. Johnston DC, Goldstein LB. Clinical carotid endarterectomy decision making: noninvasive vascular imaging versus angiography. Neurology 2001;56:1009–1015.

38. Benedetti-Valentini F, Gossetti B, Irace L, et al. Carotid surgery without angiography is possible and safe. J Cardiovasc Surg 2000;41:601–605.

39. Thusay MM, Khoury M, Greene K. Carotid endarterectomy based on duplex ultrasound in patients with and without hemispheric symptoms. Am Surgeon 2001;67:1–6.

40. Robinson ML, Sacks D, Perlmutter GS, Marinelli DL. Diagnosis criteria for carotid Duplex sonography. AJR Am J Roentgenol 1988;151:1045–1049.

41. Howard G, Baker JF, Chambless LE. An approach for the use of Doppler ultrasound as a screening tool for hemodynamically significant stenosis (despite heterogeneity of Doppler performance). A multicenter experience. Asymptomatic Carotid Atherosclerosis Study Investigators. Stroke 1996;27:1951–1957.

42. Hunink MGM, Polak JF, Barlan MM. Detection and quantification of carotid artery stenosis: efficacy of various Doppler parameters. AJR Am J Roentgenol 1993;160:619–625.

43. Kuntz KM, Polak JF, Whittemore AD, et al. Duplex ultrasound criteria for the identification of carotid stenosis should be laboratory specific. Stroke 1997;28:597–602.

44. O'Boyle MK, Vibhakar NI, Chung J, et al. Duplex sonography of the carotid arteries in patients with isolated aortic stenosis: imaging findings and relation to the severity of stenosis. AJR Am J Roentgenol 1996;166:197–202.

45. Perret RS, Sloop GD. Increased peak blood velocity in association with elevated blood pressure. Ultrasound Med Biol 2000;26:1387–1391.

46. Hayes AC, Johnston KW, Baker WH, et al. The effect of contralateral disease on carotid Doppler frequency. Surgery 1988;103:19–23.

47. Ray SA, Lockhart SJ, Dourado R, et al. Effect of contralateral disease on duplex measurements of internal carotid artery stenosis. Br J Surg 2000;87:1057–1062.

48. Bonig L, Weder B, Schott D, et al. Prediction of angiographic carotid artery stenosis indexes by colour Doppler-assisted duplex imaging. A critical appraisal of the parameters used. Eur J Neurol 2000;7:183–190.

49. Moneta GL, Edwards JM, Papanicolaou G, et al. Screening for asymptomatic internal carotid artery stenosis: duplex criteria of discriminating 60%-99% stenosis. J Vasc Surg 1995;21:989–994.

50. Faught WE, Mattos MA, van Bemmelen PS, et al. Color-flow duplex scanning of carotid arteries: new velocity criteria based on receiver operator characteristic analysis for threshold stenoses used in the symptomatic and asymptomatic carotid trials. J Vasc Surg 1994;19:818–827.

51. Neale ML, Chambers JL, Kelly AT, et al. Reappraisal of duplex criteria to assess significant carotid stenosis with special reference to reports from the North American Symptomatic Carotid Endarterectomy Trial and the European Carotid Surgery Trial. J Vasc Surg 1994;20:642–649.

52. Carpenter JP, Lexa FJ, Davis JT. Determination of duplex Doppler ultrasound criteria appropriate to the North American Symptomatic Carotid Endarterectomy Trial. Stroke 1996;27:695–699.

53. Hood DB, Mattos MA, Mansour A, et al. Prospective evaluation of new duplex criteria to identify 70% internal carotid artery stenosis. J Vasc Surg 1996;23:254–262.

54. Huston J, James EM, Brown RD, et al. Redefined duplex ultrasonographic criteria for diagnosis of carotid artery stenosis. Mayo Clin Proc 2000;75:1133–1140.

55. Carpenter JP, Lexa FJ, Davis JT. Determination of sixty percent or greater carotid artery stenosis by duplex Doppler ultrasonography. J Vasc Surg 1995;22:697–705.

56. Jackson MR, Chang AS, Robles HA. Determination of 60% or greater carotid stenosis: a prospective comparison of MRA and duplex ultrasound with conventional angiography. Ann Vasc Surg 1998;12:236–243.

57. Ballard JL, Fleig K, De Lange M, Killeen JD. The diagnostic accuracy of duplex ultrasonography for evaluating carotid bifurcation. Am J Surg 1994;169:123–126.

58. Paivansalo M, Leinonen S, Turunen J, et al. Quantification of carotid artery stenosis with various Doppler velocity parameters. Rofo Fortschr Geb Rontgenstr Neuen Bildgeb Verfahr 1996;164:108–113.

59. Wikelaar GB, Chen JC, Salvian AJ, Taylor DC. New duplex ultrasound scan criteria managing symptomatic 50% or greater carotid stenosis. J Vasc Surg 1999;29:986–994.

60. Perkins JM, Galland RB, Simmons MJ, Magee TR. Carotid duplex imaging: variation and validation. Br J Surg 2000;87:320–322.

61. Hoskins PR. Accuracy of maximum velocity estimates made using Doppler ultrasound systems. Br J Radiol 1996;69:172–177.

62. Criswell BK, Langsfeld M, Tullis MJ, Marek J. Evaluating institutional variability of duplex scanning in the detection of carotid artery stenosis. Am J Surg 1998;176:591–597.

63. Hennerici M, Rautenberg W, Trockel U, Kladezky RG. Spontaneous progression and regression of small carotid atheroma. Lancet 1985;1:1415–1419.

64. Hennerici M, Huldbomer H, Hefter H, et al. Natural history of asymptomatic extracranial arterial disease. Brain 1987;110:777–791.

65. Taylor LM, Loboa L, Porter JM. The clinical course of carotid bifurcation stenosis as determined by duplex sonographic scanning. J Vasc Surg 1988;8:255–261.

66. Lovelace TD, Moneta GL, Abou-Zamzam AM, et al. Optimizing duplex follow-up in patients with an asymptomatic internal carotid artery stenosis of less than 60%. J Vasc Surg 2001;33:56–61.

67. Zwiebel WJ. Duplex sonography of the cerebral arteries: efficacy, limitations and indications. AJR Am J Roentgenol 1992;158:29–36.

68. Kieny R, Hirsch D, Seiller C, et al. Does carotid eversion endarterectomy and reimplantation reduce the risk of restenosis? Ann Vasc Surg 1993;7:407–413.

69. O'Donnel TF, Gallow AD, Scott G, et al. Ultrasound characteristics of recurrent carotid disease: hypothesis explaining the low incidence of symptomatic recurrence. J Vasc Surg 1985;2:26–41.

70. Mattos MA, van Bemmelen PS, Barkmeirer LD, et al. Routine surveillance after carotid endarterectomy: does it affect clinical management? J Vasc Surg 1993;17:819–831.

71. Moore WS, Kempczinsky RF, Nelson JJ, Toole J. Recurrent carotid stenosis. Results from the Asymptomatic Carotid Atherosclerosis Study. Stroke 1998;29:2018–2025.

72. Frericks H, Kievit J, van Baalen JM, van Bockel JH. Carotid recurrent stenosis and risk of ipsilateral stroke. A systematic review of the literature. Stroke 1998;29:244–250.

73. Wenderhag I, Gustavsson T, Suurkula M, et al. Ultrasound measurement of wall thickness in the carotid artery: fundamental principles and description of a computerized analyzing system. Clin Physiol 1991;11:565–577.

74. Sidhu PS, Woodcock JP, Gorman S, Pugh N. Carotid Imaging and Plaque Morphology. In GM Baxter, PLP Allan, P Morley (eds), Clinical Diagnostic Ultrasound. Malden, MA: Blackwell, 1999;223–247.

75. Pauciullo P, Iannuzzi A, Sartorio R, et al. Increased intima-media thickness of the common carotid artery in hypercholesterolaemic children. Arterioscler Thromb 1994;14:1075–1079.

76. Sinclair AM, Hughes AD, Geroulakos G, et al. Structural changes in the heart and the carotid arteries associated with hypertension in humans. J Hum Hypertens 1995;7:1–13.

77. Howard G, Burke GL, Szklo M, et al. Active and passive smoking are associated with increased carotid wall thickness. The atherosclerosis risk in Communities Study. Arch Intern Med 1994;154:1277–1282.

78. Malinow MR, Nieto J, Szklo M, et al. Carotid artery intimal-medial wall thickening and plasma homocysteine in asymptomatic adults. The Atherosclerosis Risk in Communities Study. Circulation 1993;87:1107–1113.

79. Ebrahim S, Papacosta O, Whicup P, et al. Carotid plaque, intima media thickness, cardiovascular risk factors, and prevalent cardiovascular disease in men and women: the British Regional Heart Study. Stroke 1999;30:841–850.

80. Buyington RP, Furberg CD, Crouse JR 3rd, et al. Pravastatin, lipids, and atherosclerosis in the carotid arteries (PLACII). Am J Cardiol 1995;76:54C–59C.

81. Sturzenger M, Mattle HP, Rivoir A, et al. Ultrasound findings in carotid artery dissection: analysis of 43 patients. Neurology 1995;45:691–698.

82. Steinke W, Rautenberg W, Schwartz A, et al. Non-invasive monitoring of internal carotid artery dissection. Stroke 1994;25:998–1005.

83. Carroll BA. Carotid ultrasound. Neuroimaging Clin N Am 1996;6:875–897.

84. Sturzenegger M, Mattle HP, Rivoir A, et al. Ultrasound findings in spontaneous extracranial vertebral artery dissection. Stroke 1993;24:1910–1921.

85. Hoffman M, Sacco RL, Chan S, et al. Non-invasive detection of vertebral artery dissection. Stroke 1993;24:815–819.

86. Lee TH, Ryu JE, Chen ST, et al. Comparison between carotid duplex sonography and angiography in the diagnosis of extracranial internal carotid artery occlusion. J Formos Med Assoc 1992;91:575–579.

87. Gortler M, Niethammer R, Widder B. Differentiating subtotal carotid artery stenosis from occlùsions by colour-coded duplex sonography. J Neurol 1994;241:301–305.

88. Ferrer JM, Samso JJ, Serrando JR, et al. Use of ultrasound contrast in the diagnosis of carotid artery occlusion. J Vasc Surg 2000;31:736–741.

89. AbuRahma AF, Pollack JA, Robinson PA, Mullins D. The reliability of color Duplex ultrasound in diagnosing total carotid artery occlusion. Am J Surg 1997;174:185–187.

90. Bornstein NR, Zlatko GB, Norris JW. The limitations of diagnosis of carotid occlusion by Doppler ultrasound. Ann Surg 1998;207:315–317.

91. Fujitani RM, Mills JL, Wang LM, Taylor SM. The effect of unilateral internal carotid artery occlusion upon contralateral duplex study: criteria for accurate interpretation. J Vasc Surg 1992;16:459–468.

92. Baxter GM, Polak JF. Variance mapping in colour flow imaging: what does it mean? Clin Radiol 1994;49:262–265.

93. Caplan LR, Amarenco P, Lafranchise EF, et al. Embolism from the vertebral origin occlusive disease. Neurology 1992;42:1505–1512.

94. Bartels E. Vertebral Sonography. In CH Tegeler, VL Babikian, CR Gomez (eds), Neurosonology. St. Louis: Mosby, 1996;83–100.

95. Tratting S, Huebsch P, Schuster H, Poelzleitner D. Color-coded Doppler imaging of the vertebral arteries. Stroke 1990;21:1222–1225.

96. Kuhl V, Tettenborn B, Eicke BM, et al. Color-coded duplex ultrasonography of the origin of the vertebral artery: normal values of flow velocities. J Neuroimaging 2000;10:17–21.

97. Kazumi K, Yasaka M, Moriyasu H. Ultrasonographic evaluation of the vertebral artery to detect vertebrobasilar axis occlusion. Stroke 1994;25:1006–1009.

98. Touboul PJ, Bousser MG, Laplane D, Castaigne P. Duplex scanning of normal vertebral arteries. Stroke 1986;17:921–923.

99. Kotval PS, Babu SC, Shan PM. Doppler diagnosis of partial vertebral/subclavian steals convertible to full steals with physiologic maneuvers. J Ultrasound Med 1990;9:207–213.

100. Yip PK, Liu HM, Hwang BS. Subclavian steal phenomenon: correlation between duplex sonography and angiographic findings. Neuroradiology 1992;34:279–288.

101. Aaslid R, Markwalder TM, Nornes H. Noninvasive transcranial Doppler ultrasound recording of flow velocity in basal cerebral arteries. J Neurosurg 1982;57:769–774.

102. Santalucia P, Feldman E. The Basic Transcranial Doppler Examination: Technique and Anatomy. In VL Babikian, LR Wechsler (eds), Transcranial Doppler Ultrasonography. Boston: Butterworth–Heinemann, 1999;13–31.

103. Totaro R, Marini C, Cannarsa C, Prencipe M. Reproducibility of transcranial Doppler sonography: a validation study. Ultrasound Med Biol 1992;18:173–177.

104. Krejza J, Mariak Z, Walecki J, et al. Transcranial color Doppler sonography of basal cerebral arteries in 182 healthy subjects: age and sex variability and normal reference values for blood parameters. AJR Am J Roentgenol 1999;172:213–218.

105. Martin PJ, Evans DH, Naylor AR. Measurement of blood flow velocity in the basal cerebral circulation: advantages of transcranial color-coded sonography over conventional transcranial Doppler. J Clin Ultrasound 1995;23:21–26.

106. Ringelstein EB, Kahlscheuer B, Niggemeyer E, Otis SM. Transcranial Doppler sonography: anatomical landmarks and normal velocity values. Ultrasound Med Biol 1990;16:745–761.

107. Tong DC, Albers GW. Normal Values. In VL Babikian, LR Wechsler (eds), Transcranial Doppler Ultrasonography (2nd ed). Boston: Butterworth–Heinemann, 1999;33–46.

108. Lupetin AR, Davis DA, Beckman I, Dash N. Transcranial Doppler sonography. Part 1. Principles, technique and normal appearances. Radiographics 1995;15:179–191.

109. Martin PJ, Evans DH, Naylor AR. Transcranial color-coded sonography of the basal cerebral circulation. Reference data from 115 volunteers. Stroke 1994;25:390–396.

110. Zunker P, Happe S, Georgiadis AL, et al. Maternal cerebral hemodynamics in pregnancy-related hypertension. A prospective transcranial Doppler study. Ultrasound Obstet Gynecol 2000;16:179–187.

111. Krejza J, Mariak Z, Huba M, et al. Effect of endogenous estrogen on blood flow through carotid arteries. Stroke 2001;32:30–36.

112. Kaps M, Link A. Transcranial sonographic monitoring during thrombolytic therapy. Am J Neuroradiol 1998;19:758–760.

113. Christou I, Alexandrov A, Burgin WS, et al. Timing of recanalization after tissue plasminogen activator determined by transcranial Doppler correlates with clinical recovery from ischemic stroke. Stroke 2000;31:1812–1816.

114. Toni D, Fiorelli M, Zanette EM, et al. Early spontaneous improvement and deterioration of ischemic stroke patients. Stroke 1998;29:1144–1148.

115. Yasaka M, O'Keefe GJ, Chambers BR, et al., for the Australian Streptokinase Trial Study group. Streptokinase in acute stroke. Neurology 1998;50:626–632.

116. Gerriets T, Postert T, Goertler M, et al., for the DIAS Study group. DIAS I: Duplex-sonographic assessment of the cerebrovascular status in acute stroke. Stroke 2000;31:2342–2345.

117. Maurer M, Mullges W, Becker G. Diagnosis of MCA-occlusion and monitoring of systemic thrombolytic therapy with contrast enhanced transcranial Doppler sonography. J Neuroimaging 1999;9:99–101.

118. Rosenschein U, Roth A, Rassin T, et al. Analysis of coronary ultrasound thrombolysis endpoints in acute myocardial infarction (ACUTE Trial). Circulation 1997;95:1411–1416.

119. Spengos K, Behrens S, Daffertshofer M, et al. Acceleration of thrombolysis with ultrasound through the cranium in a flow model. Ultrasound Med Biol 2000;26:889–895.

120. Segura T, Serena J, Castellanos M, et al. Embolism in acute middle cerebral artery stenosis. Neurology 2001;56:497–501.

121. Lindegaard KF, Bakke SJ, Aaslid R, Nornes H. Doppler diagnosis of intracranial artery occlusive disorders. J Neurol Neurosurg Psychiatry 1986;49:510–518.

122. Giller CA, Hodges K, Batjer HH. Transcranial Doppler pulsatility in vasodilatation and stenosis. J Neurosurg 1990;72:901–906.

123. Baumgartner RW, Mattle HP, Schroth G. Assessment of >/=50% and <50% intracranial stenoses by transcranial color-coded duplex sonography. Stroke 1999;30:87–92.

124. Kimura K, Yasaka W, Wada K, et al. Diagnosis of middle cerebral artery stenosis by transcranial color-

coded real-time sonography. Am J Neuroradiol 1998;19:1893–1896.

125. Schwarze JJ, Babikian VL, De Witt LD, et al. Longitudinal monitoring of intracranial arterial stenoses with transcranial Doppler ultrasonography. J Neuroimaging 1994;4:182–187.

126. Ley-Pozo J, Ringelstein EB. Noninvasive detection of occlusive disease of the carotid siphon and middle cerebral artery. Ann Neurol 1990;28:640–647.

127. Estol CJ, De Witt LD, Tettenborn B, et al. Accuracy of transcranial Doppler in the vertebrobasilar circulation. Ann Neurol 1990;28:225–226(Abst).

128. Kenton AR, Martin PJ, Abbott RJ, Moody AR. Comparison of transcranial color-coded sonography and magnetic resonance angiography in acute stroke. Stroke 1997;28:1601–1606.

129. Kimura K, Hashimoto Y, Hirano T, et al. Diagnosis of middle cerebral artery occlusion with transcranial color-coded real-time sonography. Am J Neuroradiol 1996;17:895–899.

130. Brandt T, Knauth M, Wildermuth S, et al. CT angiography and Doppler sonography for emergency assessment in acute basilar artery ischemia. Stroke 1999;30:606–612.

131. Demchuk AM, Christou I, Wein TH, et al. Accuracy and criteria for localizing arterial occlusion with transcranial Doppler. J Neuroimaging 2000;10:1–12.

132. Seidel G, Kaps M, Gerriets T. Potential and limitation of transcranial color-coded sonography in stroke patients. Stroke 1995;26:2061–2066.

133. Postert T, Braun B, Meves S, et al. Contrast-enhanced transcranial color-coded sonography in acute hemispheric brain infarction. Stroke 1999;30:1819–1826.

134. Marti-Fabregas J, Cocho D, Lleo A, Marti-Vilalta JL. Transcranial Doppler recording in a patient with transient positional cerebral ischemia. Neurology 2000;55:731–732.

135. Mattle HP, Nirkko AC, Baumgartner RW, Sturzenegger M. Transient cerebral circulatory arrest coincides with fainting in cough syncope. Neurology 1995;45:498–501.

136. Carey BJ, Eames PJ, Panerai R, Potter JF. A case of arrhythmia-induced transient cerebral hyperaemia. Cerebrovasc Dis 2000;10:330–333.

137. Kluytmans M, van der Grond J, van Everdingen KJ, et al. Cerebral hemodynamics in relation to patterns of collateral flow. Stroke 1999;30:1432–1439.

138. Baumgartner RW, Baumgartner I, Mattle HP, Schroth G. Transcranial color-coded duplex sonography in the evaluation of collateral flow through the circle of Willis. Am J Neuroradiol 1997;18:127–133.

139. Hoksbergen AWJ, Legemate DA, Ubbink DT, Jacobs MJHM. Collateral variations in circle of Willis in atherosclerotic population assessed by means of transcranial color-coded duplex ultrasonography. Stroke 2000;31:1656–1660.

140. Demchuk AM, Christou I, Wein TH, et al. Specific transcranial Doppler flow findings related to the presence and site of arterial occlusion. Stroke 2000;31:140–144.

141. Silverstrini M, Vernieri F, Pasqualetti P, et al. Impaired cerebral vasoreactivity and risk of stroke in patients with asymptomatic carotid artery stenosis. JAMA 2000;283:2122–2127.

142. Ringelstein EB, Weiller C, Weckesser M, Weckesser S. Cerebral vasomotor reactivity is significantly reduced in low-flow as compared to thromboembolic infarctions: the key role of the circle of Willis. J Neurol Sci 1994;103–109.

143. Lipsitz LA, Mukai S, Hamner J, et al. Dynamic regulation of middle cerebral artery blood flow velocity in aging and hypertension. Stroke 2000;31:1897–1903.

144. Molina C, Sabin JA, Montaner J, et al. Impaired cerebrovascular reactivity as a risk marker for first-ever lacunar infarction. Stroke 1999;30:2296–2301.

145. Ries S, Steinke W, Neff KW, Hennerici M. Echocontrast-enhanced transcranial color-coded sonography for the diagnosis of transverse venous thrombosis. Stroke 1997;28:696–700.

146. Becker G, Bogdahn U, Gehlberg C, et al. Transcranial color-coded real-time sonography of intracranial veins. J Neuroimaging 1995;5:87–94.

147. Valdueza JM, Schultz M, Harms L, Einhaupl KM. Venous transcranial Doppler ultrasound monitoring in acute dural sinus thrombosis. Stroke 1995;26:1196–1199.

148. Schoser BG, Riemenschneider N, Hansen HC. The impact of raised intracranial pressure on cerebral venous hemodynamics: a prospective venous transcranial Doppler ultrasonography study. J Neurosurg 1999;91:744–749.

149. Steinberg HM. Management of sickle cell disease. N Engl J Med 1999;340:1021–1030.

150. Adams RJ, McKie VC, Carl EM, et al. Long-term stroke risk in children with sickle-cell disease screened with transcranial Doppler. Ann Neurol 1997;42:699–704.

151. Adams RJ, McKie VC, Hsu L, et al. Prevention of a first stroke by transfusions in children with sickle cell anemia and abnormal results on transcranial Doppler ultrasonography. N Engl J Med 1998;339:5–11.

152. National Heart, Lung, and Blood Institute (NHLBI). Clinical Alert: Periodic Transfusions Lower Stroke Risk in Children with Sickle Cell Anemia. September 18, 1997.

153. Mayberg MR, Batjer H, Dacey R, et al. Guidelines for the management of aneurysmal subarachnoid

hemorrhage: a statement for health care professionals from a special writing group of the Stroke Council. Stroke 1994;25:2315–2328.

154. Song JK, Elliott JP, Eskridge JM. Neuroradiologic diagnosis and treatment of vasospasm. Neuroimaging Clin N Am 1997;7:819–835.

155. Saito I, Shigeno T, Aritake K, et al. Vasospasm assessed by angiography and computed tomography. J Neurosurg 1979;51:466–475.

156. Heros RC, Zervas T, Varsos V. Cerebral vasospasm after subarachnoid hemorrhage: an update. Ann Neurol 1983;14:599–608.

157. Grosset DG, Straiton J, du Trevou M, Bullock R. Prediction of symptomatic vasospasm after subarachnoid hemorrhage by rapidly increasing transcranial Doppler velocity and cerebral blood flow changes. Stroke 1992;23:674–679.

158. Laumer R, Steinmeier R, Gyonner F, et al. Cerebral hemodynamics in subarachnoid hemorrhage evaluated by transcranial Doppler sonography. Part 1. Reliability of flow velocities in clinical management. Neurosurgery 1993;33:1–8.

159. Wardlaw JM, Offin R, Teasdale GM, Teasdale EM. Is routine transcranial Doppler ultrasound monitoring useful in the management of subarachnoid hemorrhage? J Neurosurg 1998;88:272–276.

160. Vora YY, Suarez-Almazor M, Steinke DE, et al. Role of transcranial Doppler monitoring in the diagnosis of cerebral vasospasm after subarachnoid hemorrhage. Neurosurgery 1999;44:1237–1248.

161. Okada Y, Shima T, Nishida M, et al. Comparison of transcranial Doppler investigation of aneurysmal vasospasm with digital subtraction angiographic and clinical findings. Neurosurgery 1999;45:443–450.

162. Bederson JB, Levy LA, Ding WH, et al. Acute vasoconstriction after subarachnoid hemorrhage. Neurosurgery 1998;42:352–362.

163. Ekelund A, Saveland H, Romner B, Brandt L. Transcranial Doppler ultrasound in hypertensive versus normotensive patients after aneurysmal subarachnoid hemorrhage. Stroke 1995;26:2071–2074.

164. Klingelhofer J, Sander D, Holzgrafe M, et al. Cerebral vasospasm evaluated by transcranial Doppler ultrasonography at different intracranial pressures. J Neurosurg 1991;75:752–758.

165. Sloan MA, Wozniak MA, Macko RF. Monitoring of Vasospasm after Subarachnoid Hemorrhage. In VL Babikian, LR Wechsler (eds), Transcranial Doppler Ultrasonography (2nd ed). Boston: Butterworth–Heinemann, 1999;109–127.

166. Lennihan L, Petty GW, Fink ME, et al. Transcranial Doppler detection of anterior cerebral artery vasospasm. J Neurol Neurosurg Psychiatry 1993;56: 906–909.

167. Compton JS, Redmond S, Symon L. Cerebral blood velocity in subarachnoid hemorrhage: a transcranial Doppler study. J Neurol Neurosurg Psychiatry 1987;50:1499–1503.

168. Lindegaard KF, Nornes H, Bakke SJ, et al. Cerebral vasospasm after subarachnoid hemorrhage investigated by means of transcranial Doppler ultrasound. Acta Neurochir Suppl (Wien) 1988;42P:81–84.

169. Lindegaard KF, Nornes H, Bakke SJ, et al. Cerebral vasospasm diagnosis by means of angiography and blood velocity measurements. Acta Neurochir (Wien) 1989;100:12–24.

170. Giller CA, Ratcliff B, Berger B, Giller A. An impedance index in normal subjects and in subarachnoid hemorrhage. Ultrasound Med Biol 1996;22:373–382.

171. Aaslid R, Huber P, Nornes H. Evaluation of cerebrovascular spasm with transcranial Doppler ultrasound. J Neurosurg 1984;60:37–41.

172. Grolimund P, Seiler W, Aaslid R, et al. Evaluation of cerebrovascular disease by combined extracranial and transcranial Doppler sonography. Experience in 1,039 patients. Stroke 1987;18: 1018–1024.

173. Sekhar LN, Wechsler LR, Luyckx K, et al. Value of transcranial Doppler examination in the diagnosis of cerebral vasospasm after subarachnoid hemorrhage. Neurosurgery 1988;22:813–821.

174. Sloan MA, Haley EC, Kassel NF, et al. Sensitivity and specificity of transcranial Doppler ultrasonography in the diagnosis of vasospasm following subarachnoid hemorrhage. Neurology 1989;39:1514–1518.

175. Burch CM, Wozniak MA, Sloan MA, et al. Detection of intracranial internal carotid artery and middle cerebral artery vasospasm following subarachnoid hemorrhage. J Neuroimaging 1996;6:8–15.

176. Proust F, Callonec F, Clavier E, et al. Usefulness of transcranial color-coded sonography in the diagnosis of cerebral vasospasm. Stroke 1999;30:1091–1098.

177. Becker G, Greiner K, Kaune B, et al. Diagnosis and monitoring of subarachnoid hemorrhage by transcranial color-coded real-time sonography. Neurosurgery 1991;30:1091–1098.

178. Baumgartner RW, Mattle HP, Kothbauer K, Schroth G. Transcranial color-coded duplex sonography in cerebral aneurysms. Stroke 1994;25:2429–2434.

179. Gerriets T, Seidel G, Modrau B, Kaps M. Contrast-enhanced transcranial color-coded duplex sonography. Efficiency and validity. Neurology 1999;52: 1133–1137.

180. Ducrocq X, Hassler W, Moritake K. Consensus opinion on diagnosis of cerebral circulatory arrest using Doppler sonography. J Neurol Sci 1998;159:145–150.

181. Bartels E, Rodiek SO, Lumenta C, Flugel KA. Evaluation of arteriovenous malformations with trans-

cranial color-coded duplex ultrasonography. J Ultrasound Med 1998;17:166–169.

182. Klotzsch C, Henkes H, Nahser HC, et al. Transcranial color-coded duplex sonography in cerebral arteriovenous malformations. Stroke 1995;12:2298–2301.

183. Krejza J, Mariak Z, Bert RJ. Transcranial color Doppler sonography in emergency management of intracerebral hemorrhage caused by arteriovenous malformation: case report. Neuroradiology 2000;42: 900–904.

184. Pasqualin A. The relevance of anatomic and hemodynamic factors to a classification of cerebral arteriovenous malformation. Neurosurgery 1991;28:370–379.

185. Baumgartner RW, Mattle HP, Schroth G. Transcranial color-coded duplex sonography of cerebral arteriovenous malformations. Neuroradiology 1996;38:734–737.

186. Chioffi F, Pasqualin A, Beltramello A, Da Pian R. Hemodynamic effects of preoperative embolization in cerebral arteriovenous malformations: evaluation with transcranial Doppler sonography. Neurosurgery 1992;31:877–885.

187. Manchola IF, De Salles AAF, Kok Foo T, et al. Arteriovenous malformation hemodynamics: a transcranial Doppler study. Neurosurgery 1993;33:556–562.

188. Padayachee TS, Gosling RG, Bishop CC, et al. Monitoring middle cerebral artery blood flow velocity during carotid endarterectomy. Br J Surg 1986;73:98–100.

189. Spencer MP, Thomas GI, Nicholls SC, Sauvage LA. Detection of middle cerebral artery emboli using transcranial Doppler ultrasonography. Stroke 1990;21: 415–423.

190. Russel D. The Detection of Cerebral Emboli Using Transcranial Doppler. Theoretical, Experimental and Clinical Aspects. In DW Newell, R Aaslid (eds), Transcranial Doppler. New York: Raven Press, 1992:207–214.

191. Berger MP, Tegeler CH. Embolus Detection Using Doppler Ultrasonography. In VL Babikian, LR Wechsler (eds), Transcranial Doppler Ultrasonography. St. Louis: Mosby, 1993;232–241.

192. Markus H, Loh A, Brown MM. Computerized detection of cerebral emboli and discrimination from artifact using Doppler ultrasound. Stroke 1993;24: 1667–1672.

193. Smith JL, Evans DH, Fan L, et al. Differentiation between emboli and artefacts using dual-gated transcranial Doppler ultrasound. Ultrasound Med Biol 1996;22:1031–1036.

194. Georgiadis D, Goeke J, Hill M, et al. A novel technique for identification of Doppler MES based on the coincidence method: in vitro and in vivo evaluation. Stroke 1996;27:683–686.

195. Droste DW, Hagedorn G, Notzold A, et al. Bigated transcranial Doppler for the detection of clinically silent circulating emboli in normal persons and patients with prosthetic cardiac valves. Stroke 1997;28: 588–592.

196. Markus HS, Brown MM. Differentiation between different pathological cerebral embolic materials using transcranial Doppler in an in vitro model. Stroke 1994;24:1–5.

197. Markus H, Loh A, Brown MM. Detection of circulating cerebral emboli using Doppler ultrasound in a sheep model. J Neurol Sci 1994;122:117–124.

198. Smith JL, Evans DH, Bell PR, Naylor AR. Time domain analysis of embolic signals can be used in place of high-resolution Wigner analysis when classifying gaseous and particulate emboli. Ultrasound Med Biol 1998;24:989–993.

199. Smith JL, Evans DH, Bell PR, Naylor AR. A comparison of four methods for distinguishing Doppler signals from gaseous and particulate emboli. Stroke 1998;29:1133–1138.

200. Healey AJ, Leeman S, Markus H. A Novel Method of Identifying Gaseous Emboli Using Fractional Harmonics. In J Klingelhofer, E Bartels, BE Ringelstein (eds), New Trends in Cerebral Hemodynamics and Neurosonology. Munster: Elsevier, 1997;380–384.

201. Moehring MA, Klepper JR. Pulse Doppler ultrasound detection, characterization and size estimation of emboli in flowing blood. Trans Biomed Eng 1994;41:35–44.

202. Markus HS, Ackerstaff R, Babikian V, et al. Intercenter agreement in reading Doppler embolic signals. A multicenter international study. Stroke 1997;28: 1307–1310.

203. Consensus Committee of the Ninth International Cerebral Hemodynamic Symposium. Basic identification criteria of Doppler microemboli. Stroke 1995;25:1123.

204. Cullinane M, Reid G, Dittrich R, et al. Evaluation of the new online automated embolic signal detection algorithm, including comparison with a panel of international experts. Stroke 2000;31:1335–1341.

205. Droste DW, Decker W, Siemens HJ, et al. Variability in occurrence of embolic signals in long term transcranial Doppler recordings. Neurol Res 1996;18: 25–30.

206. Molloy J, Khan N, Markus HS. Temporal variability of asymptomatic embolization in carotid artery stenosis and optimal recording protocols. Stroke 1998;29:1129–1132.

207. Cardiogenic brain embolism: the second report of the Cerebral Embolism Task Force. Arch Neurol 1989;46:727–743.

208. Bogusslavsky J, Hachinski VC, Boughner DR, et al. Cardiac and arterial lesions in carotid transient ischemic attacks. Arch Neurol 1986;43:223–228.

209. Bogousslavsky J, Melle GV, Regli F. The Lausanne Stroke Registry: analysis of 1000 consecutive patients with first stroke. Stroke 1988;19:1083–1092.

210. Caplan LR, Hier DB, D'Cruz I. Cerebral embolism in the Michel Reese Stroke Registry. Stroke 1983;14:530–537.

211. Babikian V, Wijman C, Hyde C, et al. Cerebral microembolism and early recurrent cerebral or retinal ischemic events. Stroke 1997;28:1314–1318.

212. Siebler M, Kleinschmidt A, Sitzer M, et al. Cerebral microembolism in symptomatic and asymptomatic high grade internal carotid artery stenosis. Neurology 1994;44:615–618.

213. Georgiadis D, Linder A, Manz M, et al. Intracranial microemboli detection in 500 patients with potential cardiac or carotid embolic source and in normal controls. Stroke 1997;28:1203–1207.

214. Srinivasan J, Newell DW, Sturzenegger M, et al. Transcranial Doppler in the evaluation of internal carotid artery dissection. Stroke 1996;27:1226–1230.

215. Babikian VL, Forteza AM, Gavrilescu T, Samaraweera R. Cerebral microembolism and extracranial internal carotid artery dissection. J Ultrasound Med 1996;15:863–866.

216. Koch S, Romano JG, Bustillo IC, et al. Anticoagulation and microembolus detection in a case of internal carotid artery dissection. J Neuroimaging 2001;11:63–66.

217. Tong D, Bolger A, Albers G. Incidence of transcranial Doppler-detected cerebral micro-emboli in patients referred for echocardiography. Stroke 1994;25:2138–2141.

218. Nadareishvili ZG, Choudary Z, Joyner C, et al. Cerebral microembolism in acute myocardial infarction. Stroke 1999;30:2679–2682.

219. Georgiadis D, Grosset D, Kilman A, et al. Prevalence and characteristics of intracranial microemboli signals in patients with different types of prosthetic cardiac valves. Stroke 1994;25:587–592.

220. Rundek T, Di Tullio MR, Sciacca RR, et al. Association between large aortic arch atheromas and high-intensity transient signals in elderly stroke patients. Stroke 1999;30:2683–2686.

221. Delcker A, Diener HC, Wilhelm H. Source of cerebral MES in occlusion of the internal carotid artery. J Neurol 1997;244:312–317.

222. Rademacher J, Sohngen D, Specker C, et al. Cerebral microembolism, a disease marker for ischemic cerebrovascular events in the antiphospholipid syndrome of systemic lupus erythematosus? Acta Neurol Scand 1999;99:356–361.

223. Forteza A, Koch S, Romano JG, et al. Transcranial Doppler detection of fat emboli. Stroke 1999;30:2687–2691.

224. Segura T, Serena J, Teruel J, Davalos A. Cerebral embolism in a patient with polycythemia rubra vera. Eur J Neurol 2000;7:87–90.

225. Sliwka U, Klotzsch C, Popescu O, et al. Do chronic middle cerebral artery stenoses represent an embolic focus? A multirange transcranial Doppler study. Stroke 1997;28:1324–1327.

226. Segura T, Serena J, Castellanos M, et al. Embolism in acute middle cerebral artery stenosis. Neurology 2001;56:497–501.

227. Georgiadis D, Braun S, Uhlmann F, et al. Doppler MES in patients with two different types of bileaflet valves. J Thorac Cardiovasc Surg 2001;121:1101–1106.

228. Sliwka U, Lingnau A, Stohlman WD, et al. Prevalence and time course of microembolic signals in patients with acute stroke. A prospective study. Stroke 1997;28:358–363.

229. Tong DC, Albers GW. Transcranial Doppler-detected microemboli in patients with acute stroke. Stroke 1995;26:1588–1592.

230. Serena J, Segura T, Castellanos M, Davalos A. Microembolic signal monitoring in hemispheric acute ischemic stroke: a prospective study. Cerebrovasc Dis 2000;10:278–282.

231. Lund C, Rygh J, Stensrod B, et al. Cerebral microembolus detection in an unselected acute ischemic stroke population. Cerebrovasc Dis 2000;10:403–408.

232. Kaposzta Z, Young E, Bath PM, Markus HS. Clinical application of asymptomatic embolic signal detection in acute stroke. A prospective study. Stroke 1999;30:1814–1818.

233. Molloy J, Markus HS. Asymptomatic embolization predicts stroke and TIA risk in patients with carotid artery stenosis. Stroke 1999;30:1440–1443.

234. Niesen W-D, Sliwka U, Lingnau A, Noth J. Cerebral emboli in cryptogenic ischemia: a reason to enforce diagnostic testing. J Stroke Cerebrovasc Dis 2001;10:44–48.

235. Alexandrov AV, Demchuk AM, Felberg RA, et al. Intracranial clot dissolution is associated with embolic signals on transcranial Doppler. J Neuroimaging 2000;10:27–32.

236. Goertler M, Baeumer M, Kross R, et al. Rapid decline of cerebral microemboli of arterial origin after intravenous acetylsalicylic acid. Stroke 1999;30:66–69.

237. Goertler M, Blaser T, Krueger S, et al. Acetylsalicylic acid and microembolic events detected by transcranial Doppler in symptomatic arterial stenoses. Cerebrovasc Dis 2001;11:324–329.

238. Nabavi DG, Arato S, Droste DW, et al. Microembolic load in asymptomatic patients with cardiac aneurysm, severe ventricular dysfunction, and atrial fibrillation. Clinical and hemorheological correlates. Cerebrovasc Dis 1998;8:214–221.

239. Lennard N, Smith J, Dumville J, et al. Prevention of postoperative thrombotic stroke after carotid

endarterectomy: the role of transcranial Doppler ultrasound. J Vasc Surg 1997;26:579–584.

240. Hayes P, Lennard N, Smith J, et al. Vascular Surgical Society of Great Britain and Ireland: transcranial Doppler-directed dextran therapy in the prevention of postoperative carotid thrombosis. Br J Surg 1999;86:692.

241. Lennard N, Smith JL, Hayes P, et al. Transcranial Doppler directed dextran therapy in the prevention of carotid thrombosis: three hour monitoring is as effective as six hours. Eur J Vasc Endovasc Surg 1999;17:301–305.

242. Lennard N, Smith J, Dumville J, et al. Prevention of postoperative thrombotic stroke after carotid endarterectomy: the role of transcranial Doppler ultrasound. J Vasc Surg 1997;26:579–584.

243. Kaposzta Z, Baskerville PA, Madge D, et al. L-arginine and S-nitrosoglutathione reduce embolization in humans. Circulation 2001;103:2371–2375.

244. Molloy J, Martin JF, Baskerville PA, et al. S-nitrosoglutathione reduces the rate of embolization in humans. Circulation 1998;98:1372–1375.

245. Bock RW, Lusby RJ. Lesions, Dynamics, and Pathogenetic Mechanisms Responsible for Ischemic Events in the Brain. In WS Moore (ed), Surgery for Cerebrovascular Disease. Philadelphia: Saunders, 1996;48–71.

246. Eicke BM, von Lorentz J, Paulus W. Embolus detection in different degrees of carotid disease. Neurol Res 1995;17:181–184.

247. Valton L, Larrue V, Arrue P, et al. Asymptomatic cerebral embolic signals in patients with carotid stenosis; correlation with appearance of plaque ulcerations on angiography. Stroke 1995;26:813–815.

248. Sitzer M, Muller W, Siebler M, et al. Plaque ulceration and lumen thrombus are the main sources of cerebral microemboli in high-grade internal carotid artery stenosis. Stroke 1995;26:1231–1233.

249. Orlandi G, Parenti G, Landucci Pellegrini L, et al. Plaque surface and microembolic signals in moderate carotid stenosis. Ital J Neurol Sci 1999;20:179–182.

250. Siebler M, Nachtman A, Sitzer M, et al. Cerebral microembolism and the risk of ischemia in asymptomatic high grade internal artery stenosis. Stroke 1995;26:2184–2186.

251. Markus HS, Thompson N, Droste DW, et al. Cerebral embolic signals in carotid artery stenosis and their temporal variability. Cerebrovasc Dis 1994;4:22.

252. Babikian VL, Hyde C, Pochay V, Winter MR. Clinical correlates of high-intensity transient signal detected on transcranial Doppler sonography in patients with cerebrovascular disease. Stroke 1994;25:1570–1573.

253. Forteza A, Babikian VL. Effect of time and cerebrovascular symptoms on the prevalence of microembolic signals in patients with cervical artery stenosis. Stroke 1996;27:687–690.

254. Executive Committee for the Asymptomatic Carotid Atherosclerosis Study. Endarterectomy for asymptomatic carotid stenosis. JAMA 1995;273:1421–1428.

255. Hartmann A, Hupp T, Koch HC, et al. Prospective study on the complication rate of carotid surgery. Cerebrovasc Dis 1999;9:152–156.

256. Halsey JH, for the International Transcranial Doppler Collaborators. Risks and benefits of shunting in carotid endarterectomy. Stroke 1992;23:1583–1587.

257. Hayes PD, Vainas T, Hartley S, et al. The Pruitt-Inahara shunt maintains mean middle cerebral artery velocities within 10% of preoperative values during carotid endarterectomy. J Vasc Surg 2000;32:299–306.

258. Kofke WA, Brauer P, Policare R, et al. Middle cerebral artery blood flow velocity and stable xenon-enhanced computed tomographic blood flow during balloon test occlusion of the internal carotid artery. Stroke 1995;26:1603–1606.

259. Babikian VL, Cantelmo NL, Wijman CAC. Neurovascular Monitoring during Carotid Endarterectomy. In VL Babikian, LR Wechsler (eds), Transcranial Doppler Ultrasonography (2nd ed). Boston: Butterworth–Heinemann, 1999;231–245.

260. Sundt TM, Sharbrough FW, Piepgras DG, et al. Correlation of cerebral blood flow and electroencephalographic changes during carotid endarterectomy. Mayo Clin Proc 1981;56:533–543.

261. Frawley JE, Hicks RG, Gray LJ, Niesche JW. Carotid endarterectomy without a shunt for symptomatic lesions associated with contralateral severe stenosis or occlusion. J Vasc Surg 1996;23:421–427.

262. Ackerstaff RGA, Moons KGM, Moll FL, et al. Association of intraoperative transcranial Doppler monitoring variables with stroke from carotid endarterectomy. Stroke 2000;31:1817–1823.

263. Cantelmo NL, Babikian VL, Samaraweera RN, et al. Cerebral microembolism and ischemic changes associated with carotid endarterectomy. J Vasc Surg 1998;27:1024–1031.

264. Levi CR, O'Malley HM, Fell G, et al. Transcranial Doppler detected cerebral microembolism following carotid endarterectomy. Brain 1997;120:621–629.

265. Spencer MP. Transcranial Doppler monitoring and causes of stroke from carotid endarterectomy. Stroke 1997;28:685–691.

266. Cao P, Giordano G, Zanetti S, et al. Transcranial Doppler monitoring during carotid endarterectomy: is it appropriate for selecting patients in need of a shunt? J Vasc Surg 1997;26:973–980.

267. Jansen C, Vriens EM, Eikelboom BC, et al. Carotid endarterectomy with transcranial Doppler and electroencephalographic monitoring. Stroke 1993;24:665–669.

268. Gaunt ME, Ratliff DA, Martin PJ, et al. On-table diagnosis of incipient carotid artery thrombosis during carotid endarterectomy. J Vasc Surg 1994;20:104–107.

269. Gaunt ME, Martin PJ, Smith JL, et al. Clinical relevance of intraoperative embolization detected by transcranial Doppler ultrasonography during carotid endarterectomy: a prospective study of 100 patients. Br J Surg 1994;81:1435–1439.

270. Jansen C, Ramos LMP, Moll FL, et al. Impact of microembolism and hemodynamic changes in the brain during carotid endarterectomy. Stroke 1994;25:992–997.

271. Jordan WD Jr, Voellinger DC, Doblar DD, et al. Microemboli detected by transcranial Doppler monitoring in patients during carotid angioplasty versus carotid endarterectomy. Cardiovasc Surg 1999;7:33–38.

272. Crawley F, Stygall J, Lunn S, et al. Comparison of microembolism detected by transcranial Doppler and neuropsychological sequelae of carotid surgery and percutaneous transluminal angioplasty. Stroke 2000;31:1329–1334.

273. Ohki T, Veith FJ. Carotid artery stenting: utility of cerebral protection devices. J Invasive Cardiol 2001;13:47–55.

274. Parodi JC, La Mura R, Ferreira LM, et al. Initial evaluation of carotid angioplasty and stenting with three different cerebral protection devices. J Vasc Surg 2000;32:1127–1136.

275. Wolf PA, Dawber TR, Thomas HEJ, et al. Epidemiologic assessment of chronic atrial fibrillation and the risk of stroke: the Framingham Study. Neurology 1978;28:973–977.

276. Peterson P. Progress reviews: thromboembolic complications in atrial fibrillation. Stroke 1990;21:4–13.

277. Tegeler CH, Burke GL, Dalley GM, et al. Carotid emboli predict poor outcome in stroke. Stroke 1993;24:186.

278. Markus HS. Doppler Embolus Detection: Stroke Treatment and Prevention. In CH Tegeler, VL Babikian, C Gomez (eds), Neurosonology. St. Louis: Mosby, 1996;239–251.

279. Nabavi DG, Allroggen A, Reinecke H, et al. Absence of circulating microemboli in patients with lone atrial fibrillation. Neurol Res 1999;21:566–568.

280. Grosset D, Georgiadis D, Kelman A, Lees KR. Quantification of ultrasound signals in patients with cardiac and carotid disease. Stroke 1993;24:1922–1924.

281. Markus HS, Droste DW, Brown M. Detection of asymptomatic cerebral embolic signal with Doppler ultrasound. Lancet 1994;343(b):1011–1112.

282. Spencer MP. Detection of Cerebral Arterial Emboli. In DW Newell, R Aaslid (eds), Transcranial Doppler. New York: Raven Press, 1992;215–230.

283. Siebler M, Nachtman A, Sitzer M, Steinmetz H. Anticoagulation monitoring and cerebral microemboli detection. Lancet 1994;344(b):555.

284. Sliwka U, Georgiadis D. Clinical correlation of Doppler microemboli signals in patients with prosthetic cardiac valves. Stroke 1998;29:140–143.

285. Sturzenegger M, Beer JH, Rihs F. Monitoring combined antithrombotic treatments in patients with prosthetic heart valves using transcranial Doppler and anticoagulation markers. Stroke 1995;26:63–69.

286. Droste D, Hansberg T, Kemeny V, et al. Oxygen inhalation can differentiate gaseous from nongaseous microemboli detected by Doppler ultrasound. Stroke 1997;28:2453–2456.

287. Nabavi DG, Georgiadis D, Mumme T, et al. Clinical relevance of intracranial microembolic signals in patients with left ventricular assist devices. A prospective study. Stroke 1996;27:891–896.

288. Di Tullio M, Sacco RL, Gopal A, et al. PFO as a risk factor for cryptogenic stroke. Ann Intern Med 1992;117:461–465.

289. Webster MW, Chancellor AM, Smith HJ, et al. Patent foramen ovale in young stroke patients. Lancet 1988;2(8601):11–12.

290. Droste DW, Kriete JU, Stypmann J, et al. Contrast transcranial Doppler ultrasound in the detection of right-to-left shunts: comparison of different procedures and different contrast agents. Stroke 1999;30: 1827–1832.

291. Albert A, Muller HR, Hetzel A. Optimized transcranial Doppler technique for the diagnosis of cardiac right-to-left shunts. J Neuroimaging 1997;7:159–163.

292. Klotzsch C, Janssen G, Berlit P. Transesophageal echocardiography and contrast-TCD in the detection of a patent foramen ovale: experiences with 111 patients. Neurology 1994;44:1603–1606.

293. Kimura K, Minematsu K, Wada K, et al. Transcranial Doppler of a paradoxical brain embolism associated with a pulmonary arteriovenous fistula. Am J Neuroradiol 1999;20:1881–1884.

294. Gilman S. Cerebral disorders after open heart operations. N Engl J Med 1965;272:489–498.

295. Newman S. The incidence and nature of neuropsychological morbidity following cardiac surgery. Perfusion 1989;4:93–100.

296. McKhann GM, Goldsborough MA, Borowicz LMJ, et al. Cognitive outcome after coronary artery bypass: a one-year prospective study. Ann Thorac Surg 1997;63:510–515.

297. Murkin JM, Farrar JK. The influence of pulsatile versus nonpulsatile cardiopulmonary bypass on cerebral blood flow and on cerebral metabolism. Anesthesiology 1989;71:A41(Abst).

298. Gravlee GP, Hudspeth AS, Toole JF. Bilateral brachial paralysis from watershed infarction following

coronary artery bypass. J Thorac Surg 1984;88:742–747.

299. Pugsley W, Klinger L, Paschalis C, et al. The impact of microemboli during cardiopulmonary bypass on neuropsychological functioning. Stroke 1994;25:1393–1399.

300. Padayachee TS, Parsous S, Theobold R, et al. The detection of microemboli in the middle cerebral artery during cardiopulmonary bypass: a transcranial Doppler ultrasound investigation using membrane and bubble oxygenators. Ann Thorac Surg 1987;44:298–302.

301. Blauth CL, Smith PL, Arnold JV, et al. Influence of oxygenator type on the prevalence and extent of microembolic retinal ischemia during cardiopulmonary bypass: assessment by digital image analysis. J Thorac Cardiovasc Surg 1990;99:61–69.

302. Vannine R, Aikia M, Kononen M, et al. Subclinical cerebral complications after coronary artery bypass grafting: prospective analysis with magnetic resonance imaging, quantitative electroencephalography and neuropsychological assessment. Arch Neurol 1998;55:618–627.

303. Wityk RJ, Goldsborough MA, Hillis A, et al. Diffusion- and perfusion-weighted brain magnetic resonance imaging in patients with neurologic complications after cardiac surgery. Arch Neurol 2001;58:571–576.

304. Clark RE, Brillman J, Davis DA, et al. Thromboemboli during coronary artery bypass grafting. J Thorac Cardiovasc Surg 1995;109:249–258.

305. Challa VR, Moody DM, Bell MA. Small Capillary and Arteriolar Dilatations (SCADs) in Brain after Cardiopulmonary Bypass. In GM McKhan, CJ Gibbs (eds), Neurological Outcomes after Coronary Bypass Surgery. New York: Thieme, 1993;330–334.

306. Moody DM, Bell MA, Challa VR, et al. Brain microemboli during cardiac surgery or aortography. Ann Neurol 1990;28:477–486.

307. Deverall PB, Padayachee TS, Parsons S, et al. Ultrasound detection of micro-emboli in the middle cerebral artery during cardiopulmonary bypass surgery. Eur J Cardiothorac Surg 1998;2:256–260.

308. Barbut D, Hinton RB, Szatrowski TP, et al. Cerebral emboli detected during bypass surgery are associated with clamp removal. Stroke 1994;25:2398–2402.

309. Van der Linden J, Casimir AH. When do cerebral emboli appear during open heart surgery? A transcranial Doppler study. Ann Thorac Surg 1991;51:237–241.

310. Barbut D, Caplan LR. Brain complications of cardiac surgery. Curr Probl Cardiol 1997;22:447–476.

311. Yao FSF, Barbut D, Hager DN, et al. Detection of aortic emboli by transesophageal echocardiography during coronary artery bypass surgery. J Cardiothorac Vasc Anesth 1996;10:314–317.

312. Barbut D, Yao FS, Hager DN, et al. Comparison of transcranial Doppler ultrasonography and transesophageal echocardiography during coronary artery bypass surgery. Stroke 1996;27:87–90.

313. Roach GW, Kanchuger M, Mangano CM, et al. Adverse cerebral outcomes after coronary bypass surgery. Multicenter Study of Perioperative Ischemia Research Group and the Ischemia Research Foundation Investigators. N Engl J Med 1996;335:1857–1863.

314. Gardner TJ, Horneffer PJ, Manolio TA, et al. Stroke following coronary artery bypass grafting: a ten-year study. Ann Thorac Surg 1985;40:574–581.

315. Marshall WG, Barziali B, Kouchoukos NT, Saffitz J. Intraoperative ultrasonic imaging of the ascending aorta. Ann Thorac Surg 1989;48:339–344.

316. Caplan LR. Protecting the brains of patients after heart surgery. Arch Neurol 2001;58:549–550.

317. Bowles BJ, Lee JD, Dang CR, et al. Coronary artery bypass performed without the use of cardiopulmonary bypass is associated with reduced cerebral microemboli and improved clinical results. Chest 2001;119:25–30.

318. Forteza AM, Koch S, Zych G, et al. Transcranial Doppler detection of cerebral fat emboli after long bone fractures. Ann Thorac Surg 2000;1:1–2(Abst).

CHAPTER

2

Magnetic Resonance Angiography

William G. Bradley, Jr.

Magnetic resonance angiography (MRA) comprises a class of MR techniques that have evolved rapidly over the last decade. In many parts of the body, MRA has largely replaced catheter angiography for most diagnostic applications, due to its lower cost and relative noninvasiveness. As MR imaging (MRI) systems have improved, so has MRA. Using the high-performance gradients that are part of every echoplanar imaging–capable MR system, contrast-enhanced MRA (CE MRA) can now be performed during the initial passage of contrast through the arterial system.

The following is a review of the various MR angiographic techniques, their principal applications, and potential pitfalls.

TIME-OF-FLIGHT MAGNETIC RESONANCE ANGIOGRAPHY

Time-of-flight (TOF) MRA is based on *flow-related enhancement*,[1] which is the entry of unsaturated (i.e., fully magnetized) spins flowing into the imaged slice. The objective of any MRA technique is to maximize signal coming from the vessel while minimizing signal coming from the background. Intraluminal signal is optimized by maximizing flow-related enhancement and minimizing intraluminal dephasing. T1-weighted, single-slice gradient echo images were initially used to maximize flow-related enhancement. These tend to enhance the high signal emanating from the vessel while minimizing the background signal.[2]

Intraluminal dephasing causes signal loss. It is reduced by using the shortest possible TEs and the smallest possible voxels. Smaller voxels decrease signal to noise, and the TE must be selected to minimize background signal by keeping fat and water out of phase. Fat precesses at a lower frequency than water, so they get out of phase and then rephase periodically with increasing TE. At 1.5 TE, they rephase every 4.2 milliseconds; thus, TEs of 2.1, 6.3, and 10.5 milliseconds produce images in which fat and water are out of phase.

To maximize image signal due to flow-related enhancement, the sections should be acquired perpendicular to the vessel of interest, progressing sequentially in the direction countercurrent to the flowing blood. This ensures that the imaged section is always meeting fresh spins head-on. Typically, a saturation pulse (i.e., a 90-degree pulse applied to a slab of tissue behind the advancing MRA slice) is applied to suppress unwanted venous (or arterial) blood. For single-slice (two-dimensional [2D] TOF) techniques, the saturation pulse travels behind the MRA slice as it advances.[3] Thus, one would acquire from the top down, in the head and neck to image normal arterial flow (Figure 2-1), while acquiring from the bottom up to image normal venous flow (Figure 2-2). For the evaluation of the superior sagittal sinus, one might also acquire from posterior to anterior to meet posteriorly flowing blood head-on.

Although the 2D TOF MRA technique is robust and relatively fast (see Figure 2-1), the slices are generally no thinner than 1.5 mm, limiting resolution in the slice dimension. Although this may be adequate for screening, it is less accurate for assessing the severity of stenoses. For this reason, the three-dimensional (3D) TOF MRA technique was developed (Figure 2-3). In this technique, signal is acquired from an entire slab of tissue, generally 5–6 cm thick, with proportionately

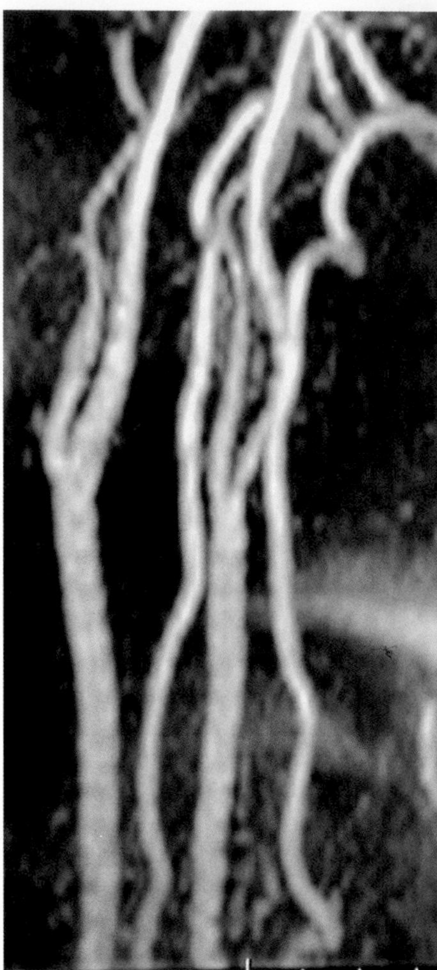

FIGURE 2-1. Two-dimensional time-of-flight magnetic resonance arteriogram. This two-dimensional time-of-flight magnetic resonance arteriogram of the carotid and vertebral arteries was acquired from the top down, countercurrent to the up-flowing arterial blood. This is 1 of 12 maximum-intensity projections. This right anterior oblique projection demonstrates the carotid bulbs in profile.

greater signal to noise ratio compared to the thin 2D TOF slice. The slab can then be subdivided into *slices* (also called *source images* or *partitions*), each 1 mm or less in thickness. Thus, the advantages of 3D TOF MRA techniques (compared with 2D TOF) are better signal to noise ratio and better spatial resolution in the slice select direction.[3]

The disadvantage of 3D TOF is the phenomenon of *saturation*. Maximum flow-related enhancement occurs when the fresh spins first enter the slab fully magnetized, or *unsaturated*. After being exposed to multiple 90-degree radiofrequency (RF) pulses as the spins traverse the slab of tissue, the magnetization is used up, and the spins are said to be *saturated*, at which point no additional signal can be elicited by an RF pulse (Figure 2-4). Visualization of vessels deeper into the slab is thus

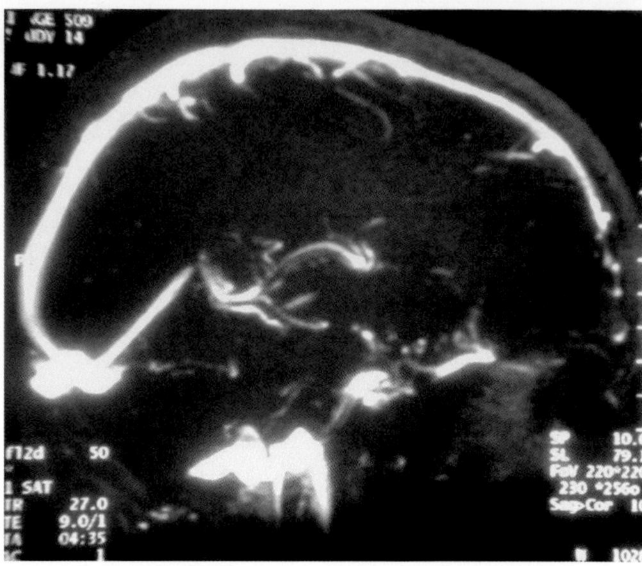

FIGURE 2-2. Two-dimensional time-of-flight magnetic resonance venogram. This normal magnetic resonance venogram of the superior sagittal sinus was acquired from bottom to top to meet the down-flowing venous blood head-on.

limited. It is saturation that limits the total 3D TOF slab thickness to approximately 6 cm for blood flowing at the velocity of vessels in the circle of Willis. Saturation tends to improve with lower flip angles, eliciting less signal per RF hit, with longer TRs, and allowing more time

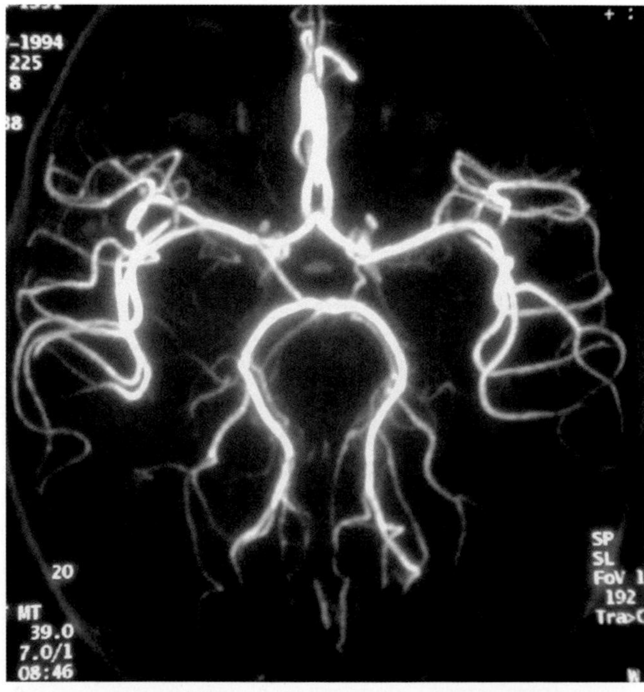

FIGURE 2-3. Normal three-dimensional time-of-flight magnetic resonance angiogram of the circle of Willis.

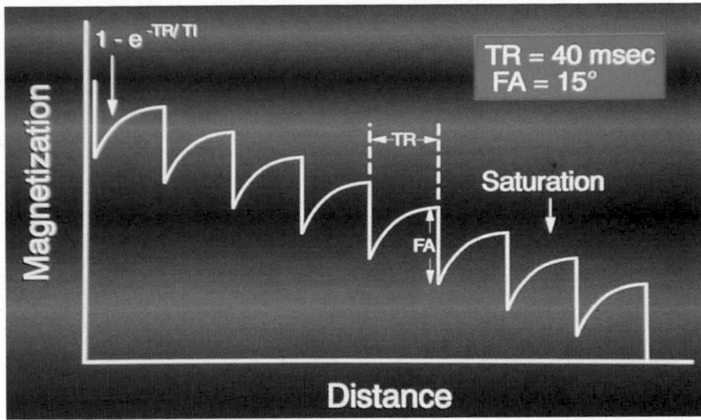

A

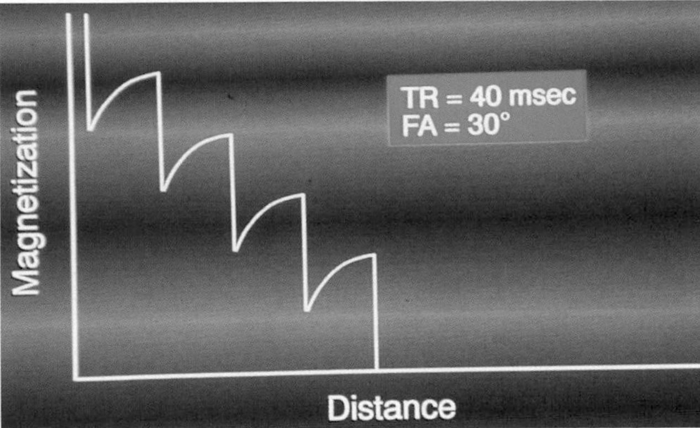

B

FIGURE 2-4. Magnetic resonance angiography saturation diagrams. **A.** Using standard three-dimensional time-of-flight magnetic resonance angiography parameters of TR = 40 milliseconds, TE = 7 milliseconds, and a flip angle (FA) of 15 degrees, this graph depicts the sawtooth decrease in magnetization as the spins are subjected to multiple radiofrequency (RF) pulses as they traverse a 6-cm-thick slab. The amount of entering magnetization at the left side of the graph depends on flow-related enhancement or entry phenomenon. Each decrease in magnetization is in proportion to the flip angle (15 degrees). The recovery of magnetization between RF pulses during the time TR occurs according to the equation $1\text{-}e^{-TR/T1}$. At some point, the signal elicited from the small amount of remaining magnetization is indistinguishable from background noise, and the spins are said to be "saturated." **B.** Increasing the FA to 30 degrees elicits more magnetization from each RF exposure, leading to earlier saturation and less penetration into the slab. This results in nonvisualization of vessels on the downstream portion of the slab.

for T1 recovery between each RF pulse. On the other hand, larger flip angles and shorter TRs use up more magnetization, resulting in decreased visualization of vessels deeper into the slab.

Thus, 2D TOF and 3D TOF MRA techniques both have certain strengths and certain weaknesses. Although the 3D TOF technique has the benefit of higher spatial resolution and greater signal to noise, it has limited coverage due to saturation effects. On the other hand, the 2D TOF technique has unlimited coverage (because there are no saturation effects), but it has lower resolution. *Multiple overlapping thin slab acquisition* (MOTSA)[4] is a hybrid technique that takes advantage of both positive features. With MOTSA, a number of relatively thin 3D TOF slabs are pasted together like thick 2D TOF slices, providing high spatial resolution and unlimited coverage. The slabs are typically 3 cm in thickness initially; however, the outer portions of the slab are discarded to minimize any remaining saturation effects that would result in "venetian blind" artifacts.[4] Although MOTSA offers the advantages of high spatial resolution and unlimited coverage (Figure 2-5), it is less efficient because of the necessity to discard the outer 10–50% of the slab.

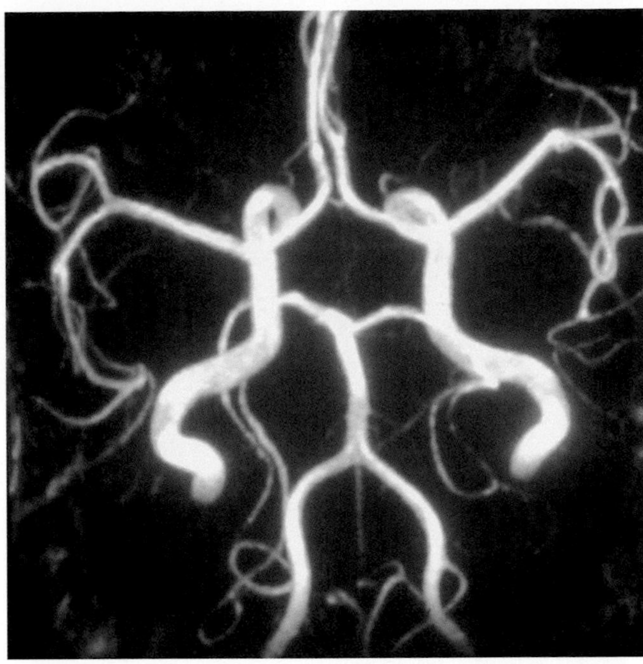

FIGURE 2-5. Multiple overlapping thin slab acquisition. This normal multiple overlapping thin slab acquisition study covers from above the circle of Willis to below the posterior inferior cerebellar artery. It is the standard technique used to screen for aneurysms.

MRA is an excellent technique for screening aneurysms in the brain. Ten years ago, using 256 × 256 matrix with 1-mm inplane spatial resolution and 1-mm slice thickness, Masaryk et al. were able to demonstrate aneurysms as small as 3 mm.[3] They also referenced two autopsy series that noted that aneurysms smaller than 3 mm tended not to rupture. Thus, there is no need to perform a catheter angiogram in an asymptomatic individual if an MR angiogram of the brain is normal.

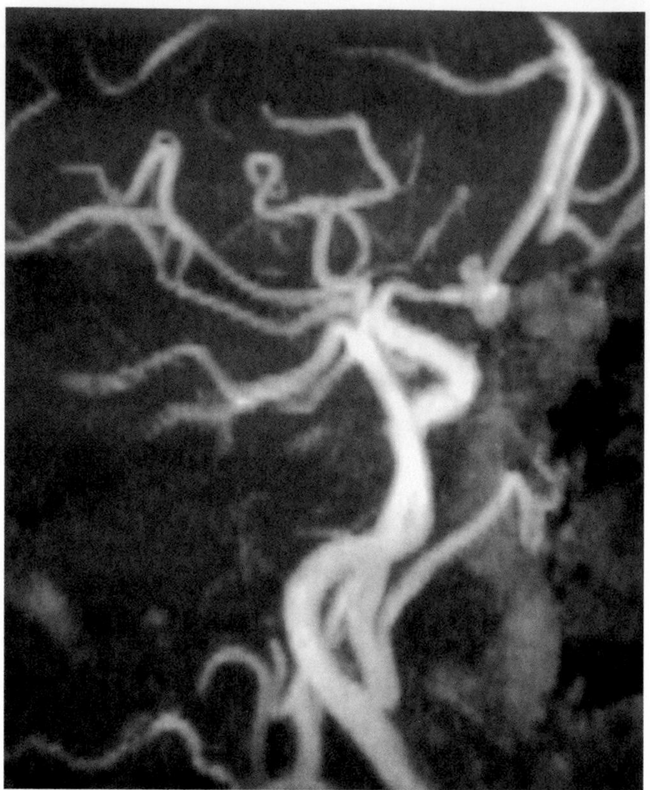

A

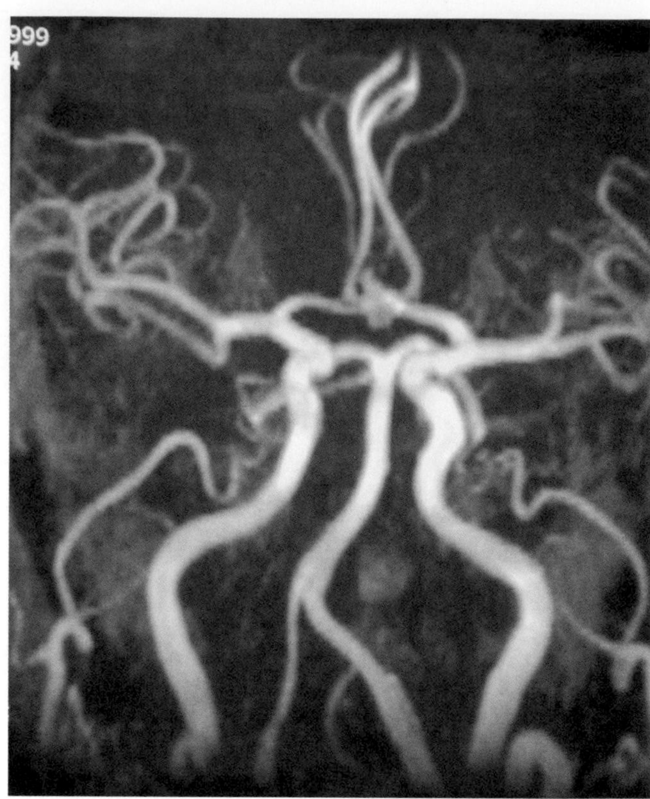

B

FIGURE 2-6. Aneurysm of the anterior communicating artery (ACOM). **A.** Lateral maximum-intensity projection from a multiple overlapping thin slab acquisition study demonstrates an ACOM aneurysm. **B.** Frontal maximum-intensity projection of the same three-dimensional data set shown in (**A**) again demonstrates the ACOM aneurysm.

The converse, however, is not true: For positive MR angiograms at the University of California, San Diego, we still perform catheter or computed tomography angiograms in addition to the MRA. In cases of acute subarachnoid hemorrhage, catheter studies are performed because spasm is currently better seen by catheter angiography than by MRA due to the relative spatial resolution. On the other hand, MRA is more sensitive to clot next to the aneurysm as well as in the dome. A study has recently documented that MRA and digital subtraction angiography are complementary for detecting aneurysms in the setting of acute subarachnoid hemorrhage.[5] It should be stated emphatically, however, that a normal examination on day 1 does not guarantee a normal examination the day after, as we have little knowledge of the natural history of aneurysms. Once they start to enlarge, they are likely to enlarge rapidly (Laplace's law). Therefore, repeat MRA should be performed if there are new cranial nerve palsies or other changing symptoms. This is particularly true in patients with an increased incidence of aneurysm (e.g., those with a positive family history, a history of polycystic kidney disease, or fibromuscular dysplasia).

We use MOTSA for our general intracranial studies, particularly if we are searching for aneurysms (Figure 2-6) and need to cover from the circle of Willis, where most aneurysms occur, through the posterior inferior cerebellar artery, which is the fourth most common location for an intracranial aneurysm. On the other hand, when we only need limited coverage, such as through the circle of Willis for a suspected infarct, we typically use a single 3D TOF slab (see Figure 2-3).

Once a series of 2D or 3D slices has been acquired, they can be viewed directly (as 64 or so separate images), scrolled consecutively on a workstation, or displayed in angiographic format. For the last option, a maximum-intensity projection (MIP) algorithm is generally used.[3] The MIP algorithm basically tells the computer to connect the bright dots of inflowing blood on the 64 source images, looking from a particular projection. We typically rotate the data around a horizontal or vertical axis, or both, acquiring 12 images every 15 degrees for a total of 180 degrees. (The back 180 degrees are the mirror image of the front 180 degrees, so it is not necessary to repeat it.) When rotating vertically, we typically cut the data set in half so the right and left sides do not overlap. This is called a *targeted MIP*. With a 512 ×

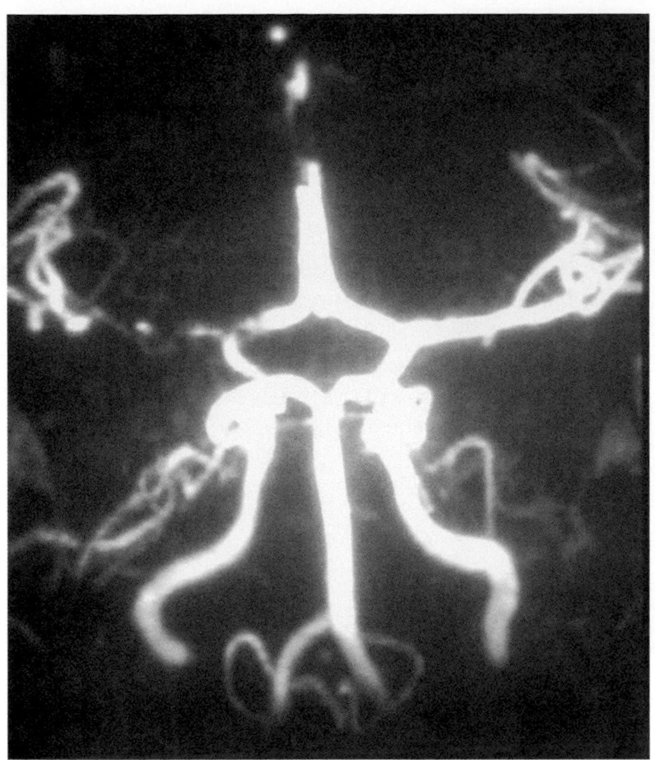

A

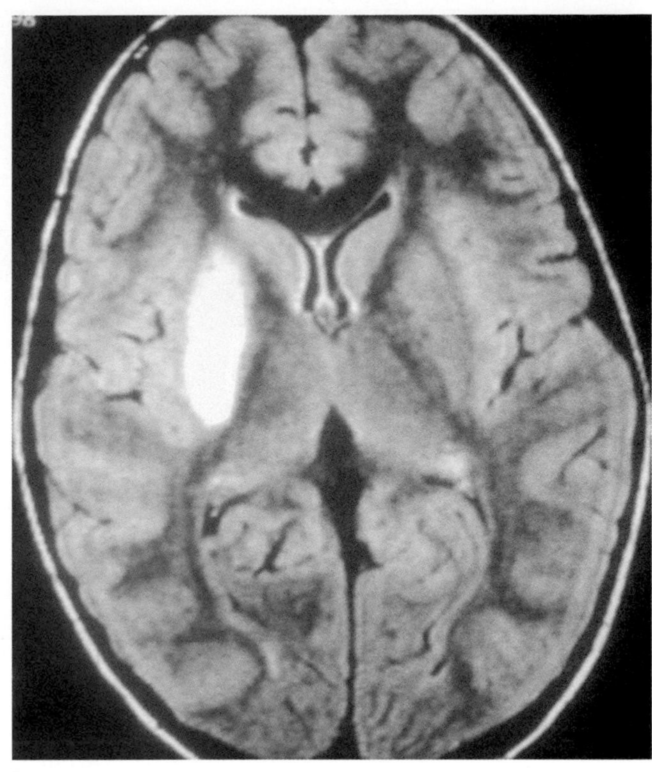

B

FIGURE 2-7. Intracranial atheroscleroses. **A.** Atherosclerotic proximal M1 segment of the middle cerebral artery is noted on this multiple overlapping thin slab acquisition study. **B.** Infarct of the right basal ganglia, resulting from occluded ostia of several lenticulostriate arteries, is demonstrated.

512 MOTSA acquisition over a 20-mm field of view (FOV), spatial resolution is approximately 0.4 mm or 400 μm. Using a 384 × 512 matrix over a 15-cm × 20-cm rectangular FOV (side-to-side × front-to-back), acquisition time can be reduced 25% without sacrificing spatial resolution. Using this technique, intracranial stenoses due to arteriosclerosis can be detected (Figure 2-7). It is also common practice to zero interpolate in k-space (i.e., before the data are reverse Fourier transformed into an image).[6] This is particularly important in the slice direction (which tends to have the lowest spatial resolution); otherwise, a "stairstep" artifact is noted during oblique MIP rotations.

With increasing gradient strength and advanced image processing, shorter repetition times are possible, making $1{,}024^2$-MRA (Figure 2-8) technically feasible.[7] Intracranial vessels appear much larger with 250-μm pixels than they do at lower resolution. This reflects the capture of pixels at the periphery of the artery, where the greatest phase dispersion occurs during laminar flow.[2] With larger voxels, this intravoxel dephasing results in nonvisualization. With higher resolution (smaller voxels), the phase differences from one edge of the voxel to the other are smaller, leading to less phase cancellation. Such improved visualization of arterial diameter at 250-μm spatial resolution will increase the applications of MRA to include vasculitis, spasm after subarachnoid hemorrhage, and detection of even smaller aneurysms. Eventually, $1{,}024^2$-MRA should replace catheter angiography for most diagnostic purposes.

One of the potential problems with the MIP algorithm is that it includes anything that is bright on the T1-weighted source images in the maximum-intensity projection image, including subacute hemorrhage, fat, or anything enhancing with gadolinium (Figure 2-9). It is therefore important to examine both MRA images and conventional MR images to determine if everything in the MIP images represents flowing blood. When bright, short T1 structures are present, it may be desirable to acquire a phase-contrast MRA that subtracts out the high-intensity stationary structures (see below).

The MIP algorithm has a signal to noise ratio threshold for what it includes in the image, so very small vessels or tight stenoses may not be visualized. For this reason, it is important to review the individual source images (Figure 2-10) before diagnosing a stenosis or complete absence of a vessel from the MIPs. The source images are also useful for diagnosing small lenticulostriate collaterals in moyamoya disease (Figure 2-11).

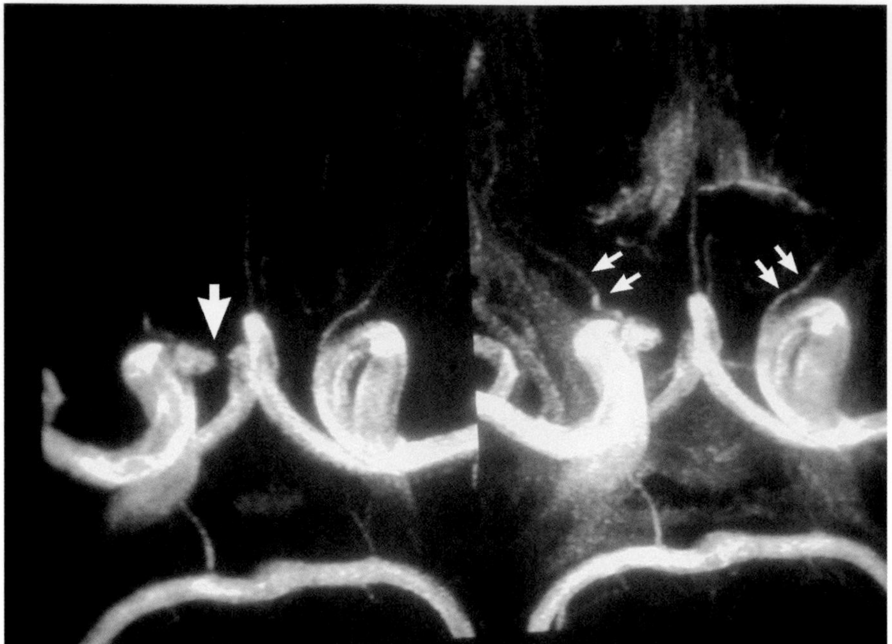

FIGURE 2-8. 1,024 × 1,024 magnetic resonance angiogram of the circle of Willis. This high-resolution acquisition through the circle of Willis demonstrates a small right cavernous carotid aneurysm (*large arrow*). By adding gadolinium (**right**), small vessels, such as the ophthalmic arteries (*small arrows*), can be seen. These images have the same spatial resolution (250 μ) as a standard digital subtraction angiography catheter study. (Courtesy of Jay Tsuruda, M.D., Salt Lake City, Utah.)

Another potential problem with TOF and other "bright blood" techniques is turbulence.[2] Turbulence leads to dephasing and irreversible signal loss. Turbulence arising from a mild to moderate stenosis can increase the apparent size of the stenosis to moderate to severe. Thus, there is a tendency for all unenhanced TOF techniques to overestimate stenosis. This tendency is increased with longer TEs (which allow greater dephasing) and larger voxels. It is markedly decreased in "black blood" MRA (see the sections Black Blood Magnetic Resonance Angiography and Contrast-Enhanced Magnetic Resonance Angiography).

BLACK BLOOD MAGNETIC RESONANCE ANGIOGRAPHY

Black blood MRA[8,9] is based on a pair of nonselective 180-degree pulses that saturate the inflowing blood

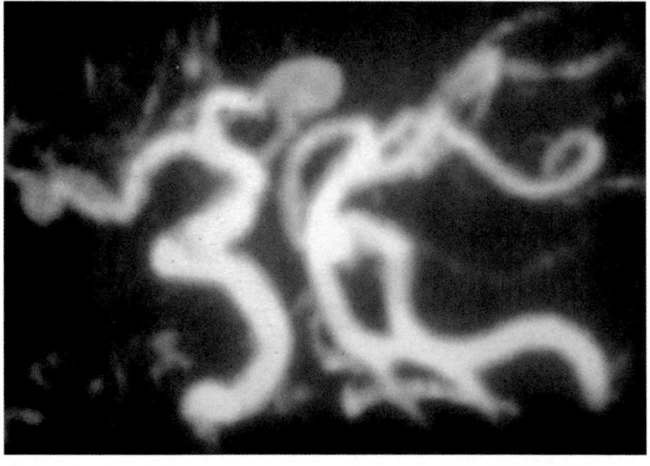

A

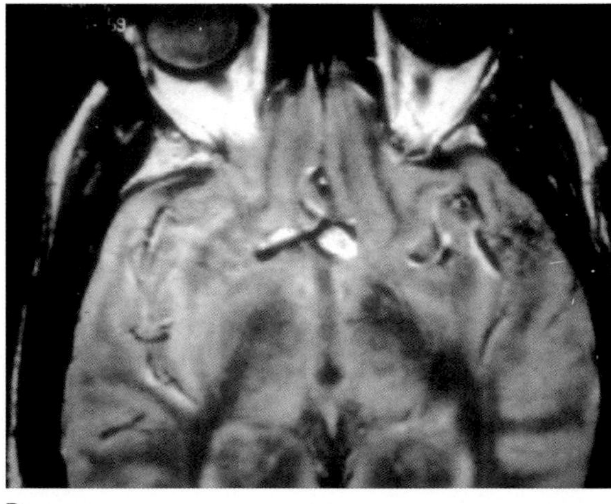

B

FIGURE 2-9. Patent aneurysm fakeout. **A.** Three-dimensional time-of-flight magnetic resonance angiogram (MRA) through the circle of Willis demonstrates presumably patent anterior communicating artery aneurysm. **B.** Conventional magnetic resonance imaging through the same level demonstrates methemoglobin within thrombosed anterior communicating artery aneurysm. Visualization on the MRA in this case is not based on flow in a patent aneurysm, but rather on the high signal from methemoglobin that is included in the maximum-intensity projection. As the objective of endovascular aneurysm therapy is to induce thrombosis, the MRA in this case is misleading. This points to the need to always evaluate the conventional images as well as the maximum-intensity projections.

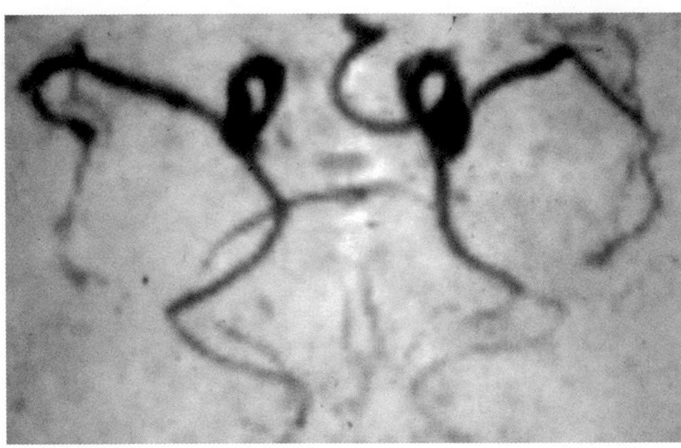

A

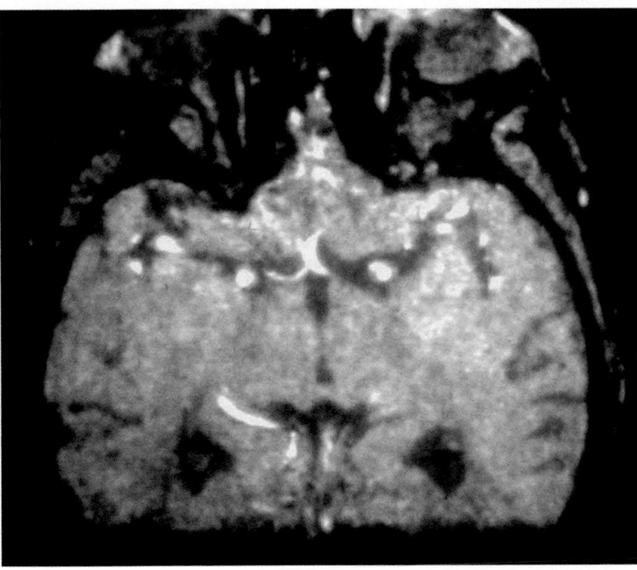

B

FIGURE 2-10. Maximum-intensity projection artifact. **A.** On this three-dimensional time-of-flight magnetic resonance angiogram through the circle of Willis, there is apparent congenital absence of the right A1 segment. **B.** On the source image through this level, the right A1 segment is clearly present but small. This case demonstrates the need to evaluate the source images as well as the maximum-intensity projected images before diagnosing absence of a vessel or complete occlusion.

before its arrival in the selected slice. Because of the two inverting pulses, *black blood MRA* (Siemens' [Iselin, New Jersey] term) is also called *double inversion recovery* by General Electric (Milwaukee, Wisconsin).

In black blood MRA, turbulence contributes to the darkness. Thus, black blood MRA does not overestimate tight stenoses like bright blood techniques.

The onset of turbulence can be predicted from the Reynolds relationship[2]:

$$\mathrm{Re} = \frac{v \cdot D}{\mu} \rho$$

Where v is the velocity, D is the vessel diameter, ρ is the density of blood, and μ is the viscosity of blood. Re is called the *Reynolds number* and is dimensionless. Ideally, if it is less than 2,200, laminar flow is present, and if it is greater than 2,200, turbulent flow is present. Figure 2-12 demonstrates the transition from laminar flow (below the line) to turbulent flow (above the line) for fluids of differing viscosity as a function of vascular diameter and velocity. Note that smaller vessels maintain laminar flow at higher velocities than larger vessels. Note also that the tendency for turbulence increases as the blood becomes less viscous (e.g., due to anemia). Turbulence is also increased where flow goes around a curve (e.g., in the carotid siphons).

Sickle cell anemia poses a particular problem for bright blood techniques. In addition to the anemia, the disease causes narrowing of the carotid siphon due to intimal hyperplasia. This is also an area affected by turbulence, which, therefore, mimics intimal hyperplasia. In this circumstance, black blood MRA can be quite useful because the turbulence contributes to the blackness. We typically acquire thin coronal sections through the carotid siphons with a black blood MRA technique and view them individually. Alternatively, they can be processed with a *minimum-intensity projection* algorithm to produce images that look like angiograms.

The minimum-intensity projection can also be used with another black blood technique known as *AVID BOLD* (*a*pplications of *v*enous *i*maging in detecting *d*isease; *b*lood *o*xygen *l*evel *d*ependent).[10] This technique is based on the increased deoxyhemoglobin content in veins compared to arteries after the oxyhemoglobin has given off its oxygen to the brain.[11] Because deoxyhemoglobin is paramagnetic and magnetically susceptible, T2*-weighted techniques show veins as dark. By prolonging the TE of the gradient echo image (to both increase the T2*-weighting and lower the bandwidth for greater signal to noise ratio), high-resolution images that are sensitive to venous structures can be produced.[10] As expected, the effect is particularly prominent at higher fields that are more sensitive to magnetic susceptibility effects.[12] AVID BOLD has been shown to be particularly sensitive for detection of venous angiomas, cavernous angiomas, and capillary telangiomas.[10,12]

CONTRAST-ENHANCED MAGNETIC RESONANCE ANGIOGRAPHY

As noted above, saturation effects increase when short TRs are used because there is not enough time for longitudinal (T1) recovery of the spins between the RF excitations. This can be rectified by injecting gadolinium, which shortens the T1 and facilitates the longitudinal recovery.[13] Adding gadolinium to a routine intracranial 3D TOF or MOTSA study can help demonstrate slow flow in a vessel that would have appeared to be totally occluded without

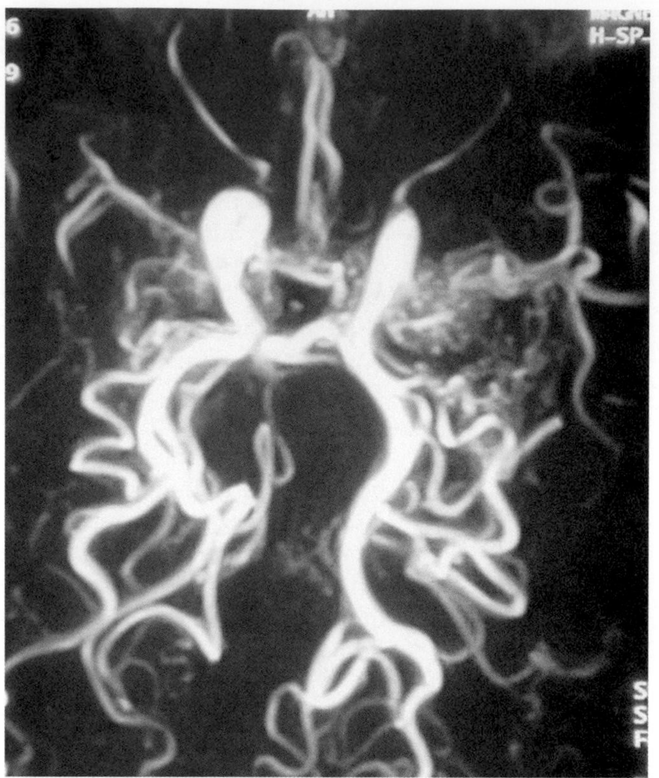

A

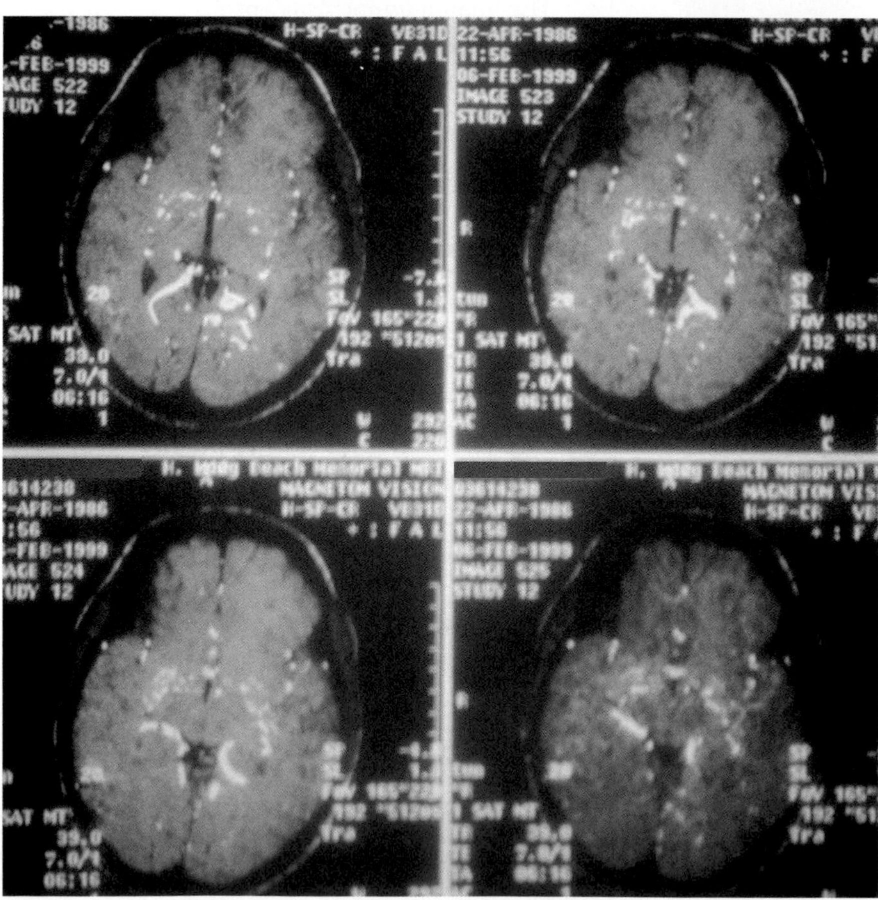

B

FIGURE 2-11. Moyamoya disease. **A.** This three-dimensional time-of-flight magnetic resonance angiogram through the circle of Willis demonstrates decreased flow in the sylvian branches of both middle cerebral arteries in this sickle cell patient with moyamoya disease. **B.** Source images through the basal ganglia demonstrate moyamoya collateral vessels (*arrows*) with much greater clarity.

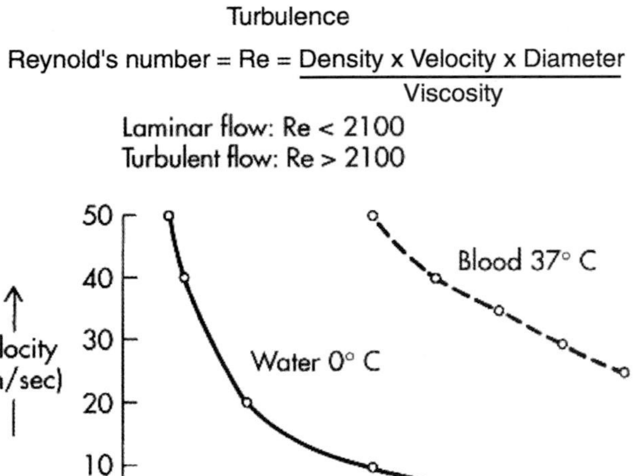

FIGURE 2-12. Reynolds relationship. These curves demonstrate the transition between laminar flow (below the line) and turbulent flow (above the line). Note that turbulence occurs at lower velocities in larger diameter vessels. Turbulence also occurs sooner in less viscous water than in blood for a vessel of given size and velocity. This becomes a factor in the evaluation of anemic patients, such as those with sickle cell anemia.

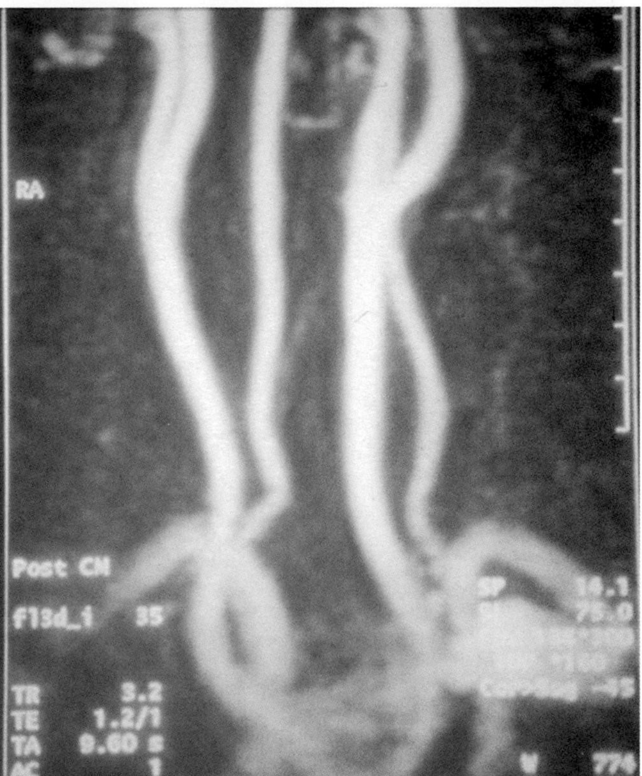

FIGURE 2-13. Multiphase contrast-enhanced magnetic resonance angiogram of the carotid arteries. After a 10-second mask acquisition, this was one of several 10-second acquisitions acquired after a bolus injection of contrast. This subtracted image caught the arterial phase without any venous contamination. Note the excellent visualization of the origins of both the carotids and the vertebral arteries, which are routinely seen with contrast-enhanced magnetic resonance angiography.

gadolinium (Figure 2-13). Thus, gadolinium can be useful in distinguishing a complete obstruction, such as from an embolus, or from a partial obstruction, such as from vasculitis or tumoral compression. One of the problems with adding gadolinium to a conventional 3D TOF or MOTSA MRA is venous enhancement. A simple method to limit venous contamination is to include only the source images that contain the desired arteries in the MIP processing (called *partial MIP*).

Another problem with gadolinium is that the contrast leaks into the adjacent soft tissues (everywhere except in the brain, assuming the blood-brain barrier is intact). This can be partially rectified by editing out the periphery of the FOV where soft tissue enhancement is greatest.

Because one of the fundamental tenets of MRA is to maximize the signal coming from the desired vessels while minimizing background signal, gadolinium that leaks into the soft tissues presents a problem. When imaging arteries, one way to solve this problem is to scan so rapidly that the bolus of gadolinium is only in the arteries, so only the arteries are seen with a minimum of venous enhancement and essentially no soft tissue enhancement. This requires very fast sequences that are feasible only on echo-planar imaging–capable MR systems with much stronger and faster gradients than previously available. Using these gradients, a complete image of the carotid arteries can be produced in less than 10 seconds (see Figure 2-13). This requires acquiring a 3D TOF slab (in the coronal plane to maximize coverage) and using extremely short TRs and TEs. With this approach, we generally acquire an unenhanced mask image and four postinjection images, one of which is always in the arterial phase. This approach is referred to as a *multiphase acquisition*.

One of the advantages of the direct coronal acquisition and contrast injection is that the origins of the carotids and vertebral arteries are now routinely visualized (see Figure 2-13). This feature was previously not possible without a separate acquisition through the upper chest.

In general, improving the spatial resolution of this technique by increasing the number of phase-encoded projections or the number of slices/partitions leads to longer imaging times and increases the risk of venous contamination. One clever way around this potential problem is to reorder the way the data are collected so that most of the signal in the image occurs during the arterial, rather than the venous, phase. When the sequence is viewed in k-space,[14,15] such techniques first fill the center of k-space (which contains most of the signal to noise)

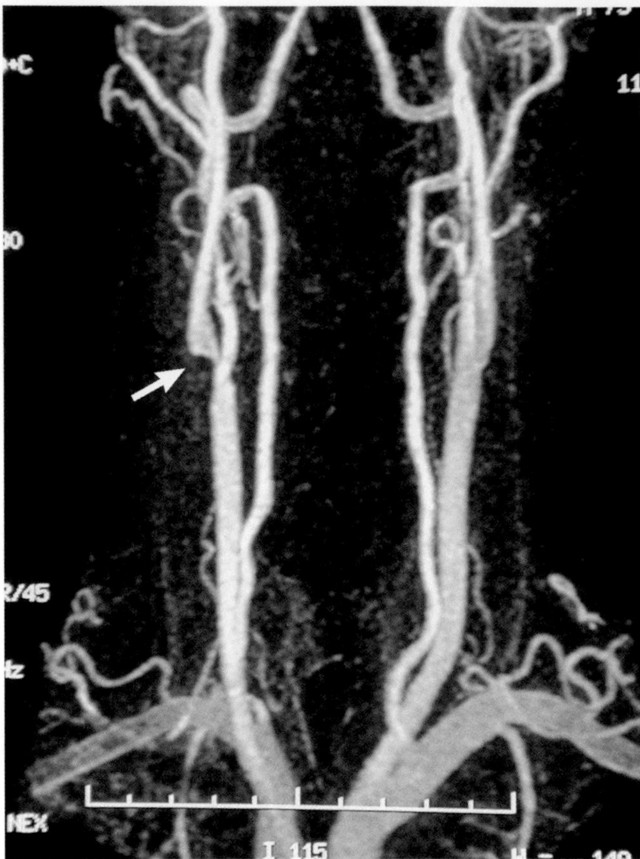

FIGURE 2-14. Elliptical centric carotid contrast-enhanced magnetic resonance angiogram. This acquisition took 1 minute to acquire; however, the center of k-space was filled during the arterial phase, minimizing any venous contamination. The longer acquisition time affords higher spatial resolution but requires a test injection to determine the timing delay. Note the excellent depiction of the proximal right internal carotid stenosis (*arrow*).

during the arterial phase and then, later, fill the periphery of k-space (low signal to noise) during the venous phase. For 2D TOF techniques, the term *centric coverage of k-space* refers to timing image acquisition so the brightest portions of the image (center of k-space) are acquired when the bolus of gadolinium arrives in the artery. For 3D TOF CE MRA techniques, the term *elliptical-centric* is used to refer to the spiral filling of the center of k-space in two dimensions along the two phase-encoding axes.[16]

The advantage of using clever k-space sampling strategies is that higher resolution can be obtained without significant venous contamination (Figure 2-14). The disadvantage is that there must be some a priori knowledge of when the contrast is going to first appear in the artery. This information can be acquired by injecting a test bolus of 2 cc of gadolinium and acquiring sequential axial, T1-weighted, gradient-echo images through the carotid bulb to determine the circulation time. It is also possible to place a voxel within the aortic arch and monitor it for increased signal, indicating arrival of gadolinium, at which point the acquisition begins. Although such automated techniques (e.g., SmartPrep [General Electric] and CareBolus [Siemens]) have demonstrated great utility for imaging the aortoiliac system or renal arteries, they are less robust for imaging the carotids.

Injection rates for gadolinium-enhanced MR angiograms depend on the location of the vessels and the specific technique used. They all require a power injector (e.g., Medrad Spectris [Pittsburgh, Pennsylvania]). For the multiphase carotid examination (see Figure 2-13), which is acquired in less than 10 seconds per image, we commonly inject 3 cc per second for a total of 15 cc and chase it with 15 cc of normal saline. This produces a tight bolus that will be captured in the arterial phase in one of the four postinjection 10-second acquisitions. For an elliptical-centric acquisition (see Figure 2-14) of the carotids that lasts 30–60 seconds, we measure the time it takes the contrast to first maximally enhance the carotid bulb with the 2-cc bolus and use that as our timing delay.

In our institution, symptomatic patients with greater than 70% stenoses by both MRA and duplex Doppler ultrasound are considered for carotid endarterectomy without a catheter study. Catheter angiography is performed only if there is a discrepancy between the MRA and the ultrasound, and there have been very few discrepancies since we began using CE MRA several years ago. It should also be noted that 70% stenosis by NASCET (North American Symptomatic Carotid Endarterectomy Trial) criteria represents the ratio of two diameters measured using cut-film catheter angiography in only two projections. Many have noted that eccentric plaques can easily over- or underestimate the true degree of luminal compromise. Better measurements of stenosis would be the absolute cross-sectional area and length of the stenosis. Such measurements are now possible with ultrasound, computed tomography angiography, and CE MRA when direct axial acquisitions are obtained.

Because first-pass CE MRA of the carotids is performed in the coronal plane, such stenosis quantification would necessitate an additional study in the axial plane through the stenosis. This might require a second injection of gadolinium or use of the new class of blood pool vascular gadolinium agents. These agents are based either on superparamagnetic iron oxide particles, such as NC 100150 by Amersham (Buckinghamshire, England), or a gadolinium–diethylenetriamine pentaacetic acid (DTPA) chelate that binds albumin, such as MS-325 by Epix (Cambridge, Massachusetts). Both agents remain in the circulation for 1 hour. Thus, additional high-resolution axial images can be acquired after the first-pass acquisition during the arterial phase to better quantify the stenosis without a second injection. In fact, with the new gadolinium blood pool agents, multiple vascular territories can be interrogated with CE MRA during a single

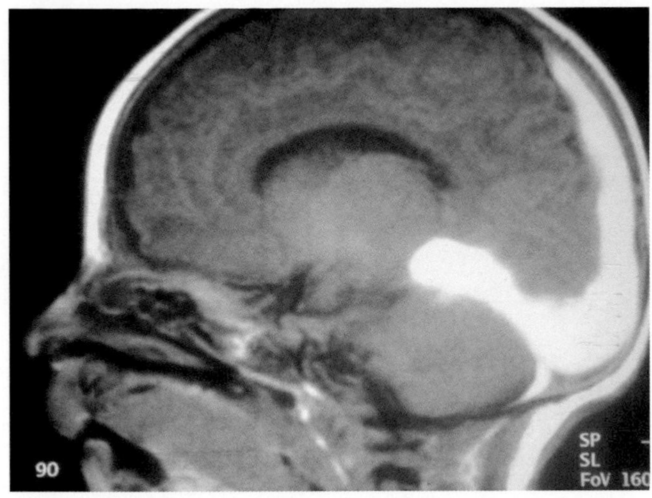

A

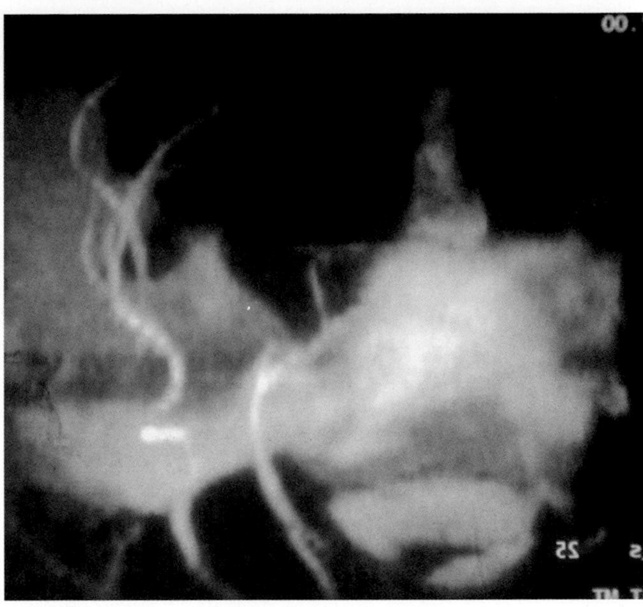

B

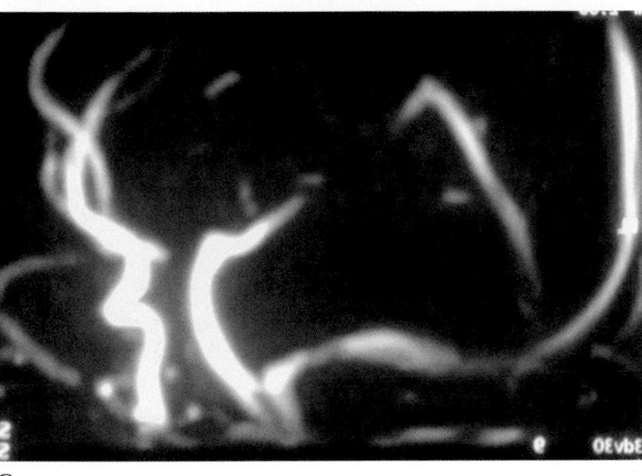

C

FIGURE 2-15. Magnetic resonance angiogram (MRA) in the presence of subacute hemorrhage. **A.** T1-weighted sagittal acquisition demonstrates a subacute subdural hematoma containing short T1, bright methemoglobin. **B.** Three-dimensional time-of-flight MRA is degraded by the presence of bright T1 hemorrhage. **C.** Phase-contrast MRA subtracts out nonmoving structures and is not contaminated by the subacute subdural hematoma.

scanning session. However, all images after the first arterial phase acquisition include veins, and, therefore, venous editing protocols or axial images are necessary.

PHASE CONTRAST

In phase-contrast MRA, signal is primarily based on the phase gain (or loss) as the spins move through a magnetic field gradient.[17] This phase change is proportional to the velocity, the strength of the gradient, and the time the gradient is applied. No more than 180 degrees of phase can be gained (or lost), or phase aliasing occurs (where the velocity appears to be maximal in one direction in one pixel and maximal in the opposite direction in the pixel next to it). For this reason, the aliasing, or encoding velocity (Venc), which is determined by the strength of the phase-sensitizing gradient, is set prospectively. A Venc of 40–60 cm per second is typically used for arterial flow, whereas 5–20 cm per second is used for venous flow.

In phase-contrast MRA, phase sensitization must be performed separately along each of the three axes and then subtracted from a reference image taken without gradient activation. Phase-contrast MRA, therefore, takes four times longer than TOF MRA techniques performed with the same TR and the same matrix. For this reason, it has not gained widespread use. Its primary indication is for MRA in the presence of subacute hemorrhage, which is bright on a T1-weighted image. Because the bright signal is found on both the base image and the flow-sensitized image in a phase-contrast technique, it subtracts out (Figure 2-15). On the TOF study, on the other hand, it remains in the image leading to image degradation and potential confusion with vascular patency (if the vessel itself is subacutely thrombosed).

Another advantage of phase-contrast techniques is that the direction and velocity of flowing blood can be determined. This capability can be used to map out the arterial supply to and the venous drainage from an arteriovenous malformation (Figure 2-16).[18] The problem is that one lengthy acquisition must be acquired with an arterial encoding velocity and then another with a venous encoding velocity. In addition, a conventional

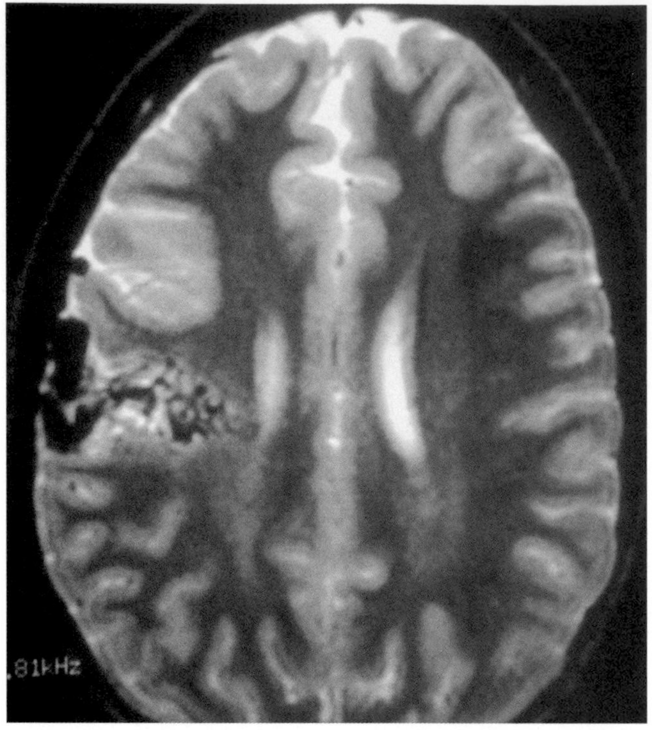

A

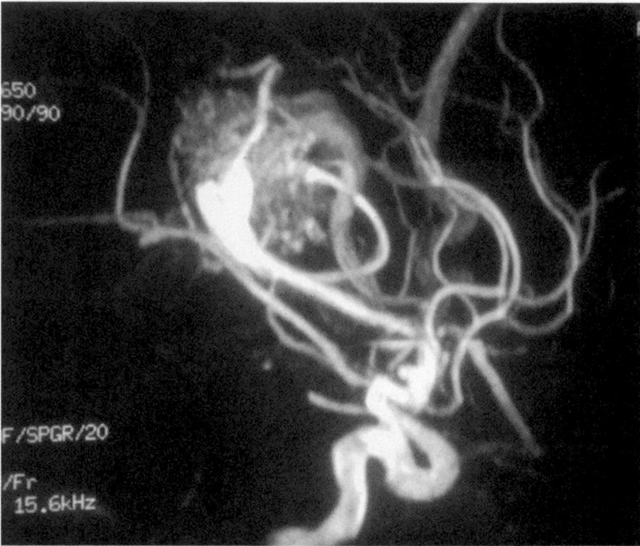

B

C

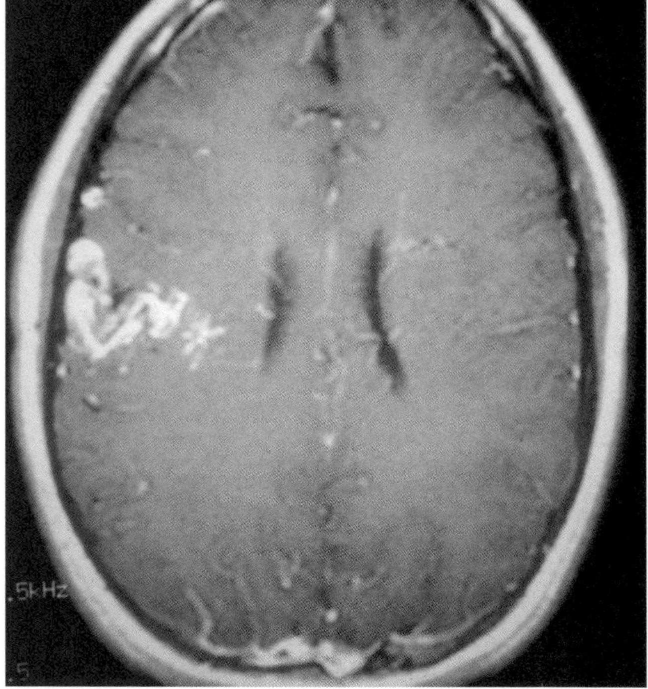

D

FIGURE 2-16. Arteriovenous malformation. **A.** T2-weighted axial acquisition demonstrates nidus and adjacent flow voids from arteriovenous malformation. **B.** Three-dimensional time-of-flight magnetic resonance angiogram demonstrates both the nidus and the abnormal vessels. **C.** Phase-contrast magnetic resonance angiogram demonstrates vessels (albeit without the nidus) and can also demonstrate the direction of flow. **D.** Gadolinium-enhanced T1-weighted image shows location and size of nidus and draining veins, which are important information for the neurosurgeon.

MRI must be acquired to best demonstrate the nidus for the Spetzler scoring. (The Spetzler score determines the likelihood of complication during surgery for arteriovenous malformations. It is based on the size of the nidus, whether it involves an eloquent part of the brain, and whether venous drainage is central or peripheral [central venous drainage increasing the chance of intraoperative bleeding].) In practice (as the catheter angiography will be performed regardless), the MR study is generally limited to a gadolinium-enhanced conventional MRI (see Figure 2-16), although new techniques like *t*ime-*r*esolved *i*maging of *c*ontrast *k*inetics

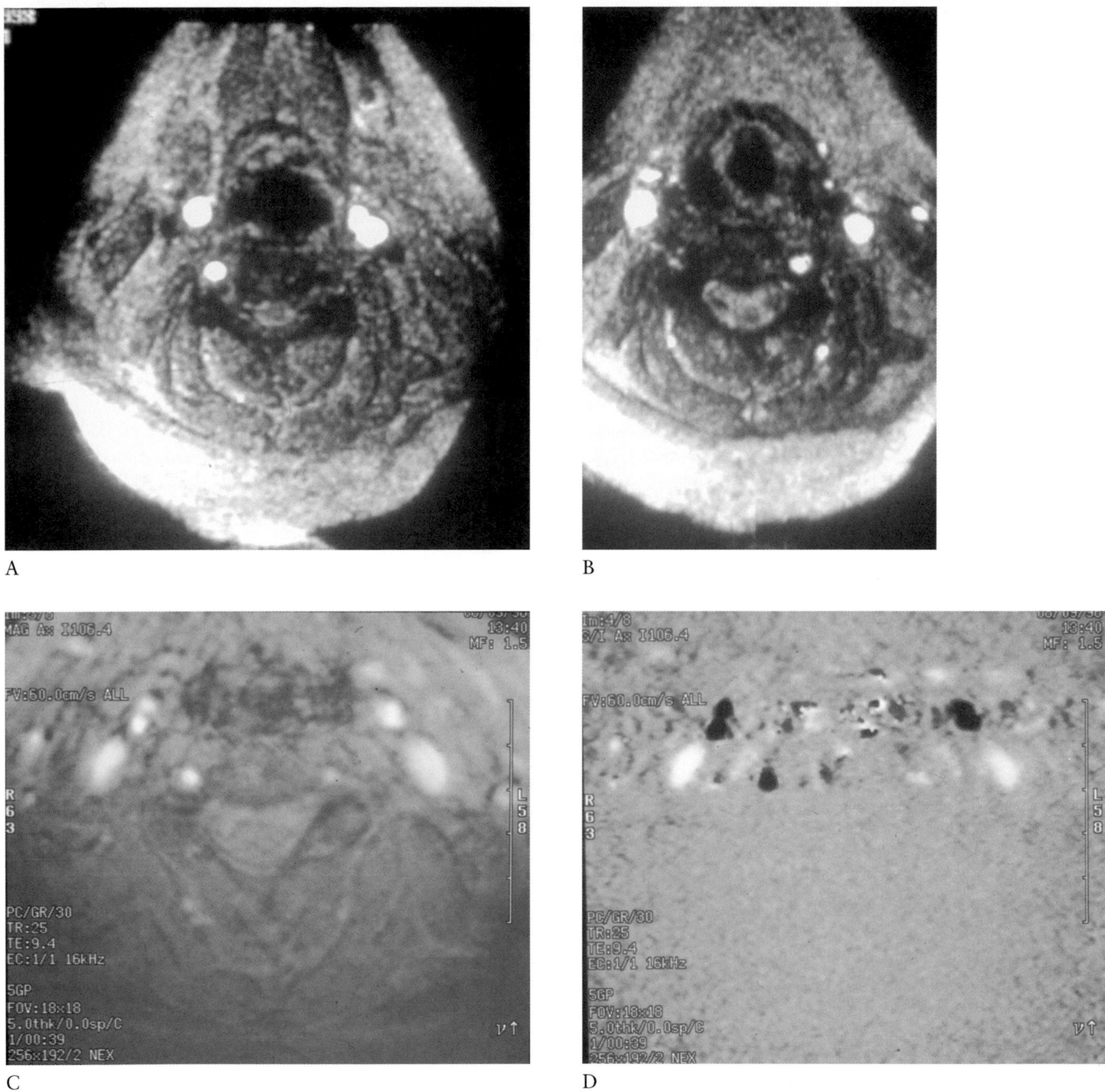

FIGURE 2-17. Two-dimensional (2D) time-of-flight and 2D phase-contrast (PC) magnetic resonance angiograms (MRA) demonstrate subclavian steal syndrome. **A.** Acquisition from superior to inferior catches up-flowing blood. In this case, the left vertebral artery is conspicuously absent. **B.** 2D time-of-flight MRA acquired from inferior to superior catches down-flowing blood. In addition to the expected signal from the jugular veins, signal is also noted from down-flowing blood in the left vertebral artery. This is due to subclavian steal syndrome from a proximal left subclavian artery stenosis. **C.** 2D PC MRA (magnitude image) demonstrates less flow-related enhancement in left vertebral artery. **D.** 2D PC MRA (phase image) demonstrates down-flowing blood (bright) in left vertebral artery.

(TRICKS), a rapid gadolinium-enhanced MRA technique showing multiple phases of enhancement, may have applications in the noninvasive evaluation of arteriovenous malformations.[19]

Phase-contrast MRA can also be used to determine if flow in the vertebral artery is cephalad or caudad in suspected subclavian steal syndrome. Of course, the latter could also be determined by comparing a 2D TOF MRA acquisition, moving superiorly with an inferior saturation pulse (to catch down-flowing blood), to one moving inferiorly with a superior saturation pulse (to catch up-flowing blood) (Figure 2-17).

Although the applicability of phase-contrast MRA may be limited at present, it is likely to increase with the introduction of the latest class of *cardiovascular* MR units with even more powerful and faster gradients. If we can perform $1{,}024^2$-MRA, we match the spatial resolution of catheter angiography (250 μm). Attempts to achieve this spatial resolution using TOF MRA have been limited by the extremely short TRs required to obtain a large number of phase views in a reasonable acquisition time. Such short TRs do not allow sufficient time for inflow of unsaturated spins to provide adequate signal to noise ratio. With phase-contrast MRA, the signal to noise ratio primarily depends on obtaining adequate phase encoding, which is determined by the strength of the gradients and the length of time they are applied. As gradients get stronger, application time decreases, decreasing the TR. Thus, phase-contrast MRA may well see a rebirth as we move toward 1,024 × 1,024 acquisitions.

Signal to noise ratio becomes problematic at 250-μm spatial resolution. Even if the slice thickness is not modified (as it should be to obtain an isotropic acquisition), every halving of inplane spatial dimension at constant acquisition time results in a 75% decrease in signal to noise ratio. Thus, in going from a 256^2 to a $1{,}024^2$ acquisition with the same slice thickness, FOV, and acquisition times, signal to noise ratio per pixel will be one-sixteenth (6.25%) of what it was originally. To achieve isotropic spatial resolution (i.e., a slice thickness of 250 μm), reduce signal to noise further to 1.5% of the original. Higher-field (e.g., 3T) scanners offer an advantage here. Gadolinium can also be used to boost signal to noise ratio, but unless the acquisition can be performed in less than 30–60 seconds, there will likely be significant venous contamination (see Figure 2-7). Although a number of editing schemes have been proposed to remove the veins, these remain labor intensive and are not likely to attain a routine clinical use until they can be automated.

REFERENCES

1. Bradley WG, Waluch V. Blood flow: magnetic resonance imaging. Radiology 1985;154:443–450.
2. Bradley WG. Flow Phenomena. In DD Stark, WG Bradley (eds), Magnetic Resonance Imaging (3rd ed). St. Louis: Mosby, 1999;231–256.
3. Masaryk TJ, Perl J 2nd, Dagirmanjiam A, et al. Magnetic Resonance Angiography: Neuroradiological Applications. In DD Stark, WG Bradley (eds), Magnetic Resonance Imaging (3rd ed). St. Louis: Mosby, 1999;1277–1316.
4. Blatter DD, Parker DL, Ahn SS, et al. Cerebral MR angiography with multiple overlapping thin slab acquisition. Part II. Early clinical experience. Radiology 1992;183:379–389.
5. Jager HR, Mansmann U, Hausmann O, et al. MRA versus digital subtraction angiography in acute subarachnoid haemorrhage: a blinded multiready study of prospectively recruited patients. Neuroradiology 2000;45(5):313–326.
6. Shigematsu Y, Korogi Y, Hirai T, et al. 3D TOF turbo MR angiography for intracranial arteries: phantom clinical studies. J Magn Reson Imaging 1999;10(6):939–944.
7. Parker DL, Goodrich KC, Alexander AL, et al. Optimized visualization of vessels in contrast enhanced intracranial MR angiography. Magn Reson Med 1998;40(6):873–882.
8. Bradley WG. Recent advances in magnetic resonance angiography of the brain. Curr Opin Neurol Neurosurg 1992;5(6):859–862.
9. Jara H, Yu BC, Caruthers SD, et al. Voxel sensitivity function description of flow induced signal loss imaging: implications for black blood MR angiography with turbo spin echo sequences. Magn Reson Med 1999;41(3):575–590.
10. Lee BCP, Vo KD, Kido DK, et al. MR high resolution blood oxygenation level dependent venography of occult (low-flow) vascular lesions. AJNR Am J Neuroradiol 1999;20:1239–1242.
11. Bradley WG. MR appearance of hemorrhage in the brain. Radiology 1993;189:15–26.
12. Reichenbach JR, Barth M, Haacke EM, et al. High resolution MR venography at 3.0 Tesla. J Comput Assist Tomogr 2000;24(6):949–957.
13. Erly WK, Zaetta J, Borders GT, et al. Gadopentetate dimeglumine as a contrast agent in common carotid arteriography. J Comput Assist Tomogr 2000;2(5):964–967.
14. Bradley WG, Chen D-Y, Atkinson DJ. Fast Spin Echo. In WG Bradley, GM Bydder (eds), Advanced MR Imaging Techniques. London: Dunitz, 1997.
15. Bradley WG, Chen D-Y, Atkinson DJ. Using High Performance Gradients. In WG Bradley, GM Bydder (eds), Advanced MR Imaging Techniques. London: Dunitz, 1997.
16. Fain SB, Riederer SJ, Bernstein MA, Huston J 3rd. Theoretical limits of spatial resolution in elliptical-centric contrast enhanced 3D MRA. Magn Reson Med 1999;42(6):1106–1116.
17. Dumoulin CL, Souza SP, Walker MF, Wagle W. Three-dimensional phase contrast angiography. Magn Reson Med 1989;9:139–149.
18. Cellerini M, Mascalchi M, Mangiafica S, et al. Phase contrast MR angiography of intracranial dural arteriovenous fistulae. Neuroradiology 1999;41(7):487–492.
19. Vigen KK, Peters DC, Grist TM, et al. Undersampled projection reconstruction imaging for time resolution contrast enhanced imaging. Magn Reson Med 2000;43(2):170–176.

CHAPTER

3

Computed Tomography Angiography

Heidi C. Roberts, Theodore J. Lee, and William P. Dillon

There are many indications for imaging the extracerebral and intracranial vasculature. These include identifying and grading vascular stenoses; diagnosing vascular diseases such as aneurysms, arteriovenous malformations, and occult vascular malformations; evaluating the dural sinuses; and diagnosing arterial dissections. Previously, vascular imaging has been the mainstay of invasive imaging techniques using catheter-based angiography. To date, digital subtraction angiography (DSA) is the accepted gold standard for imaging the cervical and cerebral arteries. However, DSA is an invasive procedure and has risks. DSA is associated with a 1% overall incidence of neurological deficits and a 0.3–0.5% incidence of stroke.[1,2] Angiographic procedures are needed when they are combined with endovascular treatments. However, the need for more noninvasive screening techniques has arisen due to the need for cost effectiveness, risk reduction, and faster imaging techniques.

Three major noninvasive modalities are now available to image the neural vasculature, which differ greatly in their availability, time requirement, applicability, and costs: Doppler ultrasound (US), magnetic resonance (MR) angiography (MRA), and computed tomography (CT) angiography (CTA).

US poses virtually no risk to the patient. Its disadvantages are its high interobserver and intermachine variability.[3] Furthermore, it is time consuming and can suffer from poor US penetration in certain patients.[4]

MRA (see Chapter 2) can be performed as a noncontrast (time-of-flight or phase-contrast) or contrast-enhanced series of images. In general, MRA yields high- quality images with increasing time required for a particular sequence, and best spatial resolution is achieved from data acquisitions that take 10 minutes or more. Data post-processing is standardized, and evaluation of the source images and display of maximum-intensity projections (MIPs) are most commonly performed to assess an examination. By using noncontrast MRA, the vessel lumens are imaged *indirectly* by using velocities or tissue saturation effects, or both, and complex flow patterns (e.g., turbulence), which may cause signal losses that can masquerade as stenoses or obscure underlying pathologic diseases.

CTA combines the intravenous injection of a contrast agent with high-speed continuous CT scanning of a volume of interest, followed by the computer-assisted generation of three-dimensional (3D) reconstructions from the original cross-sectional images. CTA is widely available and can be performed with helical or multidetector scanners, each requiring different protocols targeted to the specific clinical issues. CTA is minimally invasive, and the risks are only associated with contrast agent administration and radiation exposure. In contrast to MRA, using CTA delineates the vessel lumen in a similar manner to conventional angiography, in which contrast material outlines the vessel wall. Unlike DSA, CTA allows an assessment not only of the lumen and its size, but also of the vascular wall itself. Compared to MRA, CTA has a faster data acquisition time, which may be crucial in an emergency patient. However, post-processing is less standardized, and several approaches are offered and used in parallel.

In the cerebrovascular circulation, CTA has three major applications: (1) imaging the circle of Willis and the extracerebral carotid arteries in the assessment of an acute stroke; (2) evaluation of extracranial carotid artery occlusive disease; and (3) the detection and characterization of intracranial aneurysms. Other indications include the assessment of intracranial stenotic and occlusive disease or arterial dissections.

TECHNIQUE

CTA requires a scanner capable of rapid acquisition of numerous thin, overlapping sections during the peak of intravascular contrast enhancement. The first scanners suited for this purpose were spiral, or helical, CT scanners in 1988. The first references in the literature to the application of spiral CTA for extracranial and intracranial carotid imaging are from 1992, with progressive refinement of these techniques. The development of multidetector scanners has improved the acquisition speed and image quality of CT angiograms. Both helical and multidetector scanners are now in common use; thus, the data acquisition parameters are described separately for each of these two technologies. To maintain a high level of intravascular contrast agent throughout the acquisition, careful emphasis is placed on the appropriate timing and dosage of the contrast agent injection.

DATA ACQUISITION WITH SPIRAL OR HELICAL SCANNING

In spiral, or helical CT scanning, the slip ring technology allows the gantry to freely rotate around a full 360 degrees. CT data are acquired continuously as the table traverses through the gantry, creating a helix of data that can be reconstructed at varying slice increments and reformatted in arbitrary planes. Helical CT offers a sufficiently rapid acquisition of images during a single contrast bolus injection. This fast data acquisition allows sharper bolus geometries of contrast agent injections, giving better opacification of the blood vessels. Continuous data acquisition makes high-quality reformations possible. All of these technical advances have led to much-improved angiography-like images of the vascular territory of interest.

There is no consensus about the exact scanning parameters for an "optimal" CTA of the head and neck. Table 3-1 gives an overview from the literature on the various helical CTA parameters, both for imaging the circle of Willis and the extracerebral carotid arteries. In general, high tube currents (mA) and tube voltages (kV) are required for a sufficient signal to noise ratio. The smallest vessel size that can be resolved by spiral CTA is determined by the orientation of the vessel relative to the imaging plane. *Inplane* spatial resolution is the limiting factor for vessels perpendicular to the scanning plane. Given the typical 512 × 512 matrix of CT images, inplane resolution is sufficient for identifying even small vascular branches and may be further enhanced by using a smaller field of view than in conventional CT imaging. The *longitudinal* or *z-axis* resolution, on the other hand, is the limiting factor for vessels parallel to the scanning plane and is rather poor compared to the inplane resolution. Z-axis resolution improves with narrow collimation (i.e., slice thickness), low pitch (ratio of table speed and collimation), and reconstruction of overlapping images. Because longitudinal resolution is limited by tube-heating capacities, there is a tradeoff between collimation and pitch and the scanned CT volume. Although CTA had initial enthusiasm, spiral scanning techniques were criticized because of their limited anatomic coverage.[5]

The parameters presented in Table 3-1, with the anatomic coverage in the z-direction, are usually limited to 6 cm, which allows a spiral CT angiogram of the circle of Willis, the posterior cerebral circulation, *or* the carotid bifurcation. However, this technique is not satisfactory to assess a suspected acute stroke. Evaluation of the carotid bifurcation is only limited to the region where the majority of the disease is located, and either the scanned volume has to be placed on the presumed bifurcation location between C2-3 and C6-7,[6] or the bifurcation has to be localized on a noncontrast preceding scan.[7,8] Therefore, with only a few centimeters of coverage, complete coverage of the carotid system is not possible, and tandem lesions, which are detected in 9% of the conventional DSAs, may be missed.[9,10] As the presence of tandem lesions confers a higher stroke risk, this is a significant limitation of spiral CTA.[9,10] An increased pitch to expand the anatomic coverage area would impair the evaluation of plaque morphology, vessel lumen, and the detection of focal bands of narrowing.[8,11] A limited anatomic coverage is less critical for aneurysms, which are confined to the circle of Willis.

Further technical developments, in particular improved tube-heating capacities, could reduce, but not eliminate, the problem of limited scan volumes. A major technologic improvement was the development of CT scanners with several rows of detectors, such as the CT Twin Scanner (Elscint Ltd., Ma'alot, Israel), in 1992. Two parallel arcs of detectors simultaneously acquired two helices of volumetric data, thereby doubling the data acquisition speed. However, this scanner technology never found widespread use and was soon superseded by the evolution of multidetector CT scanners.

DATA ACQUISITION WITH MULTIDETECTOR COMPUTED TOMOGRAPHY ANGIOGRAPHY SCANNING

The primary drawback of spiral CTA has been the tube-heating capacity, resulting in an insufficient scan volume. This limitation was overcome by the development of the

TABLE 3-1. Overview of the Parameters Used in the Literature for Helical Computed Tomography Angiography for the Different Vascular Territories

Anatomic coverage	*References*	*Collimation (mm)*	*Pitch*	*Reconstruction interval (mm)*	*mA*	*kV*	*Contrast agent (ml)*	*Flow rate (ml/sec)*	*Delay (secs)*
Circle of Willis									
Floor of sella to vertex	4,27	1.5	1.25	1	125	130	130	4–5	20
1 cm below base of sella through the circle of Willis at the level of the midlateral ventricles	19	1	1:1	0.5	220	120	75–100	2.5 for 20–30 secs; 1 for 25 secs	15–20
Above the atlas vertebrae to centrum semiovale	24	1.3	1	0.6	210	120	120	2	25
3 cm covering the circle of Willis from mid-basilar artery and cavernous carotid arteries to ~2.5 cm above the genu of the anterior and middle cerebral arteries	22	1	1:1	1	165	120	60	3	18
	40	1	1.3	0.5	220–280	100	90	3	Test bolus
Floor of sella turcica	73	1	1:1	1	240–280	120	135	3	20
Extracerebral arteries									
Around bifurcation, identified on planning scan	7	3	1	—	180	120	90	3	Test dose
Started at C5-6 disk space	9	2	1:1	1	210	120	100	3	12
Started at C6-7 disk space	11	2–3	1	1	—	—	90	3	15
Carotid arteries (9 cm)	22	3	1:1	1	165	120	—	3	15
From the C6 vertebral body to the skull base	30	3	1.5	—	200–320	120	120	3	Trigger technique
From the inferior margin of the C6 vertebral body to the skull base	99	3	1:1	1.5	210	120	140	3.5	15–26
Intracranial aneurysms									
30 mm above and below the sella turcica	94	1	1:4	0.5	280–300	120	120	3	Test dose
Vertebral artery proximal to the branch of the posterior inferior cerebellar artery to the distal anterior and middle cerebral arteries	95	0.8–1.0	1:1	0.4–0.5	220	135	80–100	2–3	Trigger technique
From C2 to the bodies of the lateral ventricles	96	1	1.5	0.5	260	120	—	3	—

multidetector scanners in 1998 by several manufacturers, including the Lightspeed by General Electric (Fairfield, Connecticut); Mx8000 by Philips (Best, The Netherlands); Plus 4 Volume Zoom by Siemens (Woodbridge, New Jersey); and Aquilion by Toshiba (Tokyo, Japan). Considerable differences exist in the number and thickness of the detectors arranged along the z-axis. The length of the whole detector array ranges from 20 to 32 mm, with the minimum slice thickness ranging between 0.50 and 1.25 mm and the maximum slice thickness ranging between 8 and 10 mm. Common features among these units are a helical capability, use of a wider beam, and acquisition of several CT slices per x-ray tube rotation. Combined with an increased speed of gantry revolution compared to spiral scanners, data acquisition is eight times faster. Prior constraints due to tube cooling no longer exist with multidetector technology. This allows rapid scanning over large anatomic volumes and whole vascular territories, using only a single bolus of contrast agent.

The biggest impact of multidetector CT technology has been on CTA. It is now possible to cover not only the anterior and posterior cerebral circulation during one contrast agent bolus but also the cervical vasculature. This is done using a lower pitch for the circle of Willis and a higher pitch for the carotid arteries.[12] However, pitch switching results in a delay of several seconds' duration and a consequent drop in the contrast agent concentration, resulting in an artifact at the level where the mode was changed. Typically, a scan of the entire intra- and extracerebral volume with a low pitch yields high-quality angiograms. This volume is scanned top down, so there are no streak artifacts from high concentrations of contrast agent at the level of the subclavian vein. There are several publications on the use of multidetector scanners for CTA in neuroradiology, and these suggest tube voltages of 120–140 kV and a tube current of 170–250 mA.[12–14] Targeted protocols for multidetector CT scanners are still evolving.

CONTRAST AGENT ADMINISTRATION

To maintain a high and uniform level of intravascular contrast agent throughout the acquisition, fast data acquisition is only one requirement. The second requirement is a sharp contrast bolus geometry, injected at the appropriate preparation delay after the start of the CT scan.

Injection of a contrast agent is one of the inherent disadvantages of CTA.[5] Several early reports have indicated a possible neurotoxicity of the contrast agents.[15] However, these reports were based on the use of ionic contrast agents and were retrospective and uncontrolled. The findings could not be reproduced, and it has been shown under experimental conditions that nonionic contrast agents do not affect the volume of infarcts.[16] As of 2002, nonionic contrast media are regarded as relatively safe.[17]

A second concern with contrast agent injection, particularly in the elderly population, is the potential nephrotoxicity. In an elective situation, creatinine levels below 2.0 mg/dl confirm sufficient kidney function to handle the contrast load required for CTA. However, in an emergency situation, the contrast agent administration may be performed without the knowledge of the serum creatinine levels. A recent study from 2001 on the safety of CTA has demonstrated that serum creatinine was unchanged from baseline to hospital discharge in all study subjects given contrast for assessment of acute ischemic stroke.[14]

A third problem with contrast administration for CTA is idiosyncratic reactions to the contrast agent. However, although idiosyncratic reactions to iodinated contrast agents are still quite common, the use of nonionic agents has reduced the occurrence of moderate or severe adverse reactions.[14,18,19]

The recommended amount of contrast agent necessary for high-quality CTAs is in the range of 100–130 ml (Table 3-1). Lower volumes of 60–75 ml result in an unacceptably high rate of technically unsatisfactory CTA studies.[19,20]

Proper bolus timing and shape are very important for contrast optimization in CTA. Suboptimal timing may result in deficient or reduced vessel opacification. If the scan starts too early after injection, arterial contrast agent concentration is low, and the distal cerebral artery branches may not yet be filled. If the scan starts too late, arterial opacification might be reduced, and venous enhancement might impair image quality. If the bolus is too broad (i.e., the injection rate is too low), both of the above effects might occur.

There are two different approaches to achieve proper bolus timing: One is targeting to simplify the scanning protocol, and the other is to individualize the protocol. Ideally, scanning should start after the carotid arteries are adequately opacified but before contrast material reaches the jugular veins. The simpler approach uses an empirical fixed delay of 20–25 seconds (see Table 3-1), which has proven effective for most patients. In either case, venous opacification does not significantly impair the image quality in the neck. However, in the brain, arteries and veins are not adjacent to one another except in the area of the basal vein of Rosenthal and posterior cerebral artery within the ambient cistern. To correct for a possibly protracted contrast arrival, the delay should be increased to 30–40 seconds if a reduced cardiac output is known.

The rationale for an individualized approach is mainly based on variations in cardiac output. Such approaches use either a trigger technique or a test bolus to tailor the data acquisition to the contrast agent peak (see Table 3-1). Using the semiautomated trigger techniques, CT scanning is started when a preset enhancement threshold is reached within a preselected region of interest, typically lying just proximal to the site of clinical interest. By injecting a test bolus of 10–20 ml with continuous single-slice scanning at the level of the proximal internal carotid artery (ICA), the individual preparation delay is usually calculated based on the time to maximal test vessel opacification. Both of these techniques, however, add complexity to the protocol, further complicating image acquisition in emergency situations.

RADIATION DOSE

CTA is described as minimally invasive, not only because of the contrast agent injection but also because of the associated radiation exposure. The radiation dose for the patient is greater than with conventional CT but significantly less than with DSA. Depending on the mAs used, CTA results in a radiation dose to the patient similar to a standard cervical spine CT of approximately 3.4 cGy to the skin and thyroid gland per acquisition for spiral CT, as opposed to approximately 3.7 cGy for routine cervical spine CT.[8] Measurements of the radiation dose have been performed in a CTA study in children using a standardized CT dose index phantom[21] and mimicking study parameters with a beam collimation of 1 mm and a helical pitch of 2 to 1. Dose measurements made for 200 mA and 170 mA with 120 kV (peak) yielded 1.7 cGy and 1.4 cGy, respectively. Comparison measurements were made using the routine CT head protocols of continuous 7-mm sections with 200 mA and 120 kV(p), which resulted in a dose of 4.5 cGy. Thus, radiation exposure is not regarded as a significant concern in the predominantly older patient population.[19]

DATA POST-PROCESSING

The acquired transaxial CT images contain all of the information necessary for vascular assessment, and the sections reveal the maximum detail inherent in the data. Evaluation of source images is essential for the diagnosis of any vascular pathology. In particular, the source images are most reliable for the detection of vascular calcifications and the identification of artifacts.

Although information is present on axial source images, it might not be immediately evident, especially when vessels course parallel to the imaging plane and direct comparison with conventional angiography is difficult. Two-dimensional (2D) and 3D reconstruction images generated from the original cross-sectional images on separate work stations display the information from the axial scans in a more familiar and appealing format and, thus, help reveal pathologic findings. Reconstruction images can be accomplished in several different ways, and there is no consensus about the choice or the amount of post-processing required. All reformatting possibilities have advantages and disadvantages. In general, time, image quality, and accuracy are the tradeoffs to be considered. Post-processing time, used to obtain the reconstructed images, may vary from a few minutes to several hours.

In *MIPs*, a volume of interest is chosen from the acquired data set, and those pixels with the highest Hounsfield units (HU) are displayed. MIPs are computed from many view angles and can be displayed in a cine loop to convey 3D structure. MIP is a method that is widely used for creation of MRA displays, because the pulse sequences used for data collection are designed to result in blood vessels having high intensities relative to those of nonvascular structures. In CTA, blood vessel attenuation is maximized by administration of contrast medium, but physical constraints preclude obtaining attenuation higher than that of bone and other calcified structures. However, with appropriate window and level settings, those distinct anatomic structures can be differentiated, and calcifications can also be visualized (Figure 3-1). The higher attenuation and spatial connectivity of bone facilitates its selective removal from the data by means of the pre-processing technique of thresholding and segmentation (see Figure 3-1).[22]

There are a few caveats when using MIPs to display the cerebral vasculature. Automatic removal of bone structures or calcifications is possible using operator-defined threshold. But depending on the software, adjacent pixels also can be affected, resulting in an incorrect assessment of vessel diameter and overestimation of stenoses (Figure 3-2). Serious problems may occur when a vessel is directly adjacent to a bone, such as the vertebral artery or the petrous segment of the carotid artery. MIP displays are influenced by window and level setting (see Figure 3-1), which is influenced by the reader's experience, as well as by the viewing plane and the MIP algorithm.[23–26]

Volume-rendered algorithms offer a 3D display of the scanned anatomy.[4,27] A major disadvantage for imaging of the vasculature is that calcifications cannot be differentiated from the enhancing vessels (see Figure 3-1D). Using more effort and time, different layers can be extracted from the data set, made transparent or colored, or both, and overlain on a single image (Figure 3-3). Although this results in appealing images, it is very time consuming, and there may be overlap between adjacent structures.

In *multiplanar (volume) reformations* (MP[V]Rs), the volume is cut along an operator-defined plane, and the average Hounsfield attenuation along this cut is displayed to create an image. As indicated by the term *multiplanar*, the data set can be reconstructed in any plane (sagittal, coronal, oblique) from the axial acquired data set. Curved planes can also be created following the vascular course, and the vessel is "stretched out" along that curve. MPRs can improve the ability to detect and grade intracranial stenoses, particularly in differentiating dis-

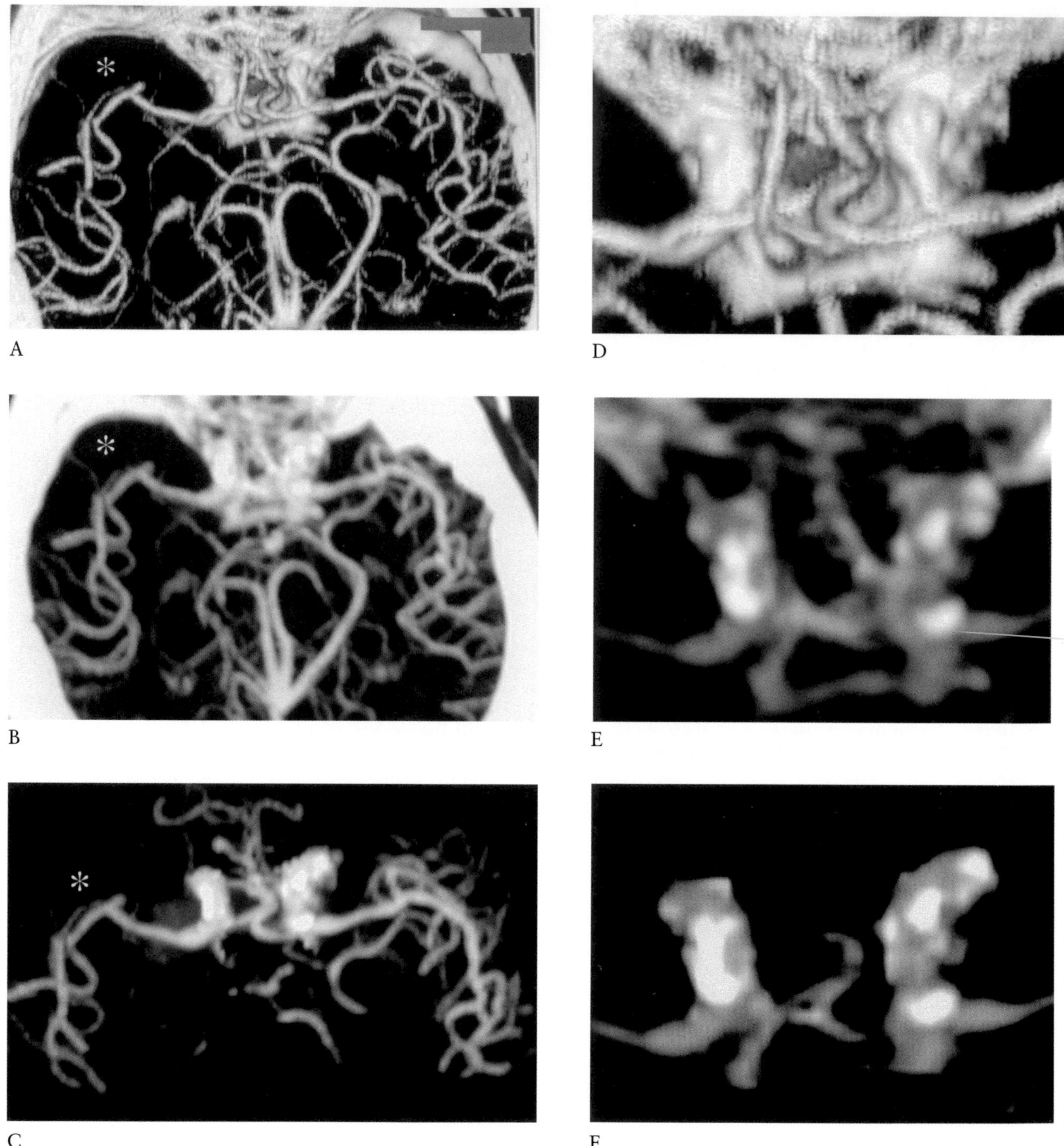

FIGURE 3-1. Three-dimensional reconstruction of the circle of Willis in a patient with a distal middle cerebral artery (M2) occlusion on the right, displayed with different techniques. **A.** Volume rendering. **B.** Maximum-intensity projection. **C.** Maximum-intensity projection after removal of the bone by segmentation. All of these displays demonstrate the lack of vascular opacification in the right middle cerebral artery territory (*asterisks*). The supraclinoid carotids are zoomed and displayed in a different window and level setting (**D–F**) to allow better visualization of the vascular calcifications. Calcifications in the supraclinoid carotid artery cannot be delineated on the volume-rendered image but can be seen on the maximum-intensity projection displays.

tal vertebral hypoplasia from stenosis and in overcoming artifacts.[24]

Curvilinear reformations, following the course of a vessel, have been used to compare rotational DSA with CTA for the detection of carotid disease.[28] Using such curved reformations, it is critical for the cutline to fit the vascular course exactly. When the cutline runs partly out of the vessel, a stenosis or occlusion is simulated. One

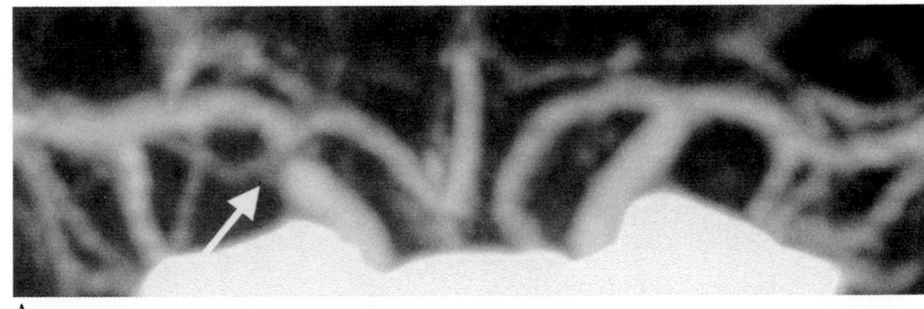

A

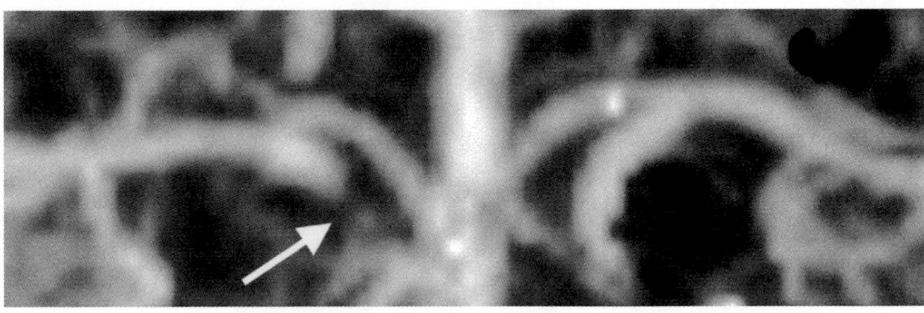

B

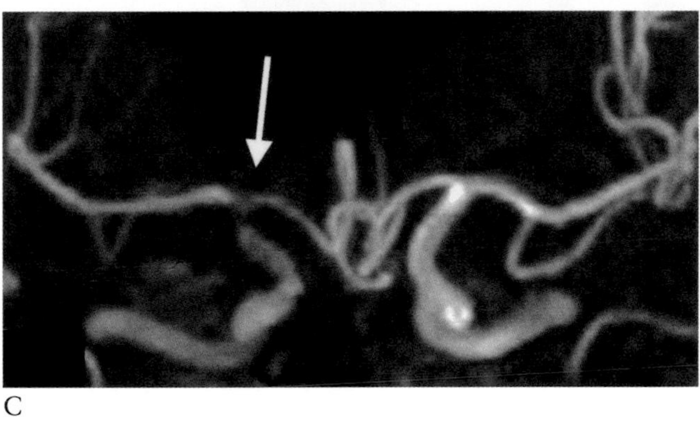

C

FIGURE 3-2. Three-dimensional reconstruction of a computed tomography angiogram of a supraclinoid carotid artery stenosis. **A.** The stenosis (*arrow*) is readily evident on the maximum-intensity projection display. **B.** After an automated, threshold-based removal of the bone (*arrow*) and high-contrast agent concentration, the vessel proximal to the stenosis has been eliminated. There is now high density in the vessel proximal to the stenosis. Without careful evaluation of the source images, such automated bone removal strategies may result in a false-positive diagnosis of an occlusion or an overestimation of stenoses. **C.** Shows the time-of-flight maximum-intensity projection reconstruction from the magnetic resonance angiogram in this patient. Due to the presence of turbulent flow around the stenosis (*arrow*), signal intensity is decreased in the vessel surrounding the stenosis.

way to overcome this problem is to create curved cutlines in different orientations (e.g., coronal, oblique) and to assess them separately, with the tradeoff of an increased time for data post-processing and analysis (Figure 3-4).

Shaded surface displays (SSDs) are generated by computing a mathematic model of a surface that connects all pixels with HU greater than a predetermined threshold. This threshold must be carefully picked on the basis of contrast material attenuation in the area of interest. Depending on the degree of luminal contrast, a value of 80–300 HU is suitable, such that only bone, contrast-filled vessels, and calcifications are visible.[29,30] In many cases, these displays result in clear depiction of vessel morphology,[22] and they provide excellent anatomic detail without visualization of the overlapping structures.

SSDs are not the preferred algorithms used to display the cerebral or cervical vasculature. This technique works best for vessels that run perpendicular through the CT scanning plane. Because this algorithm rejects voxels with attenuations below the threshold, it may not show vessels of the circle of Willis that run parallel to the scanning plane and, thus, may have reduced intensities caused by partial volume averaging. Similarly, SSDs experience suboptimal bolus timing, reduced flow distal to stenoses, or noise.[11,22,29] Display of the carotids and their perpendicular course suffers from the fact that the gray scale of the slice sensitivity profile is unrelated to x-ray attenuation. It is based on the computed reflection of a hypothetical light source from the surface. Calcified or high-density atherosclerotic plaques are averaged with contrast medium and, therefore, cannot be distinguished from their high-density intraluminal contents.[8,11]

To summarize, assessment of the carotid arteries is facilitated on source images, because they run perpendicular through the imaging plane. Stenoses and clots can be found and evaluated. 2D or 3D reconstructions display the anatomy and pathology in a more appealing and familiar way, and the craniocaudal extent of a find-

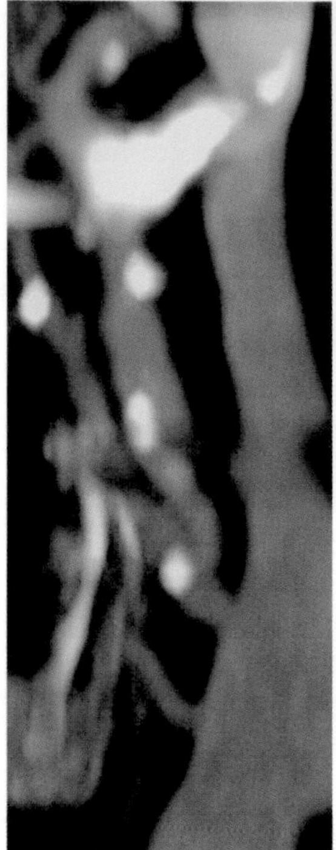

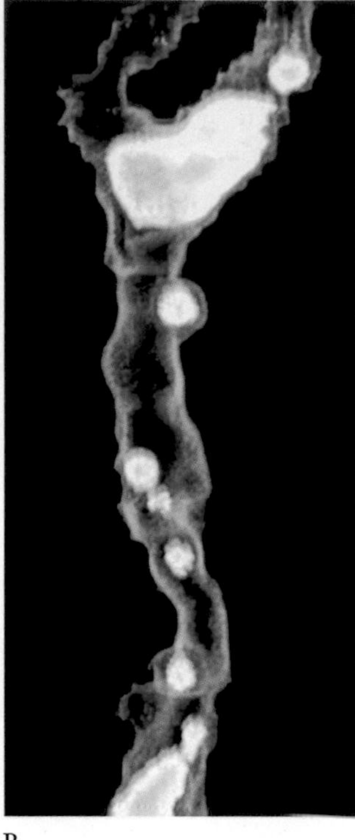

A B

FIGURE 3-3. Three-dimensional reconstruction of a computed tomography angiogram of the extracranial carotid artery in a patient with multiple calcifications. **A.** Maximum-intensity projection display. **B.** Volume-rendered image. For the latter, different layers have been identified from the data set, the vessel has been made transparent, and the calcifications have been made dense white. This results in an appealing view of the carotid artery and its calcifications.

ing might become more evident. Assessment of calcifications and clot morphology is worse on volume-rendered images, possible on MIPs or multiplanar reformations, and best on source images. The relatively horizontal course of the circle of Willis, which is parallel to the imaging plane, makes the assessment on source images more difficult. MIPs are most commonly performed to display the anatomy, and they are quickly created and reveal vascular anatomy. Source images are the most reliable for the detection of calcifications.

INDICATIONS FOR COMPUTED TOMOGRAPHY ANGIOGRAPHY

Acute Stroke

Critical questions that arise during the early stages of a suspected acute ischemic stroke include whether a hemorrhagic or nonhemorrhagic infarct is present, if the ischemic insult is reversible or permanent, and the underlying cause of the ischemic insult.[5] A nonenhanced CT scan can easily exclude hemorrhage, and new CT perfusion techniques provide information on the state of the injured tissue (see Chapter 21). The lack of imaging documentation for the site of vascular occlusion has been an inherent methodologic flaw[31] for both the National Institute of Neurological Disorders and Stroke (NINDS) trial[32] and the European Cooperative Acute Stroke Study (ECASS I).[33] The natural history and treatment may be different, depending on the site of the clot. Recanalization rates are much better in middle cerebral artery (MCA) occlusions compared to ICA occlusions.[34–36] Carotid terminus occlusions, in general, have a very poor outcome with thrombolysis.[37] Clinically, it is not usually possible to identify those two vascular occlusions or predict whether a patient has a proximal or distal vascular occlusion. Up to 20% of patients with suspected cerebral ischemia have a negative angiogram, possibly due to early spontaneous clot lysis, and another 10–20% have other angiographic exclusion criteria.[38,39]

Since the approval of intravenous recombinant tissue plasminogen activator in June 1996 for the acute treatment of ischemic stroke in the United States, the need for a noninvasive study has become important. A diagnostic goal in suspected acute stroke is to identify, as quickly as possible, patients who may benefit from intra-arterial thrombolysis (in clinical studies), intravenous thrombolysis, or other available acute stroke therapies. In addition, it should be used to exclude those patients with stroke mimics (e.g., transient ischemic attacks, complex migraines, seizures) who will not benefit from a lytic agent and who may be harmed from such therapies. Because emphasis is on efficient decision making, MR imaging has serious limitations for such patients in most institutions.

CTA may be the ideal tool in this clinical situation, as patients always undergo a noncontrast CT scan for the exclusion of hemorrhage. Several articles have demonstrated the strong potential of CTA in documenting intracranial vessel anatomy and occlusive disease. The sensitivity of CTA for the anatomy of the circle of Willis has been documented by a study by Katz et al.[40] Wildermuth et al.[4] performed a CTA study of the circle of Willis with suspected occlusions. CTA was technically successful in all 40 patients, and a vascular occlusion could be determined in 34 patients. However, this study lacked angiographic confirmation of the clot location. Only in a subgroup of seven patients was DSA available for comparison, and the CTA diagnosis was confirmed in six of them. In one case, CTA showed an ICA occlusion not confirmed by DSA 1 hour later. The authors attribute this to a spontaneous lysis between the two studies. However, another explanation for such a false-positive finding might be the presence of slow flow in the ICA proximal to a more distal occlusion (Figure 3-5). In such an instance (i.e., a complete ICA occlusion on a CTA), it is recommended to obtain a delayed CT scan to identify slow or late contrast arrival. In a study by Shrier

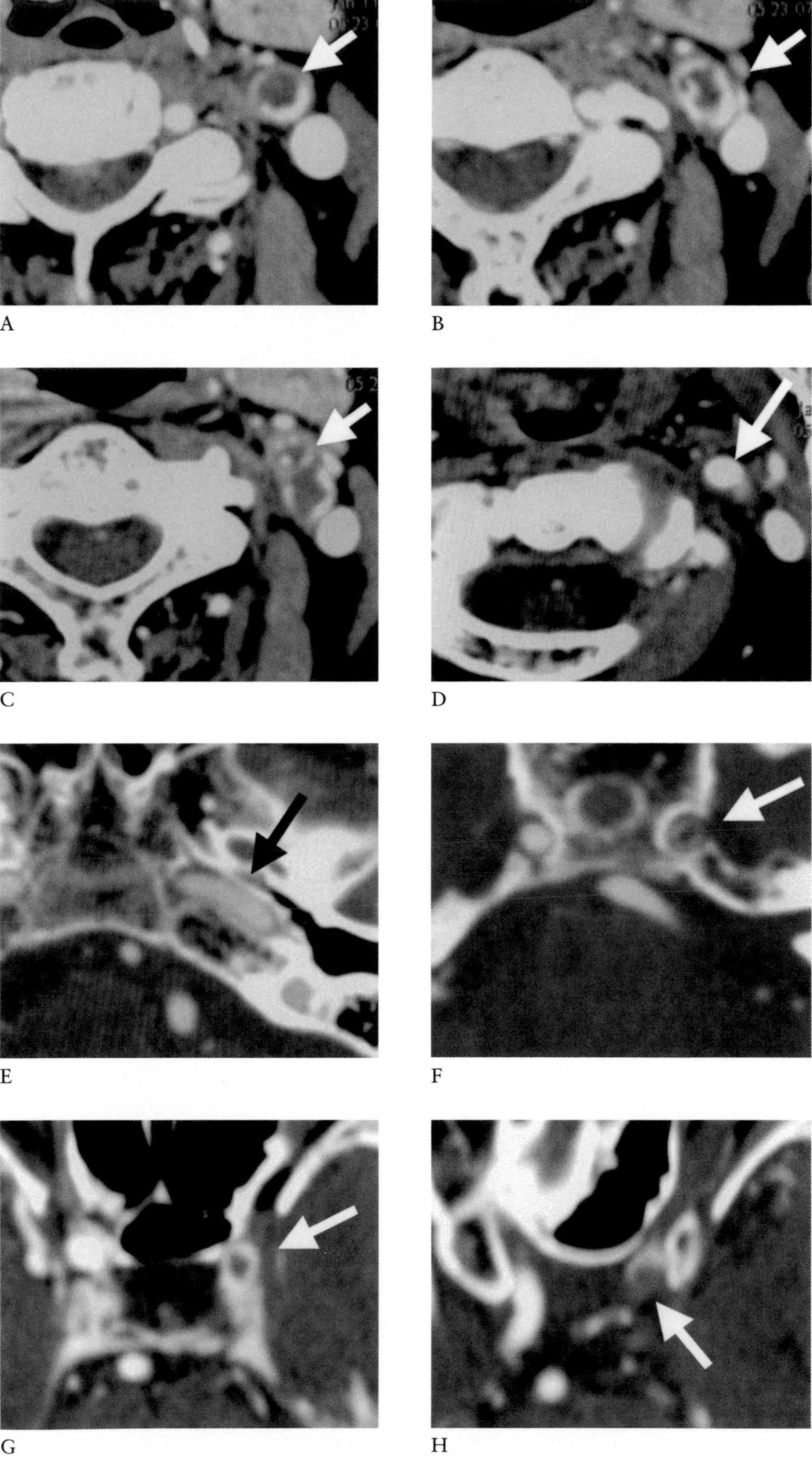

FIGURE 3-4. Computed tomography angiogram in a patient with an acute ischemic stroke. The combined assessment of the extra- and intracranial carotid vasculature reveals two lesions at the level of the bifurcation and the cavernous/supraclinoid carotid artery. The source images (**A–H**) demonstrate a hypodense (i.e., lipid-containing) clot in the distal common carotid artery (*arrow* in **A**), which extends into the bifurcation (*arrow* in **B**) and both the internal carotid artery (ICA) and external carotid artery (*arrow* in **C**). More cranially, the proximal ICA (*arrow* in **D**) and the petrous ICA (*arrow* in **E**) are patent. The second hypodense clot is found in the cavernous (*arrow* in **F**) carotid, extending into the supraclinoid (*arrow* in **G**) carotid, which is finally occluded (*arrow* in **H**). The diagnosis and detailed clot evaluation are possible from the source data. A more evident and appealing view of the patient's clots is achieved with reconstructions. (*Continued*)

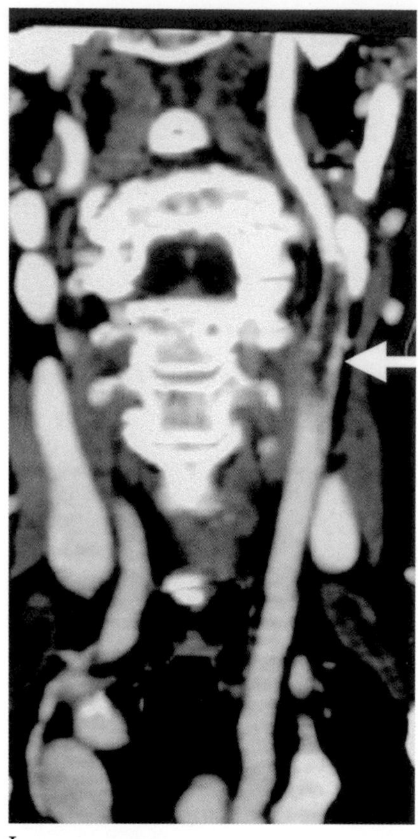

I

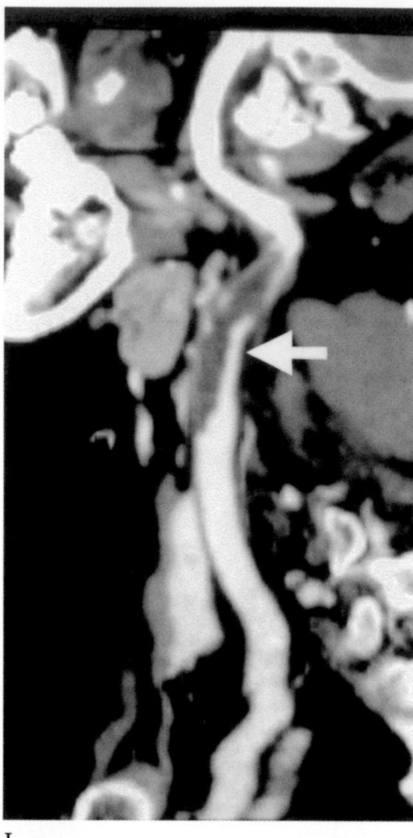

J

FIGURE 3-4. *Continued.* Coronal (I) and sagittal (J) curved reformations, following the course of the common carotid artery and ICA, reveal the complete extent of the clot (*arrows*). Both curved reformations are reconstructed from the same three-dimensional data set. Note that the coronal curved reformation (I) appears "longer" because the carotid artery has more curves in the sagittal plane (J) that are "stretched out" on a coronal plane for the coronal curved reformations. The clot in the supraclinoid carotid artery and the vascular occlusion are displayed best using the maximum-intensity projection algorithm (*arrow*) (**K**).

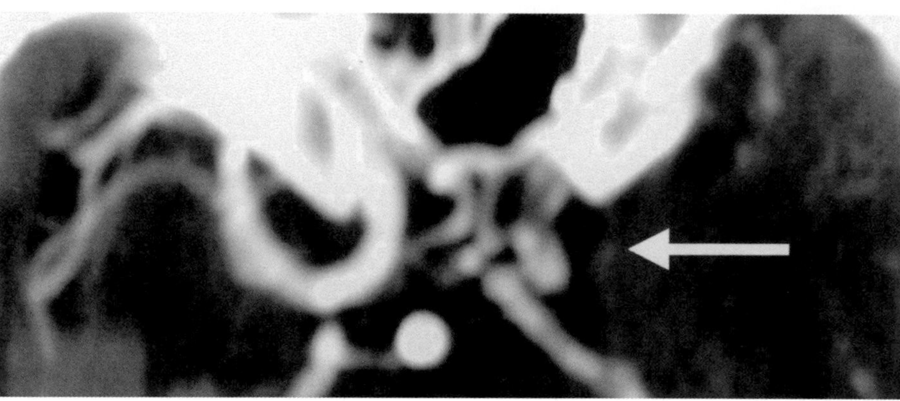

K

et al.,[19] 89% of the CTAs were rated as good or excellent. Technically unsatisfactory CT angiograms were attributed to a low contrast agent dose of 75 ml. Compared to DSA, CTA had a sensitivity of 89% and a specificity of 100% in the detection of arterial stenoses or occlusions around the circle of Willis. Shrier et al. also compared CTA with MRA for the detection of intracranial stenoses and occlusions and found a high agreement, with a CTA sensitivity of 83% and a specificity of 99% compared to MRA. In a series of 16 patients[27] presenting within 6 hours of a suspected acute occlusion in the anterior circulation, CTA of the intracerebral vasculature correctly demonstrated all occlusions of the ICA and the MCA. The assessment of branch occlusions of the MCA was less reliable. In 11 patients, the occlusion site was confirmed angiographically.

In suspected acute occlusions, a CTA study for intracranial stenotic and occlusive disease also supports the utility of CTA in the assessment of a suspected acute stroke.[24] The closest correlation between CTA and DSA results was found in cases of occlusion and high-grade stenoses. These pathologies are most important to identify in the acute setting.

From all publications on acute and chronic disease, CTA of the circle of Willis has reliably shown the clinically relevant occlusions of the major cerebral arter-

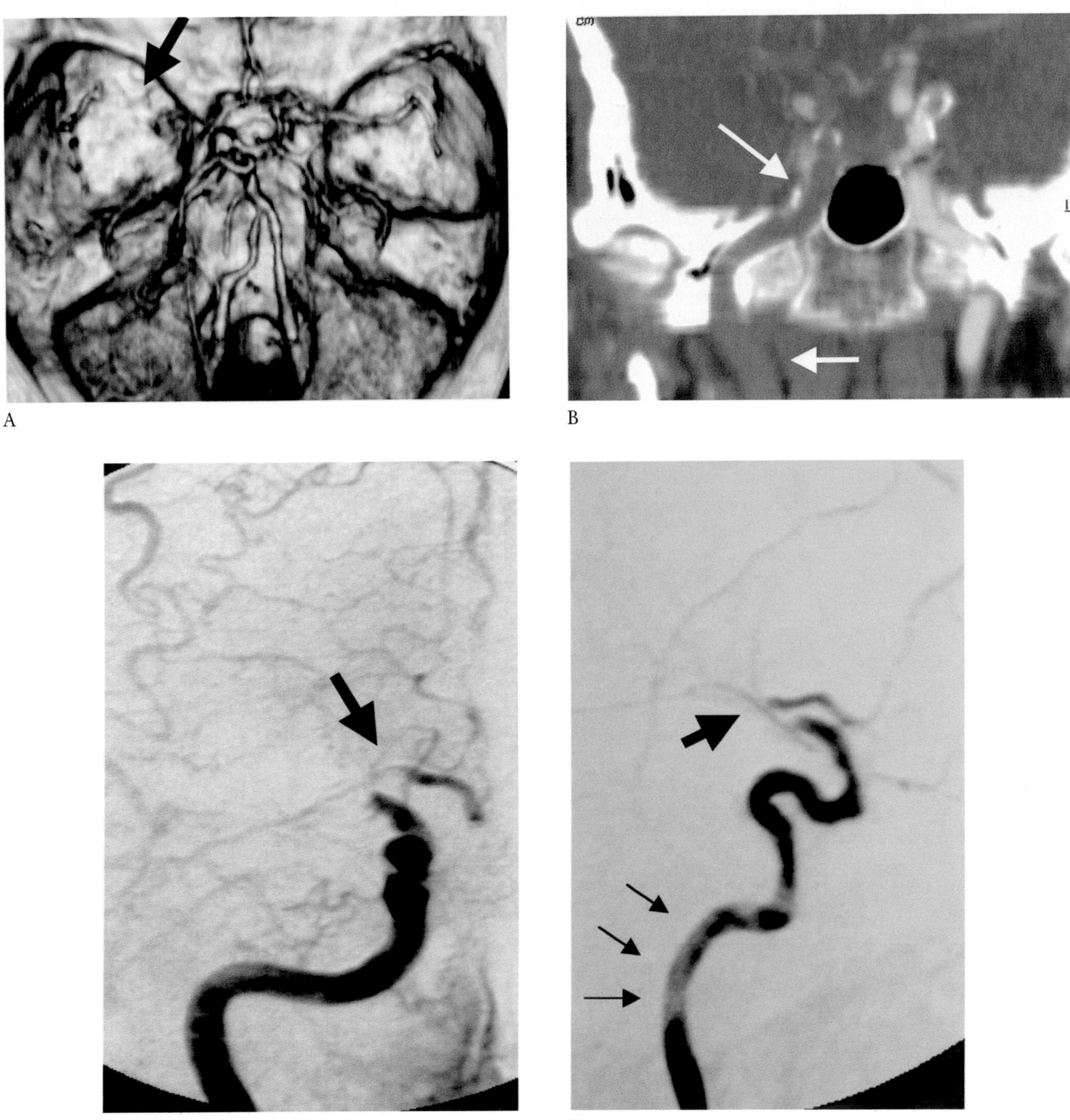

FIGURE 3-5. Computed tomography angiography (CTA) reconstructions (**A,B**) and anterior-posterior (**C**) and lateral (**D**) angiography of a patient with an acute right-hemispheric stroke. The volume-rendered reconstruction of the circle of Willis documents the missing opacification of the right middle cerebral artery (*arrow* in **A**). The coronal curved reconstruction, along the course of the internal carotid artery, suggests that the embolus extends proximally into the internal carotid artery, which appears occluded (*arrows* in **B**). Immediately after the computed tomography scan, an angiogram was performed and, surprisingly, showed a patent internal carotid artery and a distal vascular occlusion at the level of the carotid terminus (*arrows* in **C,D**). An explanation for this false-positive CTA diagnosis of an internal carotid artery occlusion is the slow flow and, thus, late (i.e., after the CTA data acquisition) contrast arrival in the internal carotid artery caused by the more distal occlusion. An indication for the slow flow is given by the "layered" appearance of the contrast agent in the internal carotid artery (*small arrows* in **D**). These density differences result from different precipitation of blood and contrast agent that may occur in slow flow scenarios. Note that the patient is actually lying supine, and the images are for convenience commonly displayed in the craniocaudal direction.

ies. However, CTA is less reliable in showing MCA branch occlusions. The natural course of MCA branch occlusions is usually more benign, whereas occlusions of the MCA trunk, intracranial ICA, and basilar artery are associated with much higher morbidity and mortality and are, therefore, considered the targets of thrombolytic treatment.[41,42]

The final infarct size, patient prognosis, and benefit from thrombolytic treatment depends not only on the site of the occlusion but also on the *collateral blood supply.*[33,43,44] It has been tried, with varying success, to assess the extent of collateral flow from CT angiographic scans.

Wildermuth et al.[4] graded the collateral supply in patients presenting with an acute ischemic stroke, based on the source images and 3D reconstruction images. It was possible to determine the extent of leptomeningeal collateral circulation in patients with an acute hemispheric stroke and to use this parameter to predict outcome after thrombolytic therapy. Skutta et al.[24] found that CTA enables good visualization of the poststenotic vasculature, which is important for assessing collateral blood flow. However, the capacity of collateral flow could not be determined because of CTA's inability to measure flow velocities or flow volumes. Thus, according to their results, a predictive value of the collateral flow for the extent of the infarction, as seen with CTA, cannot be reliably established. Similarly disappointing are the results from Knauth et al.[27] Based on the site of the occlusion and the collateral flow estimation, a successful prediction of the extent of the cerebral infarction, as determined on a follow-up CT scan, was possible in only 62% of those patients studied.

One reason for the difficult assessment of collateral flow with CTA is that this technique gives no information of the direction of flow. Thus, it may be impossible to differentiate antegrade flow through a stenosis from retrograde flow through collaterals. A major improvement on the assessment of collateral flow is achieved by adding a CT perfusion study to the stroke CT protocol (see Chapter 21).

Currently, the window of opportunity for intravenous thrombolytic treatment is 3 hours and 6 hours for intra-arterial treatment after symptom onset. Therefore, special consideration has to be given for a rapid reconstruction algorithm. For vessels running perpendicular to the imaging plane (e.g., ICA, anterior cerebral artery, basilar artery), examination of the axial source image data is diagnostic (see Figure 3-4) and might still reveal diagnostic information in sufficiently large vessels with a horizontal course (e.g., proximal M1 [see Figure 3-4]). Source images have been shown to be most accurate in the diagnosis of *extracervical* carotid artery disease.[30] The fastest and most reliable way to reconstruct and display the intracerebral vasculature is with the creation of MIPs (see Figures 3-1, 3-2, and 3-4).[12]

Acute basilar artery occlusion is a frequent but often difficult differential diagnosis in patients with rapid onset of decreasing consciousness and progressive brain system dysfunction. Intra-arterial thrombolysis is a potentially lifesaving procedure in selected cases of acute basilar artery occlusion.[45,46] Although DSA is the gold standard for the diagnosis, CTA has been evaluated as a noninvasive screening technique.[47] Using a helical scanner, a 2-mm slice thickness, with a 1.5-mm index, is recommended to increase the anatomic coverage.[27] In a series of five patients with suspected basilar artery occlusion, CTA correctly demonstrated all trunk occlusions of the basilar artery.[27] In a larger series of 19 patients, definite diagnosis or exclusion of basilar artery occlusion was possible in all but one patient. CTA provided reliable information on basilar artery patency on the exact site and extent of the basilar artery occlusion and on collateral pathways. Due to severe basilar artery calcification, CTA results were inconclusive in one patient. It appears reasonable to rely on CTA results in decisions concerning thrombolytic therapy in clinically suspected basilar artery occlusion in the preliminary setting.[47]

Dissections of the extracranial ICA are increasingly recognized as causes of stroke, accounting for up to 20% of ischemic strokes in young adults.[48] Helical CT was found to be valuable in the diagnosis of extracranial ICA dissection in the acute stage and to be in close agreement with angiography. In one study,[9] two dissections of the ICA could be well demonstrated in a typical location extending from the bifurcation to the upper cervical portion of the ICA. The presence of a narrowed, eccentric lumen in association with enlargement of the overall diameter of the ICA was the best criterion for the diagnosis of an acute carotid dissection. A hyperdense hematoma surrounding a narrowed vascular lumen might also be seen (Figure 3-6). The combined assessment of both the extra- and intracerebral vasculature is possible with multidetector scanning. This now offers the possibility to diagnose a carotid dissection as the cause for an acute stroke (see Figure 3-6). Helical CTA is also useful for depicting arterial luminal patency after carotid dissection and for showing residual arterial abnormalities (e.g., pseudoaneurysms).[49] CTA may be more suitable than angiography for the diagnosis and follow-up of arterial dissections, because it provides additional information on the arterial wall itself.[50]

In summary, CTA can be regarded as a safe, convenient, and accurate technique for the evaluation of vessel patency around the circle of Willis in patients with symptoms of an acute stroke. The new multidetector scanners can now be extended to visualize the extracerebral carotid arteries as well. Only limited information is available on the use of such a protocol combining intra- and extracerebral vasculature in suspected acute ischemia. Pettiti et al.[13] scanned 20 consecutive patients using extended imaging for anatomic coverage. In their

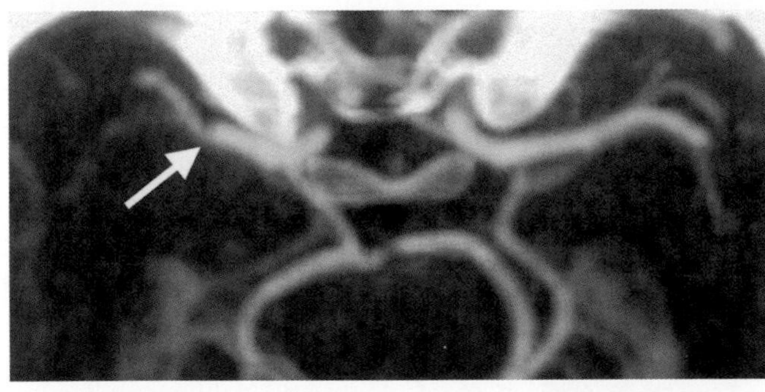
A

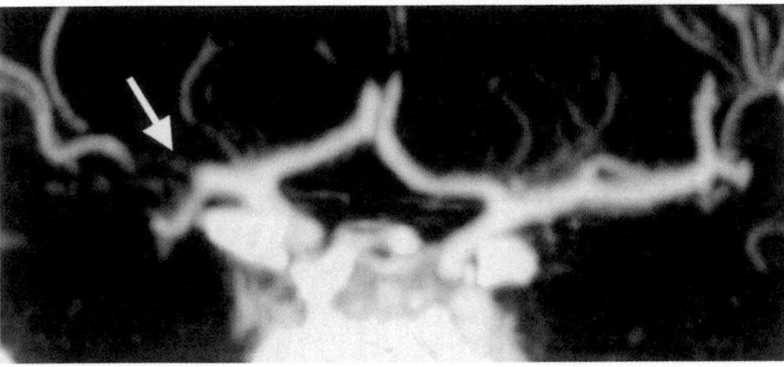
B

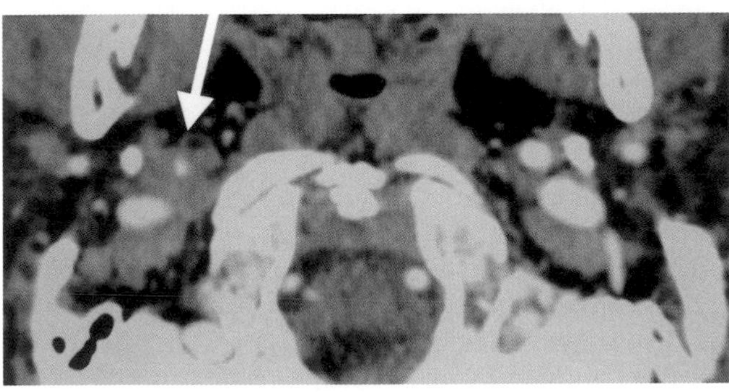
C

FIGURE 3-6. Computed tomography angiogram (CTA) of a patient with an acute right-hemispheric stroke. A multidetector CTA covering the circle of Willis and the extracerebral carotid arteries is performed. Axial (**A**) and coronal maximum-intensity projections (**B**) reveal the embolus in the middle cerebral artery M1 segment (*arrows*). The cause of the embolus is documented on the axial source image that shows a dissection of the carotid artery (**C**), which manifests as hyperdense tissue surrounding a narrowed vascular lumen (*arrow*).

series, multidetector CTA clarified or confirmed the findings of all other imaging modalities. CTA could eliminate the need for other imaging studies in four cases. In another series of 38 patients with an acute stroke,[14] image quality was degraded by motion in three studies.

Multidetector CTA was 91% sensitive and 89% specific for carotid disease compared with duplex, MRA, or conventional angiography. All carotid occlusions were correctly identified by CTA. Multidetector scanning protocols allow, during a single contrast agent injection, a "one-stop" imaging of the great vessel origins, the carotid artery bifurcations, the vertebrobasilar system, and the circle of Willis; they also yield a measurement of the perfused blood volume with whole-brain coverage. Multidetector CT scanning has the potential to become the screening method of choice for evaluating patients with significant vascular lesions amenable to acute intracranial thrombolytic therapy, so that a DSA may be limited to those patients in whom CT examinations are inconclusive. In the future, CTA may allow differentiation of reversible ischemia from infarction or at least optimal selection of patients for potential endovascular thrombolytic therapy.[51]

EXTRACRANIAL CAROTID ARTERY OCCLUSIVE DISEASE

Clinical trials have demonstrated the effectiveness of carotid endarterectomy over medical therapy in reducing stroke risk from carotid stenosis in neurologically symptomatic patients with carotid arterial stenoses greater than 70%.[52,53] The North American Symptomatic Carotid Endarterectomy Trial collaborators also demonstrated that for those patients with stenoses in the 50–69% range, carotid endarterectomy lowered the overall stroke risk significantly, but the benefit was less than for the severe stenosis group.[54] For patients with asymptomatic carotid stenosis, only those with greater than 60% stenosis by angiographic measurement benefited from prophylactic endarterectomy in the Asymptomatic Carotid Atherosclerosis Study.[55] Those trials employed catheter-based angiographic determinations of carotid narrowing. However, for screening purposes, a noninvasive method is required to stratify patients for treatment management.

Spiral CTA of the carotid arteries has been evaluated in several studies, using different means of data post-processing, mainly using MIPs[9,11,20,22] or SSDs.[8,29,56] One early study reported poor results in which both overestimation and underestimation of stenoses occurred.[20] However, their results were based on only a 60-ml contrast agent injection with a 2-ml-per-second injection flow rate and a section thickness of 5 mm.

Later studies on spiral CTA with more optimal parameters have consistently reported good overall agreement between CTA and DSA for the detection of carotid artery disease. Schwartz et al., using SSD for stenosis calculation, found a perfect agreement between CTA and DSA for occlusion and for moderate and severe stenosis.[8] More recent publications have also found near-perfect sensitivity and accuracy for occlusion and high-grade stenosis but a poorer result for the detection of moderate stenosis by CTA.[9,11,29,30,56–60] A very complete study was published in 2000 by Anderson et al.[30] They tested the accuracy of CTA to distinguish

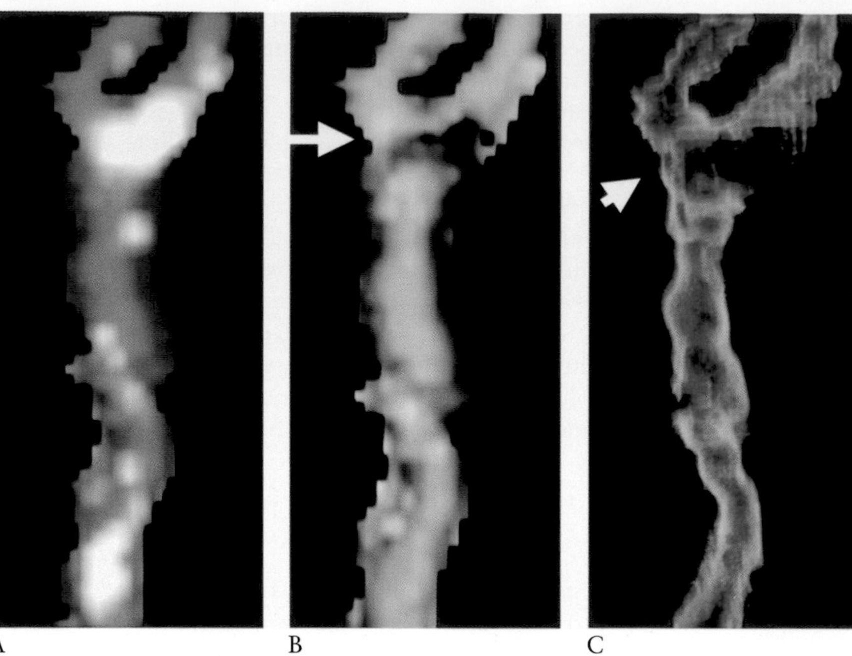

FIGURE 3-7. Further post-processing of the carotid computed tomography angiogram of the patient in Figure 3-3. **A.** Shows a maximum-intensity projection display from the internal carotid artery and carotid bifurcation, after exclusion of the surrounding tissue from the reconstructed data set. In (**B**), the calcifications have been removed based on an operator-defined threshold. **C.** Shows the volume-rendered display from Figure 3-3B after threshold-based removal of the calcifications. The narrow residual lumen becomes obvious both in the maximum-intensity projection and volume-rendered display (*arrows* in **B,C**).

between clinically important degrees of stenosis. They compared CTA with the gold standard of DSA, and also US, by viewing the source images and creating MIPs and SSDs. Their results indicate that the CTA source axial images correlate with DSA more closely than MIP or SSD images for all degrees of stenosis. Furthermore, the correlation between US and DSA was poorer than between CTA and DSA. Anderson et al. concluded that CTA is an excellent examination for the detection of carotid occlusion (99% accuracy compared to DSA) and categorization of stenosis in either the 0–29% (96% accuracy) or greater than 50% (90% accuracy) ranges. However, CTA was unable to reliably distinguish between moderate (50–69%) and severe (70–99%) stenosis, which is an important limitation in the investigation and treatment of carotid stenosis. Thus, the authors do not believe that CTA, in its present form, is an adequate replacement for DSA in the investigation of carotid stenoses.

A major problem in CTA of the carotid arteries is the assessment of the arterial lumen in the presence of mural calcifications. In general, calcifications can be removed by using segmentation with connectivity algorithms or with subtraction techniques, resulting in an image that reflects the contrast medium column alone.[30] However, these procedures substantially increase the processing time. There are several approaches, but no reliable method, for removing mural calcifications from 3D reconstruction images (Figure 3-7). Every technique performed to eliminate high-attenuation mural calcifications may lead to overestimation of stenosis because it involves removal of the neighboring voxels.[8,9] It is especially difficult to assess circumferential plaques due to the inability to differentiate calcification from contrast material.[9] Signal intensities within circumferential plaques may be depressed because of beam hardening, and the plaques may be erroneously interpreted as stenotic regions.[11]

Other artifacts other than calcifications might impair image quality. Beam-hardening artifacts from teeth are often seen.[9] Our experience has been that these types of artifacts may obscure the area around the bifurcation in a considerable number of cases. Schwartz et al.[8] suggested angling the gantry a few degrees to limit artifact within the image plane.

The presence of calcifications represents a pathology that makes it difficult to assess the vascular lumen; however, it yields important information on the composition of a given atherosclerotic plaque. Observations that only a small proportion of stroke patients have severe carotid stenosis[61,62] and that many elderly people have severe carotid stenosis but no symptoms[63] suggest that the degree of stenosis is not the sole variable in predicting the natural history and stroke risk. Thus, the nature of the plaque is important, and histologic studies have identified patterns of carotid artery plaque composition associated with stroke symptoms.[64,65] The presence of plaque irregularity on DSA is associated with an increased risk of early stroke.[66] Moreover, severe stenosis, combined with plaque ulceration, is associated with an increased stroke rate when treated with medical therapy alone, indicating a greater benefit from surgery in this patient group.[67] Compared to angiography, CTA has the advantage of allowing not only assessment of the vascular lumen and its size, but also the morphology of the vascular wall—in particular, calcification or lipid content (see Figure 3-4) that cannot be obtained with conventional angiography.[9,56,58] A study correlating CTA of the carotid bifurcation with histology[7] found correlation between histologic appearance and plaque density on CT angiograms, which has important implications for the prediction of plaque stability. These preliminary results suggest that the presence of low density on CT angiograms may predict plaque that is histologically unstable.[7] Whereas CTA gives information both on vessel lumen and the atheromatous vessel wall, it has demonstrated poor results regarding the detection of plaque ulceration[7–9] owing to limitations in spatial resolution. However, ulcerations are problematic for MR, US, and angiography as well. Smaller areas of ulceration that may act as sources of embolic material are very difficult to identify by conventional angiography.[68,69]

In chronic vascular disease, time for data post-processing and creation of reconstructions is not as critical as in the emergency situation of an acute stroke. Axial source images are the most accurate CTA images for carotid diagnosis.[30] Window width and center level settings of 550–700 HU and 200 HU, respectively, have been suggested to provide the best contrast between vessel opacification and adjacent structures. The border between soft tissue or calcified plaque is approximately halfway between the maximum HU of the two objects. As in other vascular areas, 3D reconstruction images are more visually appealing and provide a sense of the location and length of the carotid plaque and the location and orientation of calcifications (see Figures 3-3 and 3-4).

In the assessment of an acute stroke compared to MRA, CTA has the inherent advantage of being immediately available, a short examination time, and clear depiction of vascular occlusions. In emergency situations, CTA thus is the first examination method of choice. Under elective conditions and in chronic carotid diseases, MRA has its advantages (see Chapter 2), such as complete noninvasiveness, high image quality, and diagnostic accuracy, which improves with increasing scanning time (e.g., multiple repetitions, high inplane resolution, etc.). In these instances, CTA as the method of choice is limited to these indications:

1. Clarifying disagreements and conflicting data between US and MRA (e.g., vascular loops, possible vascular dissection, low US velocities due to critical stenoses, and pre-endarterectomy evaluation of retrograde flow).
2. When US and MRA combined are unable to answer the clinical question before an invasive angiogram is performed.
3. Demonstrating calcifications and clot morphology.
4. Demonstrating important anatomic data such as carotid artery hyoid bone compression not evident on other modalities.
5. Accurate determination of the residual lumen diameter in the case of moderate and severe stenosis because of flow artifacts in MRA.
6. Distinguishing small residual lumen from complete occlusion. An important pitfall, contributing to the false-positive interpretation of a totally occluded carotid artery as patent, is mistaking the ascending pharyngeal artery or muscular branches for a small residual carotid lumen. This is of critical importance, because a small residual carotid lumen generally requires endarterectomy, whereas a totally occluded vessel does not.
7. Demonstrating kinks and loops without flow-related artifacts.
8. General contraindications for MR.

INTRACRANIAL STENOTIC-OCCLUSIVE DISEASE

Carotid stenosis is a common disease, and numerous studies on prevalence, natural history, and treatment have been performed. Much less is known about the prognosis of intracranial stenotic-occlusive disease. Intracranial stenoses are, however, more common than extracranial stenoses in Hispanics, Japanese, and Chinese.[70,71] The Warfarin-Aspirin Symptomatic Intracranial Disease study[72] showed that symptomatic patients with 50–99% stenosis of an intracranial artery (carotid, anterior, middle, posterior, vertebral, or basilar) benefited from treatment with warfarin compared to a control group treated with aspirin. Therefore, a noninvasive technique to correctly depict the degree of a vascular stenosis would be of great use.

Early studies comparing spiral CT scanning with MRA (3D time-of-flight) concluded that MRA is more reliable than CTA to determine MCA stenosis.[73] Skutta et al.[24] found that CTA acquired with a double-detector CT scanner and post-processed with advanced algorithms is as reliable as MRA in depicting the vasculature of the anterior and posterior cerebral circulation and in grading intracranial stenotic-occlusive lesions. Their CTA assessments could be performed by a radiologist in approximately 15–20 minutes. The rate of complete agreement between DSA and CTA for the degree of stenosis was 70% on the basis of MIP images alone and could be increased to 80% by viewing source images. Approximately one-third of wrong assessments were related to the petrous segment of the carotid artery. This problematic area can potentially be visualized better with the use of subtraction techniques.[74,75] First efforts in this direction were disappointing as a result of motion artifacts between the two examinations. Registration software might help, but the post-processing time is still too long for routine use.[9]

INTRACRANIAL ANEURYSMS

As for other cerebral pathologies, the gold standard for imaging intracranial aneurysms is selective catheter angiography.[76] However, for screening purposes in patients with subarachnoid hemorrhage, as well as in high-risk patients (with a strong family history or autosomal-dominant polycystic kidney disease), a less invasive method may be useful. The use of screening for familial intracranial aneurysms was questioned in 1999.[77] Using MRA (which has a similar sensitivity and specificity to CTA), screening is not an effective way of reducing morbidity and mortality from ruptured intracranial aneurysms in individuals with a history of greater than or equal to two affected first-degree relatives with a ruptured intracranial aneurysm, unless the expected incidence of asymptomatic aneurysm is greater than 10%.

Both CTA and MRA have been evaluated for the detection of intracerebral aneurysms in numerous studies. CT has the advantage of immediate availability and is a key part of the initial diagnostic evaluation in subarachnoid hemorrhage.

Meta-analysis of information on CTA, MRA, and transcranial Doppler US, published between 1988 and 1998, was performed by White et al.[78] They found 14 eligible studies that compared CTA with angiography[75,79–91] and two additional studies that compared MRA with CTA and angiography.[92,93] The median sample size of the CT studies was 30 subjects, and the median prevalence of aneurysms was 79.5%. In more than 50% of the studies, the assessment was confined to the circle of Willis. Complications were mentioned in only two CTA studies. The overall diagnostic accuracy of CTA and MRA was similar, approaching 90%. Both on a per patient basis and on a per aneurysm basis, there was no significant difference between CTA and MRA. Both CTA and MRA were marginally more accurate at depicting posterior circulation aneurysms than depicting anterior circulation aneurysms, but the differences were small. The sensitivity for the detection of other anterior circulation aneurysms was relatively poor, because in cases in which the circle of Willis was examined, the aneurysms could have been outside the examined volume. In this meta-analysis, there was a trend toward a greater accuracy of the more recently performed CTA studies (i.e., after spiral technology had been well established). The results of this meta-analysis support the size of 3 mm as a practical cutoff point for the detection of aneurysms, beneath which the sensitivity of aneurysm detection with CTA decreased sharply from 96% to 61%. This limitation might be overcome with the introduction of multidetector CT scanners, in particular from those manufacturers who allow the collimation to be reduced to 0.5 mm while still assuring a sufficient anatomic coverage. This might also improve the more detailed demonstration of the neck and the relationship of the aneurysm to the feeding artery, information that is necessary for surgical and interventional treatment planning.

Although sensitivities and specificities seem to be similar for CTA and MRA, a few characteristics deserve mentioning. Given the nonuniform flow in and around aneurysms, time-of-flight MRA is limited by its insensitivity to slow, turbulent, limited, or complex flow. The most important limitation of CTA for the assessment of aneurysms is its inability to visualize very small arteries arising from an aneurysm.

Following the enrollment period of the meta-analysis, more studies on the use of CTA for the detection of intracranial aneurysms have been published. The scanning parameters of those studies are summarized in Table 3-1.

Korogi et al.[95] reported a sensitivity of 64% for small aneurysms less than 4 mm in size, which may be attributed to methodologic problems such as a low flow rate of 2–3 ml per second. Villablanca et al.[96] could decrease the detection threshold to an aneurysm as small as 1.7 mm. In their series, CTA was a valuable tool for the detection and characterization of both patent and nonpatent intracranial aneurysm components. Information provided by CTA about mural calcifications in an intraluminal thrombus is not available by using other imaging modalities. In a large series of 173 patients, spiral CT scanning resulted in a sensitivity and specificity of CTA for the detection of all aneurysms, ruptured and unruptured, of 84% and 100%, respectively. Missed aneurysms were always small (<4 mm) and were usually found in patients with multiple aneurysms in whom the larger, ruptured aneurysm was identified by CTA.

Similar to other indications, there is no consensus as to optimal reconstruction technique. Volume-rendering techniques have been advocated to be superior to surface shaded display and MIP techniques[95] (Figure 3-8). SSD techniques do not allow differentiation between blood clot and a patent aneurysm,[79,83] and the use of MIPs has been shown to lead to extensive loss of image information.[97] Additionally, orthogonal and curved oblique reformatted MPRs have been shown to be useful.[96]

SUMMARY

CTA using spiral technology has been established for several indications, has proven its utility, and has its limitations. The advent of multidetector technology promises higher anatomic coverage with identical collimation. This is important for the simultaneous assessment of the intracranial and extracranial vasculature or higher spatial resolution with identical anatomic coverage and is relevant for the detection of small intracranial aneurysms. However, this new multidetector technique

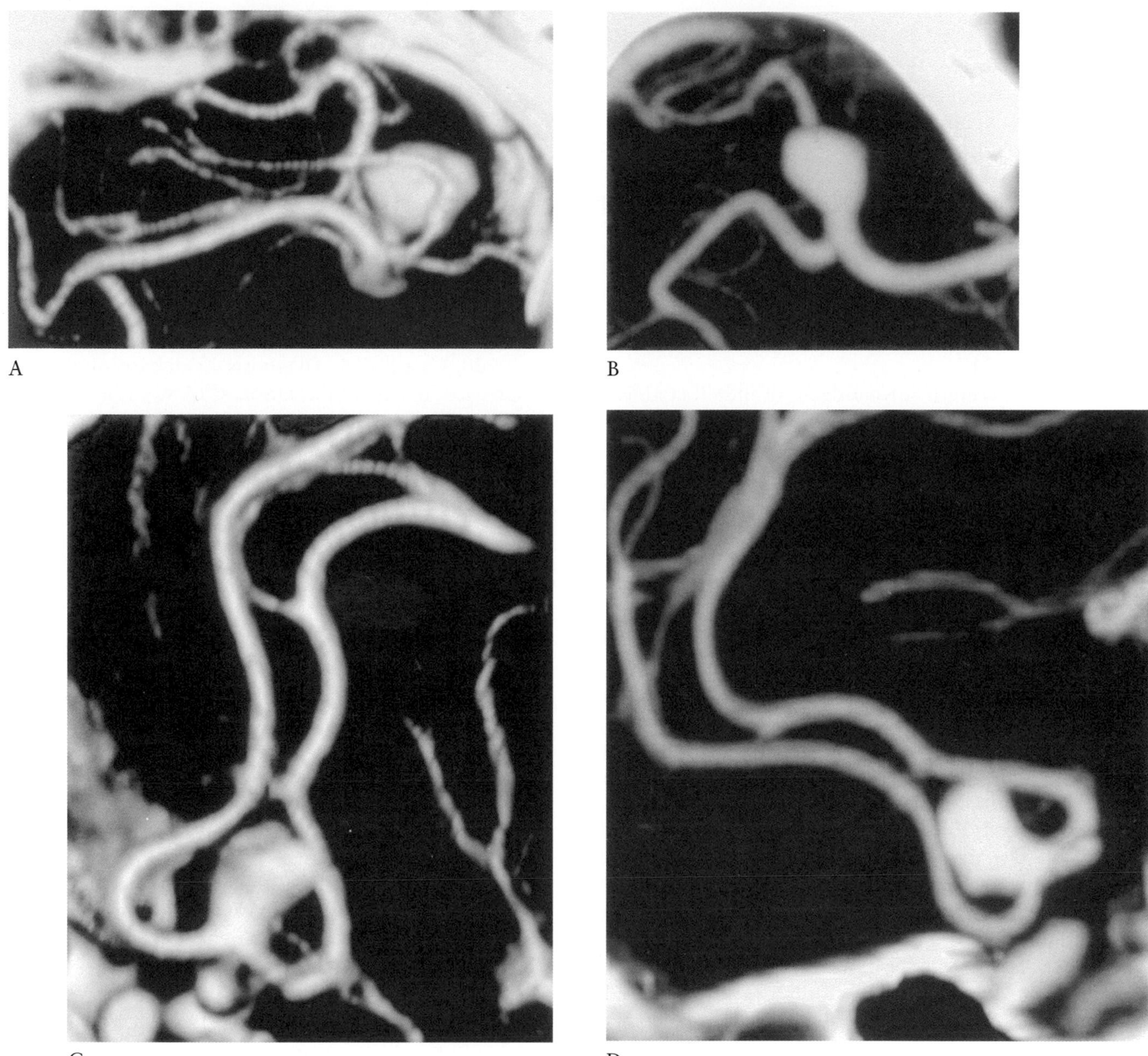

FIGURE 3-8. Computed tomography angiogram of a patient with two aneurysms: one arising from the right middle cerebral artery (**A,B**) and the other from the anterior communicating artery (**C,D**). For both aneurysms, the volume-rendered algorithm (**A,C**) displays the complex three-dimensional anatomy better than the maximum-intensity projection algorithm (**B,D**).

for CTA still has to prove that it has improved performance sufficient to supplant other imaging, especially MRA.

To date, the only inherent advantages of CTA, compared to MRA, are its easy accessibility and performance in an emergency situation. This is extremely important, however, for the evaluation of acute stroke patients. This indication remains the mainstay for CTA. Although there is no consensus on the optimal scanning parameters for spiral CTA, there is even less agreement on the evolving multidetector CTA protocols. Further technical development is ongoing, and, increasingly, this must occur in the form of developments in computational analysis. This refers mainly to the time-consuming and often difficult 3D post-processing of the acquired data.

It would be advantageous if post-processing algorithms for CTA could become as automated and user-friendly as the programs for MRA so that the reconstructions can be generated by the technologist in a timely fashion. In time, multidetector CTA may be as competitive as MRA for visualization of the extracranial and intracranial cerebral vasculature.[98]

REFERENCES

1. Heiserman JE, Dean BL, Hodak JA, et al. Neurologic complications of cerebral angiography. AJNR Am J Neuroradiol 1994;15:1401–1407; discussion 1408–1411.

2. Waugh JR, Sacharias N. Arteriographic complications in the DSA era. Radiology 1992;182:243–246.

3. Schwartz SW, Chambless LE, Baker WH, et al. Consistency of Doppler parameters in predicting arteriographically confirmed carotid stenosis. Asymptomatic Carotid Atherosclerosis Study Investigators. Stroke 1997;28:343–347.

4. Wildermuth S, Knauth M, Brandt T, et al. Role of CTA in patient selection for thrombolytic therapy in acute hemispheric stroke. Stroke 1998;29:935–938.

5. Brant-Zawadzki M. CTA in acute ischemic stroke: the right tool for the job? AJNR Am J Neuroradiol 1997;18:1021–1023.

6. Lasjaunias P, Berenstein A. Arterial Anatomy: Introduction. In P Lasjaunias, A Berenstein (eds), Surgical Neuroangiography, Vol. 1. Berlin: Springer, 1980;1–32.

7. Oliver TB, Lammie GA, Wright AR, et al. Atherosclerotic plaque at the carotid bifurcation: CT angiographic appearance with histopathologic correlation. AJNR Am J Neuroradiol 1999;20:897–901.

8. Schwartz RB, Jones KM, Chernoff DM, et al. Common carotid artery bifurcation: evaluation with spiral CT. Radiology 1992;185:513–519.

9. Link J, Brossmann J, Grabener M, et al. Spiral CTA and selective digital subtraction angiography of ICA stenosis. AJNR Am J Neuroradiol 1996;17:89–94.

10. Marzewski DJ, Furlan AJ, St. Louis P, et al. Intracranial internal carotid artery stenosis: long-term prognosis. Stroke 1982;13:821–824.

11. Marks MP, Napel S, Jordan JE, Enzmann DR. Diagnosis of carotid artery disease: preliminary experience with maximum-intensity-projection spiral CTA. AJR Am J Roentgenol 1993;160:1267–1271.

12. Berzin TM, Lev MH, Gonzales G. CT offers early view of hyperacute stroke. Diagn Imaging 2000;11–14.

13. Petitti N, Lev MH, Ackerman RH, et al. Multidetector Helical CTA—Rapid Evaluation of the Complete Neurovascular System. Proceedings of the American Society of Neuroradiology 38th Annual Meeting; April 3–8, 2000; Atlanta. Abstract 48.

14. Smith W, Johnston S, Tsao J, et al. Safety and Speed of a CT Imaging Protocol for the Entire Cerebrovascular Axis During Acute Stroke. 26th International Stroke Conference. February 4–16, 2001; Fort Lauderdale, FL. Abstract.

15. Kendall BE, Pullicino P. Intravascular contrast injection in ischaemic lesions. II. Effect on prognosis. Neuroradiology 1980;19:241–243.

16. Doerfler A, Engelhorn T, von Kummer R, et al. Are iodinated contrast agents detrimental in acute cerebral ischemia? An experimental study in rats. Radiology 1998;206:211–217.

17. Velaj R, Drayer B, Albright R, Fram E. Comparative neurotoxicity of angiographic contrast media. Neurology 1985;35:1290–1298.

18. Grzyska U, Freitag J, Zeumer H. Selective cerebral intraarterial DSA. Complication rate and control of risk factors. Neuroradiology 1990;32:296–299.

19. Shrier DA, Tanaka H, Numaguchi Y, et al. CTA in the evaluation of acute stroke. AJNR Am J Neuroradiol 1997;18:1011–1020.

20. Castillo M. Diagnosis of disease of the common carotid artery bifurcation: CTA vs catheter angiography. AJR Am J Roentgenol 1993;161:395–398.

21. Alberico RA, Barnes P, Robertson RL, Burrows PE. Helical CTA: dynamic cerebrovascular imaging in children. AJNR Am J Neuroradiol 1999;20:328–334.

22. Napel S, Marks MP, Rubin GD, et al. CTA with spiral CT and maximum intensity projection. Radiology 1992;185:607–610.

23. Diederichs CG, Keating DP, Glatting G, Oestmann JW. Blurring of vessels in spiral CTA: effects of collimation width, pitch, viewing plane, and windowing in maximum intensity projection. J Comput Assist Tomogr 1996;20:965–974.

24. Skutta B, Fürst G, Eilers J, et al. Intracranial stenoocclusive disease: double-detector helical CTA versus digital subtraction angiography. AJNR Am J Neuroradiol 1999;20:791–799.

25. Anderson CM, Saloner D, Tsuruda JS, et al. Artifacts in maximum-intensity-projection display of MR angiograms. AJR Am J Roentgenol 1990;154:623–639.

26. Cline HE, Dumoulin CL, Lorensen WE, et al. Volume rendering and connectivity algorithms for MR angiography. Magn Reson Med 1991;18:384–394.

27. Knauth M, von Kummer R, Jansen O, et al. Potential of CTA in acute ischemic stroke. AJNR Am J Neuroradiol 1997;18:1001–1010.

28. Pozza C, Sebben R, Kew J, Fitridge R. Comparison of multi-slice CTA against digital subtraction angiography in patients with symptomatic, ultrasonographically significant stenosis of the extracranial carotid arteries. Radiology 2000;217(Suppl P):245.

29. Dillon EH, van Leeuwen MS, Fernandez MA, et al. CTA: application to the evaluation of carotid artery stenosis. Radiology 1993;189:211–219.

30. Anderson GB, Ashforth R, Steinke DE, et al. CTA for the detection and characterization of carotid artery bifurcation disease. Stroke 2000;31:2168–2174.

31. Nichols DA. Thrombolytic treatment for acute stroke should be individualized for each patient. AJNR Am J Neuroradiol 1998;19:993–994.

32. The National Institute of Neurological Disorders and Stroke rt-PA Stroke Study Group. Tissue plasminogen activator for acute ischemic stroke. N Engl J Med 1995;333:1581–1587.

33. Hacke W, Kaste M, Fieschi C, et al. Intravenous thrombolysis with recombinant tissue plasminogen activator for acute hemispheric stroke. The European Cooperative Acute Stroke Study (ECASS). JAMA 1995;274:1017–1025.

34. Jansen O, von Kummer R, Forsting M, et al. Thrombolytic therapy in acute occlusion of the intracranial internal carotid artery bifurcation. AJNR Am J Neuroradiol 1995;16:1977–1986.

35. von Kummer R, Hacke W. Safety and efficacy of intravenous tissue plasminogen activator and heparin in acute middle cerebral artery stroke. Stroke 1992;23:646–652.

36. Mori E, Yoneda Y, Tabuchi M, et al. Intravenous recombinant tissue plasminogen activator in acute carotid artery territory stroke. Neurology 1992;42: 976–982.

37. Kucinski T, Koch C, Grzyska U, et al. The predictive value of early CT and angiography for fatal hemispheric swelling in acute stroke. AJNR Am J Neuroradiol 1998;19:839–846.

38. Fisher M, Pessin MS, Furian AJ. ECASS: lessons for future thrombolytic stroke trials. European Cooperative Acute Stroke Study. JAMA 1995;274: 1058–1059.

39. Furlan AJ, Higashida R, Wechsler L, et al. Intra-arterial prourokinase for acute ischemic stroke. The PROACT II Study: a randomized controlled trial. JAMA 1999;282:2003–2011.

40. Katz DA, Marks MP, Napel SA, et al. Circle of Willis: evaluation with spiral CTA, MR angiography, and conventional angiography. Radiology 1995;195: 445–449.

41. Saito I, Segawa H, Shiokawa Y, et al. Middle cerebral artery occlusion: correlation of computed tomography and angiography with clinical outcome. Stroke 1987;18:863–868.

42. von Kummer R, Holle R, Rosin L, et al. Does arterial recanalization improve outcome in carotid territory stroke? Stroke 1995;26:581–587.

43. Forsting M, Krieger D, von Kummer R, et al. The Prognostic Value of Collateral Blood Flow in Acute Middle Cerebral Artery Occlusion. In GJ del Zoppo, E Mori, W Hackes (eds), Thrombolytic Therapy in Acute Ischemic Stroke II. New York: Springer, 1993;160–167.

44. Roberts HC, Dillon WP, Furlan AJ, et al. Angiographic Collaterals in Acute Stroke—Relationship to Clinical Presentation and Outcome: The PROACT II trial. 26th International Stroke Conference, February 4–16, 2001; Fort Lauderdale, FL. Abstract 4.

45. Hacke W, Zeumer H, Ferbert A, et al. Intraarterial thrombolytic therapy improves outcome in patients with acute vertebrobasilar occlusive disease. Stroke 1988;19:1216–1222.

46. Brandt T, von Kummer R, Müller-Küppers M, Hacke W. Thrombolytic therapy of acute basilar artery occlusion. Variables affecting recanalization and outcome. Stroke 1996;27:875–881.

47. Brandt T, Knauth M, Wildermuth S, et al. CTA and Doppler sonography for emergency assessment in acute basilar artery ischemia. Stroke 1999; 30:606–612.

48. Leys D, Moulin T, Stojkovic T, et al. Follow-up of patients with history of cervical artery dissection. Cerebrovasc Dis 1995;5:43–49.

49. Leclerc X, Lucas C, Godefroy O, et al. Helical CT for the follow-up of cervical internal carotid artery dissections. AJNR Am J Neuroradiol 1998;19:831–837.

50. Latchaw RE. The role of CTA in the long-term management of cerebrovascular dissection. AJNR Am J Neuroradiol 1998;19:992–993.

51. Dillon WP. CT techniques for detecting acute stroke and collateral circulation: in search of the Holy Grail. AJNR Am J Neuroradiol 1998;19:191–192.

52. North American Symptomatic Carotid Endarterectomy Trial. Methods, patient characteristics, and progress. Stroke 1991;22:711–720.

53. MRC European Carotid Surgery Trial: interim results for symptomatic patients with severe (70–99%) or with mild (0–29%) carotid stenosis. European Carotid Surgery Trialists' Collaborative Group. Lancet 1991;337:1235–1243.

54. Barnett HJ, Taylor DW, Eliasziw M, et al. Benefit of carotid endarterectomy in patients with symptomatic moderate or severe stenosis. North American Symptomatic Carotid Endarterectomy Trial Collaborators. N Engl J Med 1998;339:1415–1425.

55. Endarterectomy for asymptomatic carotid artery stenosis. Executive Committee for the Asymptomatic Carotid Atherosclerosis Study. JAMA 1995; 273:1421–1428.

56. Cumming MJ, Morrow IM. Carotid artery stenosis: a prospective comparison of CTA and conventional angiography. AJR Am J Roentgenol 1994;163: 517–523.

57. Magarelli N, Scarabino T, Simeone AL, et al. Carotid stenosis: a comparison between MR and spiral CTA. Neuroradiology 1998;40:367–373.

58. Sugahara T, Korogi Y, Hirai T, et al. CTA in vascular intervention for steno-occlusive diseases: role of multiplanar reconstruction and source images. Br J Radiol 1998;71:601–611.

59. Simeone A, Carriero A, Armillotta M, et al. Spiral CTA in the study of the carotid stenoses. J Neuroradiol 1997;24:18–22.

60. Sameshima T, Futami S, Morita Y, et al. Clinical usefulness of and problems with three-dimensional

CTA for the evaluation of arteriosclerotic stenosis of the carotid artery: comparison with conventional angiography, MRA, and ultrasound sonography. Surg Neurol 1999;51:301–308.

61. Brown PB, Zwiebel WJ, Call GK. Degree of cervical carotid artery stenosis and hemispheric stroke: duplex US findings. Radiology 1989;170:541–543.

62. Weinstein R. Noninvasive carotid duplex ultrasound imaging for the evaluation and management of carotid atherosclerotic disease. Hematol Oncol Clin North Am 1992;6:1131–1139.

63. Salonen R, Seppänen K, Rauramaa R, Salonen JT. Prevalence of carotid atherosclerosis and serum cholesterol levels in eastern Finland. Arteriosclerosis 1988;8:788–792.

64. Seeger JM, Barratt E, Lawson GA, Klingman N. The relationship between carotid plaque composition, plaque morphology, and neurologic symptoms. J Surg Res 1995;58:330–336.

65. Carotid artery plaque composition—relationship to clinical presentation and ultrasound B-mode imaging. European Carotid Plaque Study Group. Eur J Vasc Endovasc Surg 1995;10:23–30.

66. Rothwell P, Villagra J, Fox A, et al. The role of carotid atherosclerosis in the etiology of ischemic stroke. Cerebrovasc Dis 1996;6:S1.

67. Eliasziw M, Streifler J, Fox A, et al. Significance of plaque ulceration in symptomatic patients with high-grade carotid stenosis. North American Symptomatic Carotid Endarterectomy Trial. Stroke 1994;25:304–308.

68. Edwards JH, Kricheff II, Riles T, Imparato A. Angiographically undetected ulceration of the carotid bifurcation as a cause of embolic stroke. Radiology 1979;132:369–373.

69. Streifler J, Eliasziw M, Fox A, et al. Angiographic detection of carotid plaque ulceration. Comparison with surgical observations in a multicenter study. North American Symptomatic Carotid Endarterectomy Trial. Stroke 1994;25:1130–1132.

70. Caplan LR, Gorelick PB, Hier DB. Race, sex and occlusive cerebrovascular disease: a review. Stroke 1986;17:648–655.

71. Leung SY, Ng TH, Yuen ST, et al. Pattern of cerebral atherosclerosis in Hong Kong Chinese. Severity in intracranial and extracranial vessels. Stroke 1993;24:779–786.

72. Chimowitz MI, Kokkinos J, Strong J, et al. The Warfarin-Aspirin Symptomatic Intracranial Disease Study. Neurology 1995;45:1488–1493.

73. Wong KS, Lam WW, Liang E, et al. Variability of magnetic resonance angiography and computed tomography angiography in grading middle cerebral artery stenosis. Stroke 1996;27:1084–1087.

74. Görzer H, Heimberger K, Schindler E. Spiral CTA with digital subtraction of extra- and intracranial vessels. J Comput Assist Tomogr 1994;18:839–841.

75. Imakita S, Onishi Y, Hashimoto T, et al. Subtraction CTA with controlled-orbit helical scanning for detection of intracranial aneurysms. AJNR Am J Neuroradiol 1998;19:291–295.

76. Broderick JP, Adams HP Jr, Barsan W, et al. Guidelines for the management of spontaneous intracerebral hemorrhage: a statement for healthcare professionals from a special writing group of the stroke council, American Heart Association. Stroke 1999;30:905–915.

77. Crawley F, Clifton A, Brown MM. Should we screen for familial intracranial aneurysm? Stroke 1999;30:312–316.

78. White PM, Wardlaw JM, Easton V. Can noninvasive imaging accurately depict intracranial aneurysm? A systematic review. Radiology 2000;217:361–370.

79. Hope JK, Wilson JL, Thomson FJ. Three-dimensional CTA in the detection and characterization of intracranial berry aneurysms. AJNR Am J Neuroradiol 1996;17:439–445.

80. Liang EY, Chan M, Hsiang JH, et al. Detection and assessment of intracranial aneurysms: value of CTA with shaded-surface display. AJR Am J Roentgenol 1995;165:1497–1502.

81. Alberico RA, Patel M, Casey S, et al. Evaluation of the circle of Willis with three-dimensional CTA in patients with suspected intracranial aneurysms. AJNR Am J Neuroradiol 1995;16:1571–1578.

82. Anderson GB, Findlay JM, Steinke DE, Ashforth R. Experience with computed tomographic angiography for the detection of intracranial aneurysms in the setting of acute subarachnoid hemorrhage. Neurosurgery 1997;41:522–527.

83. Hsiang JN, Liang EY, Lam JM, et al. The role of computed tomographic angiography in the diagnosis of intracranial aneurysms and emergent aneurysm clipping. Neurosurgery 1996;38:481–487.

84. Lenhart M, Bretschneider T, Gmeinwieser J, et al. Cerebral CTA in the diagnosis of acute subarachnoid hemorrhage. Acta Radiol 1997;38:791–796.

85. Ng SH, Wong HF, Ko SF, et al. CTA of intracranial aneurysms: advantages and pitfalls. Eur J Radiol 1997;25:14–19.

86. Ogawa T, Okudera T, Noguchi K, et al. Cerebral aneurysms: evaluation with three-dimensional CTA. AJNR Am J Neuroradiol 1996;17:447–454.

87. Preda L, Gaetani P, Rodriguez y Baena R, et al. Spiral CTA and surgical correlations in the evaluation of intracranial aneurysms. Eur Radiol 1998;8:739–745.

88. Röhnert W, Hänig V, Hietschold V, Abolmaali N. Detection of aneurysm in subarachnoid hemorrhage—CTA vs. digital subtraction angiography. Aktuelle Radiol 1998;8:63–70.

89. Strayle-Batra M, Skalej M, Wakhloo AK, et al. Three-dimensional spiral CTA in the detection of cerebral aneurysm. Acta Radiol 1998;39:233–238.

90. Velthuis BK, Rinkel GJ, Ramos LM, et al. Subarachnoid hemorrhage: aneurysm detection and preoperative evaluation with CTA. Radiology 1998;208:423–430.

91. Vieco PT, Shuman WP, Alsofrom GF, Gross CE. Detection of circle of Willis aneurysms in patients with acute subarachnoid hemorrhage: a comparison of CTA and digital subtraction angiography. AJR Am J Roentgenol 1995;165:425–430.

92. Schwartz RB, Tice HM, Hooten SM, et al. Evaluation of cerebral aneurysms with helical CT: correlation with conventional angiography and MR angiography. Radiology 1994;192:717–722.

93. Tsuchiya K, Makita K, Furui S. 3D-CT angiography of cerebral aneurysms with spiral scanning: comparison with 3D-time-of-flight MR angiography. Radiat Med 1994;12:161–166.

94. Anderson GB, Steinke DE, Petruk KC, et al. Computed tomographic angiography versus digital subtraction angiography for the diagnosis and early treatment of ruptured intracranial aneurysms. Neurosurgery 1999;45:1315–1320.

95. Korogi Y, Takahashi M, Katada K, et al. Intracranial aneurysms: detection with three-dimensional CTA with volume rendering—comparison with conventional angiographic and surgical findings. Radiology 1999;211:497–506.

96. Villablanca JP, Martin N, Jahan R, et al. Volume-rendered helical computerized tomography angiography in the detection and characterization of intracranial aneurysms. J Neurosurg 2000;93:254–264.

97. Fishman EK, Drebin B, Magid D, et al. Volumetric rendering techniques: applications for three-dimensional imaging of the hip. Radiology 1987;163:737–738.

98. Lane B. Multi-detector helical CTA: poor cousin or contender. AJNR Am J Neuroradiol 1999;20:731.

99. Marcus CD, Ladam-Marcus VJ, Bigot JL, et al. Carotid arterial stenosis: evaluation at CTA with the volume-rendering technique. Radiology 1999;211:775–780.

CHAPTER

4

Catheter Angiography

Tjhi Wen Tjauw and Gary M. Nesbit

Conventional catheter-based neuroangiography remains the gold standard in the evaluation of various intracranial and extracranial vascular abnormalities despite the advances in computed tomography angiography (CTA) and magnetic resonance angiography (MRA). Although the initial diagnosis is often made on MRA or CTA, catheter angiography is important in planning cerebrovascular surgical or endovascular therapy in diseases such as stroke, atheromatous stenosis, aneurysms, vascular malformations, and vascular tumors.

The combination of high-resolution anatomic evaluation and the physiologic information obtained during the passage of a contrast bolus through the arterial, capillary, and venous cerebral vasculature cannot currently be equaled with other imaging techniques. The quality and safety of neuroangiography have greatly improved over the past decade with the introduction of newer diagnostic catheters, guide wires, nonionic contrast media, and improved imaging instruments. Diagnostic neuroangiography remains a relatively safe procedure and continues to be an integral part in the evaluation of the majority of cerebrovascular disorders.

TECHNIQUE OF CATHETER ANGIOGRAPHY

The quality of digital subtraction angiography (DSA) has improved so that it has surpassed conventional cut-film techniques in evaluating cerebrovascular diseases. The basic concepts for the performance of safe and high-quality angiography are presented.

The Seldinger technique, with either a double-wall or single-wall puncture into the common femoral artery, is the standard method for vessel entry. Meticulous site location over the femoral head is necessary if a closure device is to be used.

Catheter and wire selections vary depending on the preference of the neuroangiographer. A 70-degree cerebral curve is often used with a soft distal guidewire. Reverse curved catheters (e.g., Simmons) or sidewinder catheters (e.g., Newton or Kerber) are often helpful in patients with severely tortuous vessels. Good guidelines to follow to avoid vasospasm, dissection, and catheter-related emboli include always leading with the guidewire, approaching carefully with gentle manipulation of the wire and catheter, and keeping the system below the carotid bifurcation. It is important to monitor for thrombus problems, and double-flushing or using constant perfusion systems are also important practice techniques to avoid emboli. Fluoroscopic monitoring of the tip, removal of excess torque or catheter redundancy, and a small hand test injection before the angiographic run will also avoid creating a dissection during the angiographic filming or converting a small dissection into an occlusive one.

Standard digital subtraction angiography is performed with variable rates and usually with a 1.5-second injection time (Table 4-1). Standard flow rates are as follows:

1. Linear rise of 0.2–0.3 ml per second is applied to prevent the catheter from dislodging.
2. With DSA imaging, a 75% dilution of regular-strength contrast is adequate to opacify the vessel.

TABLE 4-1. Suggested Contrast Injection Rates and Volumes

Vessel	*Rate (ml/sec)*	*Total volume (ml)*
Aortic arch	20–25	40–50
Common carotid artery	6–7	6–10
Internal carotid artery	6	8
External carotid artery	2–3	3–5
Vertebral	4–5	6–8

The flow rates may need to be adjusted in the setting of diseases in which the flow is altered. Flow rates as high as 10–12 ml per second may be needed with arteriovenous malformations (AVMs) and as low as 3 ml per second with internal carotid artery occlusions or a critical stenosis. In slow-flow states, an injection time of 3 seconds or longer may better delineate collateral blood flow; with newer techniques, such as rotational or three-dimensional DSA, longer injection times with normal rates are needed.

Angiographic projections are also important. The standard angiographic anterior-posterior (AP) and lateral projections usually suffice with Waters' angulation used for imaging the vertebrobasilar system.

NORMAL ANATOMY OF THE AORTIC ARCH AND ITS BRANCHES

Understanding the normal anatomy, its variants, and abnormalities of the aortic branches and their tributaries is important in safe and efficient catheterization and evaluation of the cerebral blood vessels.

The proximal aortic arch gives rise to three major branches: the brachiocephalic trunk (also called the *innominate artery*), the left common carotid artery, and the left subclavian artery. Arch aortographic images are best obtained perpendicular to the plane of the arch with 30–60 degrees in the left anterolateral oblique projection, depending on the degree of tortuosity.

The brachiocephalic artery is the first and the largest branch of the aortic arch. It ascends posterolaterally to the right at first anterior to the trachea, then to its right. Near the right sternoclavicular joint, the brachiocephalic artery bifurcates into the right common carotid artery and the subclavian artery. The right subclavian artery gives rise to the right vertebral, internal mamillary, thyrocervical, and costocervical trunks. The relative anatomic relationships can change dramatically in elderly or hypertensive patients with significant tortuosity.

The left common carotid artery is the second major vessel that arises from the aortic arch. Its origin is typically immediately distal, left, and slightly anterior to the brachiocephalic artery's origin. Both common carotid arteries travel alongside the trachea in a vertical direction toward the cranium without any branches, although significant tortuosity of the proximal common carotid arteries may occur. At the midcervical spine, typically between C3 and C5, the common carotid arteries bifurcate into the internal and external carotid arteries. The internal carotid artery (ICA) supplies the cranial and orbital contents, whereas the external carotid artery (ECA) supplies the exterior of the head, the face, and the anterior neck.

The left subclavian artery is the third and last major vessel that arises from the aortic arch. The left subclavian artery gives rise to the left vertebral artery and the internal thoracic artery along with the left thyrocervical and costocervical trunks. In the majority of cases, the left vertebral artery is equal to, or significantly larger than, the right vertebral artery.

The typical origin of the cerebral arteries from the aortic arch is present in 65% of patients. The most common normal variant is a shared origin of the left common carotid artery and brachiocephalic trunk occurring in 27% of cases. In 2.5%, the four large arteries may branch separately. The remaining 5% show a variety of other branching patterns.[1]

Anterior Circulation

The ICAs provide approximately 90% of the blood supply to the brain parenchyma. From the carotid bifurcation, the ICA ascends to the skull base and enters the cranial cavity via the carotid canal. The ICA is commonly described in four segments.[2] In ascending order, it consists of the cervical, petrous, cavernous, and supraclinoid segments (Figure 4-1). The cervical carotid segment extends from the common carotid bifurcation to the skull base. This segment of the ICA is enclosed by the carotid sheath, which contains the ninth, tenth, eleventh, and twelfth cranial nerves, sympathetic nerves, and the internal jugular vein. The petrous segment begins at the skull base at the extracranial opening of the carotid canal, ascends approximately 1 cm, turns anteromedially at the genu, and enters the intracranial space and cavernous sinus above the foramen lacerum. The end of this segment lies at approximately the meningohypophyseal trunk.

The cavernous segment enters the cavernous sinus at the petrolingual ligament and courses superiorly and then anteriorly through the cavernous sinus. Anteriorly, the vessel makes a 180-degree turn and pierces the proximal dural ring. Within the cavernous sinus, the ICA is surrounded by endothelial-lined venous sinusoids. The lateral cavernous sinus wall contains cranial nerves III, IV, V1, and V2; cranial nerve VI lies within the sinus inferolateral to this carotid segment. The cavernous segment ends at the distal dural ring where the ICA enters

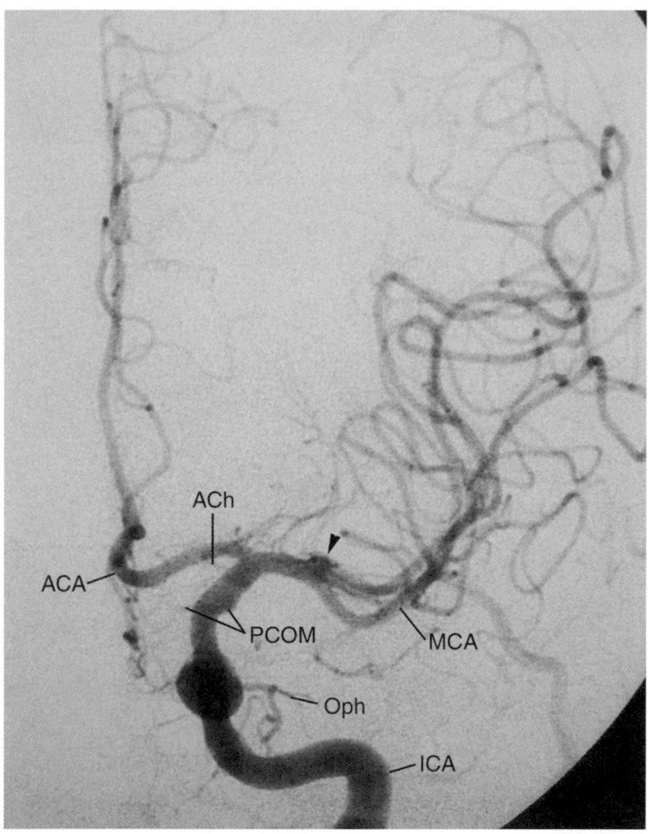

A

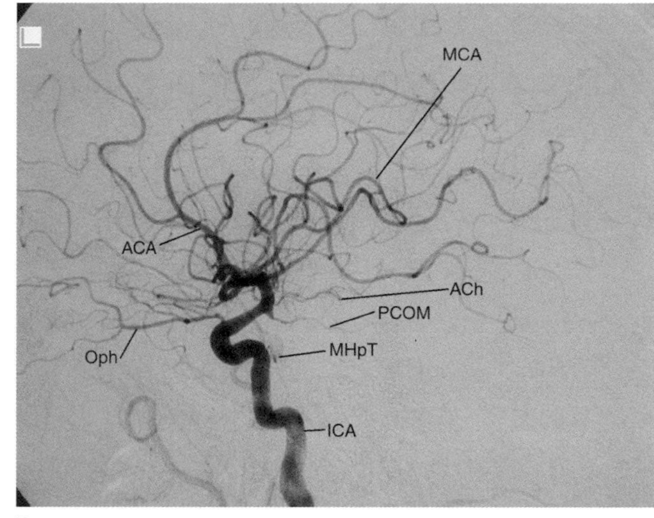

B

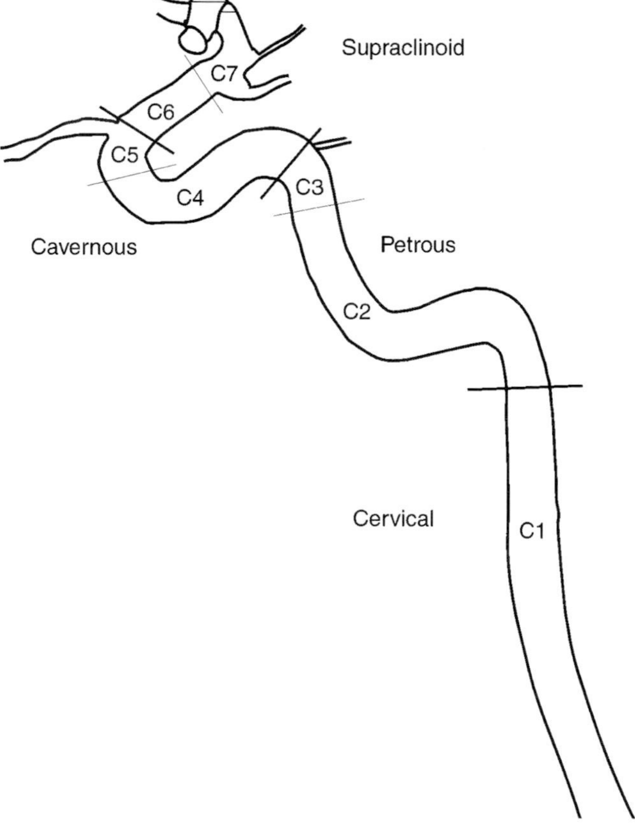

C

FIGURE 4-1. Normal internal carotid artery (ICA) angiogram. Anterior-posterior (**A**) and lateral (**B**) projections demonstrate the left ICA with its branches: the meningohypophyseal trunk (MHpT), ophthalmic artery (Oph), posterior communicating artery (PCOM), and anterior choroidal artery (ACh). The ICA then divides into the M1 and its sylvian M2 branches of the middle cerebral artery (MCA), and the A1 and its A2 segments of the anterior cerebral artery (ACA). The anterior-posterior view demonstrates a prominence (*arrowhead*) of the distal M1 segment at the lateral lenticulostriate arteries. **C.** The four major segments of the ICA and the seven numbered segments, C1–C7.[2] The four major segments all have different locations, physiology, pathology, and clinical sequelae. (*Continued*)

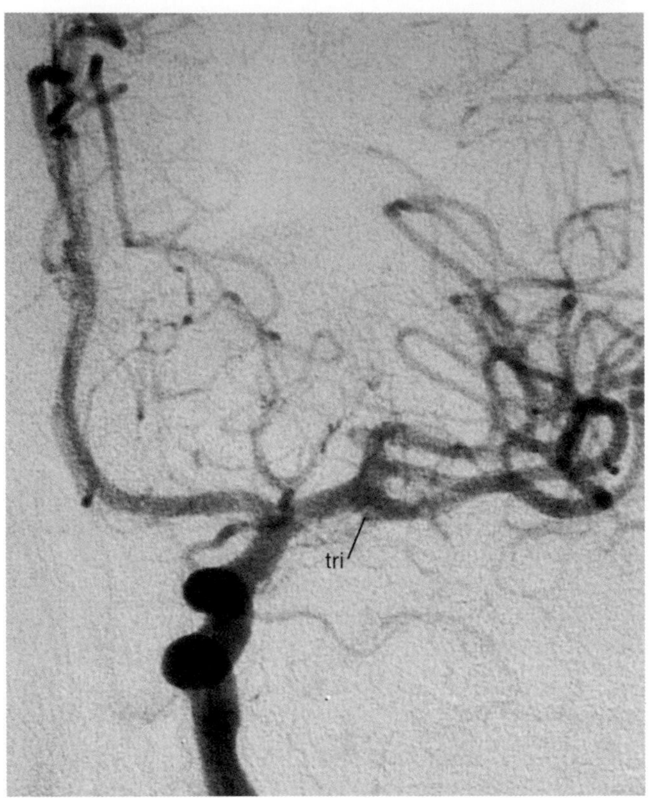

D

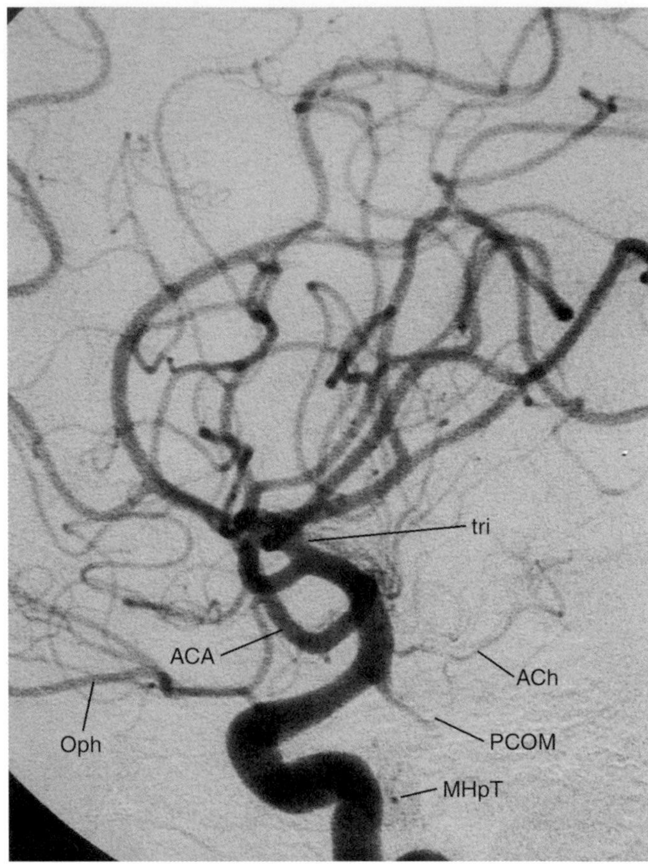

E

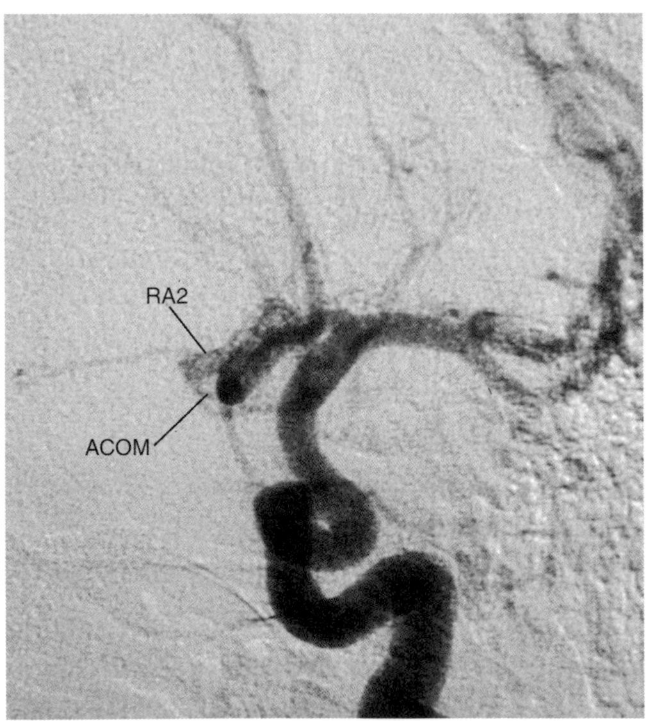

F

FIGURE 4-1. *Continued.* A semi-Waters' (**D**) and Schueller's (**E**) (caudal left lateral) projection reveals a normal MCA trifurcation (tri) without aneurysm. The small anterior communicating artery (ACOM) and A2 segment of the right ACA (RA2) are delineated only with a right transorbital oblique (**F**) and right carotid compression.

the subarachnoid space. On lateral projections, the curving portion of the cavernous and the supraclinoid segments form the S-shaped curve of the carotid siphon.

The supraclinoid segment runs from the distal dural ring to the intracranial ICA bifurcation. Before its division into the anterior and middle cerebral arteries, the ICA sends out three branches in the following order: the ophthalmic, the posterior communicating, and the anterior choroidal arteries. The ophthalmic artery originates near the dural ring and courses anteriorly, accompanied by the optic nerve into the optic canal. The posterior communicating artery (PCOM) originates at the posterior aspect of the supraclinoid ICA. It courses above the oculomotor nerves (cranial nerve III) and then joins the horizontal, or P1, segment of the ipsilateral posterior cerebral artery. Not only is the PCOM a significant portion of the circle of Willis, providing collateral supply between the carotid and vertebrobasilar systems, but it also has small anterior thalamoperforating arteries that supply the medial and anterior thalamus along with the adjacent internal capsule and optic tracts.

A short distance distal to the PCOM, the anterior choroidal artery arises from the posterior medial aspect of the supraclinoid ICA. It courses through the choroidal fissure and continues into the choroid plexus. The anterior choroidal artery is crucial, supplying the posterior limb of the internal capsule, lower lentiform nucleus, and lateral thalamus. Lying just lateral to the anterior thalamoperforating arteries, it also supplies the optic tracts.

In the suprasellar cistern, the ICA divides into the anterior and middle cerebral arteries. The anterior cerebral artery (ACA) courses anteromedially above the optic nerve and then turns vertically to travel in the interhemispheric fissure curving along the genu of the corpus callosum. The horizontal segment of the ACA is called the *A1 (precommunicating) segment*, and the vertical portion of the ACA is called the *A2 (postcommunicating) segment*. As it curves along the corpus callosum, the A2 gives rise to several cortical branches that are named according to the structures that they supply: the orbitofrontal artery, the frontopolar artery, the pericallosal artery, and callosomarginal artery.

In addition to the major cortical branches, the ACA gives rise to small perforator arteries such as the medial lenticulostriate arteries and the recurrent artery of Huebner. These arteries supply important structures such as the caudate head nucleus, the anteromedial aspect of the putamen, the globus pallidus, the anterior limb of the internal capsule, and rostrum of the corpus callosum.

The middle cerebral artery (MCA) supplies large and important territories, including the motor and sensory cortex. It also covers many eloquent areas including those controlling receptive and expressive components of language and higher cognitive functions. The MCA has been classically described as dividing from its horizontal trunk, the M1 segment, into an anterior temporal artery, supplying the anterior and lateral temporal lobe, and anterior and posterior divisions. These later divisions supply the anterior and lateral aspects of the frontal lobe, the majority of the parietal lobe, and the posterior and lateral aspects of the temporal lobes, respectively. However, the branching pattern of the MCA is often quite variable, and branches extend from the anterior sylvian fissure in a radial pattern from the M1 segment. Viewed from the left, these branches radiate out in a clockwise fashion to supply the inferolateral and superolateral frontal lobe, the frontoparietal (rolandic) junction, the mid-parietal lobe, the angular region of the sylvian fissure, and the posterolateral temporal lobe.

The sylvian portions of the MCA course along the insula in a parasagittal fashion before making a right angle to extend underneath the frontoparietal operculum. These insular branches give rise to very small perforating arteries that supply the insular cortex and subinsular white matter and collaterally supply the lateral aspects of the basal ganglia along with the lenticulostriates and thalamoperforators. Beyond this portion, MCA branches extend over the cerebral convexity, providing perforating arteries that extend into the sulci and directly into the brain parenchyma. Collateral anastomoses between the ACAs and MCAs occur predominantly on the surface of the brain in a parasagittal location approximately 1.5–3.0 cm off midline. This creates a zone of distal-most branches known as the *watershed* or *border zone* that not only run along the parasagittal surface but also run in the deep white matter in a paraventricular location.[3,4]

Posterior Circulation

The vertebral arteries continue their cephalad course and enter the foramen transversarium, usually at the C6 vertebral segment, and exit from C1. They course posteromedially after crossing the dural ring above C1 and turn anterosuperiorly to enter the skull via the foramen magnum. The intracranial vertebral artery gives rise to the posterior inferior cerebellar artery (PICA), which supplies the medulla before coursing to supply the tonsils, fourth ventricle, and inferior cerebellar hemispheres.

The vertebral artery distal to the PICA has numerous perforating branches that supply the medulla and upper spinal cord. The bilateral vertebral arteries unite to form the midline basilar artery at the pontomedullary junction. The basilar artery also has numerous perforating arteries that supply the pons. The basilar artery gives rise to two important cerebellar branches: the anterior inferior cerebellar arteries that supply the pons, brachium pontis, and anterolateral cerebellum, and the superior cerebellar arteries that supply the superior cerebellum and vermis (Figure 4-2).

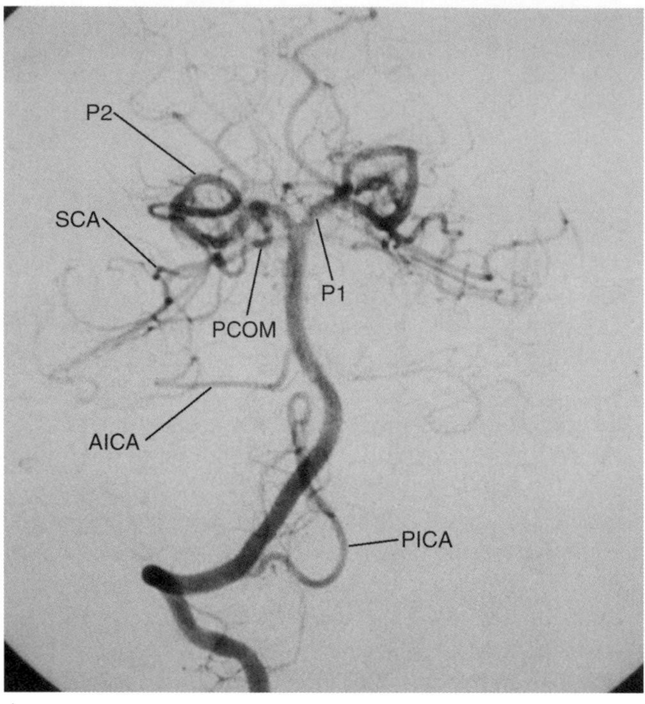

A

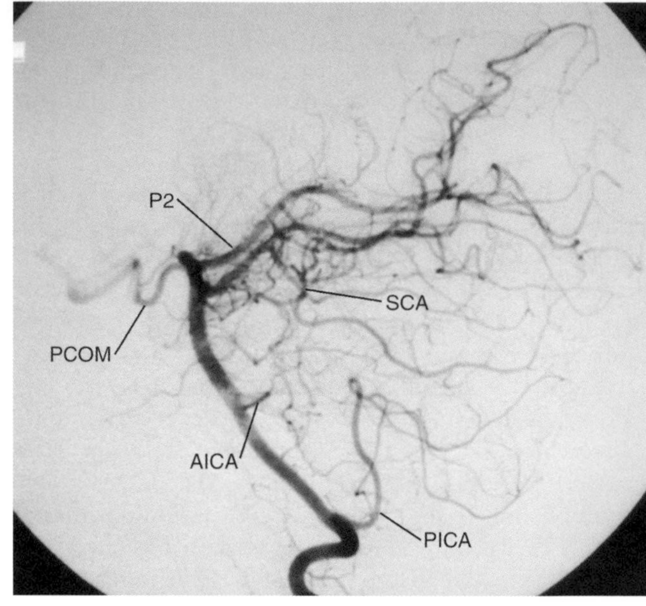

B

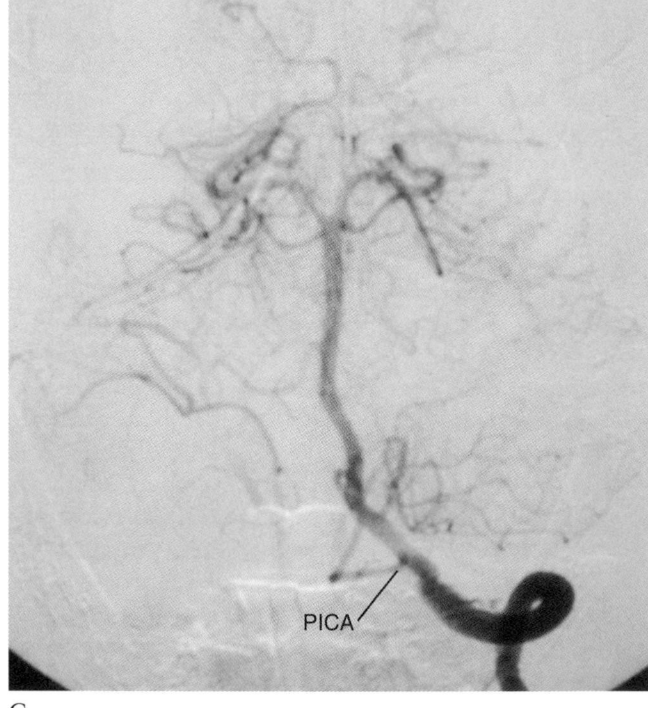

C

FIGURE 4-2. Normal right and left vertebral artery. A semi-Waters' (**A**) and lateral (**B**) projection demonstrate the major branches of the vertebrobasilar system, including the posterior inferior cerebellar artery (PICA), anterior inferior cerebellar artery (AICA), superior cerebellar artery (SCA), and posterior cerebral artery (P1 and P2 segments). The right posterior communicating artery (PCOM) is also seen. In this subarachnoid hemorrhage evaluation, the left vertebral artery injection (Waters' projection) (**C**) was performed to demonstrate the left PICA origin.

At the midbrain level, the basilar artery divides into two posterior cerebral arteries (PCAs). The proximal segment of the PCA is called the *P1 (precommunicating) segment*. The PCA extends from the basilar bifurcation to its junction with the PCOM. Also arising from the distal basilar artery and the P1 segment are a number of small perforating arteries, the posterior thalamoperforators. These thalamoperforating arteries supply the upper midbrain and central medial aspects of the thalamus and may also occasionally supply the contralateral thalamus. The *P2 (postcommunicating) segment* of the PCA then courses around the cerebral peduncle to supply a portion of the peduncle and the medial aspect of the temporal lobe at, and posterior to, the uncus. This segment then divides into its three main branches, the lateral temporal, parieto-occipital, and calcarine arteries.

Circle of Willis

The circle of Willis provides important anastomoses that connect the anterior and posterior circulation and is a crucial source of collateral supply in proximal artery cerebral occlusions. The circle of Willis is located in the suprasellar cistern above the optic chiasm and oculomotor nerves. It consists of the paired distal ICAs, the A1 segments of the ACAs, the P1 segments of the PCAs, and the anterior communicating arteries (ACOM) and PCOM.

The ACOM connects the paired A1 segments and has several perforator branches to supply the optic chiasm, anterior hypothalamus, and medial frontal lobes. The PCOMs connect the supraclinoid segment of the ICA and PCA at the P1-P2 junction.

A complete circle of Willis is present in only 20–25% of cases. Common variants are hypoplastic or absent PCOM, ACOM, or A1 segments and fetal origin of the PCA from the ICA with a hypoplastic or absent P1 segment.

Venous System

Evaluation of the venous system is important for understanding the pathophysiology of many vascular diseases. The anatomy of the dural sinuses is best seen in AP and lateral projections, although a Towne's projection can delineate the transverse and sigmoid sinuses (Figure 4-3).

The superior sagittal sinus originates near the crista galli and courses posteriorly along the superior margin of the falx, joining the straight sinus to form the torcular Herophili. The superior sagittal sinus drains the superficial cerebral veins from the lateral and medial surfaces of the cerebral hemisphere. The largest named vein is the vein of Trolard in the parietal region. The inferior sagittal sinus is located along the inferior free margin of the falx. The pair of internal cerebral veins joins the perimesencephalic veins to form the vein of Galen, which joins the inferior sagittal sinus to become the straight sinus. The straight sinus then courses along the falcine-tentorial junction to join the torcula.

From the torcula, the transverse sinuses course laterally along the posterior margin of the tentorium and turns inferiorly to form the sigmoid sinus. The sigmoid sinus continues inferiorly and becomes the internal jugular vein as it enters the jugular foramen. The transverse sinus receives many tributaries from the cerebellum and temporal and occipital lobes, most notably, the vein of Labbé.

The cavernous sinuses lie on either side of the sella turcica. They are the most important means of communication of the intracranial and extracranial venous system. Anteriorly, the cavernous sinus receives tributaries from the superior and inferior ophthalmic veins as well as the sphenoparietal sinus, which receives its supply from the great sylvian veins. Posteriorly, the cavernous sinus receives draining channels from the temporal lobe—specifically, the uncal or the middle cerebral vein. Posteriorly, the cavernous sinus drains into the superior petrosal and inferior petrosal sinuses that join the sigmoid sinus and jugular vein, respectively.

ANGIOGRAPHY IN CEREBROVASCULAR DISEASE

Atherosclerotic Vascular Disease

Atherosclerotic disease of the aortic arch and cervical and intracranial arteries is a common cause of cerebrovascular insufficiency. The treatment plan for atherosclerotic disease depends on the patient's clinical status and angiographic findings. The goals of angiography in patients with atherosclerotic disease are numerous. The first goal is to confirm and determine the location, extent, and degree of atherosclerotic stenosis, often by ultrasonography or MRA (Figure 4-4). This can significantly alter the medical management or surgical approach, especially if there is intracranial disease or if the cervical stenosis extends superiorly above the mandible. Another goal of angiography is to detect unsuspected tandem lesions either distal (e.g., carotid siphon) or proximal (e.g., brachiocephalic) to the cervical lesion.

Proximal aortic and brachiocephalic atheromatous stenosis, cervical carotid disease, and intracranial stenosis are all independent risk factors for cerebral ischemia.[5] In the angiographic assessment of carotid stenosis, one study found 15% concomitant severe intracranial stenosis.[6] Therefore, angiographic evaluation of atherosclerotic disease must include an arch aortogram and selective studies of the cervical carotid arteries with intracranial projections. Tandem lesions may lead to ineffective treatment and possibly increase the risk of stroke during surgery (Figure 4-5). The tandem lesion may also be treated at the same time if it is in an appropriate location. Analysis of arch anatomy, tortuosity, and other features that may increase the risk of guide catheter navigation, angioplasty, and stent placement is also important.

The third goal of angiography in patients with atherosclerotic disease is to detect risk factors, such as near complete occlusion or intraluminal thrombus, that may lead to urgent treatment. The fourth is to evaluate existing and potential pathways for collateral circulation. The lack of significant collateral circulation may lead to hypoperfusion and significant stroke while cross-clamping during a carotid endarterectomy. The fifth goal is exclusion of other incidental cerebrovascular lesions (e.g., aneurysm, AVM) that may increase risk and require treatment before revascularization.

The angiographic findings of atherosclerosis are vascular stenosis and occlusion. Less commonly, atherosclerosis may cause damage to the blood vessel wall of the media and result in fusiform dilatation. Stenosis may be smooth and circumferential or eccentric and even ulcerated. The degree of stenosis at the carotid bifurcation and its clinical implications have been studied extensively but continue to be debated. There are three commonly used methods to calculate the degree of stenosis: the North American Symptomatic Carotid Endarterectomy Trial (NASCET), the European Carotid

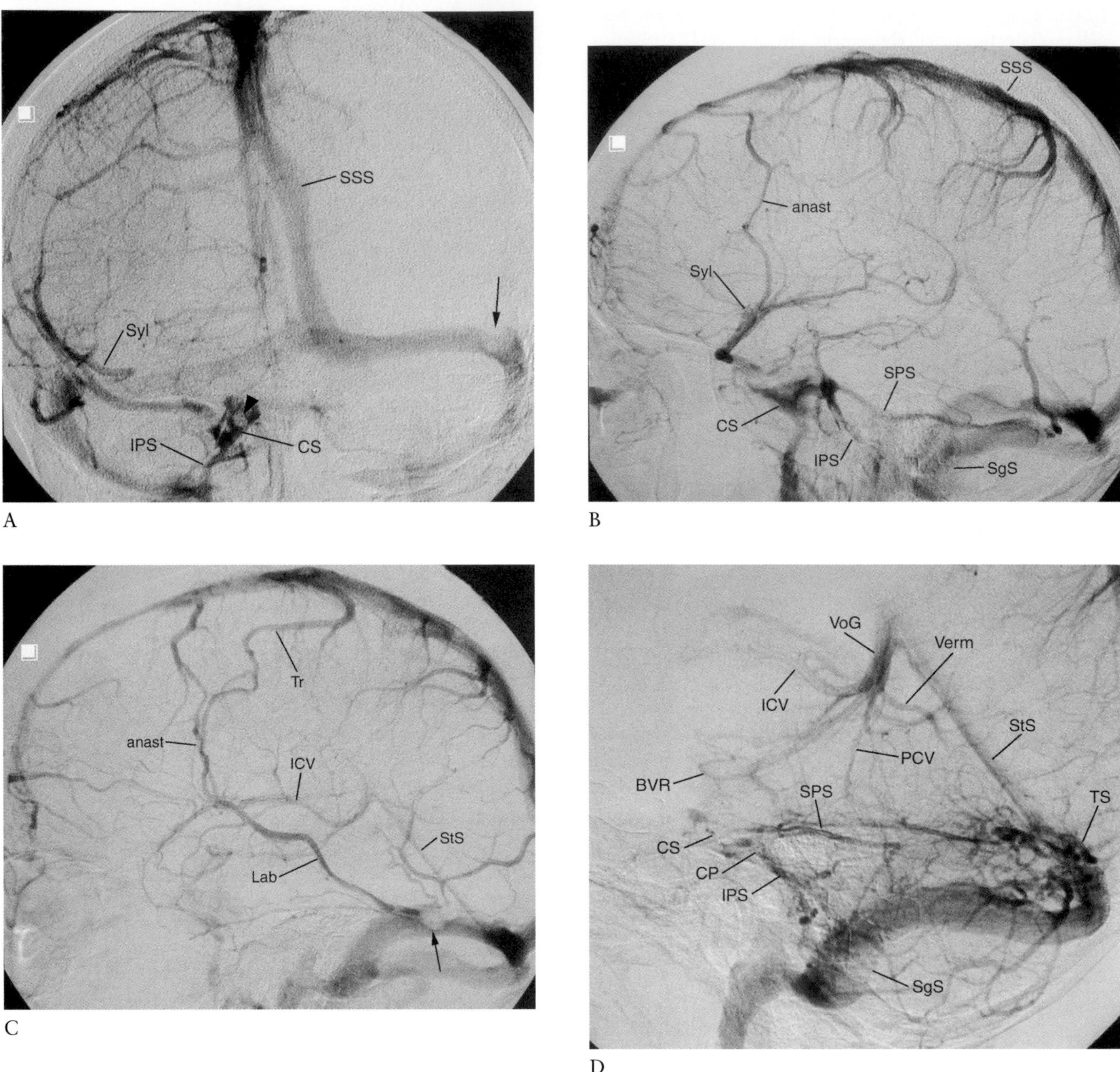

FIGURE 4-3. Normal venous phase. Anterior-posterior venous phases of the right internal carotid artery (RICA) (**A**) and lateral venous phases of the RICA (**B**). Left internal carotid artery (LICA) (**C**) demonstrates the superior sagittal sinus (SSS), transverse sinus, and sigmoid sinus (SgS) well. The straight sinus (StS) is only faintly filled due to significant flow from the nonopacified posterior circulation. On the right (**A,B**), the dominant sylvian vein (Syl) drains into the cavernous sinus (CS) and inferior petrosal sinus (IPS). Note the oval filling defect in the left transverse sinus (*arrow* in **A,C**) due to a normal arachnoid granulation and the round filling defect of the right internal carotid artery (*arrowhead* in **A**). Direct cortical venous anastomoses (anast) are common. On the left (**C**), a dominant vein of Trolard (Tr) and Labbé (Lab) are seen. The lateral projection of the vertebral venous phase (**D**) demonstrates the deep venous system, including the internal cerebral veins (ICV), basal vein of Rosenthal (BVR), vermian vein (Verm), and precentral cerebellar vein (PCV), which lead to the vein of Galen (VoG) and StS. The various cerebellar veins drain into the transverse sinus (TS) and may join pontine and brachial veins, which cross the cistern into the superior petrosal sinus (SPS), clival plexus (CP), CS, and IPS.

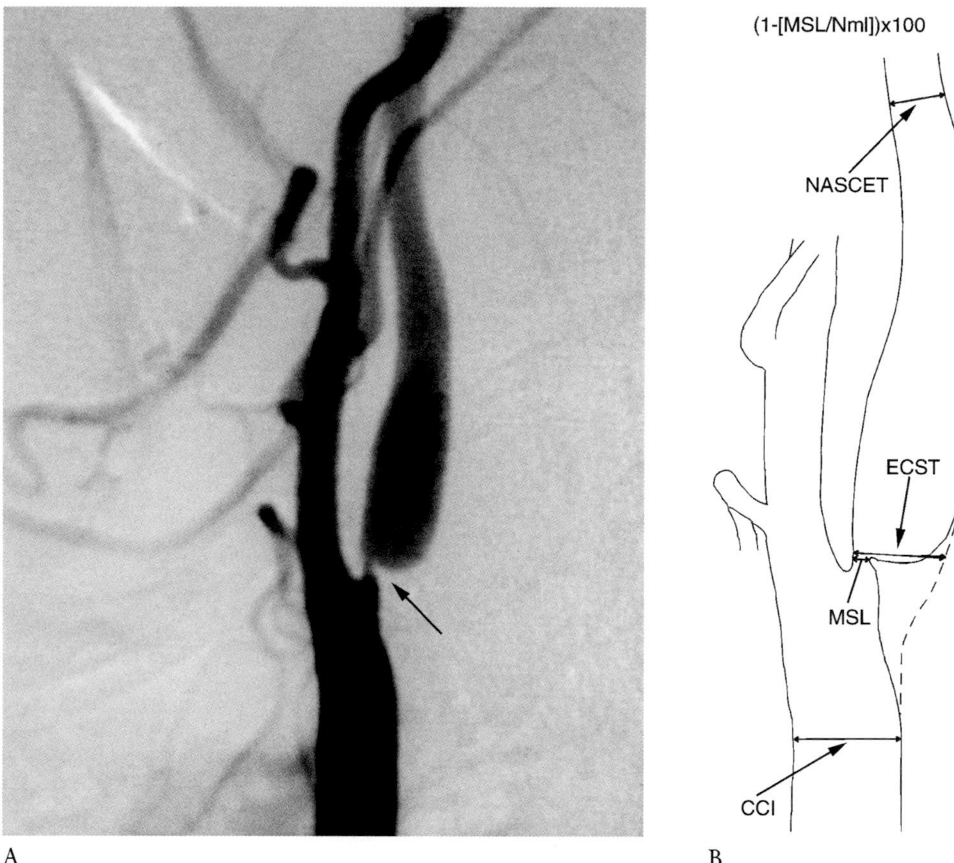

FIGURE 4-4. Internal carotid stenosis. **A.** Lateral projection demonstrates a high-grade stenosis at the origin of the left internal carotid artery (*arrow*). **B.** The three common methods for measuring carotid stenosis. The maximal stenotic lumen (MSL) and the normal (Nml) denominator for the various methods (North American Symptomatic Carotid Endarterectomy Trial [NASCET], European Carotid Surgery Trial [ECST], Common Carotid Index [CCI]) are marked. The percent stenosis is calculated using the formula noted at the top of the figure. This specific stenosis measures approximately 75% by NASCET, 87% by ECST, and 93% by the CCI method.

Surgery Trial (ECST), and the Common Carotid Index methods. All three methods use a ratio of the luminal diameter at the point of greatest stenosis (the maximal stenotic lumen) but differ in the choice of denominator, the normal reference lumen (see Figure 4-4B).

The NASCET method is the most commonly used method to measure stenosis in North America. The NASCET method calculates the degree of stenosis using the ratio of the maximal stenotic lumen and the normal nontapering ICA, the normal part of the cervical ICA beyond the carotid bulb. This method is based on the concept that the nontapered ICA is more reproducibly measured, but it gives a lower percentage stenosis than the other two methods. The NASCET study concluded that carotid endarterectomy is highly beneficial in symptomatic groups who had stenosis from 70% to 99%. Carotid endarterectomy reduces the risk of ipsilateral stroke from 26% to 9%—an absolute risk reduction of 17%.[7] A subsequent study under the Asymptomatic Carotid Atherosclerotic Study (ACAS), using a measuring method similar to NASCET, indicated that asymptomatic patients with carotid artery stenosis of 60% or greater also benefit from carotid endarterectomy when compared to medical management alone (daily aspirin administration). The aggregate risk over 5 years for ipsilateral stroke in postendarterectomy patients was estimated at 5.1% compared to 11.0% for patients treated only medically.[8]

The ECST method bases the calculation on the presumed normal lumen of the same site, requiring an estimation of the size and shape of the carotid bulb. The ECST data concluded that there was little risk of ipsilateral stroke in patients with only mild (0–29%) stenosis. The risk of the surgery is outweighed by the small natural risk of stroke. For patients with moderate (30–69%) stenosis, the balance of surgical risk and eventual benefit remain uncertain. However, for patients with severe (70–99%) stenosis, carotid endarterectomy was significantly beneficial, with a 2.8% risk of ipsilateral stroke in postendarterectomy patients compared to 16.8% in the control group.[9]

The Common Carotid Index method calculates stenosis based on the diameter of the common carotid artery.[10] Because of different methods of calculation, the

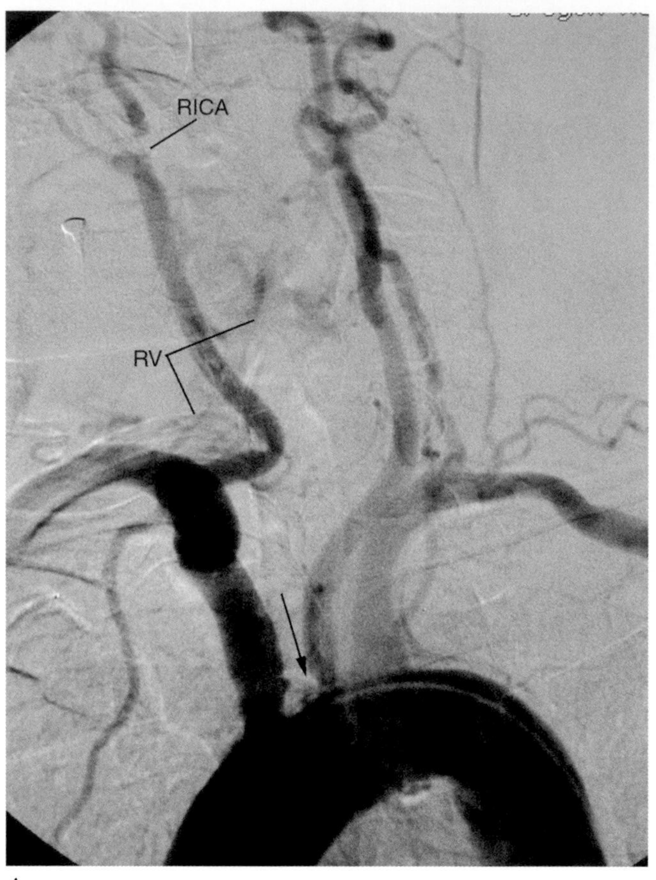

A

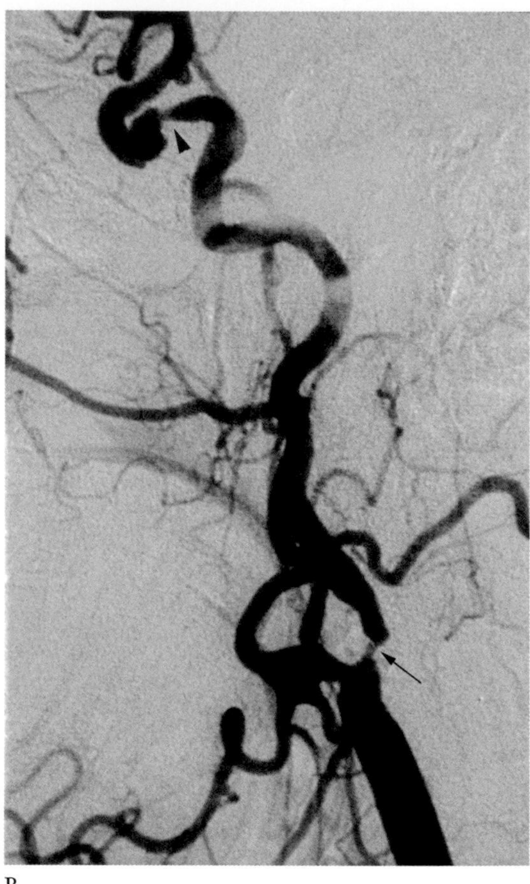

B

FIGURE 4-5. Tandem atherosclerotic stenosis. **A.** Left anterior oblique arch aortogram demonstrates irregular atheromatous disease at the origin of the right innominate artery and the origin of the left common carotid artery (*arrow*). The left carotid lesion results in approximately 40% stenosis. The significant right internal carotid artery (RICA) stenosis is also noted. The right vertebral artery (RV) shows only filling of the proximal cervical segment and is occluded distally. The right common carotid artery lateral projection (**B**) demonstrates a 70% RICA origin stenosis (*arrow*) with a second approximately 70% stenosis of the cavernous portion of the RICA (*arrowhead*) with poststenotic dilatation. This patient underwent right carotid endarterectomy but had recurrent right carotid symptoms and ultimately went for treatment by angioplasty and stent placement of the RICA cavernous lesion.

same stenosis has a higher percentage of narrowing using the ECST and Common Carotid Index methods compared to the NASCET approach. In cases of severe stenosis with decreased distal lumen, the NASCET method, and possibly the ECST method, tends to underestimate the degree of stenosis.

Acute Stroke

Stroke is a major cause of death in the United States and a significant cause of long-term morbidity and dependence. More than 700,000 strokes occur annually in the United States, of which 85% are ischemic, posing a large health care problem that costs more than $30 billion annually.[11] Until recently, cerebral angiography has had a very limited role in acute stroke evaluation. However, with the emergence of acute intervention and endovascular treatment, this is rapidly changing. The goal of acute stroke therapy is to accurately establish the diagnosis and quickly reperfuse the ischemic area.

Intravenous systemic fibrinolytic treatment using recombinant tissue plasminogen activator (alteplase) has shown success in the acute treatment of stroke if administered within 3 hours of the initiation of symptoms,[12] and intra-arterial (IA) thrombolysis has also shown success if initiated within 6 hours.[13] The initial diagnostic modality of stroke has been, and continues to be, noncontrast-enhanced CT, primarily to exclude hemorrhage and a mass lesion, although diffusion and perfusion magnetic resonance imaging (MRI) may also have potential advantages and play a greater role in the future. Cerebral angiography is not required for intravenous fibrinolytic treatment and, given the degree of the systemic fibrinolytic state, may carry some increased risk.

In the setting of acute stroke, cerebral angiography may be necessary in determining further stroke risk that

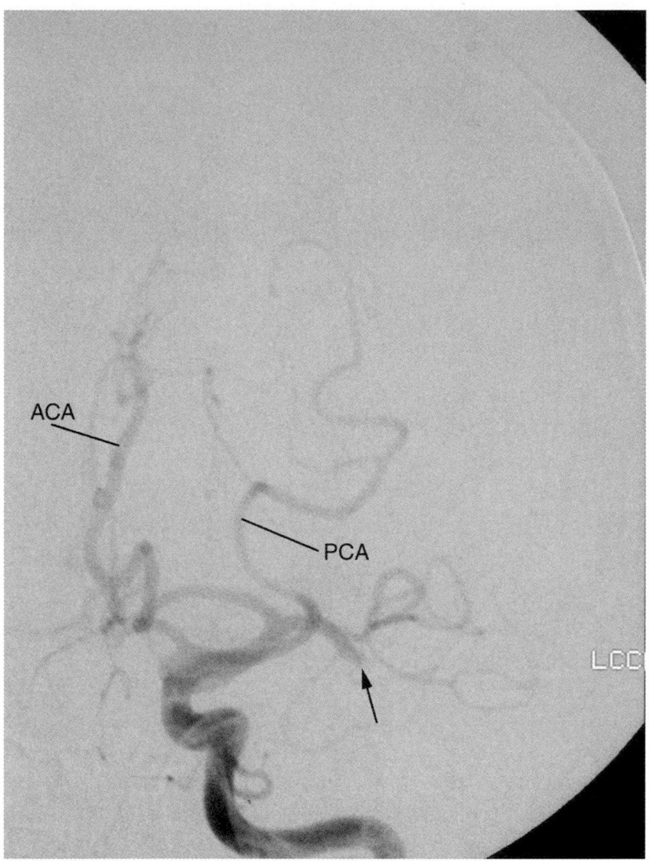

A

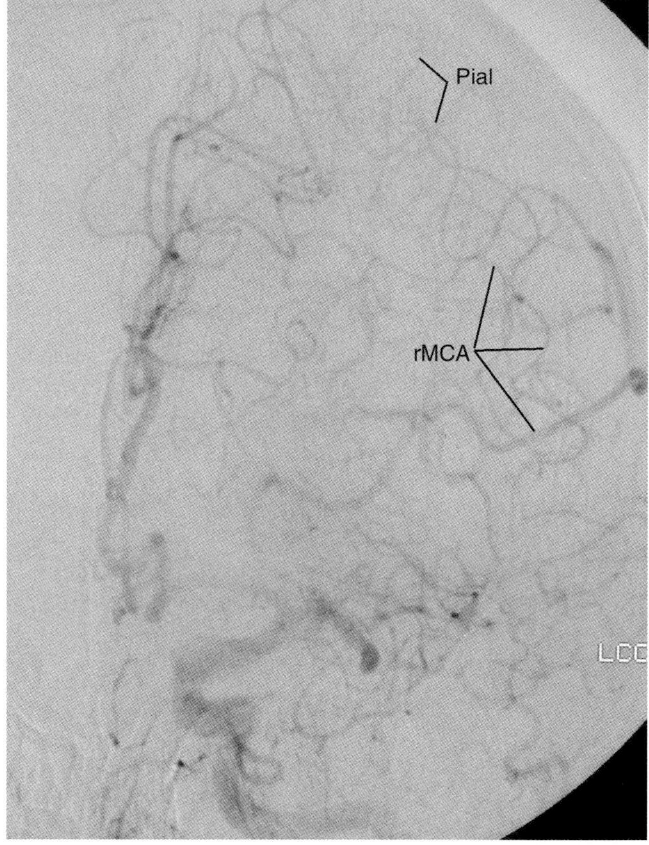

B

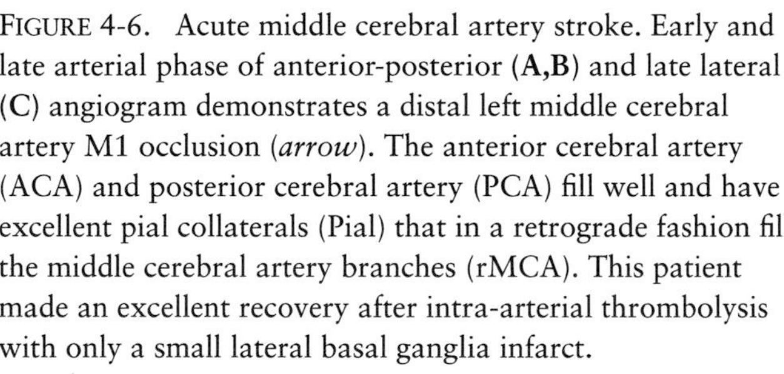

FIGURE 4-6. Acute middle cerebral artery stroke. Early and late arterial phase of anterior-posterior (**A,B**) and late lateral (**C**) angiogram demonstrates a distal left middle cerebral artery M1 occlusion (*arrow*). The anterior cerebral artery (ACA) and posterior cerebral artery (PCA) fill well and have excellent pial collaterals (Pial) that in a retrograde fashion fill the middle cerebral artery branches (rMCA). This patient made an excellent recovery after intra-arterial thrombolysis with only a small lateral basal ganglia infarct.

C

requires immediate assessment and cannot be accurately delineated by noninvasive means. More critically, angiography is the initial assessment method used to determine an appropriate occlusive lesion site and type for potential IA thrombolysis. In patients who do not fit the emergent treatment criteria, the evaluation can be performed on a more semiurgent or elective basis, depending on the clinical status of the patient and the risk of recurrent stroke as determined by the findings of noninvasive studies.

The goals of angiographic evaluation for IA thrombolysis are to determine the location and extent of the occlusion, the degree and source of collateral supply, the amount of residual perfusion to the ischemic area, and the potential cause of thromboembolism (Figure 4-6). Angiographic evaluation of the symptomatic vessel should be performed first, followed by a study of the remaining cerebral vasculature. For example, if an M1 occlusion is found, and the ACA fills appropriately, further angiography is not necessary before initiating thrombolysis. On the other hand, if an ICA terminus occlusion is found, then the contralateral ICA, and possibly the vertebral artery, will need angiographic evaluation.

The location of the occlusion is identified as an intravascular filling defect or abrupt termination of the column of the contrast. Other findings include slow antegrade flow and delayed "washout" time in the arterial phase. Collateral supply can arise from the circle of Willis, pial arterial anastomoses, or perforator anastomotic channels. Evidence of prominent pial collaterals presents as retrograde filling of more proximally occluded vessels. A paucity of vessels and lack of capillary blush are usually observed in the nonperfused, or poorly perfused, brain parenchyma. The degree of collateral supply to the ischemic region gives an estimation of the amount of residual perfusion and may be helpful in predicting the outcome. The pial collaterals can be evaluated by degree of retrograde filling, which can extend back to the level of the occlusion. The degree of capillary blush can be assessed during the capillary phase. Increasing the image contrast when reviewing the angiographic run is helpful in assessing the capillary phase.

There are numerous causes of ischemic stroke, including cardiac or systemic emboli, small vessel disease, hypercoagulable states, and cerebrovascular disease. Although atherosclerotic disease is a significant contributor to thromboembolism, other causes may be encountered and must be evaluated. Carotid or vertebral dissection, either spontaneous or traumatic, can result in stroke due to thromboemboli or poor perfusion from an occlusive or near-occlusive proximal lesion (Figure 4-7). They are seen most commonly in the internal carotid or vertebral arteries but can also be seen in the common carotid arteries or intracranial vessels. Cerebrovascular dissections usually appear as a long, tapered, undulating stenosis with a possible pseudoaneurysm or as an intimal flap, which may be seen only when tangential to the x-ray beam. An associated intraluminal thrombus in dissections may lead to devastating consequences of stroke. Its discovery can be crucial in the determination of risk of further emboli, especially if one is planning on navigating catheters beyond the dissection for IA therapy.

Vasculitis involving the central nervous system (CNS) presents in a variety of types: isolated angiitis of the CNS; giant cell or temporal arteritis; systemic vasculitides such as polyarteritis nodosa, Wegener's granulomatosis, or Churg-Strauss syndrome; and secondary vasculitis from infection, drugs, or neoplasm. Intracranial involvement with vasculitis carries a higher risk of hemorrhage—parenchymal or subarachnoid—and is usually considered a contraindication to thrombolysis.[14] Steroid or more aggressive anti-inflammatory immunosuppressive therapy is part of the treatment regimen; therefore, a prompt and correct diagnosis will have significant clinical impact.

Intracranial vasculitis usually presents with multiple, concentric, long, tapered stenoses, with possible occlusion in the medium-sized arteries such as M2 or the distal branches of the MCA. Differential considerations include subacute vasospasm or, more commonly, intracranial atheromatous disease, which can be virtually indistinguishable from vasculitis. High-resolution angiography is necessary to evaluate the findings in these medium-sized arteries, and the external carotid arteries should also be evaluated for the possibility of involvement, especially in giant cell or temporal arteritis.[15] Takayasu's arteritis[16] involves the aorta and its great vessels and the innominate, common carotid, and subclavian arteries and rarely extends into the ICA.

Fibromuscular dysplasia (FMD) is a disorder that involves the smooth muscle and elastic tissues of large arteries, most commonly the cervical internal carotid and vertebral arteries as well as the renal arteries.[17] There are rare reported instances of intracranial and external carotid involvement.[18] FMD typically presents with hypertension due to renal involvement, and the cerebrovascular involvement is, in most cases, asymptomatic. Cerebrovascular symptoms and complications, such as transient ischemic attack, dissection, pseudoaneurysm, and arteriovenous fistula, are the second most common presentations of FMD.

FMD appears as multiple band-like narrowings with areas of dilation, the so-called string of beads appearance. In rare instances, the degree of stenosis may

FIGURE 4-7. ▶ Various nonatheromatous causes for stroke. **A.** Right internal carotid artery dissection from motor vehicle accident. The irregular and somewhat narrowed lumen (*arrows*) of the cervical carotid artery is noted along with a right middle cerebral artery M1 occlusion (*black arrowhead*). There is a subtle U-shaped filling defect in the internal carotid artery distal to the dissection (*white arrowhead*) representing intraluminal thrombus. **B.** Left internal carotid artery fibromuscular dysplasia. Note the multiple band-like areas of stenosis throughout the mid-cervical segment of the left internal carotid artery, resulting in areas of narrowing and slight dilation (*arrows*) that are rather typical for fibromuscular dysplasia. This is symptomatic with recurrent transient ischemic attacks. **C.** Isolated angiitis of the central nervous system with multiple concentric areas of stenosis in the anterior and middle cerebral arteries (*arrowheads*). This patient responded to steroid therapy, although intracranial atheromatous disease and unusual vasospasm could also have this appearance. **D.** Takayasu's arteritis. The left internal carotid artery is occluded with a tapered occlusion (*long arrow*). A long, tapered high-grade stenosis of the right common carotid artery is noted from its origin to the carotid bifurcation (*curved arrows*). There is also some mild stenosis of the right subclavian origin. Note the relative sparing of both vertebral arteries. (LV = left vertebral artery; RV = right vertebral artery.)

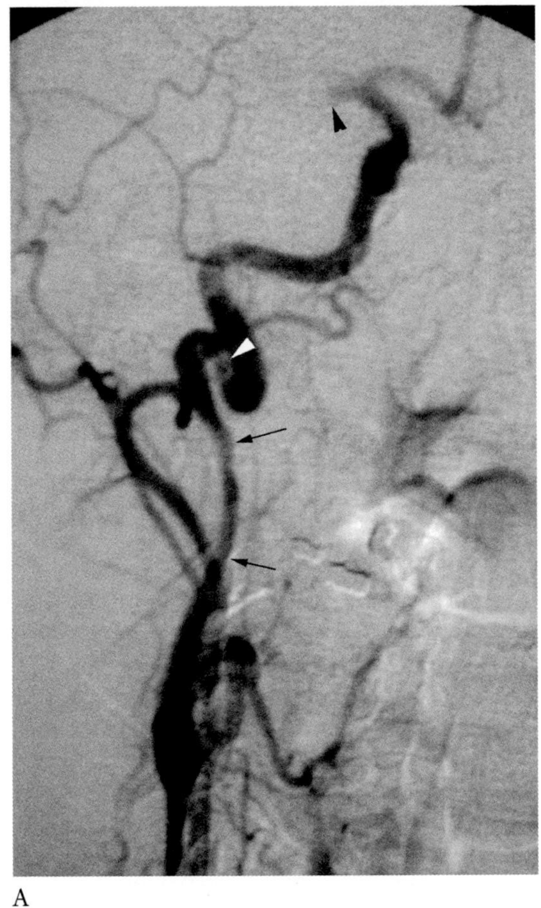

A

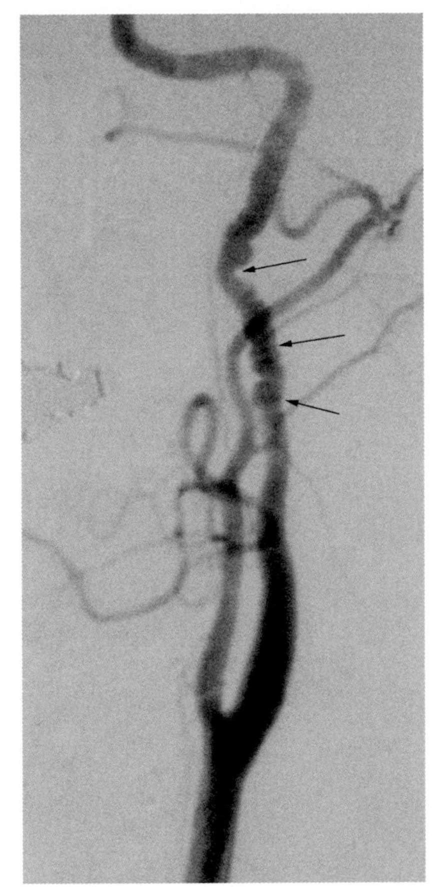

B

C

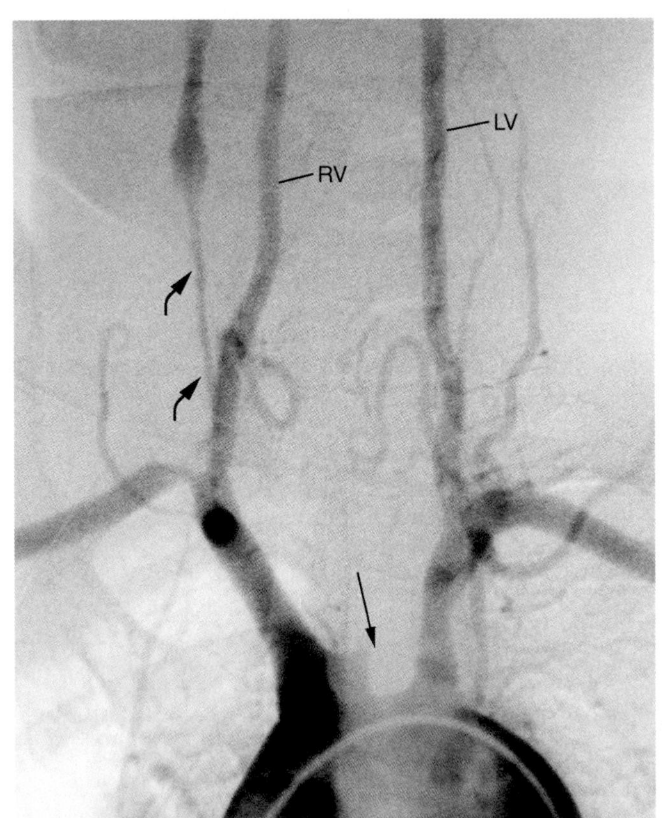

D

be significant enough to result in flow-limiting ischemia, and antiplatelet or antithrombotic therapy is the primary treatment for presumed microembolic emboli causing these transient ischemic attacks. Revascularization techniques may favor stent therapy over endarterectomy because of the difficulties in surgically assessing the typically involved upper cervical segment of the ICA.

Other connective tissue diseases, such as Ehlers-Danlos syndrome and Marfan's syndrome, can also lead to vessel dissection and acute stroke. Moyamoya and sickle cell disease can also produce stroke due to intracranial cerebrovascular stenosis or occlusion.

Cerebral Aneurysms

Cerebral aneurysm is a focal pathologic dilation of an arterial wall. The majority of aneurysms arises from a congenital anomaly, creating a relative weakness of the vessel wall in the elastic and muscular layers. Over time, the pulsation pressures on this weakness result in acute or progressive stretching, and an aneurysm is formed. The most common clinical presentation of a cerebral aneurysm is headache related to subarachnoid hemorrhage (SAH), with 80–90% of spontaneous SAH due to aneurysmal rupture. The size of the aneurysm and the patient's age are the major predictors of the risk of aneurysm rupture. Unruptured aneurysms that have a diameter less than 10 mm carry a 0.5–2.0% rate of rupture per year. Aneurysms measuring 10–15 mm have a 3–4% rate of rupture per year, and aneurysms measuring more than 25 mm have an 8–9% rate of rupture per year.[19]

The clinical outcome of aneurysmal SAH is generally poor, with approximately 17% of individuals dead before or on arrival at the hospital. In those who do reach the hospital, the greatest risk is aneurysm rehemorrhage, although cerebral vasospasm significantly contributes to overall morbidity and mortality. As many as 50% of SAH patients eventually die as a result of their hemorrhage, and an additional 25% experience permanent neurologic injury.[20] The clinical status of patients who are able to reach medical attention is commonly graded by the Hunt and Hess scale.[18]

Grade	Clinical Condition
I	Asymptomatic, minimal headache, or slight nuchal rigidity
II	Moderate to severe headache, nuchal rigidity, neurologic deficit confined to cranial nerve palsy
III	Drowsiness, confusion, or mild focal deficit
IV	Stupor, moderate to severe hemiparesis, possible early decerebrate rigidity, and vegetative disturbances
V	Deep coma, decerebrate rigidity, moribund appearance

Many studies have used the Hunt and Hess clinical grading to stratify the clinical outcome of aneurysmal SAH. Grades I–III are predictors of good outcome. In a 10-year retrospective study of patients with a ruptured anterior circulation aneurysm, there was a 97% favorable outcome for patients with Hunt and Hess grade I, 88% with grade II, and 81% with grade III. The chance of rehemorrhage in the first month is very high, with an approximately 20% aneurysmal rebleed rate in the first 2 weeks and 35% over the first month if the aneurysm is left untreated. After the first 30 days, the risk of rehemorrhage drops back to 1–2% per year.[21,22]

Occasionally, aneurysms present as cranial nerve palsies or other signs of mass effect. Eighteen percent of acute third nerve palsy are due to a PCOM aneurysm.[23] Cavernous sinus syndrome, often beginning with a sixth nerve palsy, can be seen with a cavernous ICA aneurysm, and visual loss due to optic nerve compression can be seen with cavernous or, more likely, supraclinoid ICA aneurysms. Larger aneurysms can also present with parenchymal compression symptoms, especially in the midbrain and pons. With the increasing use of MRI, incidental asymptomatic aneurysms are found more often.

The pattern of SAH can predict the location of an aneurysm and may assist in selecting the order of vessels to be examined during cerebral angiography. Interhemispheric SAH suggests an aneurysm in the ACOM, whereas a hematoma in the sylvian fissure is often associated with aneurysmal rupture in the MCA at the trifurcation. Perimesencephalic and prepontine hemorrhage is often caused by rupture of a basilar tip or PCOM aneurysm. The cerebellopontine angle and fourth ventricle SAH are commonly associated with the rupture of a PICA aneurysm. Intraventricular hemorrhage is associated with a PCOM (temporal horn), ACOM (frontal horn), or basilar tip (third ventricle) aneurysm.

A properly performed diagnostic cerebral angiogram in a patient with suspected aneurysmal SAH requires a bilateral carotid and at least one vertebral artery injection. The study must visualize the entire component of the circle of Willis, MCA bifurcation, vertebrobasilar system, and both PICA origins. At minimum, this study should be performed in AP and lateral projections. Other projections, such as a transorbital oblique, Waters', submentovertex, and Towne's, may also help in select cases (see Figure 4-1; Figure 4-8). The goal of performing a study in these other projections is to demonstrate the aneurysm neck and parent vessel relationship, which can be critical in planning either the surgical approach or endovascular technique for treatment (Figure 4-9).

If the ACOM is not visualized on routine injection, injection of one carotid artery during temporary cross-compression of the contralateral carotid artery should opacify this vessel, if present. Temporary compression of the ipsilateral carotid artery may also help opacification

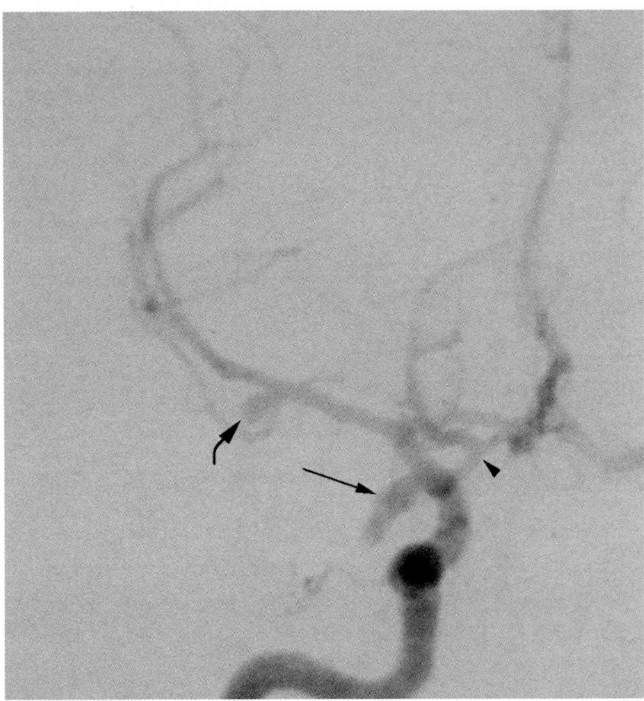

A

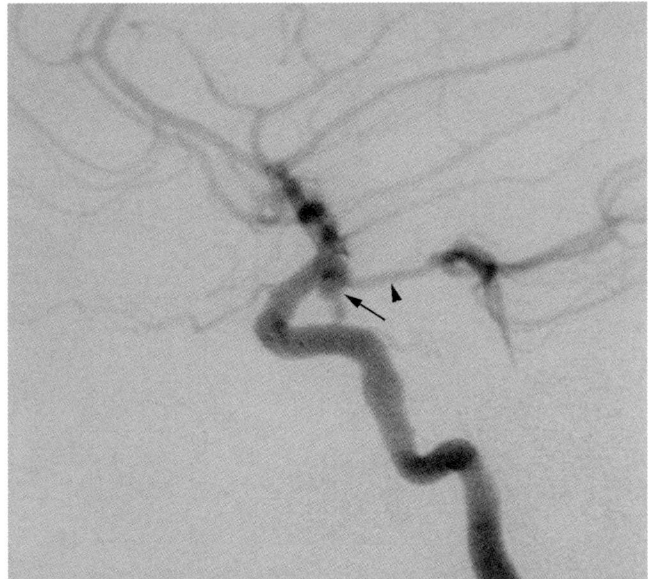

B

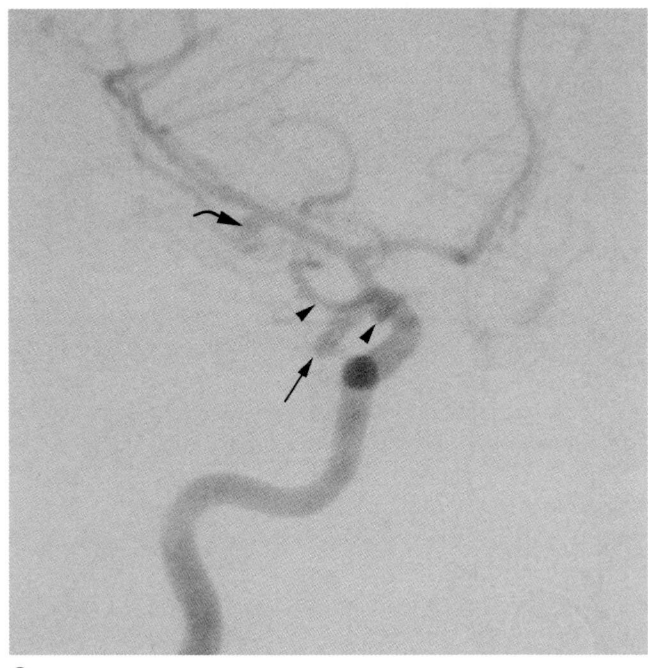

C

FIGURE 4-8. Cerebral aneurysms. **A.** Anterior-posterior projection of the right common carotid artery. A somewhat elongated aneurysm (*arrow*) arises from the origin of the posterior communicating artery (*arrowhead*) and internal carotid artery. A smaller right middle cerebral artery aneurysm (*curved arrow*) is also noted on this projection. **B.** Lateral projection again demonstrates the posterior communicating artery aneurysm (*arrow*) with its inferior daughter aneurysm. However, the exact relationship of the aneurysm neck to the posterior communicating artery (*arrowhead*) is not well delineated in this study. The daughter aneurysm indicates that this is an aneurysm that has ruptured. **C.** The right transorbital oblique projection nicely delineates the aneurysm (*arrow*) and the posterior communicating artery (*arrowheads*) arising from the medial aspect of the neck of the aneurysm and its junction with the internal carotid artery. The middle cerebral artery aneurysm is also delineated on this projection (*curved arrow*).

of the PCOM during vertebral artery injection. This maneuver can also help in differentiating a PCOM infundibulum (a funnel-shaped origin of the PCOM with small hemorrhage risk) from an aneurysm, as the infundibulum opacification should precede that of the ICA, whereas aneurysm opacification should follow the ICA. In the posterior circulation, the entire intracranial circulation of both vertebral arteries should be demonstrated. This usually can be achieved with injection of the dominant, usually left, vertebral artery. The contrast should reflux from the ipsilateral vertebral artery down into the contralateral vertebral artery to at least a few centimeters below the PICA to allow filling of the peri-PICA segment from the physiologic direction. If it does not, a separate injection of the contralateral vertebral artery is required.

The goals of angiographic evaluation of aneurysmal SAH are (1) evaluating the aneurysm in detail, including delineating the size and position of the aneurysm neck, the direction of the dome, and the presence of branches or perforating vessels at the neck; (2) imaging the entire intracranial circulation to search for other aneurysms because 20–33% of patients with an intracranial aneurysm have multiple aneurysms;[24] and (3) iden-

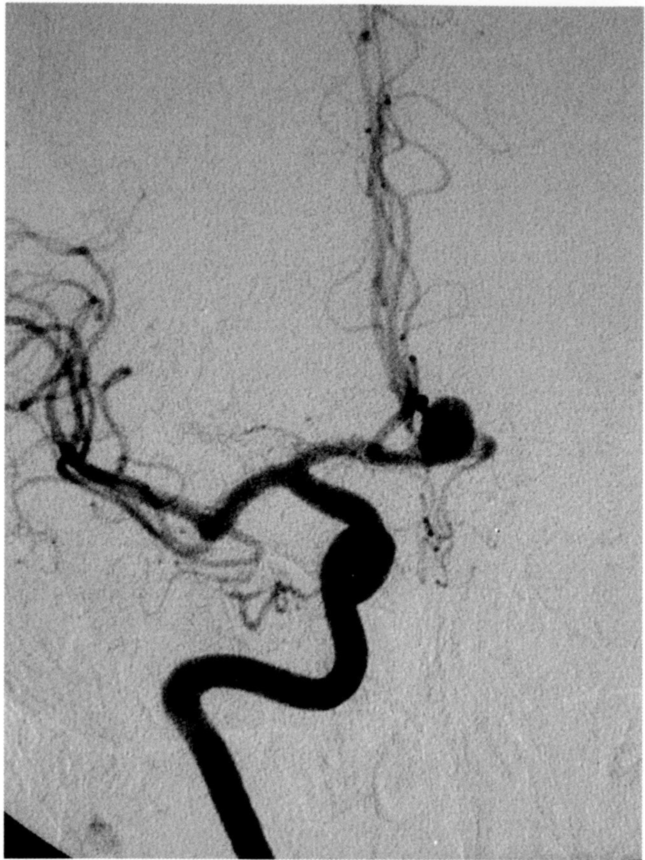

A

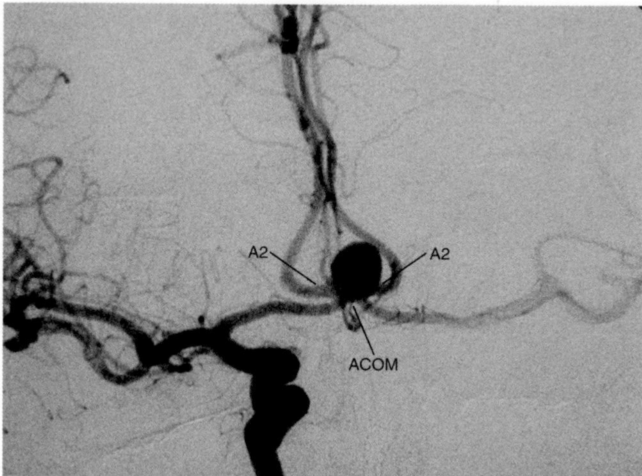

B

FIGURE 4-9. Unruptured anterior communicating artery aneurysm. **A.** The anterior-posterior view demonstrates the aneurysm involving the anterior communicating artery but does not delineate the neck or its relationship to its apparent vessels. In the Waters' projection (**B**), this relationship is well demonstrated, showing this aneurysm to have a wide neck involving the entire anterior communicating artery (ACOM) along with the origins of the A2 segments of both anterior cerebral arteries (A2). Often, unusual oblique angles are necessary to delineate aneurysm necks such as this, which favor surgical clipping over endovascular therapy.

tifying other associated abnormalities such as vasospasm, mass effect from associated hematoma, or herniation from diffuse swelling or hydrocephalus.

In the cases in which no aneurysm is visualized due to thrombosis or vasospasm, a repeat angiogram is often performed in several days if there is a high clinical suspicion as a result of the type or amount of SAH. On the follow-up angiogram, external carotid angiography should also be performed when no aneurysm is detected to evaluate for a dural arteriovenous fistula (DAVF). An MRI study can also detect subtle abnormalities in the subarachnoid space that may direct the follow-up angiographic study. In patients with a very high clinical suspicion, a third angiogram at approximately 6 weeks after SAH may detect an occult aneurysm not initially seen.

Some centers use CTA for initial screening in SAH. Due to its rapid availability and minimal risk, CTA can provide important information a few minutes after diagnosing SAH. The sensitivity of CTA is less than that of catheter angiography, so a formal follow-up catheter angiogram is recommended with an initially negative high-quality CT angiogram (Figure 4-10).

Aneurysms are commonly classified by their configuration (saccular and fusiform), their etiology (mycotic, traumatic, high flow related), and their size. Saccular aneurysms are round, oval, or sometimes irregular-shaped outpouchings that usually arise from arterial bifurcations. Anatomically, saccular aneurysms are commonly found in the circle of Willis and the bifurcation of the MCA. Approximately 90% of aneurysms are located on the anterior circulation, whereas the remaining 10% occur in the vertebrobasilar system. Common locations are the ACOM (30–35%), the junction of the internal carotid artery and PCOMs (30–35%), and the MCA bifurcation (20%).[25,26]

Unlike saccular aneurysms, fusiform aneurysms involve the entire circumference of the vessel wall, are usually large, and may be tortuous. They do not have a definable neck and can arise from congenital weakness (e.g., saccular aneurysms) or dissection, but they are most commonly associated with atherosclerotic vascular disease. In the basilar artery, atherosclerosis can result in dolichoectasia of the entire vessel. The atherosclerotic aneurysms are thought to carry a lower risk of SAH and often present with mass effect or embolic symptoms; however, the dissecting aneurysm type may have a very high hemorrhage rate (Figure 4-11).

Mycotic aneurysms are associated with various bacterial and fungal infections. Several authors have described an increased rate of aneurysms in immunocompromised patients that are thought to be directly caused by necrotizing vasculitis from the human immu-

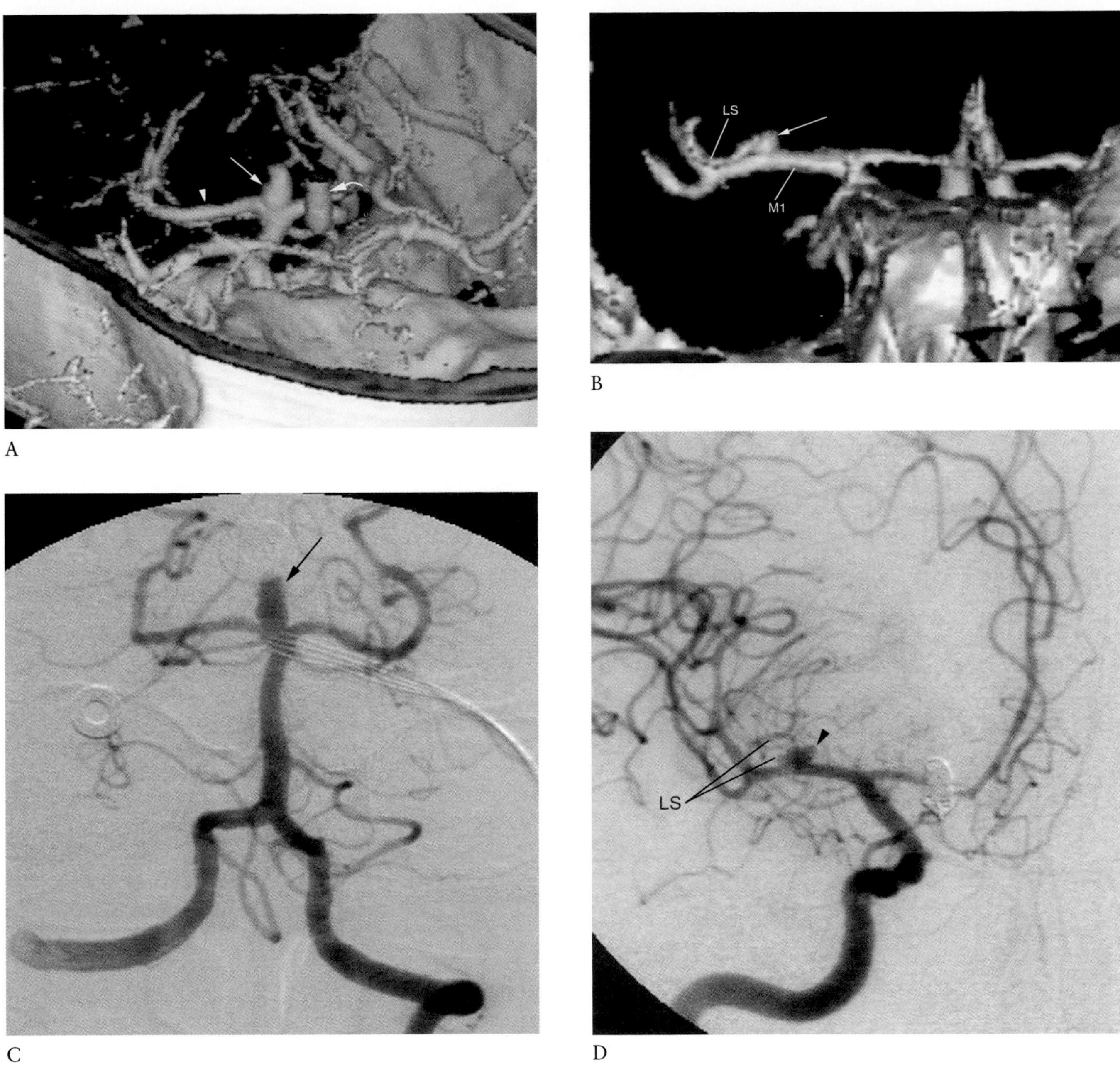

FIGURE 4-10. Computed tomographic angiogram (CTA) in a patient with a cerebral aneurysm. **A.** CTA in the Towne's right anterior oblique projection demonstrates a bilobed aneurysm of the basilar tip (*arrow*) and nicely delineates its relationship to the posterior cerebral arteries (*arrowhead*). A tip of the ventricular shunt catheter is also included (*curved arrow*). A Waters' projection (**B**) also demonstrates a small aneurysm (*arrow*) arising from a prominent right middle cerebral artery (M1) lenticulostriate branch (LS). Its relationship to this small lenticulostriate artery is not well delineated, and it appears as though this vessel arises from the dome. **C,D.** The catheter angiogram again demonstrates the basilar tip aneurysm (*arrow*), and after endovascular coil embolization of this aneurysm, the lenticulostriate aneurysm (*arrowhead*) is again demonstrated. The lenticulostriate artery (LS) is superimposed on the aneurysm but appears to arise from a lateral aspect of the aneurysm neck. This relationship allowed for successful coil embolization of this aneurysm. Three-dimensional catheter angiography may better delineate these more complex relationships than lower-resolution CTA or limited two-dimensional digital subtraction angiography.

nodeficiency virus or other acquired, possibly subclinical, infections such as syphilis and tuberculosis.[27,28] Mycotic aneurysms are due to impaction of a septic embolism in the intima of the vessel, resulting in arteritis, focal mural necrosis, and, ultimately, aneurysmal formation.[29] This explains the friable nature of the wall of these aneurysms and their propensity to rupture spontaneously or during surgery. Mycotic aneurysms are typ-

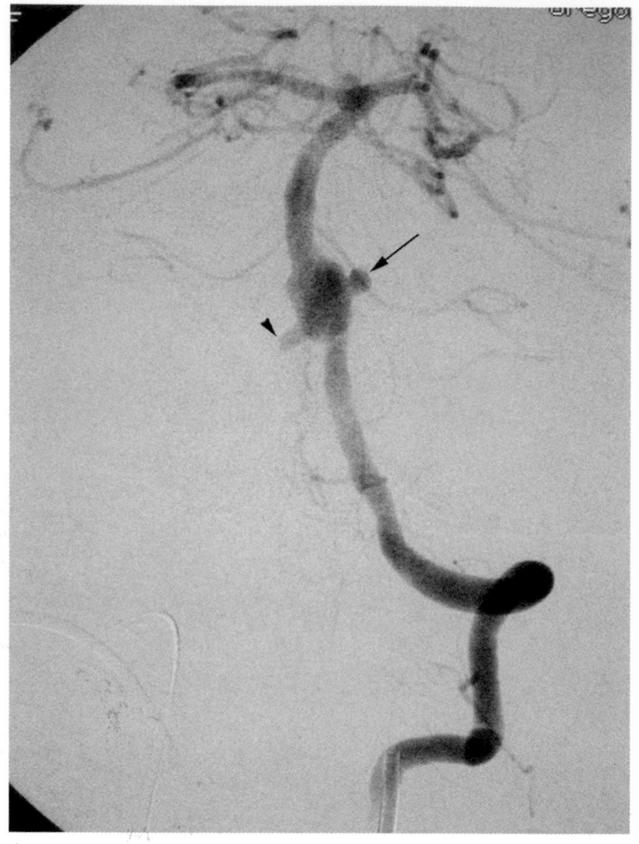

A

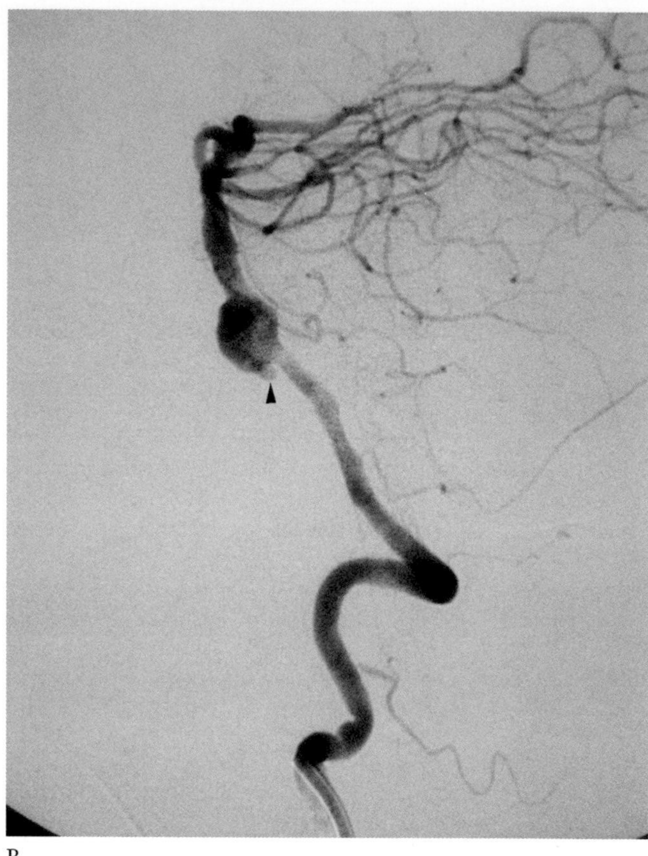

B

FIGURE 4-11. Fusiform dissecting aneurysm. Anterior-posterior (**A**) and lateral (**B**) projections demonstrate a fusiform irregular aneurysm arising from the vertebrobasilar junction. This aneurysm involves the entire wall and has a daughter aneurysm (*arrow*) along its left lateral margin. The slight filling of the right vertebral artery (*arrowheads*) is also noted. Its fusiform shape and the patient's presentation suggested this may represent a dissecting aneurysm or merely a fusiform aneurysm with a secondary daughter sac, the most likely rupture site.

ically found in the distal vessels, are often multiple in number, and are often irregular in shape. Unlike congenital aneurysms, they are not commonly located in vessel bifurcations (Figure 4-12). Patients with mycotic aneurysms may develop new aneurysms during the initial month after antibiotic treatment, as the initial necrosis may have set in. Follow-up angiography at 2-week intervals during this period is recommended.

Traumatic aneurysms are caused by direct penetrating or nonpenetrating high-velocity trauma as well as after surgical injury. Penetrating traumatic aneurysms are commonly associated with multiple bone or metal fragments near the aneurysm. These are often false aneurysms or pseudoaneurysms and are contained by a hematoma or parenchyma rather than the vessel wall. Nonpenetrating traumatic aneurysms can also occur as a result of shear injury, most commonly at the collosomarginal branches against the falx cerebri or the MCA against the sphenoid ridge.[30]

Flow-related aneurysms are thought to result from vascular response to a high flow state, which may lead to generalized dilation and focal aneurysmal formation in areas of weakness. The incidence of aneurysms is increased within AVMs, with most studies reporting a 5–15% association of an aneurysm and AVM.[31] These aneurysms are found in the circle of Willis, along the feeding vessel to the AVM, in the nidus, or, less commonly, in a remote site hemodynamically unrelated to the AVM. A majority of AVM patients demonstrate multiple aneurysms (Figure 4-13).

Vascular Malformations of the Brain

Conceptually, there are five types of vascular malformations of the CNS:

1. AVM
2. Cavernous malformation
3. Capillary telangiectasia
4. Developmental venous anomaly (venous angioma)
5. DAVF

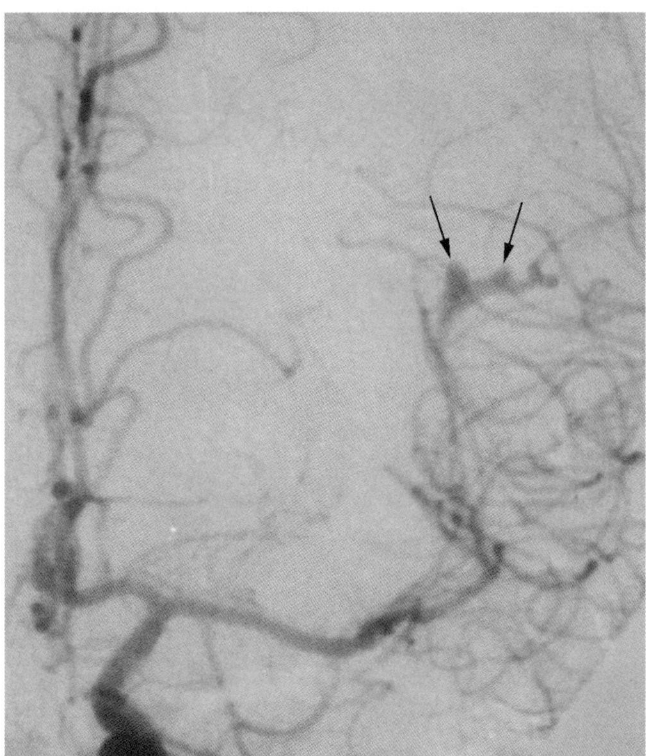

FIGURE 4-12. Mycotic aneurysm. Left middle cerebral anterior-posterior projection demonstrates an irregular enlargement of the distal sylvian portion of the left angular artery consistent with mycotic aneurysm (*arrows*). This patient presented with an adjacent intraparenchymal hemorrhage.

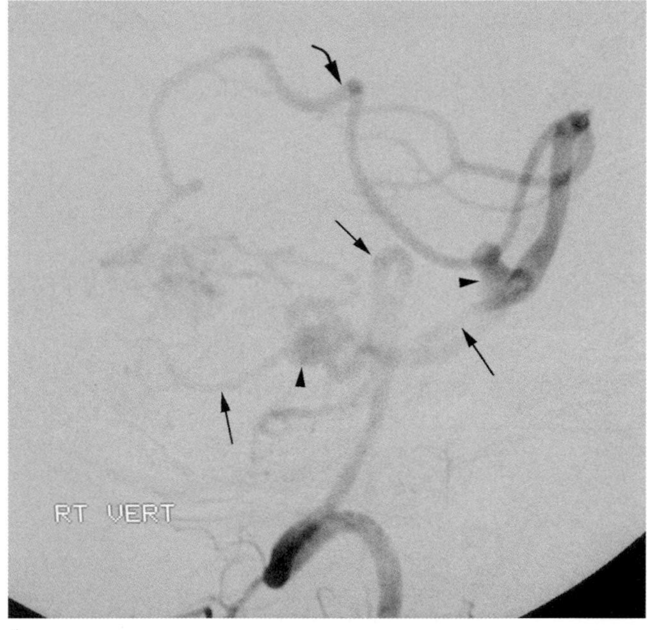

A

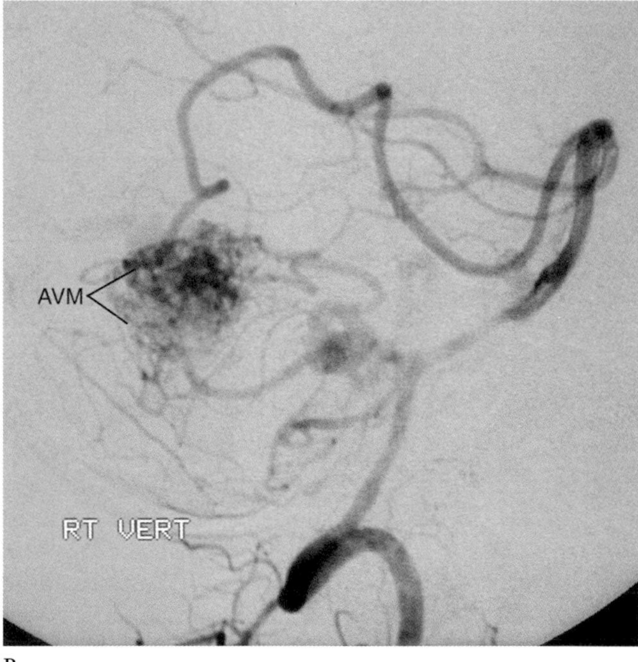

B

FIGURE 4-13. Cerebellar arteriovenous malformation with aneurysms. Early (**A**) and mid- (**B**) arterial phase demonstrates a modest-sized arteriovenous malformation (AVM) in the right cerebellar hemisphere being supplied by an anterior inferior cerebellar artery branch (*arrows*) that has two feeding pedicle aneurysms (*arrowheads*). There is also supply from the superior cerebellar artery (*curved arrow*). The presence of these aneurysms can significantly alter the endovascular treatment and the surgical approach, especially aneurysms in the region of the nidus. (RT VERT = right vertebral artery.)

An AVM of the brain is the product of abnormal angiogenesis of the cerebral vasculature consisting of an abnormal tangle of vessels (nidus) that permit artery-to-vein shunting with no intervening capillaries. The afferent artery and efferent vein are abnormally dilated. Microscopically, there may be small amounts of intervening neural tissue that are often gliotic and can potentially become a seizure focus. AVMs are thought to be sporadic in occurrence and nonfamilial or not inherited, except in rare vascular malformations associated with hereditary hemorrhagic telangiectasia (Rendu-Osler-Weber syndrome) or Wyburn-Mason's syndrome.

Spontaneous hemorrhage is the most common presentation of an AVM, accounting for 41–79% of cases. The second most common presentation of an AVM is seizures, which occur in 11–33% of cases.[32] Both classic and common migraines have been reported in association with an AVM. In contrast to patients with classic or common migraine headaches, patients who are diagnosed with an AVM often complain of headaches and unilateral visual symptomatology that are consistently referable to the side of the lesion; however, significant overlap exists.

A CT or MRI brain scan commonly establishes the diagnosis of an AVM. Hence, cerebral angiography supports an analytic rather than a diagnostic role in evaluation

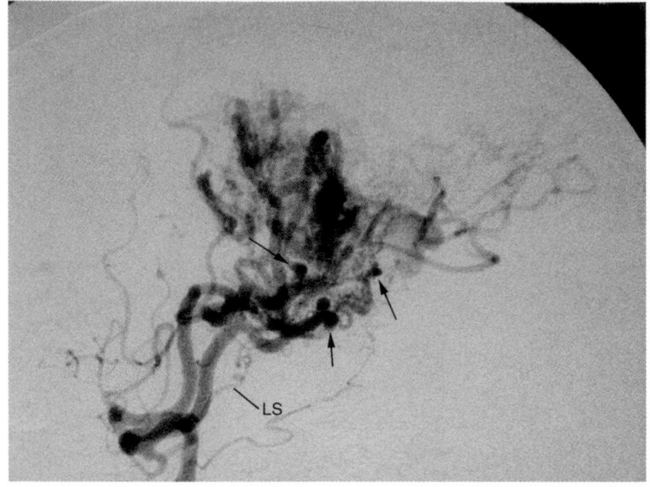

A

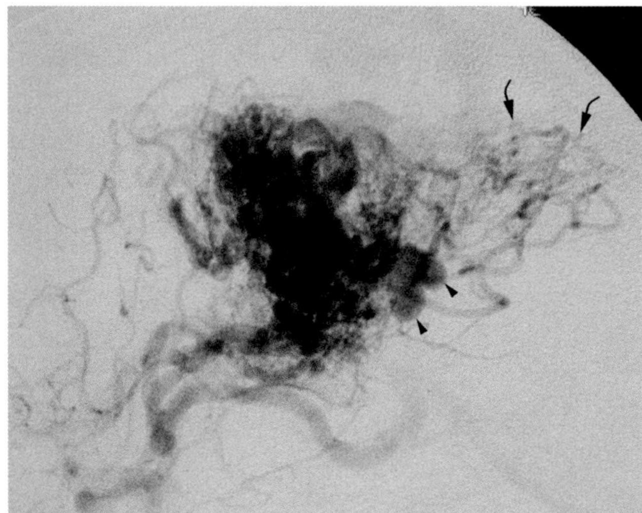

B

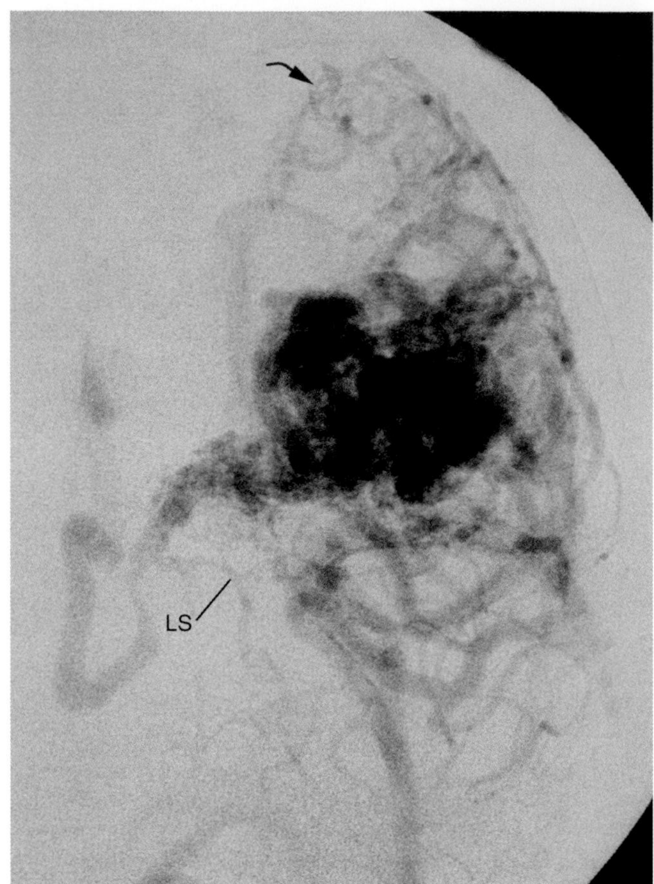

C

FIGURE 4-14. Parietal arteriovenous malformation (AVM) with nidus aneurysms and angiomatous change. Lateral early (**A**) and late (**B**) arterial phases of the left internal carotid artery angiogram demonstrate enlarged middle cerebral artery–feeding pedicles with small aneurysms (*arrows*) within and adjacent to the nidus along with an early draining varix (*arrowheads*). The angular parietal branch fills the AVM via angiomatous change (*curved arrows*) with a network of numerous small vascular channels collateral to and filling the posterior aspect of the AVM. On the Towne's projection (**C**), this angiomatous change is also demonstrated along with lenticulostriate supply (LS) to the portion of this AVM.

of an AVM (see Figure 4-13). The goals of angiographic evaluation of an AVM are (1) identifying the individual feeding arteries and draining veins; (2) determining the size of the nidus; (3) detecting the presence of any aneurysms; (4) identifying angiomatous changes and high flow angiopathy; (5) detecting the presence of an arteriovenous fistula; and (6) determining the degree of venous restrictive disease.

The most challenging technical aspect of cerebral angiography of an AVM is achieving adequate opacification of the lesion. Based on prior diagnostic information on the AVM, few technical modifications may be required during the cerebral angiogram, such as (1) increasing the rate and volume of injection; (2) increasing the filming rate beyond the standard two or three films per second to four films per second or higher; (3) filming until the entire shunted and normal venous drainage system is opacified; and (4) using size markers to improve estimation of the nidus size and to correct magnification.

Over time, an AVM induces secondary changes in the surrounding vascular structure. Angiomatous changes may occur with recruitment of collateral vessels that should not be considered part of the AVM. Angiomatous *change* is different from angiomatous *nidus* (Figure 4-14). An angiomatous nidus is a morphologic feature of a fine, nodular, mass-like network of vessels rather than a fistulous nidus, which has a larger portion of direct arteriovenous fistulas. High-resolution and high-speed imaging often distinguish the angiomatous change from the actual nidus. Angiomatous change is usually a reticulated fine network of collateral vessels that ultimately fill the feeding vessels. If this is adjacent to the nidus and supplies small feeders, it can be very difficult to differentiate and often cannot be seen until superselective angiography at the time of an embolization treatment. Features of angiomatous change include a more normal velocity of flow and subsequent opacification in the collateral vessels, compared to the higher velocity in the directly feeding vessels.

High flow angiopathy is a variable degree of vascular dilatation associated with a high flow state. Microscopically, it is caused by necrosis and vacuolization of the media muscle and by invasion of adventitia by foreign cells and small blood vessels. Aneurysms may develop in the weakened vessel wall. These dysplastic changes often reverse after the AVM is obliterated.[33]

Hemorrhage is the most serious complication of a cerebral AVM. An unruptured AVM has a 2–4% chance of bleeding per year. The mortality rate increases with the number of hemorrhages. Clinical factors such as systemic hypertension and morphologic features such as large size, large arteriovenous fistulas, and venous drainage are associated with a higher rate of hemorrhage in AVMs. A single draining vein, deep venous drainage alone, or severely impaired venous drainage increases the rate of hemorrhage.[34]

Although it is difficult to predict the natural risk of an AVM, Spetzler and Martin have developed a grading system to guide decision making in the therapy of an AVM. The grading system is based on the nidus size, eloquent location, and type of venous drainage. The nidus size is measured angiographically and corrected for magnification. The eloquent location includes the sensory, motor, language, and visual cortices; hypothalamus; thalamus; internal capsule; brain stem; cerebellar peduncles; and deep cerebellar nuclei. The deep venous drainage is comprised of vessels that drain into the internal cerebral vein, basal veins of Rosenthal, vein of Galen, and straight sinus. Each criterion is assigned a point. Each patient is categorized into grade I–V based on the sum of the point values of size, location, and venous drainage.[35]

Spetzler-Martin AVM Grading System	Point
Size	
Small <3 cm	1
Medium 3–6 cm	2
Large >6 cm	3
Location	
Noneloquent	0
Eloquent	1
Pattern of venous drainage	
Superficial vein	0
Deep draining vein	1

Grades I, II, and III are considered low grade, whereas grades IV and V are high grade. The lower-grade AVM is associated with better prognosis. In a study of 100 patients with a cerebral AVM who received microsurgical resection, the permanent major neurologic morbidity for grades I–III was 0%, increasing to 17% in grade IV and 22% in grade V.[36,37]

Cavernous malformations (hemangioma) represent discrete venous sinusoids with variable thrombosis. Capillary telangiectasias are microscopically dilated capillaries commonly seen pathologically but usually barely perceptible with gadolinium-enhanced MR brain scans. Both are angiographically occult; therefore, angiography is not usually performed unless adjacent vessels or atypical MR features require exclusion of an associated AVM.

A developmental venous anomaly (venous angioma) is a collection of veins draining normal parenchyma in an abnormal way, such as the cortex draining into the internal cerebral veins or the basal ganglia draining to the surface. They rarely hemorrhage but usually are associated with cavernous malformations that bleed. The venous anomaly has a typical "caput medusae" appearance on enhanced CT or MR brain scans. Angiography is usually only necessary if unusual features are present.

DAVFs are almost always acquired lesions and, therefore, are not true congenital malformations. They consist of numerous channels in the wall of a dural sinus being supplied by dural arteries such as the middle meningeal, ascending pharyngeal, and occipital arteries. Depending on their venous drainage pattern, DAVFs may present with pulse-synchronous bruit, signs and symptoms of carotid cavernous fistula, or hemorrhage. The risk of hemorrhage is variable and related to retrograde sinus or cortical venous drainage (Figure 4-15). Numerous classification schemes have been described; conceptually, however, five drainage patterns exist[38]:

1. Patent sinus, antegrade drainage
2. Patent sinus, antegrade and retrograde drainage
3. Occluded sinus, retrograde sinus drainage
4. Cortical and sinus drainage
5. Cortical venous drainage only

In descending order, the degree of venous hypertension and, hence, risk of stroke and hemorrhage increase.

Treatment depends on the type of lesion. The lower-risk lesions may require no treatment, whereas the higher-risk lesions with cortical venous drainage require endovascular, surgical, or combined treatments, depending on venous access. Angiographic assessment usually requires selective ICA and ECA injections and evaluation of both vertebral arteries.

Vascular Tumors

Angiography plays an important role in the evaluation of vascular intracranial, skull base, and head and neck

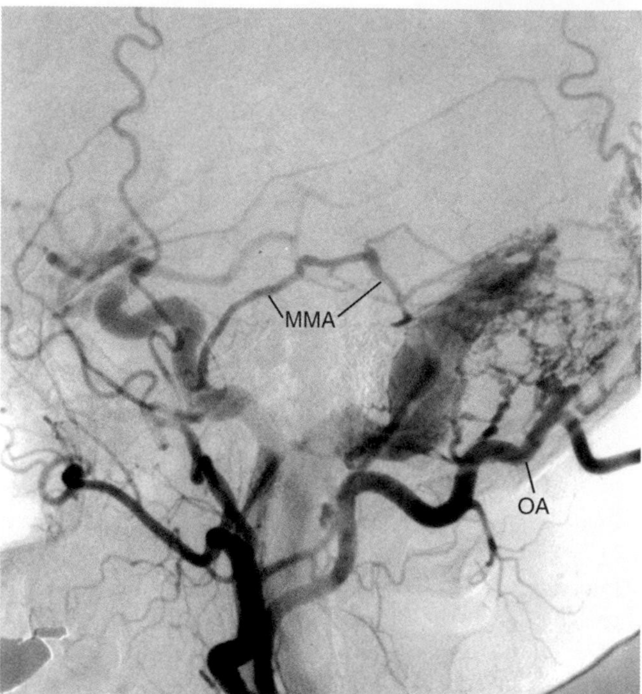

FIGURE 4-15. Type I dural arteriovenous fistula. This right external carotid artery angiogram with some reflux into the internal carotid artery vessels demonstrates numerous dural branches from the occipital artery (OA) and posterior division of the middle meningeal artery (MMA), which supply this transverse sigmoid sinus dural arteriovenous fistula with antegrade venous drainage. This patient had a modest pulse-synchronous bruit that was tolerable and did not require therapy.

tumors, including hemangioblastoma, meningioma, paraganglioma, and some vascular schwannomas. The goals of angiography in vascular tumors include (1) determining the arterial supply and venous drainage; (2) evaluating the degree of vascular blush and overall tumor neovascularity; (3) evaluating the displacement, compression, or occlusion of adjacent or encompassed normal vessels; (4) determining the degree of collateral supply in cases in which cerebral vascular sacrifice is anticipated; and (5) assisting other imaging studies in a preoperative diagnosis. These goals are primarily designed for presurgical evaluation and to assist in the surgical approach, expected complications, and adjunctive measures such as surgical bypass or preoperative embolization.

In the evaluation of vascularity and vascular supply of tumors, it is very important to differentiate the internal and external carotid vascular supply, which can alter management. A meningioma with significant pial to meningeal collateral supply likely will have a higher hemorrhage rate, and the surgeon may leave a cap of tissue to avoid risk of injury to the adjacent brain. This pial supply does not indicate brain invasion or malignancy. Knowing the degree of ECA supply versus ICA supply is also helpful in determining the expected degree of devascularization from transarterial embolization. Therefore, selective internal and external carotid angiography are recommended if it is safe to catheterize the ICA. If catheterization is not safe, then common carotid and external carotid angiography suffices, and the differential vessels and blush estimate the internal supply. The vertebral arteries usually need evaluation, and the skull base evaluation of the ascending pharyngeal artery may also require a common carotid artery study. In head and neck tumors, other vessels such as the thyrocervical trunk, which includes the inferior thyroidal artery and ascending cervical artery, may need evaluation.

Meningiomas have highly variable vascularity, and, although there is no correlation with the degree of gadolinium or contrast enhancement, there is correlation with the presence of central flow voids. Meningiomas typically have a central core of meningeal vessels in a radiating pattern (the "sunburst" pattern) and often have a peripheral cap of draining veins (see Figure 4-15). The vascular blush is usually a homogeneous, fine, and persistent blush that stays long after the venous phase. Meningiomas, along with other vascular tumors of the skull and skull base, are supplied primarily by the middle, anterior, and posterior meningeal arteries, depending on location, but also are supplied by other vessels to the skull such as the occipital, ascending pharyngeal, ophthalmic, and petrous branches of the ICA. As mentioned previously, meningiomas may recruit pial vascular supply, which increases the risk of surgical resection (Figure 4-16).

Paragangliomas (glomus tumors), vascular schwannomas, and hemangioblastomas usually have a much coarser vascular blush and often show early draining veins indicative of arteriovenous shunting (Figures 4-17 and 4-18). As such, they often look more like a vascular malformation, although their well-defined, usually rounded margins are indicative of a mass lesion. It is helpful to extend the angiogram throughout the normal venous phase to determine the patency and position of the internal jugular veins. Malignant squamous cell carcinoma is almost always angiographically hypovascular; however, it can have a modest vascular blush. Such tumors are rarely evaluated angiographically, as imaging studies are usually specific, and angiography is not necessary except in cases of persistent hemorrhage.

Spinal Angiography

Spinal angiography is performed for evaluation of spinal vascular malformations, vascular spinal column or spinal cord tumors, or preoperative localization of spinal cord vascular supply; however, it is not commonly performed even at neurointerventional centers. Depending on the indication, spinal angiography can be limited to a few intercostals or lumbar pedicles or can extend to selective evaluation of all of the intercostals and lumbar pedicles,

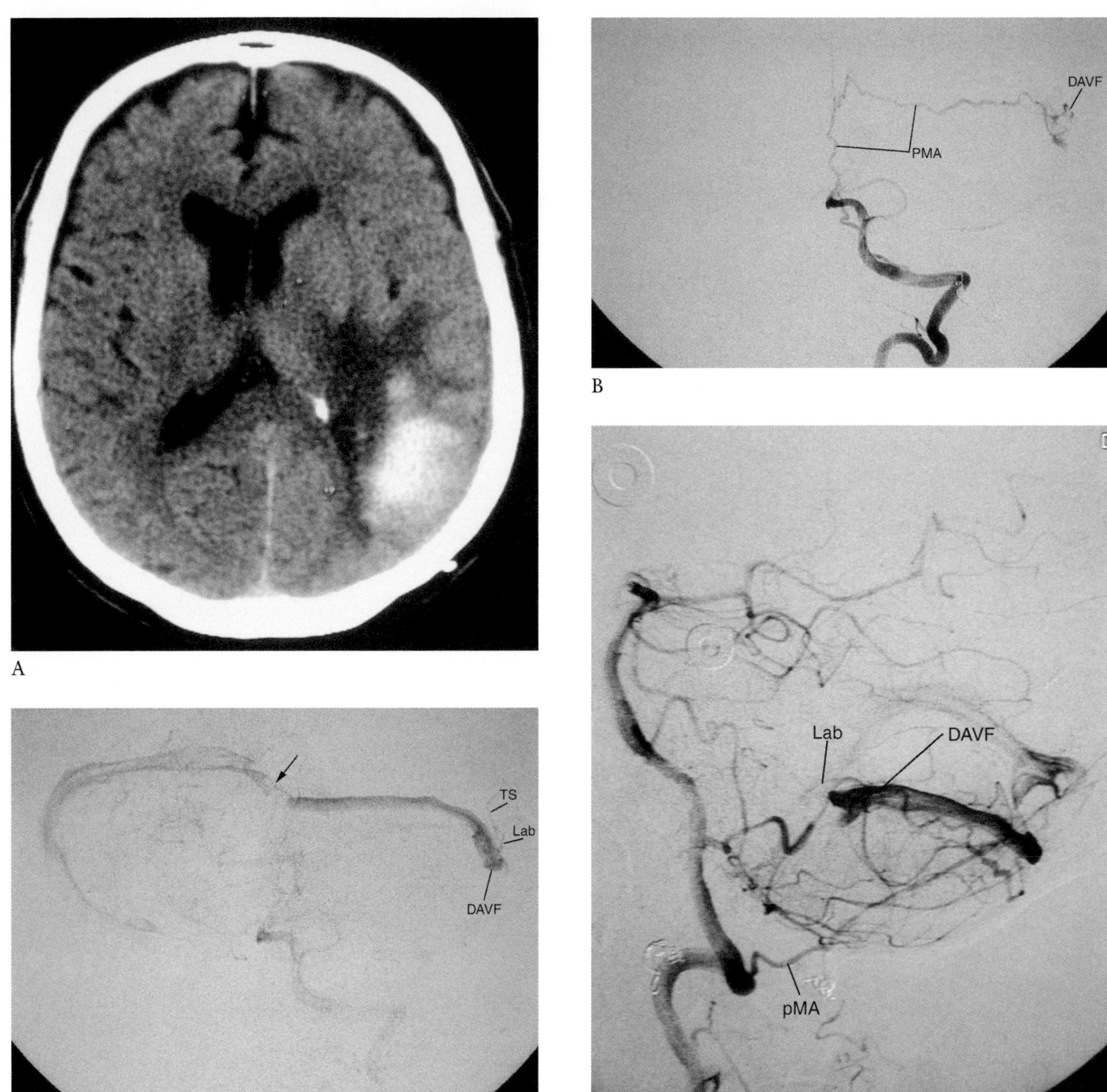

A B C D

FIGURE 4-16. Type IV dural arteriovenous fistula. This patient presented with a left posterolateral temporal parietal hematoma as demonstrated on the computed tomography scan (**A**). The early (**B**) and late (**C**) arterial phases of the left vertebral artery angiogram and mid-arterial lateral view (**D**) demonstrate an enlarged posterior meningeal artery (PMA; pMA) that fills this short segment dural arteriovenous fistula (DAVF) at the transverse sigmoid junction (TS). The sigmoid sinus on this side is occluded, and there is retrograde filling across the torcula to the right transverse sigmoid sinus. There is also some mild retrograde filling of the vein of Labbé (Lab); however, only the proximal segment filled, suggesting that the occlusion most likely resulted in the hemorrhage. This was treated with transfemoral transvenous coil embolization of the involved segment via the right jugular venous system. Navigation through the small collateral channel at the torcula (*arrow*) was difficult and required good angiographic demonstration of this channel versus the normal venous channels.

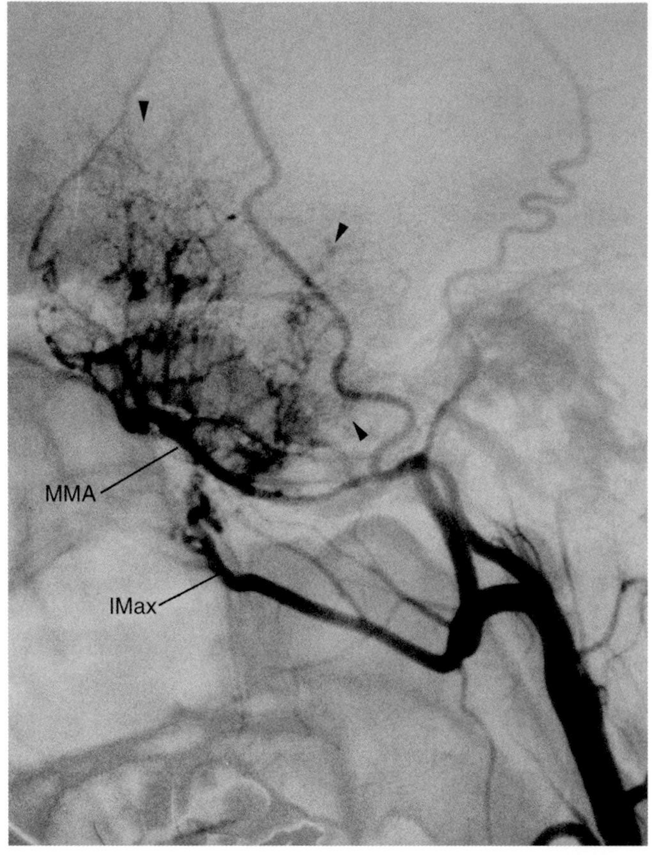

A

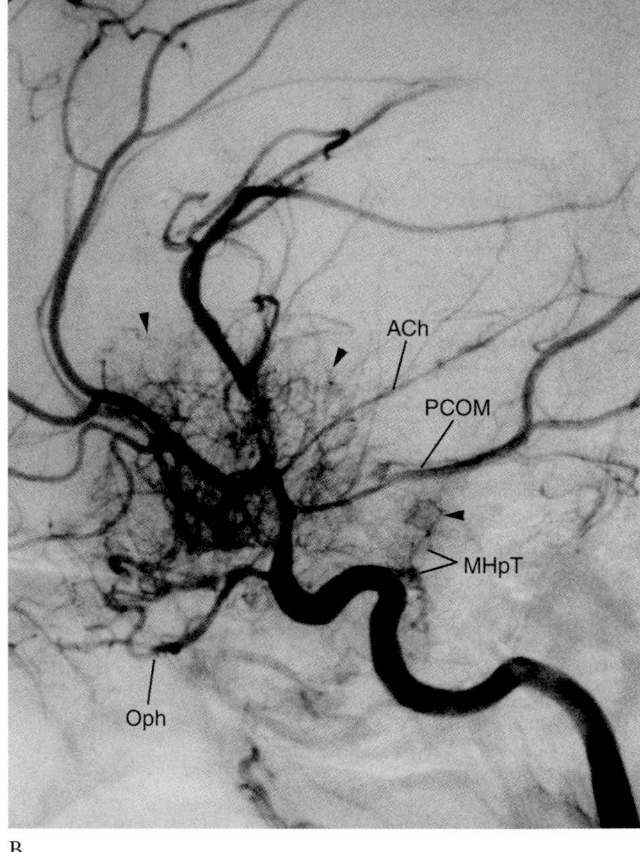

B

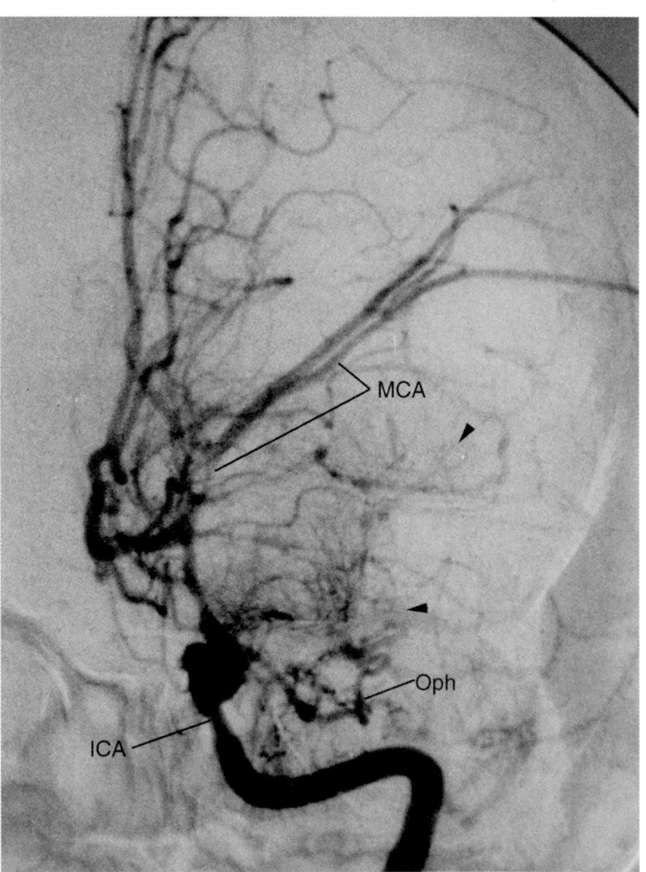

C

FIGURE 4-17. Sphenoid wing meningioma. Lateral external carotid artery (**A**), internal carotid artery (ICA) (**B**), and anterior-posterior internal carotid artery (**C**) angiograms demonstrate a typical radiating pattern of arterial supply (*arrowheads*) to a large sphenoid wing meningioma. This is supplied by the middle meningeal artery (MMA) along with collateral branches of the internal maxillary (IMax) and ophthalmic (Oph) arteries. There is also supply of the posterior aspect via the meningohypophyseal trunk artery (MHpT). This mass extends medially to involve and encase the supraclinoid ICA with narrowing of the posterior communicating artery (PCOM), displacement and stretching of the anterior choroidal artery (ACh), and marked uplifting displacement and narrowing of the left middle cerebral artery (MCA).

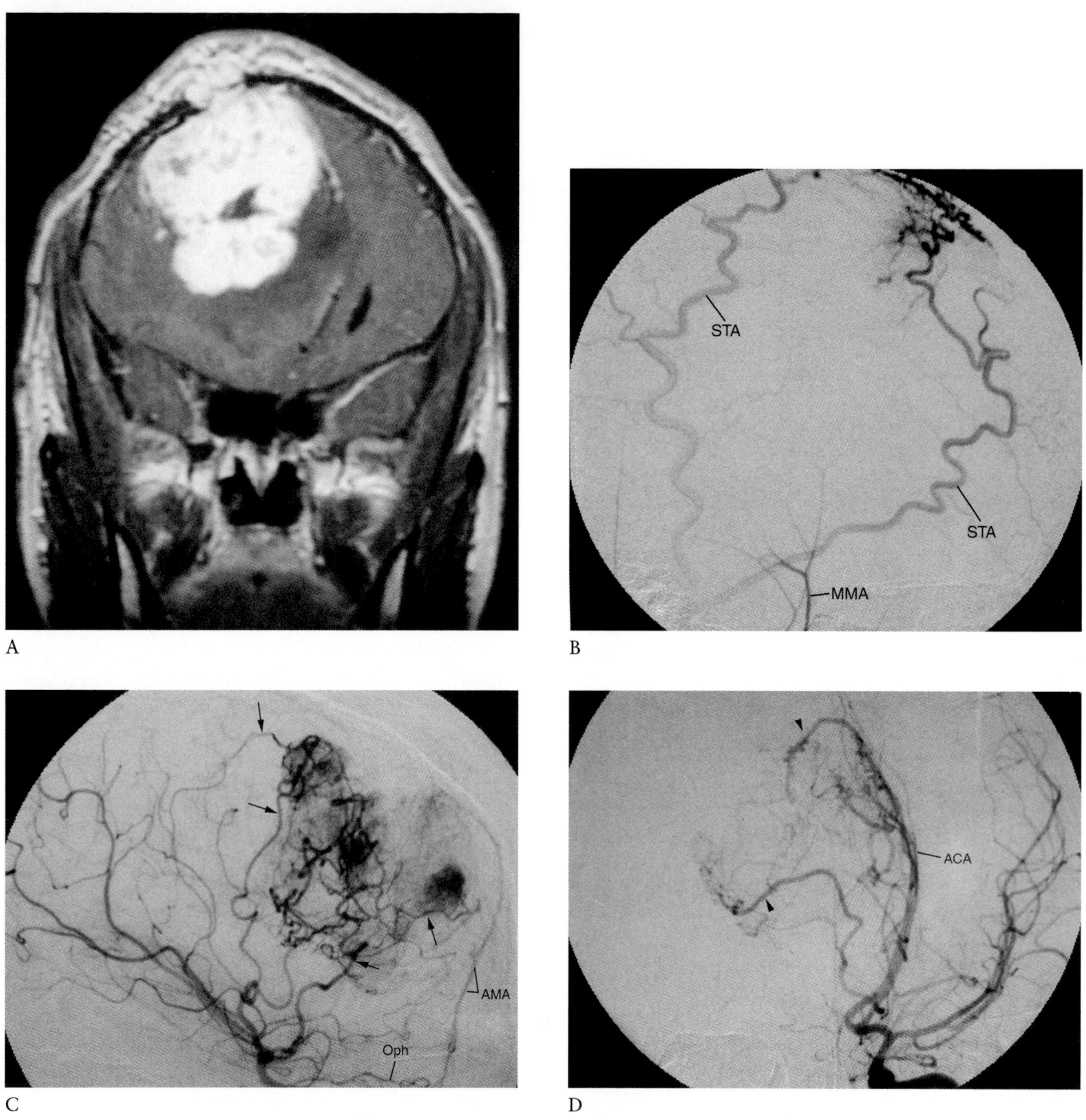

FIGURE 4-18. Aggressive meningioma with pial vascular supply. A large, enhancing right frontal meningioma that extends through the skull into the subcutaneous tissues as seen on the coronal magnetic resonance image (**A**). Lateral right external carotid (**B**) and internal carotid (**C**) artery angiograms. There is significant supply from dilated branches of the superficial temporal artery (STA) with no significant supply from the middle meningeal artery (MMA) on the external carotid artery study. On the internal carotid artery angiogram, there is pial vascular supply from multiple frontal branches of the right middle cerebral artery (*arrows*) and supply from the anterior meningeal artery (AMA) arising from the ophthalmic artery (Oph). The anterior-posterior left carotid artery angiogram (**D**) demonstrates the significant mass effect with frontal shift of the anterior cerebral arteries (ACAs) with pial vascular supply from the right ACA branches (*arrowheads*).

both vertebral arteries, subclavian arteries, internal iliacs, and other vessels that may supply the spinal canal. Selective catheterization of the right and left segmental intercostal and lumbar arteries is usually necessary, although flush aortograms are sometimes needed. In the lower thoracic and lumbar aorta, a retrograde flush aortogram with a straight end-hole catheter will selectively opacify the posterior spinal vessels over the anterior splanchnic vessels and may improve detection. Because the aortic spinal vessels arise as side branches, a wide-arched side-pointing catheter (Cobra C-2, Mikkelson) is usually effective in selecting vessels for angiography. The lumbar vessels tend to project inferiorly, and a reverse-curved catheter, such as a Simmons, may be more effective. Techniques to minimize the patient's diaphragmatic (general anesthesia and chemical paralysis) and gastrointestinal motion (glucagon) are often required.

Spinal vascular malformation is a rare disease compared to intracranial AVM. Spinal vascular malformations can be conceptually divided into two simple categories: intradural spinal cord malformation and DAVF.[39] Intradural spinal cord AVMs are congenital lesions in which the nidus may be located within the spinal cord (intramedullary) or on the spinal cord surface (perimedullary) (Figure 4-19). They can have an angiomatous nidus (glomus) or a single arteriovenous fistula. The arterial supply for both types arises from the anterior and posterior spinal arteries and drains into dilated, ascending, and descending veins located dorsal and ventral to the spinal cord. Approximately 20% of the spinal AVMs are associated with aneurysms and constitute a significant risk of acute intramedullary hemorrhage or SAH. As such, the patients usually present at an earlier age with more acute symptoms than DAVF, although they can present with a slowly progressive myelopathy. Angiography in patients with a suspected spinal cord AVM involves selective studies for finding the artery of Adamkiewicz and anterior spinal artery. The anterior spinal artery will almost always supply the thoracic spinal cord AVMs (Figure 4-20). Other selective studies are necessary to uncover vascular supply from the posterior spinal arteries. As in the brain, angiographically occult cavernous malformations and complex mixed spinal column intradural malformations can also exist.

A spinal DAVF, like its intracranial counterpart, is an acquired arteriovenous vascular communication situated in the dura of the spinal canal and is usually supplied by one or more dural branches of a radicular artery (Figure 4-21). They almost always lie in the dural thecal sac immediately below a pedicle. The fistula then drains into arterialized radicular, medullary, and spinal perimedullary veins. The arterialized veins may extend for several segments above or below the level of the feeder and may even extend the entire length of the spinal column (Figure 4-22). The resultant venous hypertension results in capillary hypertension and presents with a slow, progressive onset of myelopathy. MRI usually demonstrates dilated tortuous vessels dorsal, and sometimes ventral, to the spinal cord and may show multilevel central increased T2-cord signal and possible enhancement. Spinal DAVFs are usually supplied by a single radicular artery that does not usually supply the spinal cord. As such, they are notoriously elusive lesions. The angiographic evaluation may require injection of all of the thoracic, lumbar, vertebral, internal iliac, and even bronchial arteries until the correct pedicle is found.

Spinal vascular tumor evaluation is similar to that in the head and neck and usually requires a more limited evaluation of the abnormal intercostal or lumbar level and one or two levels above and below the lesion site. This may be performed in conjunction with preoperative embolization and may also include evaluation of the pedicle supplying the artery of Adamkiewicz to help in surgical planning. As expected, spinal cord vascular tumors, such as a hemangioblastoma, are supplied by a pedicle that may also supply the spinal cord.

CONCLUSION

Due to a wide range of treatment options available to patients with neurovascular diseases, including surgical, radiation, or endovascular therapy, a detailed diagnostic angiographic study is a critical factor in determining appropriate treatment for a patient. The various cerebrovascular diseases often require unique projections and techniques to be adequately evaluated. A thorough understanding of neurovascular diseases and knowledge of available technical modifications are critical in performing thorough and safe neuroangiography.

FIGURE 4-19. ▶ Spinal cord arteriovenous malformation. **A.** Sagittal T2-weighted image demonstrates multiple irregular vascular channels in the spinal canal. The small tuft or glomus is noted at the T11-T12 interspace (*arrowhead*). This small tuft appears to lie within the parenchyma of the conus on the magnetic resonance image and is consistent with an intramedullary spinal arteriovenous malformation. A small draining vein (*arrow*) is noted. **B.** Lateral spinal angiogram with injection of the right T10 intercostal artery demonstrates supply to the anterior spinal artery (ASA), which descends to supply the small nidus (*arrowhead*) and then the initial draining of vein (*arrow*), which correlates well with the magnetic resonance image. On the early anterior-posterior view (**C**), one can see the ASA, the arteriovenous malformation glomus (*arrowhead*) and draining vein (*arrow*), and, slightly later (**D**), an ascending draining vein (*curved arrow*).

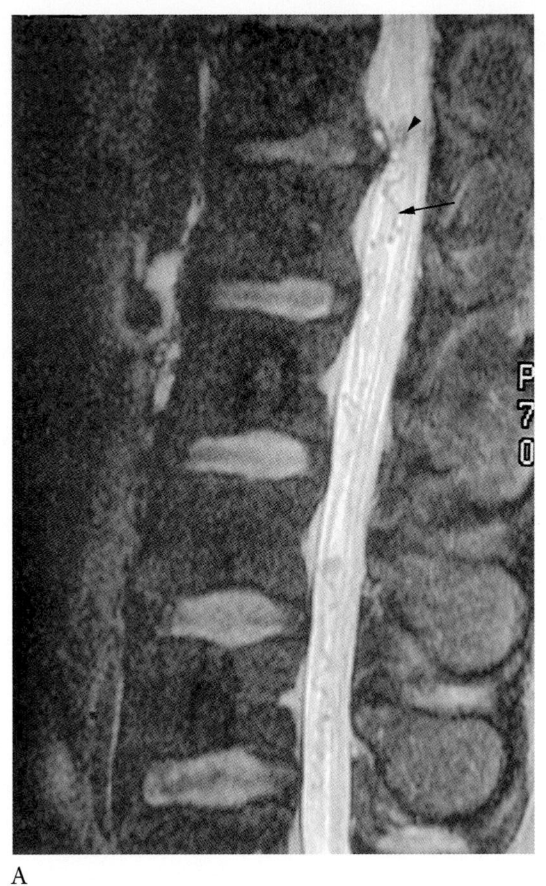

A

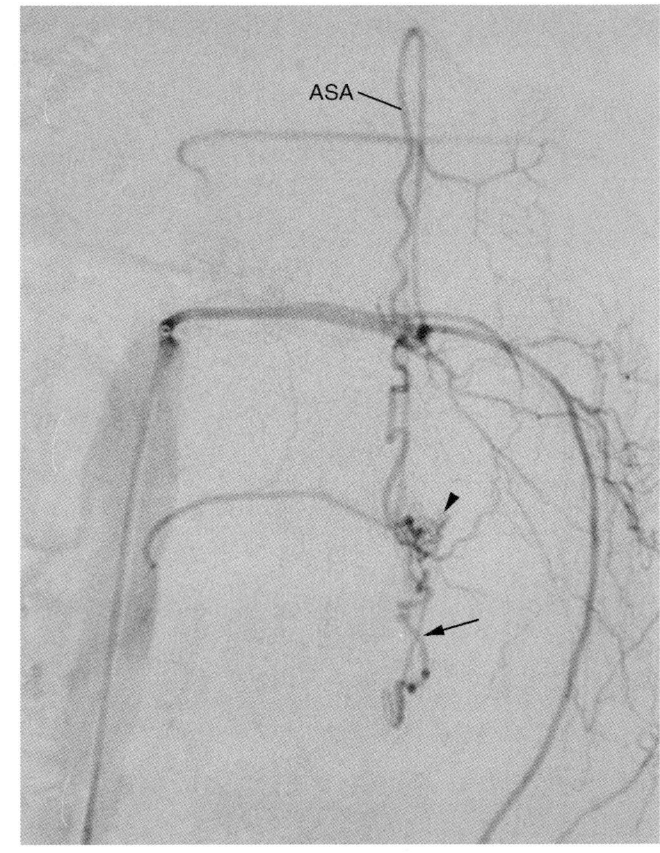

B

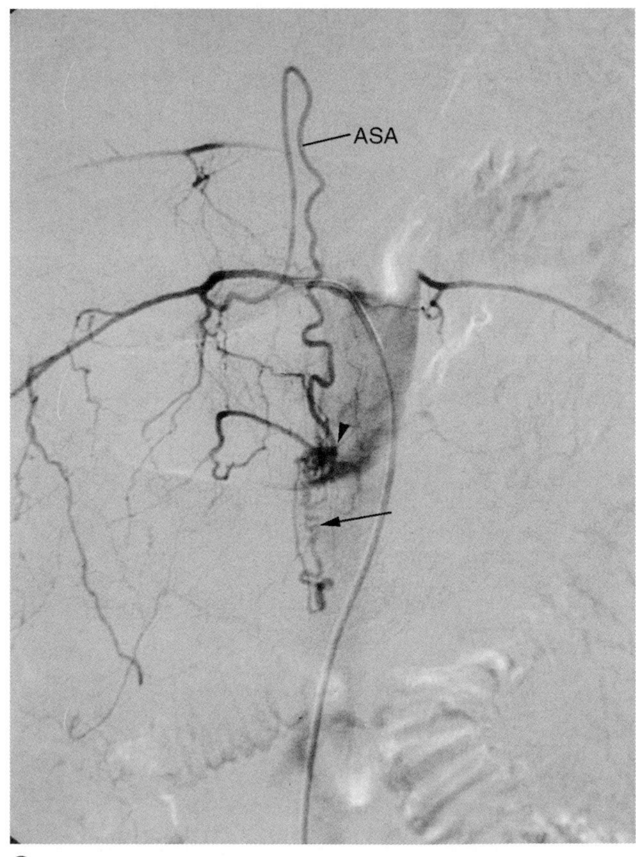

C

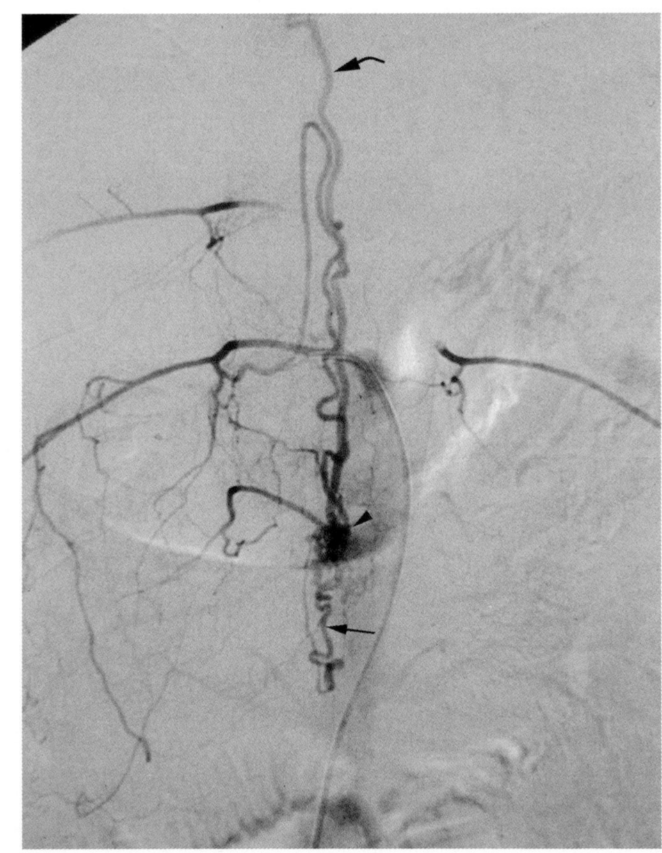
D

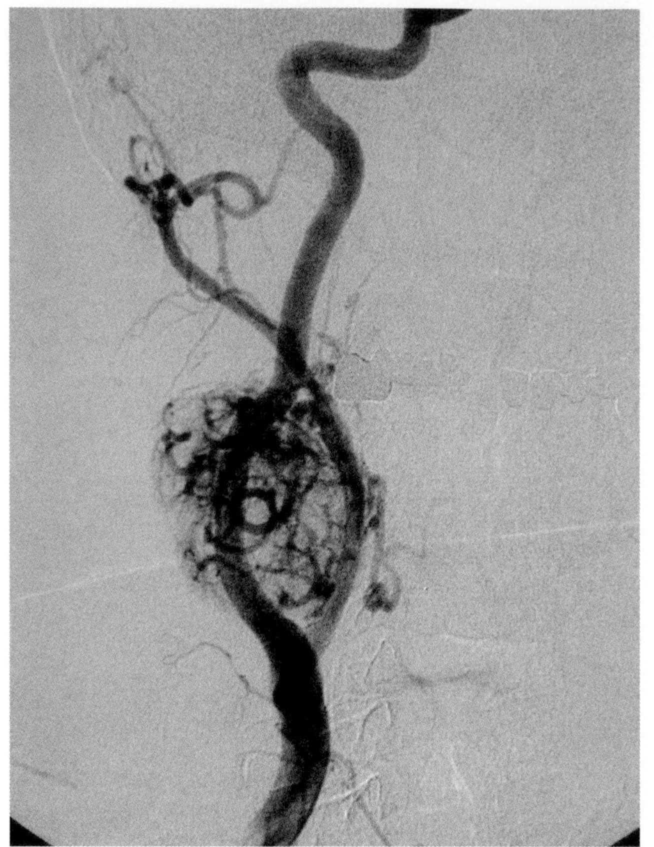
A

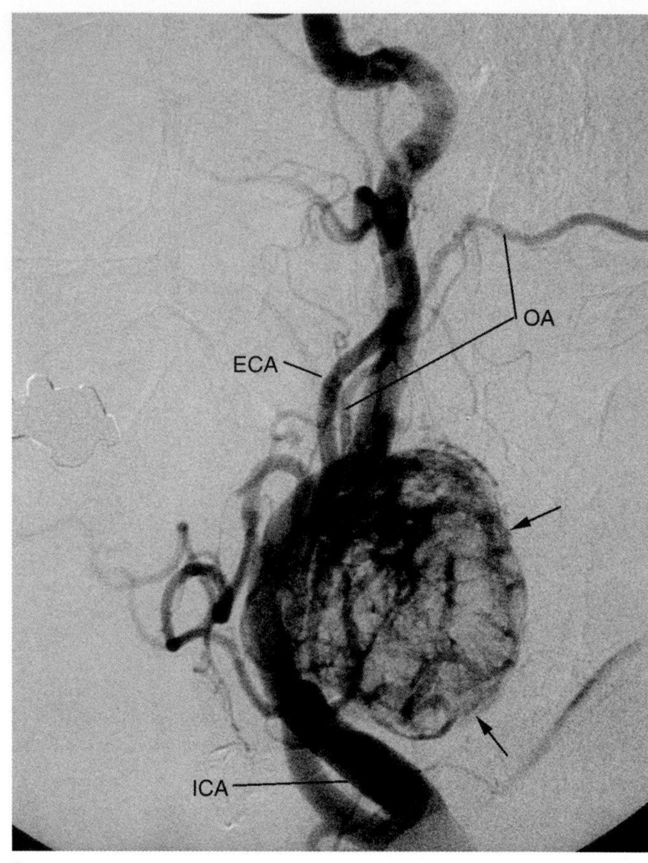

B

FIGURE 4-20. Paraganglioma. Anterior-posterior (**A**) and lateral (**B**) right common carotid artery angiograms demonstrate a markedly hypervascular mass (*arrows*) in the common carotid artery bifurcation. This is supplied by numerous small branches of the right external carotid artery (ECA), including the occipital artery (OA) and ascending pharyngeal artery. On the anterior-posterior view, this appears to splay the carotid bifurcation, which suggests that it might represent a carotid body tumor; however, on the lateral view, it is better delineated and lies posterior to both the ECAs and internal carotid arteries (ICAs) and is above the bifurcation, typical of a glomus vagale or vagal paraganglioma. Evaluation of the other vascular distributions is required to detect the multifocal paragangliomas.

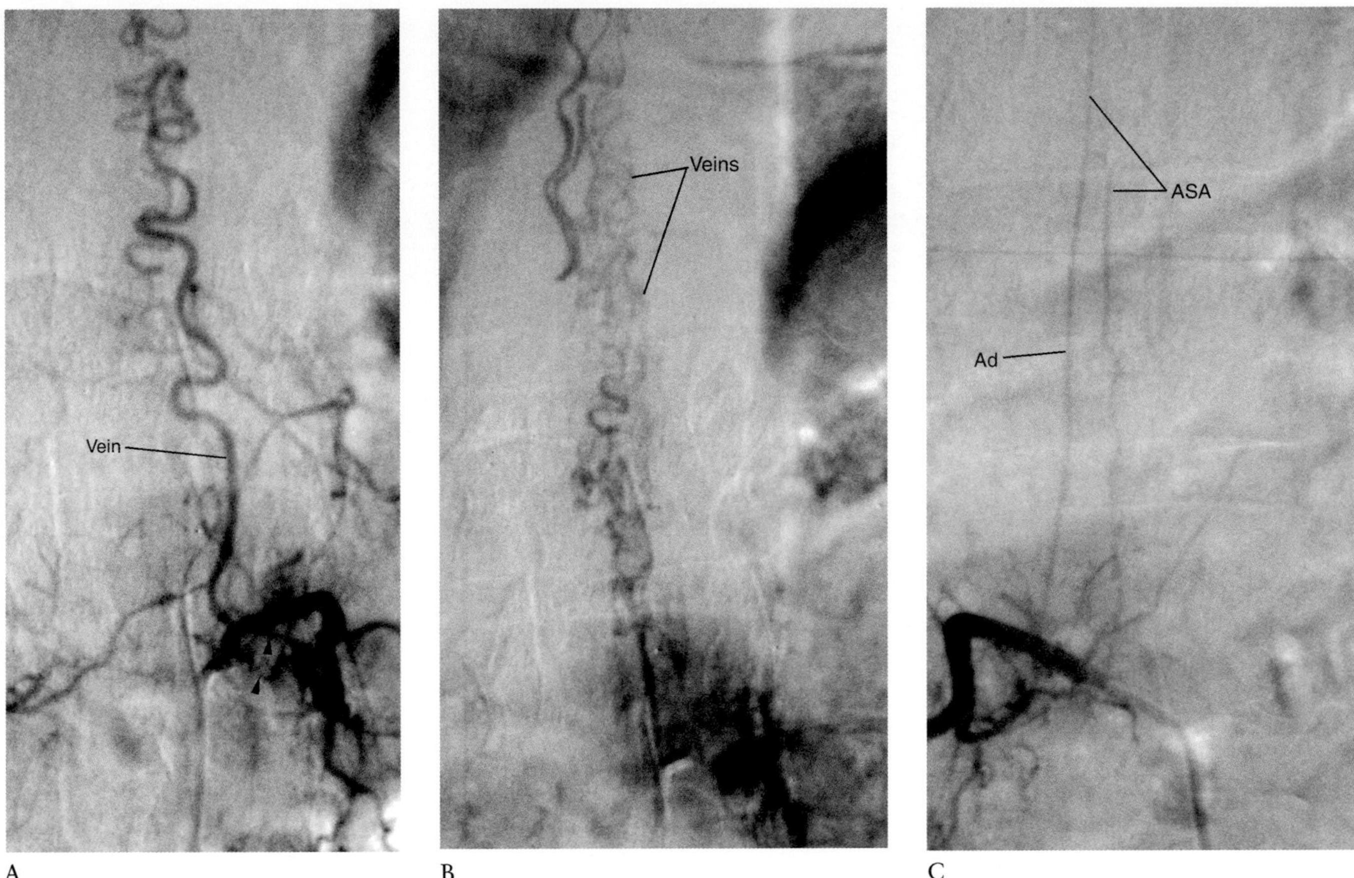

FIGURE 4-21. Spinal dural arteriovenous fistula. Early (**A**) and late left L1 lumbar injection demonstrate a very irregular and tortuous vessel in the spinal canal. Note the significant tortuosity of the ascending portion of this vessel compared to the artery of Adamkiewicz (Ad) seen in Figure 4-19. This tortuous ascending vessel represents a draining vein (Vein); on the later phase (**B**), there is filling of other numerous venous channels (Veins) along the spinal cord. The actual fistula arises at, or immediately within, the dura at L12, consisting of a small network of channels (*arrowheads*) leading to the draining vein seen in (**A**). The right L1 lumbar angiogram (**C**) pedicle fills the Ad and the anterior spinal artery (ASA) but does not supply this fistula.

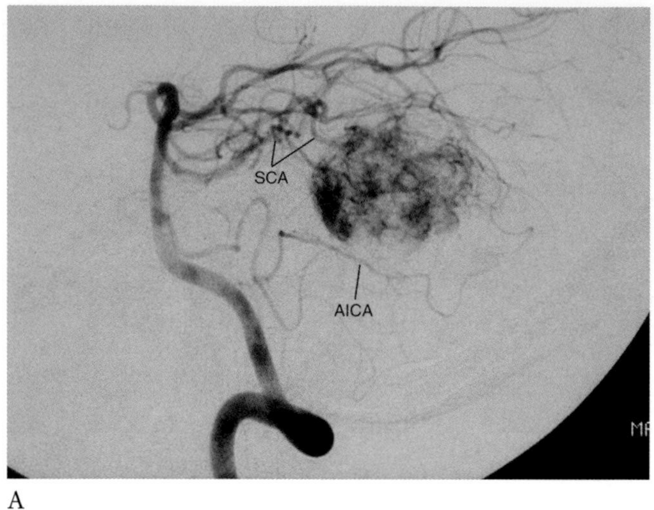

A

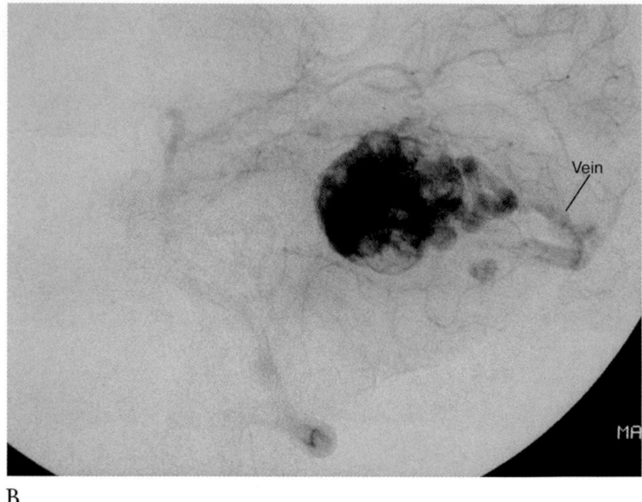

B

FIGURE 4-22. Hemangioblastoma. Mid-arterial (**A**) and late arterial to capillary phase (**B**) from the lateral right vertebral artery angiograms demonstrate a fine network of vessels with a hypervascular mass supplied predominantly by the branches of the right superior cerebellar artery (SCA) and minimally from the anterior inferior cerebellar artery (AICA). On the later venous phase, note the dense capillary blush of this mass and the early venous drainage (Vein), indicating some mild arteriovenous shunting. This arteriovenous shunting is commonly seen in these various hypervascular masses and is not specific. The degree of vascularity can sometimes be confused with an arteriovenous malformation; however, the degree of shunting is usually much less pronounced.

REFERENCES

1. Anson BH. The Aortic Arch and Its Branches. In AA Luisada (ed), Cardiology (Vol. I). New York: McGraw-Hill, 1963;119.

2. Bouthiller A, van Loveren HR, Keller JT. Segments of the internal carotid artery: a new classification. Neurosurgery 1996;38:425–433.

3. Gibo H, Carver CC, Rhoton AL Jr, et al. Microsurgical anatomy of the middle cerebral artery. J Neurosurg 1981;54:151–169.

4. Osborn AG. The Posterior Cerebral Artery. In Diagnostic Cerebral Angiography. Philadelphia: Lippincott–Raven, 1999;153–171.

5. Jones EF, Kalman JM, Calafiore P, et al. Proximal aortic atheroma: an independent risk factor for cerebral ischemia. Stroke 1995;26:218c–224c.

6. Griffiths PD, Worth S, Gholkar A. Incidental intracranial vascular pathology in patients investigated for carotid stenosis. Neuroradiology 1996;38: 25–30.

7. North American Symptomatic Carotid Endarterectomy Trial Collaborators. Beneficial effect of carotid endarterectomy in symptomatic patients with high-grade stenosis. N Engl J Med 1991;325:445–453.

8. Executive Committee for ACAS Study. Endarterectomy for asymptomatic carotid artery stenosis. JAMA 1995;273:1421–1428.

9. MRC European Carotid Surgery trial: interim results for symptomatic patients with severe (70–99%) or with mild (0–29%) carotid stenosis. European Carotid Surgery Trial Collaborative Group. Lancet 1991;337:1235–1243.

10. Rothwell PM, Gibson RJ, Slattery J, et al. Equivalence of measurement of carotid stenosis. Stroke 1994;25:2435–2439.

11. Guidelines for medical treatment of stroke prevention. American College of Physicians. Ann Intern Med 1994;121:44–55.

12. Furlan A, Higashida R, Wechsler LR, et al. Intra-arterial prourokinase for acute ischemic stroke. The PROACT II study: a randomized controlled trial. Prolyse in Acute Cerebral Thromboembolism. JAMA 1999, 282(21):2003–2011.

13. National Institute of Neurological Disorders and Stroke rTPA Stroke Study Group. Generalized efficacy of tPA for acute stroke subgroup analysis of the NINDS tPA Stroke Trial. Stroke 1997;28:2119–2125.

14. Moore PM. Diagnosis and management of isolated angiitis of the central nervous system. Neurology 1989;39:167–173.

15. Klein R, Hunder G, Stanson A, et al. Large artery involement in giant cell (temporal) arteritis. Ann Intern Med 1975;83:806–811.

16. Stanson A. Roentgenographic findings in major vasculitic syndromes. Rheum Dis Clin North Am 1990;16:293–308.

17. Mettinger K, Erickson K. Fibromuscular dysplasia and the brain: observations on angiographic, clinical, and genetic characteristics. Stroke 1982;13:46–50.

18. Rinaldi I, Harris W, Kopp J. Intracranial fibromuscular dysplasia: report of two cases, one with autopsy verification. Stroke 1976;7:511–516.

19. Ljunggren B, Saveland H, Brandt L, Zygmunt S. Early operation and overall outcome in aneurysmal subarachnoid hemorrhage. J Neurosurg 1985;62(4): 547–551.

20. Hunt WE, Hess RM. Surgical risk as related to time of intervention in repair of intracranial aneurysms. J Neurosurg 1968;28:14–20.

21. Le Roux PD, Elliott JP, Downey L, et al. Improved outcome after rupture of anterior circulation aneurysm: a retrospective 10-year review of 224 good-grade patients. J Neurosurg 1995;83(3):394–402.

22. Wiebers DO, Whisnant JP, Sundt TM, et al. The significance of unruptured intracranial saccular intracranial aneurysm. J Neurosurg 1987;66:23–29.

23. Mcfadzean RM, Teasdale EM. Computerized tomography angiography in isolated third nerve palsies. J Neurosurg 1998;88:679–684.

24. Pierot L, Boulin A, Castaings L, et al. The endovascular approach in the management of patients with multiple intracranial aneurysms. Neuroradiology 1997;39:361–366.

25. Osborn AG. Intracranial Aneurysm. In AG Osborn (ed), Diagnostic Cerebral Angiography. Philadelphia: Lippincott–Raven, 1999;277–283.

26. Stebhen WE. Aneurysm and anatomical variations in cerebral arteries. Arch Pathol 1963;75:45–64.

27. Sinzobahamvya N, Kalangu K, Hamel-Kalinowski W. Arterial aneurysm associated with human immunodeficiency virus (HIV). Acta Chir Belg 1989; 89(4):185–188.

28. Marks C, Kuskov S. Pattern of arterial aneurysm in acquired immunodeficiency disease. World J Surg 1995;19(1):127–132.

29. Scotti G, Li MH, Righi C, et al. Endovascular treatment of bacterial intracranial aneurysms. Neuroradiology 1996;38:186–189.

30. Naskad P, Normes H, Hauge HN. Traumatic aneurysms of pericallosal arteries. Neuroradiology 1986;28:335–338.

31. Gao E, Young WL, Pile-Spellman J, et al. Cerebral arteriovenous feeding artery aneurysm. Neurosurgery 1997;41:1345–1358.

32. Ojemann RG, Heros RC, Crowell RM. Arteriovenous Malformation of the Brain. In RG Ojemann, RC Heros, RM Crowell (eds), Surgical Management of Cerebrovascular Disease (2nd ed). Baltimore: Williams & Wilkins, 1988;347.

33. Pile-Spellman JMD, Baker KF, Liszczak TM, et al. High-flow angiopathy: cerebral blood vessel change in chronic arteriovenous fistula. AJNR Am J Neuroradiol 1986;7:811–815.

34. Pollock BE, Flickinger JC, Lundsford LD, et al. Factors that predict the bleeding risk of cerebral arteriovenous malformations. Stroke 1996;27:1–6.

35. Spetzler RF, Martin NA. A proposed grading system for arteriovenous malformations. J Neurosurg 1986;65:476–483.

36. Spetzler RF, Hamilton MG. The prospective application of a grading system for arteriovenous malformations. Neurosurgery 1994;34:2–7.

37. Spetzler RF, Anson JA. Classification of spinal arteriovenous malformations and implications for treatment. BNI Q 1992;8(2):2–8.

38. Higashida RT, Malek AM, Halbach VV, et al. Diagnosis and treatment of dural arteriovenous fistulas. Neuroimaging Clin North Am 1998;8(2):445–468.

39. Muraszko K, Oldfield E. Vascular malformations of the spinal cord and dura. Neurosurg Clin N Am 1990:1:631–652.

Section

II

Cerebral Blood Flow and Physiology

CHAPTER

5

Regional Cerebral Blood Flow by Xenon-133 Clearance

Walter D. Obrist

Historically, determination of regional cerebral blood flow (rCBF) by two-dimensional xenon-133 (^{133}Xe) clearance has contributed significantly to our understanding of brain pathophysiology. For three decades (1960–1990), ^{133}Xe clearance was the most widely used method of CBF measurement in humans. Even with the advent of tomographic (three-dimensional) technology, this approach continues to provide useful quantitative data in clinical investigations.

rCBF measurement by ^{133}Xe clearance is based on the same principle as the pioneer nitrous oxide method of Kety and Schmidt[1]—namely, that the rate of uptake and clearance of an inert diffusible gas is proportional to blood flow in the tissue. Whereas the nitrous oxide technique yields global estimates of CBF based on the concentration of gas in arterial and jugular venous blood, the use of a radioactive tracer permits direct monitoring of tissue clearance by external detection, thus providing estimates for a particular brain region.

Lassen and Ingvar[2] were the first to use radioisotopes for assessment of rCBF when they introduced the intracarotid (IC) injection method in 1961. Because of the risk entailed by IC injection, Veall and Mallett[3] proposed inhalation of ^{133}Xe, whereas Austin and coworkers[4] proposed intravenous injection. Although the two noninvasive techniques (inhalation and intravenous injection) are theoretically the same and give equivalent results, they differ from the classic IC injection method in several respects. The present chapter describes the methodology and summarizes the clinical research findings for both the IC and noninvasive ^{133}Xe methods. A more extensive review has been published elsewhere.[5]

METHODOLOGY

Intracarotid Xenon-133 Method

The IC ^{133}Xe method involves a bolus injection of ^{133}Xe in saline into one internal carotid artery (ICA). Extracranial monitoring of gamma radiation is performed by multiple collimated detectors placed over the injected hemisphere.[2] As shown in Figure 5-1, a rapid rise in count rate occurs as the bolus enters the brain, followed by a slower decline over the next 10–15 minutes as the isotope clears. Little recirculation of ^{133}Xe occurs because the cerebral venous blood is diluted by isotope-free blood from the rest of the body and because of efficient elimination of the gas by the lungs. Analysis of the clearance curves assumes that CBF does not change during the 10-minute measurement interval (i.e., a steady state prevails).

Calculation of CBF is performed by a simple height-over-area formula derived by Zierler[6] from mean transit time concepts. Estimates of mean flow are obtained by dividing the initial height of the curve by the area under it,[2,7] as illustrated in Figure 5-1. Basic to this methodology is the assumption that all of the ^{133}Xe seen by a detector arrives before any appreciable amount leaves.

Because the brain contains two tissues (gray and white matter) that have distinctly different clearance rates, it is possible to perform a biexponential analysis in which separate estimates of flow are obtained for the fast (gray) and slow (white) clearing compartments.[7] An alternative approach for estimating gray matter flow is to determine the initial slope of the curve, which over the first minute is dominated by the fast clearing compartment and approximates a single exponential.[8] This procedure is illustrated in Figure 5-1.

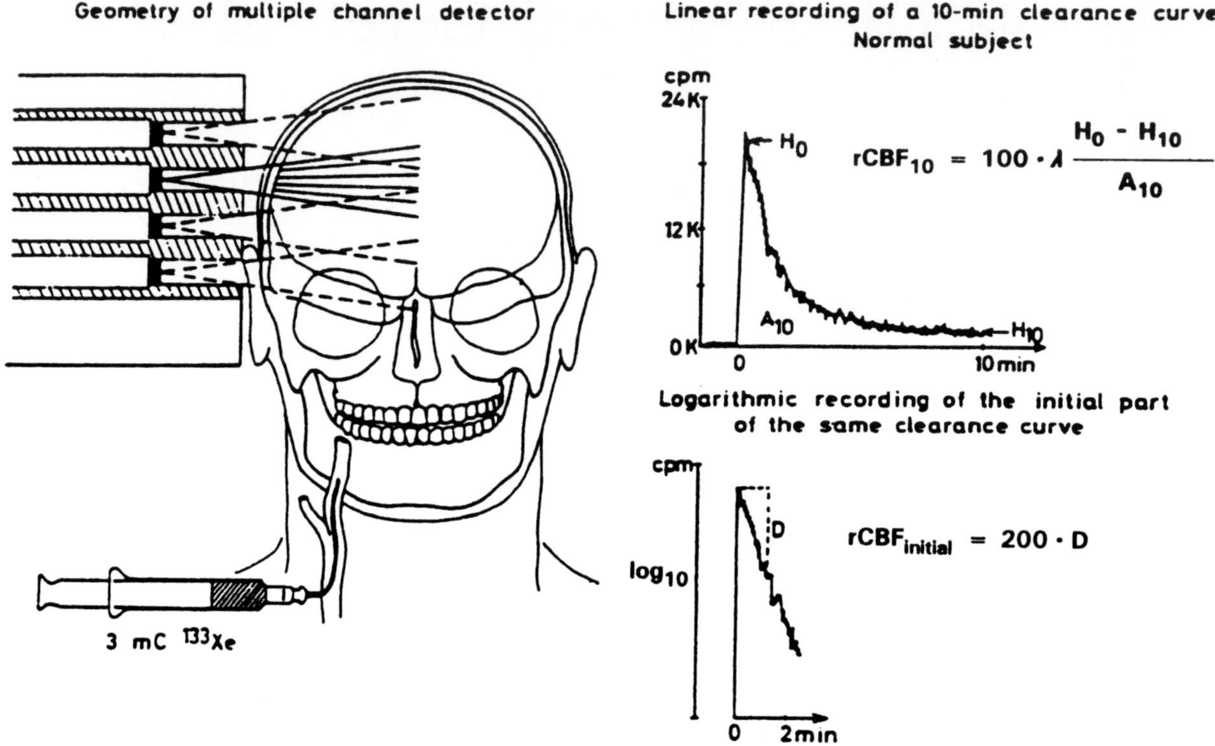

FIGURE 5-1. **Left:** Collimated scintillation detectors placed over the hemisphere ipsilateral to an intracarotid xenon-133 (^{133}Xe) injection. **Upper right:** Clearance curve showing the height-over-area calculation. **Lower right:** Logarithmic recording reveals a linear "initial slope" over the first minute of the curve. (λ = brain-blood partition coefficient for ^{133}Xe; A_{10} = area under the curve from time 0 to 10 minutes; D = initial slope of curve; H_0 = initial height; H_{10} = ordinate value at 10 minutes; rCBF = regional cerebral blood flow.) (Modified from OB Paulson. Regional cerebral blood flow in apoplexy due to occlusion of the middle cerebral artery. Neurology 1970;20:63–77.)

Owing to the difficulty of separating fast and slow tissue compartments in pathologic conditions, the more reliable height-over-area method has generally been used in preference to biexponential analysis. Height-over-area estimates of CBF are in excellent agreement with those obtained by the Kety-Schmidt technique, yielding comparable normal values of 50 ml/100 g per minute.

Noninvasive Xenon-133 Method

The noninvasive ^{133}Xe method is an extension and modification of the IC method, using multiple detectors over each hemisphere. Rather than a selective injection into one ICA, the isotope is introduced into the systemic circulation, either by a brief (1- to 2-minute) inhalation or by intravenous injection. These two noninvasive routes differ from the IC method in a very important respect—the duration of isotope input. Instead of a rapid bolus that directly enters the brain and clears with minimal recirculation, the input from either inhalation or intravenous injection is distributed over time and includes considerable recirculation. Clearance curve analysis must, therefore, take account of the arterial input that can be estimated noninvasively by continuous monitoring of the expired end-tidal air.[3]

Based on the Fick principle, Kety[9] derived a generalized equation for the uptake and clearance of an inert diffusible gas in which the arterial input is convoluted with an exponential function. This convolution was first applied to human CBF studies by Obrist and coworkers,[10] who proposed a two-compartment model that contains both fast and slow clearing tissue components. Thus,

$$C(t) = \sum_{i=1}^{2} P_i \int_0^t C_A(u) e^{-K(t-u)} \, du$$

where $C(t)$ and $C_A(t)$ are the measured cerebral and end-tidal ^{133}Xe concentrations, respectively; P_1 and P_2 are weighting coefficients; and K_1 and K_2 are the clearance rates for the two compartments. Computer solutions for the linear coefficients and nonlinear clearance rates are easily obtained by a least-squares curve-fitting procedure.[10]

Multiplying the rate constant of the fast clearing compartment, K_1, by the assumed ^{133}Xe partition coefficient for gray matter, λ_1, yields an estimate of gray mat-

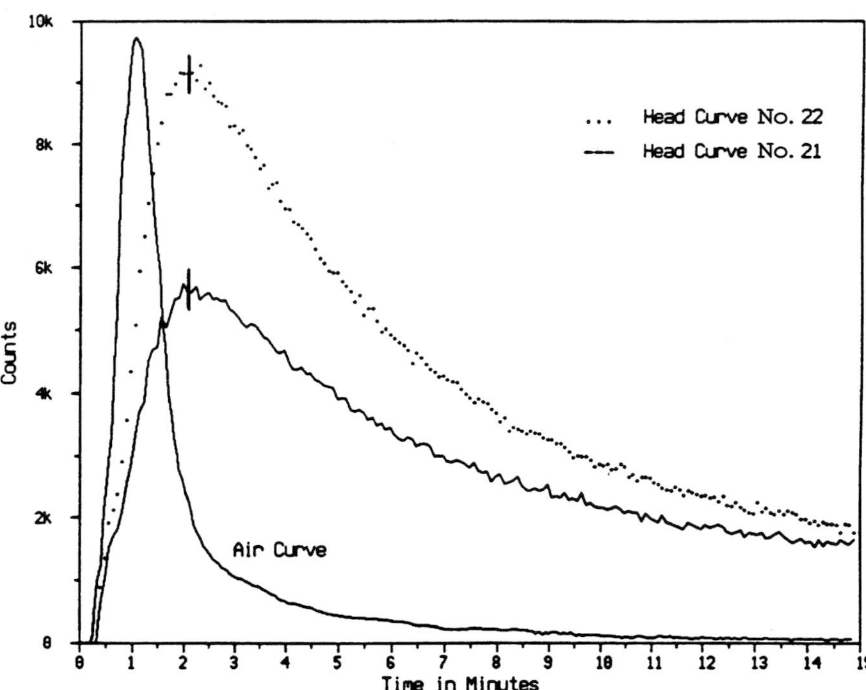

FIGURE 5-2. Two xenon-133 clearance curves superimposed on the end-tidal air curve of a patient with a left frontoparietal infarction. Detector No. 21 was located directly over the infarct; No. 22 was placed over the homologous noninfarcted region on the right. The vertical lines on each curve represent the start of curve fitting. (Reprinted with permission from WD Obrist, WE Wilkinson. Regional cerebral blood flow measurement in humans by xenon-133 clearance. Cerebrovasc Brain Metab Rev 1990;2:283–327.)

ter blood flow: $f_1 = \lambda_1 K_1$. Such estimates, which approximate 80 ml/100 g per minute in normals, are highly correlated with those obtained by the IC method. In severe pathologic conditions, however, f_1 becomes unstable owing to shifts in compartment size. More reliable estimates can be obtained from noncompartmental indices based on slope or height-over-area determinations. The most commonly used indices are the slope between 2 and 3 minutes on the curve[11] and CBF_{15}, a height-over-area estimate of mean gray and white matter flow[5] comparable to that of the IC technique.

Figure 5-2 illustrates ^{133}Xe clearance curves obtained by intravenous injection in a stroke patient studied with 32-detector instrumentation. The end-tidal air curve, representing arterial input, is superimposed. Detector No. 21 was positioned over a left frontoparietal infarct observed on computed tomography (CT) scan, whereas No. 22 was located symmetrically over the noninfarcted right hemisphere. The two clearance curves have a distinctly different time course, with the infarcted region showing less ^{133}Xe uptake and much slower clearance. The occurrence of uptake and clearance on the infarcted side can be attributed to tissue perfusion adjacent to the lesion, which was in the detector's field of view.

CLINICAL RESEARCH FINDINGS

Intracarotid Xenon-133 Method

By the time the IC method was introduced in the early 1960s, more than a decade of human CBF studies had been performed by the nitrous oxide technique. The latter provided a wealth of new information on global CBF in both health and disease as well as insight into its regulatory mechanisms.[12] It remained for the IC method to determine regional blood flow variations and their relationship to normal and abnormal brain function. Because of its association with carotid angiography—widely practiced at the time—the IC method was particularly suited to investigations of acute pathophysiology. An increased number of detectors (up to 254) permitted more precise delineation and imaging of regional flow.

Three areas of investigation stand out in which pioneer contributions were made by the IC method: (1) correlation of rCBF variations with focal neurologic and anatomic findings; (2) disturbances of CBF regulation in acute illnesses, particularly cerebrovascular disorders and brain trauma; and (3) relationship of rCBF patterns to cerebral function in chronic dementia and during functional cortical activation.

Derangement of Regional Cerebral Blood Flow Regulation

This is perhaps the most important contribution of the IC method. Stimulated by parallel animal studies that defined CBF responses to alterations in blood pressure and carbon dioxide (CO_2), emphasis was placed on disturbances in blood flow regulation in acute cerebrovascular disorders. Back-to-back measurements permitted observations before and after either blood pressure manipulation or changes in arterial partial pressure of CO_2 (P_{CO_2}). Deviations from normal autoregulation (constant CBF with blood pressure change), as well as impairment of the usual responses to hyper- and hypocapnia, were observed in a high proportion of stroke and transient ischemic attack (TIA) patients.[13–15] Of particular interest were the findings of dissociated vasoparalysis (impaired pressure autoregulation with preserved CO_2 reactivity) and paradoxic CO_2 responses. The latter consisted of an intracerebral steal (focal CBF decrease with hypercapnia) and an inverse steal (focal increase with hypocapnia). With the observation by Paulson et al.[16] that hypocapnia could restore autoregulation, these findings had clear therapeutic implications.

Occurrence of Hyperemia

In 1966, Lassen[17] proposed the concept of "luxury perfusion," defined as a relative hyperemia in which blood flow exceeds the metabolic requirement of the brain. He attributed it to tissue acidosis secondary to accumulation of lactic acid. Although suggested by earlier observations of narrow arteriojugular venous oxygen differences, the occurrence of luxury perfusion was first demonstrated in humans by the IC ^{133}Xe technique.[18] Focal hyperemia was found in approximately half of acute stroke cases, particularly in those with cortical infarcts.[19]

Intraoperative Studies

A special application of the IC method is rCBF monitoring during carotid endarterectomy.[20,21] Extensive intraoperative observations have provided physiologic information on pressure-flow dynamics, relation to electroencephalography, influence of anesthesia, and correlation with outcome. rCBF monitoring has contributed to the safety of the procedure by guiding decisions on preocclusion shunting.

Intraoperative studies have also been performed during hypothermic cardiopulmonary bypass in open heart surgery,[22,23] in which the technique has been modified for intra-aortic or common carotid injection. This research has addressed the important issue of optimal $PaCO_2$ and blood pressure management during the bypass procedure.

Noninvasive Xenon-133 Method

The noninvasive method was widely used in the 1970s and 1980s. Interest in it derived from the ability to examine patients and control subjects who were not candidates for IC injection. Because of its noninvasiveness, the method has made unique contributions in several areas: (1) cross-sectional CBF studies that define age and sex differences and their relationship to risk factors; (2) longitudinal studies that describe the natural history of pathologic CBF changes; and (3) investigation of special subgroups such as children and patients undergoing intensive care. In each of these applications, the ability to acquire large samples, to use normal controls, and to make repeated measurements has facilitated statistical treatment of the results. Being able to view both hemispheres simultaneously was a particular advantage, because both regional and hemispheric asymmetries are sensitive indicators of unilateral alterations in flow.

Normal Aging and Risk Factors

Consistent with earlier findings by the nitrous oxide method, a gradual and progressive reduction of global CBF was found between 20 and 80 years of age. Significant sex differences were also observed. Of special interest is the observation by Shaw and coworkers[24] that age-related declines in flow are accelerated by risk factors for cerebrovascular disease.

Cerebrovascular Disease

Patients with unilateral carotid occlusion show regional and hemispheric CBF reductions on the ipsilateral side. Carotid stenosis is less likely to be associated with reductions except in symptomatic cases.[25] Extensive areas of flow reduction have been found in patients with small subcortical infarcts, suggesting a remote effect.[26] Following TIAs, blood flow tends to normalize but with varying individual time courses.[27]

Cerebrovascular Reserve

Using the ^{133}Xe inhalation method, a landmark observation was made by Norrving et al.[28] on rCBF responses to hypercapnia in patients with unilateral carotid occlusion. A normal CBF increase occurred in patients with adequate collateral flow demonstrated angiographically. Patients with poor collateral circulation had impaired CO_2 reactivity and an exacerbation of CBF asymmetries. This was the first report of reduced cerebrovascular reserve in such patients, a phenomenon subsequently confirmed by positron emission tomography and stable Xe/CT. Similar results have been obtained with acetazolamide using the ^{133}Xe intravenous method in candidates for carotid endartectomy.[29]

Figure 5-3 illustrates a reduction of cerebrovascular reserve in a 62-year-old man (studied by the author) who had a complete occlusion of the right ICA and a 50% stenosis on the left. Clinically, the patient had TIAs involving left upper extremity weakness and numbness. A CT scan was negative for infarction. CBF images were obtained by intravenous ^{133}Xe injection with 32-detector equipment. As seen in Figure 5-3, a normocapnic baseline (PCO_2 = 36.9 mm Hg) was followed by 5% CO_2 inhalation (PCO_2 = 47.6 mm Hg). Relative to the expected regional variation in normal controls, baseline CBF_{15} values were 10% lower in the right hemisphere (*green*). During CO_2 inhalation, there was a significant enhancement of this right-

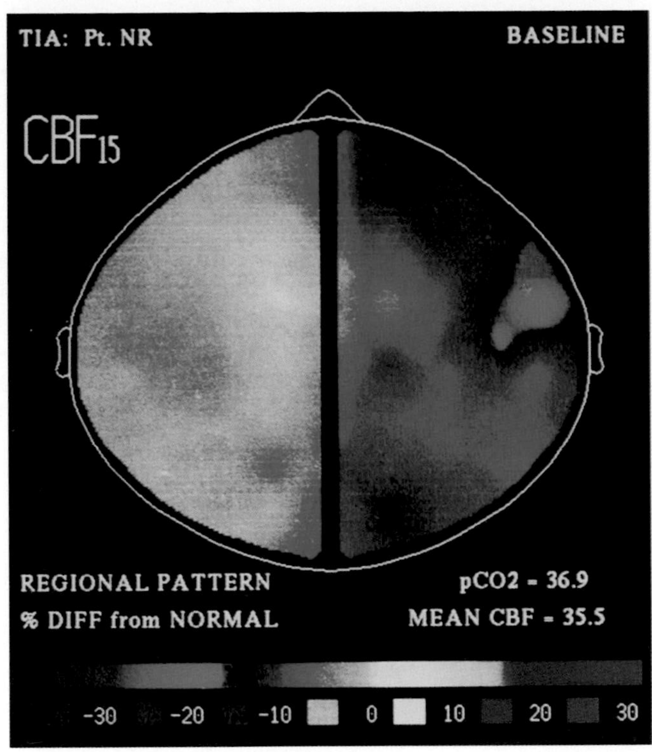

A

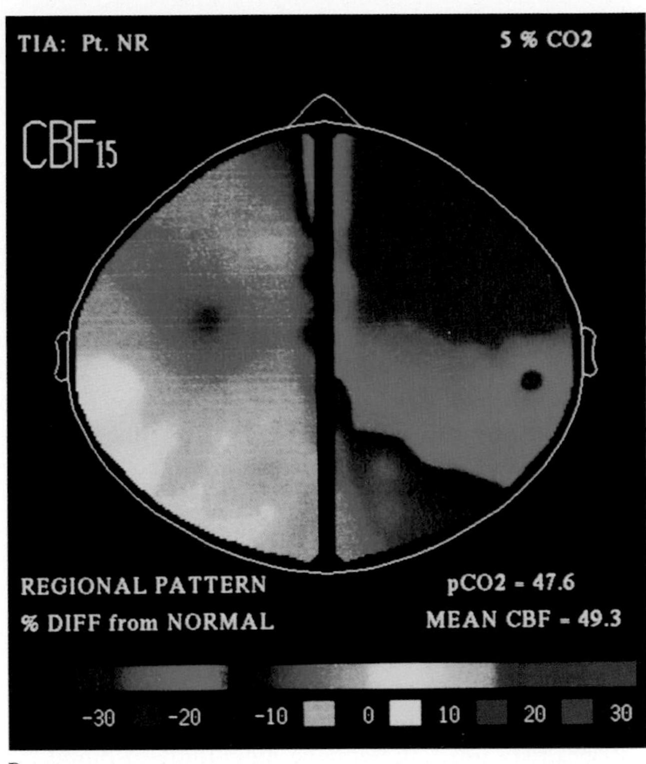

B

FIGURE 5-3. **A,B.** Images obtained with 32-detector instrumentation (intravenous xenon-133 method) in a patient with right internal carotid artery occlusion and transient ischemic attacks (TIAs). Hypercapnia induced by 5% carbon dioxide (CO_2) inhalation is compared with a baseline normocapnic condition. Two-dimensional images of the brain surface are displayed, as viewed by external detectors. Color coding indicates percent deviation from cerebral blood flow (CBF_{15}) values in normal control subjects. CO_2 inhalation produced a relative regional CBF decrease (*blue*) in the anterior and central regions of the right hemisphere, consistent with a reduction in cerebrovascular reserve. See text for details. (DIFF = difference.)

sided reduction, with the more anterior regions approaching minus 30% (*dark blue*). Calculated CO_2 reactivity (CBF increase per mm P_{CO_2} change) was 1% in the right frontotemporal region, compared with a normal 4% contralaterally. Sixteen days later, the patient suffered a stroke from a right frontoparietal infarct.

Cerebral Vasospasm

The noninvasive method is particularly suited to the intensive care environment, where serial rCBF measurements at bedside are desirable for detection of clinically relevant blood flow changes. Vasospasm, secondary to aneurysmal subarachnoid hemorrhage, is one of the conditions in which such monitoring has provided useful information. Blood flow level is well correlated with neurologic grade[30] and has been used to evaluate the effects of treatment, particularly "triple-H" therapy.[31]

Because transcranial Doppler flow velocity measurements are a function of CBF as well as vessel diameter, Jakobsen and coworkers[32] devised a *spasm index* (i.e., the ratio of blood velocity to blood flow). Increases in this index were associated with both clinical deterioration and widened (ischemic) arteriojugular venous oxygen differences. Comparable findings have been obtained in post-traumatic vasospasm, in which this index was a significant predictor of outcome.[33]

Rheologic Factors

There has been considerable interest in the rheologic parameters affecting CBF. Studies on polycythemic patients undergoing venesection have shown significant increases in blood flow attributed to lowered blood viscosity. Indeed, direct measurements of whole blood viscosity are inversely related to CBF. However, a series of studies by Brown and associates[34] convincingly demonstrated that the observed CBF changes depend on arterial oxygen content rather than on blood viscosity. These findings have implications for hemodilution therapy in acute stroke and vasospasm.

Intraoperative Studies

Portable rCBF instrumentation is readily used in the operating room, where blood flow measurements have been obtained during surgery for intracranial aneurysms and arteriovenous malformations.[35] The effects of anesthesia on CBF have also been studied in this setting.

ADVANTAGES AND LIMITATIONS OF TWO-DIMENSIONAL XENON-133 METHODS

The IC and noninvasive methods have several advantages in common: (1) low radiation dose; (2) relatively low cost; (3) repeatable in a brief time interval; (4) good counting statistics and signal to noise ratio; (5) well-developed quantitative analyses; and (6) the ability to separate fast- and slow-clearing compartments. These methods are particularly valuable when combined with other physiologic measurements (arteriojugular venous oxygen differences, intracranial and arterial pressures), thus providing a more comprehensive picture of cerebral hemodynamic and metabolic alterations.

The primary limitation of both methods is an insensitivity to local alterations of flow due to averaging of multiple tissues in view of the detector (i.e., the "look-through phenomenon"). This means that the computed values may not represent the magnitude of blood flow changes in and around a lesion, and areas of zero flow may go unrecognized. Even so, significant rCBF increases and decreases can be found that bear a meaningful relationship to neurologic, anatomic, and physiologic findings.

Intracarotid Method

Owing to the weak gamma radiation of ^{133}Xe, the underlying cortex is seen better than tissues at the depth. Extraction of the fast component of the clearance curve provides a good estimate of cortical flow and, with an array of small detectors, permits high-resolution cortical topography. This is a major advantage of the IC technique.

The primary disadvantage derives from the invasiveness of the procedure, so that only a limited population is available for study, and sample sizes are restricted. Simultaneous bilateral observations are not obtainable.

Noninvasive Method

Distinct advantages of the noninvasive method are the broad population and large samples available for study and the ease of making repeated measurements. Portable instrumentation permits bedside studies and special examinations in the intensive care unit and operating room.

A specific limitation of the noninvasive method is extracerebral contamination from underlying tissues (scalp, bone) plus scattered radiation originating in the airways (nasopharynx, throat). These effects can be minimized by appropriate recording and analysis of the clearance curves, as described elsewhere.[5,10]

CONCLUSION

Newer imaging techniques such as xenon CT, magnetic resonance imaging, single-photon emission CT, and positron emission tomography have largely replaced ^{133}Xe CBF measurements in most clinical settings. The pioneering information obtained using this technique provided important insights into human cerebrovascular physiology and paved the way for the clinical application of CBF measurements. ^{133}Xe CBF studies demonstrate the importance of quantitative CBF information in understanding both normal human physiology and pathophysiology of disease states affecting the cerebral circulation, and they continue to provide a benchmark for other methods of measuring CBF.

REFERENCES

1. Kety SS, Schmidt CF. The nitrous oxide method for the quantitative determination of cerebral blood flow in man: theory, procedure, and normal values. J Clin Invest 1948;27:476–483.

2. Lassen NA, Ingvar DH. Radioisotopic assessment of regional cerebral blood flow. Prog Nucl Med 1972;1:376–409.

3. Veall N, Mallett BL. Regional cerebral blood flow determination by ^{133}Xe inhalation and external recording: the effect of arterial recirculation. Clin Sci 1966;30:353–369.

4. Austin G, Horn N, Rouhe S, Hayward W. Description and early results of an intravenous radioisotope technique for measuring regional cerebral blood flow in man. Eur Neurol 1972;8:43–51.

5. Obrist WD, Wilkinson WE. Regional cerebral blood flow measurement in humans by xenon-133 clearance. Cerebrovasc Brain Metab Rev 1990;2:283–327.

6. Zierler KL. Equations for measuring blood flow by external monitoring of radioisotopes. Circ Res 1965;16:309–321.

7. Hoedt-Rasmussen K, Sveinsdottir E, Lassen NA. Regional cerebral blood flow in man determined by intra-arterial injection of radioactive inert gas. Circ Res 1966;18:237–247.

8. Olesen J, Paulson OB, Lassen NA. Regional cerebral blood flow in man determined by the initial slope of the clearance of intra-arterially injected ^{133}Xe. Stroke 1971;2:519–540.

9. Kety SS. The theory and applications of the exchange of inert gas at the lungs and tissues. Pharmacol Rev 1951;3:1–41.

10. Obrist WD, Thompson HK, Wang HS, Wilkinson WE. Regional cerebral blood flow estimated by ^{133}xenon inhalation. Stroke 1975;6:245–256.

11. Risberg J, Ali Z, Wilson EM, et al. Regional cerebral blood flow by ^{133}xenon inhalation: preliminary

evaluation of an initial slope index in patients with unstable flow compartments. Stroke 1975;6:142–148.

12. Lassen NA. Cerebral blood flow and oxygen consumption in man. Physiol Rev 1959;39:183–238.

13. Paulson OB. Regional cerebral blood flow in apoplexy due to occlusion of the middle cerebral artery. Neurology 1970;20:63–77.

14. Fieschi C, Agnoli A, Battistini N, et al. Derangement of regional cerebral blood flow and its regulatory mechanisms in acute cerebrovascular lesions. Neurology 1968;18:1166–1179.

15. Skinhoj E, Hoedt-Rasmussen K, Paulson OB, Lassen NA. Regional cerebral blood flow and its autoregulation in patients with transient focal ischemic attacks. Neurology 1970;20:485–493.

16. Paulson OB, Olesen J, Christensen MS. Restoration of autoregulation of cerebral blood flow by hypocapnia. Neurology 1972;22:286–293.

17. Lassen NA. The luxury-perfusion syndrome and its possible relation to acute metabolic acidosis localized within the brain. Lancet 1966;2:1113–1115.

18. Hoedt-Rasmussen K, Skinhoj E, Paulson O, et al. Regional cerebral blood flow in acute apoplexy: the "luxury perfusion syndrome" of brain tissue. Arch Neurol 1967;17:271–281.

19. Olsen TS, Larsen B, Skriver EB, et al. Focal cerebral hyperemia in acute stroke. Incidence, pathophysiology and clinical significance. Stroke 1981;12: 598–607.

20. Boysen G. Cerebral hemodynamics in carotid surgery. Acta Neurol Scand 1973;49(Suppl 52):1–84.

21. Sundt TM, Sharbrough FW, Anderson RE, Michenfelder JD. Cerebral blood flow measurements and electroencephalograms during carotid endarterectomy. J Neurosurg 1974;41:310–320.

22. Prough DS, Stump DA, Roy RC, et al. Response of cerebral blood flow to changes in carbon dioxide tension during hypothermic cardiopulmonary bypass. Anesthesiology 1986;64:576–581.

23. Murkin JM, Farrar JK, Tweed WA, et al. Cerebral autoregulation and flow/metabolism coupling during cardiopulmonary bypass: the influence of Pa_{CO_2}. Anesth Analg 1987;66:825–832.

24. Shaw TG, Mortel KF, Meyer JS, et al. Cerebral blood flow changes in benign aging and cerebrovascular disease. Neurology 1984;34:855–862.

25. Yanagihara T, Wahner HW. Cerebral blood flow measurement in cerebrovascular occlusive diseases. Stroke 1984;15:816–822.

26. Hojer-Pedersen E, Petersen OF. Changes of blood flow in the cerebral cortex after subcortical ischemic infarction. Stroke 1989;20:211–216.

27. Hartmann A. Prolonged disturbances of regional cerebral blood flow in transient ischemic attacks. Stroke 1985;16:932–939.

28. Norrving B, Nilsson B, Risberg J. rCBF in patients with carotid occlusion: resting and hypercapnic flow related to collateral pattern. Stroke 1982;13:155–162.

29. Schroeder T. Cerebrovascular reactivity to acetazolamide in carotid artery disease: enhancement of side-to-side CBF asymmetry indicates critically reduced perfusion pressure. Neurol Res 1986;8:231–236.

30. Rosenstein J, Suzuki M, Symon L, Redmond S. Clinical use of a portable bedside cerebral blood flow machine in the management of aneurysmal subarachnoid hemorrhage. Neurosurgery 1984;15:519–525.

31. Origitano TC, Wascher TM, Reichman OH, Anderson DE. Sustained increased cerebral blood flow with prophylactic hypertensive hypervolemic hemodilution ("triple-H" therapy) after subarachnoid hemorrhage. Neurosurgery 1990;27:729–740.

32. Jakobsen M, Enevoldsen E, Dalager T. Spasm index in subarachnoid haemorrhage: consequences of vasospasm upon cerebral blood flow and oxygen extraction. Acta Neurol Scand 1990;82:311–320.

33. Lee JH, Martin NE, Alsina G, et al. Hemodynamically significant cerebral vasospasm and outcome after head injury: a prospective study. J Neurosurg 1997;87:221–233.

34. Brown MM, Wade JPH, Marshall J. Fundamental importance of arterial oxygen content in the regulation of cerebral blood flow in man. Brain 1985; 108:81–93.

35. Young WL, Prohovnik I, Ornstein E, et al. Monitoring of intraoperative cerebral hemodynamics before and after arteriovenous malformation resection. Anesth Analg 1988;67:1011–1014.

CHAPTER

6

Positron Emission Tomography

Jean-Claude Baron

Imaging brain perfusion and energy metabolism by means of positron emission tomography (PET) affords unique insights into the pathophysiology of cerebrovascular diseases with major implications for patient management. The main points are briefly demonstrated in this chapter.

TECHNIQUES

Using oxygen-15–labeled tracers such as water, carbon dioxide (CO_2), carbon monoxide, and oxygen, and the glucose analogue fluorine-18 (^{18}F)–fluoro-2-deoxy-D-glucose, quantitative mapping of the cerebral blood flow (CBF), cerebral blood volume (CBV), cerebral metabolic rate of oxygen ($CMRO_2$), oxygen extraction fraction (OEF), and brain glucose utilization (CMRglc) can be obtained.[1] In addition, access to CBF and CBV allows computing the CBV/CBF ratio, which represents the mean transit time; the reverse CBF/CBV ratio is an index of the local cerebral perfusion pressure (CPP).[2–4] There are three specific markers of interest for cerebrovascular disease: (1) carbon-11 (^{11}C)–flumazenil (^{11}C-FMZ), a benzodiazepine receptor radioligand[5] that has been used as a marker of neuronal integrity; (2) ^{11}C-PK 11-195 (^{11}C-PK), a peripheral benzodiazepine radioligand that has been used as a marker of glial inflammation[5,6]; and (3) ^{18}F–fluoro-misonidazole (^{18}F-MISO), a marker of tissue hypoxia.[7]

The main limitations of PET are its cost and complexity, especially in absolute quantitation and radioligand investigations. These limitations have hampered the clinical applications of PET in cerebrovascular diseases, but successful transfer of physiologic and pathophysiologic concepts and investigational techniques and models from PET to other more accessible techniques, such as single-photon emission computed tomography and magnetic resonance imaging (MRI), has been effective for over a decade.

BASIC PATHOPHYSIOLOGIC CONCEPTS AND TERMINOLOGY

In physiologic conditions, metabolic regulation of the cerebral circulation translates into a matching of CBF, CMRglc, $CMRO_2$, and CBV, according to linearly proportional relationships.[3,8]

Table 6-1 summarizes the changes, subdivided into four stages of increasing severity, that occur in response to a fall in the CPP distal to an arterial obstruction.[9–11] Initially, the CBF remains unchanged (autoregulation change) thanks to a marked increase in CBV, reflecting dilatation of the resistance vessels (hemodynamic reserve). The autoregulation can also be identified by means of a CO_2 inhalation test or an intravenous acetazolamide vasoreactivity stress test, revealing partial or complete loss of CBF reactivity or paradoxic CBF decreases (steal phenomenon) (Figure 6-1). With further CPP decreases, the CBF starts to decline, whereas the $CMRO_2$, at first, remains unaltered (oligemia stage). This CBF-$CMRO_2$ mismatch translates as a focal increase in the OEF and has been termed *misery perfusion* (Figure 6-2).[12] With further reductions in the CPP, the $CMRO_2$ decreases despite maximal OEF. This stage, therefore, signals neuronal dysfunction that at first is still reversible (ischemic penumbra) but ultimately becomes irreversible (ischemic core) (Figure 6-3).

TABLE 6-1. Four Stages of Brain Hemodynamic and Metabolic Impairment as a Function of Severity in Cerebral Perfusion Pressure Drop[a]

Stage	*Cerebral perfusion pressure (%)*	*Cerebral blood volume*	*Cerebral blood flow*	*Oxygen extraction fraction*	*Cerebral metabolic rate of oxygen*
1. Autoregulation	60–100	↑	N	N	N
2. Oligemia	40–60	↑↑	17–50 ml/100 ml/min[b]	↑	N
3. Ischemic penumbra	20–40	↑	7–17 ml/100 ml/min[b]	↑↑	>0.76 ml/100 ml/min[c]
4. Impending necrosis	<40	↓	<8.4 ml/100 ml/min[c]	↑ to ↓	<0.76 ml/100 ml/min[c]

↑ = increased; ↓ = decreased; N = unchanged.

[a]Measurements are given here in brain units of milliliters rather than the usual grams. As with positron emission tomography, it is the tissue volume that is assessed rather than its weight.

[b]Data from M Furlan, G Marchal, F Viader, et al. Spontaneous neurological recovery after stroke and the fate of the ischemic penumbra. Ann Neurol 1996;40:216–226.

[c]Data from G Marchal, V Beaudouin, P Rioux, et al. Prolonged persistence of substantial volumes of potentially viable brain tissue after stroke: a correlative PET-CT study with voxel-based data analysis. Stroke 1996;27:599–606.

Luxury perfusion describes a situation in which the oxygen supply is in excess of demand,[13] and it occurs when there is reperfusion within the previously ischemic tissue (see Figure 6-3). Its hallmark is a focal reduction of the OEF.[9] The CBF (which represents nutritional perfusion) may be increased (hyperperfusion), in the normal range, or even decreased though still in excess of prevailing $CMRO_2$ (relative luxury perfusion).

CHRONIC HEMODYNAMIC FAILURE

Pathophysiologic Observations

The first account of misery perfusion was in a patient with internal carotid artery (ICA) occlusion and continued reversible ischemic attacks despite optimal medical treatment.[12] Subsequent studies have repeatedly documented that severe ICA disease is prone to induce distal hemodynamic consequences.[14–20] Across all patients, the severity of hemodynamic disturbance is related to the degree of ICA obstruction, with more than 50% stenosis or occlusion having measurable effects, but at the single-subject level the effects are unpredictable. Likewise, the extent of compensation via the circle of Willis seems to determine the degree of brain hemodynamic changes, with maximal disturbances observed in association with reversed ophthalmic artery flow, but, again, this relationship may not always hold at the individual level.[21] Similar observations apply to long-standing middle cerebral artery (MCA) stem stenosis or occlusion.[22–24]

When present, the hemodynamic alterations that are observed distal to ICA or MCA obstruction range from

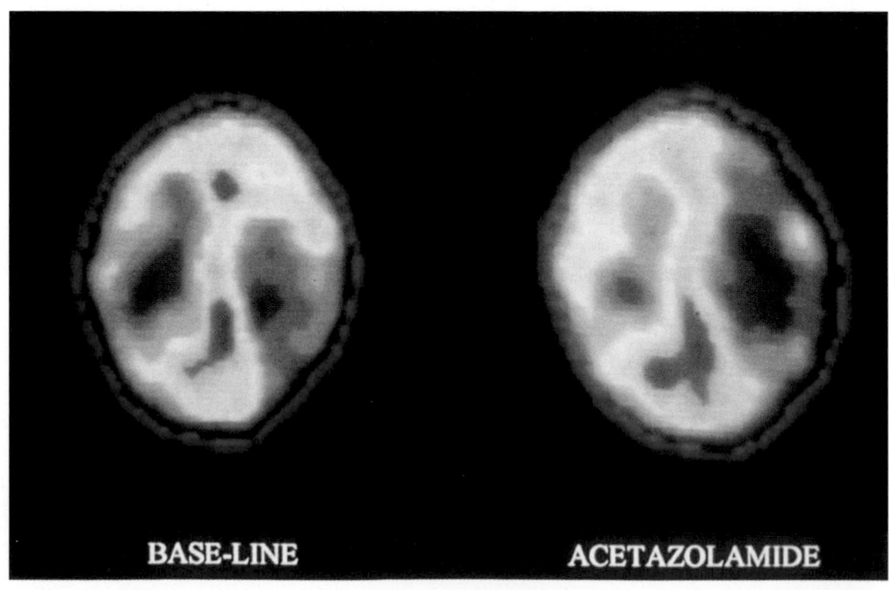

FIGURE 6-1. Impaired hemodynamic reserve. Resting and postacetazolamide positron emission tomography of cerebral blood flow (CBF) in a patient with repeated transient ischemic attacks due to left internal carotid artery occlusion with revascularization through the ipsilateral ophthalmic artery and the contralateral internal carotid artery. The resting scan (**left**) showed little or no alteration in CBF in the affected hemisphere. The vasodilatation challenge (**right**) induced a marked increase in CBF on the unoccluded side, but no increase in CBF on the occluded side with a decrease in the posterior and anterior parts of the left carotid territory, suggesting hemodynamic steal.

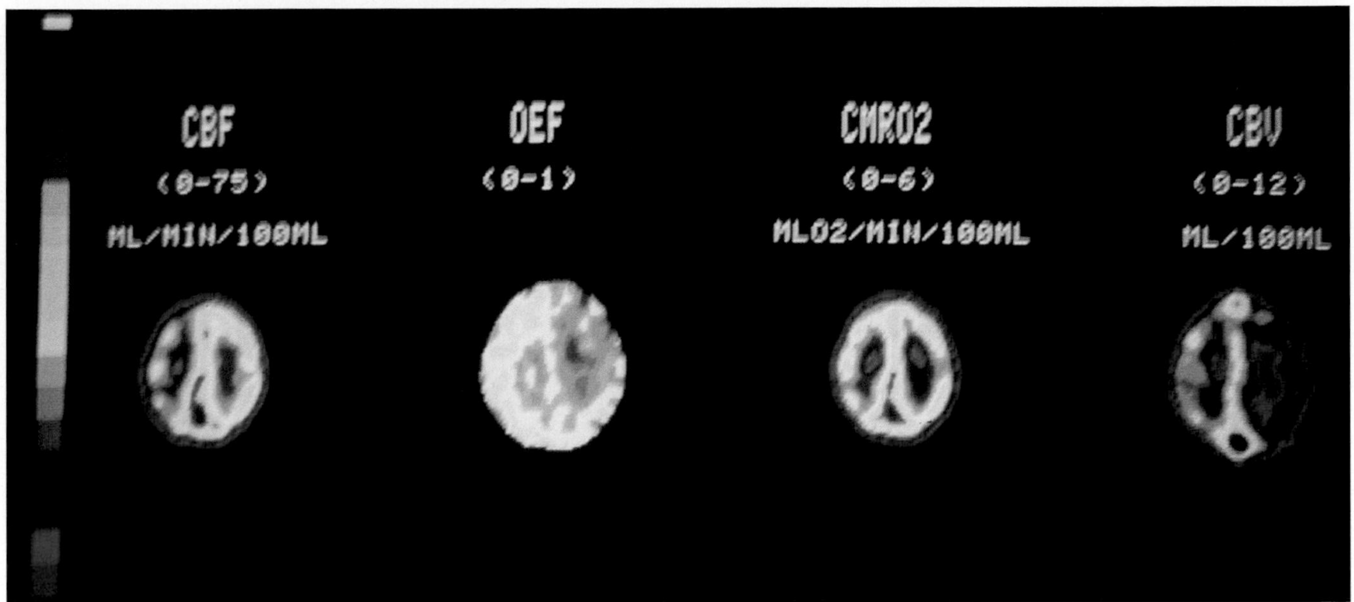

FIGURE 6-2. Misery perfusion in chronic symptomatic carotid artery occlusion. Stage 2 of hemodynamic failure. Occlusion of the right internal carotid artery was diagnosed when this patient presented with a transient ischemic attack ipsilateral to the occlusion. Transient ischemic attacks continued despite antiplatelet agents and subsequently warfarin, some of them being clearly postural. Positron emission tomography showed moderate hypoperfusion in the territory of the right internal carotid artery with a completely normal cerebral metabolic rate of oxygen (CMRO2). As a result, the oxygen extraction fraction (OEF) was increased (i.e., misery perfusion). This pattern suggests inability of the collateral circulation to compensate for the internal carotid artery occlusion, with the local autoregulation being overridden. Accordingly, there is a marked increase in cerebral blood volume (CBV) of the occluded side. (CBF = cerebral blood flow.)

autoregulated (i.e., with normal resting CBF but increased CBV, reduced CBF/CBV ratio, and reduced vasodilatory capacity to CO_2 or acetazolamide stress) to chronic oligemia (i.e., reduced resting CBF, increased OEF, increased CBV, markedly reduced CBF/CBV ratio, and abolished vasodilatory capacity with occasional hemodynamic steal) (see Figures 6-1 and 6-2).[2,25–27] Whatever their severity, these changes tend to predominate in watershed territories.[14,17,28] Misery perfusion is important to identify because it may forerun the occurrence of watershed infarction in patients with tight stenosis or occlusion of the ICA.[29,30]

Regarding moyamoya disease, the limited data[31–34] point to clear-cut hemodynamic insufficiency—be it in the pediatric type (with transient ischemic attacks [TIAs] and ischemic strokes as sole clinical manifestations) or in the adult type (with TIAs and brain hemorrhages). Impaired vasoreactivity, especially affecting the cerebral cortex, is the main observation, whereas misery perfusion is reported in a fraction of the cases only and particularly in children.

Very few PET studies of vertebrobasilar insufficiency have been published, possibly because of both the lack of clear operational clinical criteria and limitations of physiologic imaging in the posterior fossa. One study of eight patients reported significant reductions in CBF and increases in OEF with significant improvement after posterior fossa bypass surgery, but these changes were widespread to the whole brain and were interpreted by the authors as reflecting chronic ischemia of autonomic brain stem centers.[35] In a patient with subclavian steal and multiple arterial obstructions due to Takayasu's arteritis, a PET study revealed hemodynamic effects of left arm exercise on CBF and OEF, but, again, these effects were not confined to the posterior circulation.[36] In a patient with bilateral vertebral artery disease, posterior-circulation TIAs, and impaired vasodilatory response in the right cerebellum and occipital cortices at the time of PET, an infarct subsequently developed in these physiologically impaired areas,[37] making this the single proven example of vertebrobasilar hemodynamic impairment to date.

Clinical Correlates and Implications for Therapy

Clinical correlates of hemodynamic changes can be straightforward, as in the rare instance of orthostatic TIAs,[12] but in many situations, they are difficult to ascertain, as substantial hemodynamic abnormalities can exist in asymptomatic hemispheres or even in asymptomatic subjects. Across patients, however, there is a significant relationship between the finding of high OEF and ipsilateral ischemic symptoms.[38,39]

Following Baron's original report,[12] it has been consistently documented that successful cerebral revas-

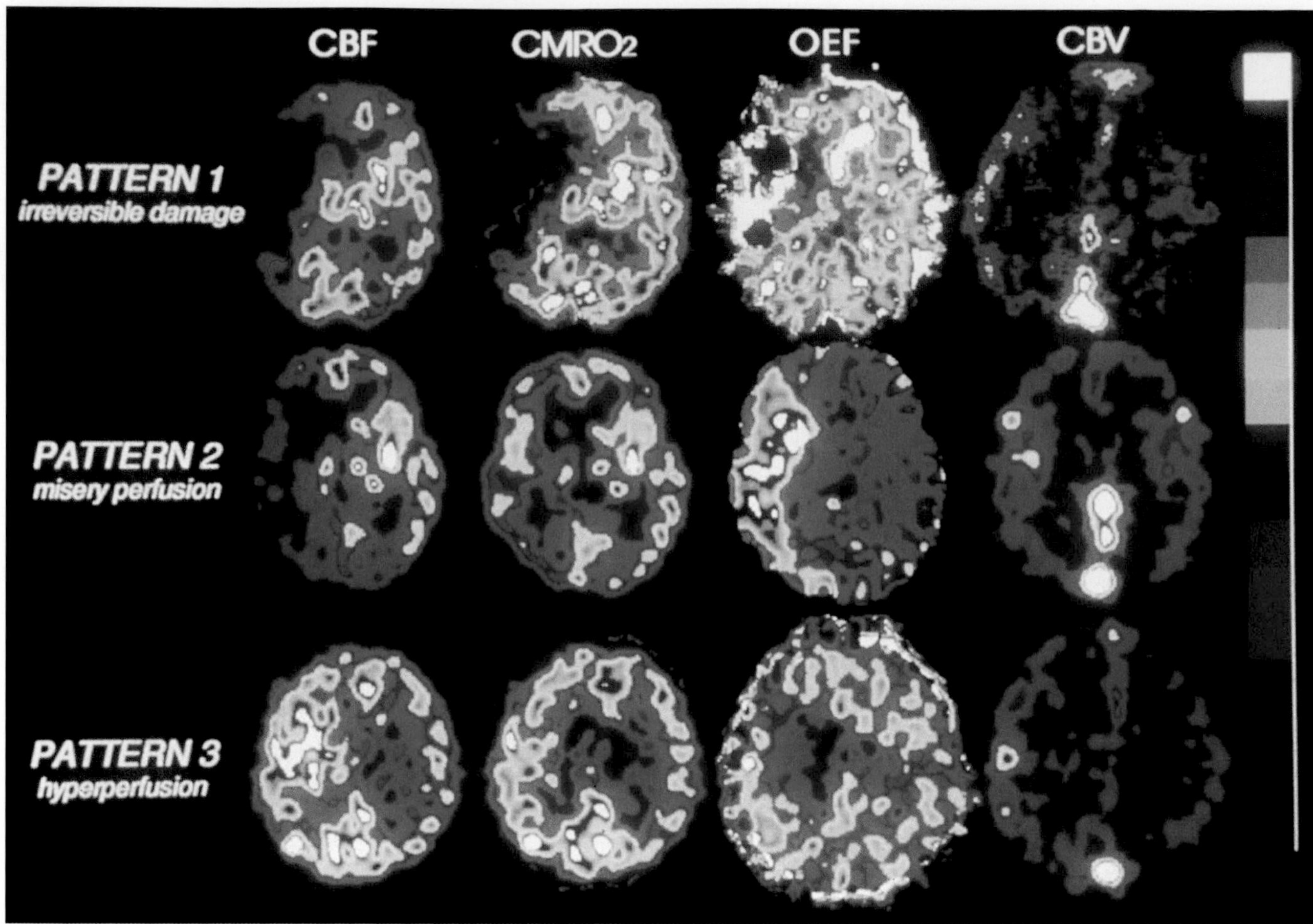

FIGURE 6-3. Illustrative positron emission tomography (PET) patterns in acute middle cerebral artery (MCA) territory stroke. This figure illustrates the three PET patterns of cerebral blood flow (CBF) and cerebral metabolic rate of oxygen ($CMRO_2$) changes observed within 18 hours from onset of stroke. **Top:** An example of early extensive irreversible damage in a patient with right-sided MCA territory stroke studied with PET 17 hours after symptom onset. There was a near-zero CBF and $CMRO_2$ in the whole right MCA territory (pattern 1), together with patchy oxygen extraction fraction (OEF) (black pixels represent immeasurable OEF). The patient survived, but outcome was poor, and the whole MCA territory was infarcted at follow-up computed tomography. **Middle:** Misery perfusion. In this patient, the PET study, performed 12 hours after onset, revealed a markedly reduced CBF in the whole right MCA territory, associated with relatively preserved $CMRO_2$ (except in the lenticulostriate area, which represents the core) and extremely elevated OEF. This example corresponds to a typical pattern 2 of PET changes. **Bottom:** Images illustrate an example of early luxury perfusion (pattern 3) in a patient studied with PET 13 hours after onset of stroke. There is markedly increased CBF in the central right MCA territory, associated with normal or slightly increased $CMRO_2$ and decreased OEF. This patient made a full recovery, and the follow-up computed tomography scan showed a small periventricular infarct. (CBV = cerebral blood volume.)

cularization—be it by means of carotid endarterectomy, superficial temporal-MCA extracranial-intracranial (EC-IC) bypass, or encephalo-duro-arterio synangiosis—at least partially reverses the hemodynamic compromise observed preoperatively.[12,14,15,40–45] This also applies to moyamoya disease.[46,47] In the early 1980s, documentation of a high OEF distal to ICA occlusion in a symptomatic patient became advocated as the sole rational basis for EC-IC bypass.[12] However, this surgical procedure was subsequently shown to lack significant clinical benefit in a randomized study and was criticized for not having used physiologic imaging as an entry criterion.[48] Apparently consistent with this finding, two retrospective nonrandomized studies by the St. Louis PET group[49,50] concluded that hemodynamic compromise accurately predicted neither poor outcome if medical therapy was elected nor good outcome if a bypass was performed. In contrast, several similarly open studies concluded that severely impaired cerebrovascular reactivity carried a significantly increased risk of ipsilateral stroke despite the best medical treatment.[15,51–56] This observation was subsequently replicated in a prospective study of 81 patients with symptomatic ICA occlusion carried out by the St. Louis group[57] that showed an increased risk of ipsilateral stroke at follow-up in the subgroup with misery perfusion with an odds ratio of 7.3 ($p = .004$). Yamauchi et al.[24] reported similar findings from a prospective study of symptomatic patients with tight stenosis or occlusion of the ICA or the MCA. They found that the risk of subsequent ipsilateral ischemic stroke was considerably higher in those patients with increased OEF with an odds ratio of 7.2, strikingly similar to the data reported by the St. Louis group. The latter group published the results of yet another prospective study, this time on patients with never-symptomatic ICA occlusion, that showed a very low risk of subsequent stroke in association with normal OEF.[39] All this accumulated evidence prompted the results from the EC-IC bypass study to be contested anew,[11,58] and a new multicenter trial, in which patient inclusion requires the finding of a high OEF, is presently under way. It appears, however, that those patients with the most compromised cerebrovascular physiology may be the most at risk for perioperative complications such as low-pressure breakthrough of autoregulation as a result of protracted microvascular dysregulation.[14,15,59] A significant association has been shown between the degree of preoperative impairment of cerebrovascular reactivity and the risk of postoperative cerebral hyperperfusion, which carries a high risk of intracerebral hemorrhage and seizures,[59,60] suggesting that in patients with severely compromised cerebrovascular physiology, special preventive measures such as strict blood pressure monitoring and control are necessary in the perioperative period. When making management decisions, it should also be borne in mind that hemodynamic disturbances have a spontaneous tendency to gradually resolve, probably from development of collaterals[61]; in some patients, however, the hemodynamic situation actually deteriorates even without new clinical symptoms.[62]

Medical management should also be planned in patients with carotid artery disease and impaired brain hemodynamics. For instance, systemic hypotension (as a result of drug therapy or any surgical procedure, especially cardiac) should be carefully avoided. Furthermore, because embolic events may have more serious tissue consequences in a dysregulated vascular bed than they would in normal brain, medical measures to prevent embolism should be implemented whenever necessary.

ARTERIOVENOUS MALFORMATIONS

As reviewed elsewhere,[63] although the hemodynamic hypothesis for the occurrence of either transient/fluctuating neurologic deficits or postoperative "hyperperfusion syndrome" in arteriovenous malformations (AVMs) has received some support from direct intraoperative measurements, studies of CBF performed outside the operating theater have been inconclusive or have even produced paradoxic results.[64] Although PET should in principle be ideally suited to identify with confidence any hemodynamic impairment in the surrounds of the nidus, it unfortunately suffers from serious limitations for the assessment of AVMs. All PET models assume that the blood pool in the voxels is either negligible or small enough to be corrected accurately,[1] but in the case of AVMs, this assumption may be incorrect due to dilated draining veins, causing errors in the estimation of not only CBV but also CBF, the CBF/CBV ratio, the OEF, and the $CMRO_2$.[1] This problem presumably accounts for the unphysiologic CBV values reported in some AVM PET studies. Although it is in principle possible to exclude all the voxels above a given CBV cutoff from the analysis, doing this may lead to excluding effectively large parts of the parenchyma, especially those surrounding the AVM itself. Despite these caveats, all PET studies published to date tend to indicate the presence of hemodynamic disturbances in AVMs.[65–67] In one study, an increased CBV/CBF ratio was observed in the hemisphere ipsilateral to small lesions and in both hemispheres in large lesions.[65] In another study, a similar finding was observed in the tissue adjacent to the nidus, but the available data were interpreted as inconsistent with a steal mechanism.[67] Thus, although reductions in CBF have been consistently observed in the surrounding tissue, they may go along with a normal or even reduced OEF as well as with reduced $CMRO_2$ and CMRglc. The latter can actually spread to the whole affected hemisphere and even to the opposite hemisphere, which may represent extensive synapse or neuron loss due to long-standing reductions in CPP.

ACUTE ISCHEMIC STROKE

In this section, the *acute stage of stroke* is defined as the first 24 hours after onset of clinical symptoms. Only a brief summary of the events that occur after this initial period are given here (see Baron[68,69] for further details). Being the most common subtype, MCA territory stroke has been the almost exclusive topic of research to date and is the only stroke subtype discussed.

As detailed previously, the following classification of four brain tissue subtypes allows us to operationally characterize the pathophysiologic situation in acute ischemic stroke: (1) the *core* (defined as the irreversibly damaged tissue already present at time of imaging); (2) the *penumbra* (defined as that severely hypoperfused tissue at risk for, but that can still be saved from, infarction); (3) the *oligemia* (defined as mildly hypoperfused tissue and not at risk for infarction under normal circumstances); and (4) the *hyperperfused tissue* (defined as tissue with CBF higher than that in the contralateral homologous tissue and taken to represent effective reperfusion).

Mapping the Core

Mapping the ischemic core is one major goal of acute stroke imaging because it depicts the extent of tissue already beyond therapeutic reach and potentially at risk for hemorrhagic transformation spontaneously or after the use of thrombolytics. To implement core mapping, however, validated infarction thresholds for the variables under study need to be determined first. Early PET studies using gray matter regions of interest reported a $CMRO_2$ threshold for irreversibility of approximately 1.4 ml/100 ml per minute.[8,70,71] More recently, a threshold value of approximately 0.9 ml/100 ml per minute for any voxel in brain tissue has been reported from PET studies done in the 5- to 18-hour interval,[72] a cut point applicable for core mapping purposes. Corresponding values for CBF have been reported as approximately 12.0 and 8.5 ml/100 ml per minute, respectively. However, contrary to oxygen consumption that is likely to be time independent, the CBF threshold is expected to depend on time since occlusion.[73] Accordingly, a CBF infarction threshold approximately 5 ml/100 ml per minute has been reported from studies performed within 6 hours of stroke onset[74]; for methodologic reasons detailed elsewhere, this value should be taken with some caution.[75] Finally, Heiss et al.[74,76,77] recently computed an irreversibility threshold for ^{11}C-FMZ for cortical tissue within 12 hours of stroke onset that was less than 3.4 times the white matter value.

In many patients, and consistent with its end-artery vascular system, the striatocapsular area exhibits irreversible damage very early, in striking contrast with the cortical ribbon that demonstrates misery perfusion (see Figure 6-3).[78,79] In some patients, the core extends to include part of the central MCA cortical territory surrounded by the penumbra. In a subset of patients, however, the entire MCA cortical territory exhibits irreversible damage as early as 4–6 hours after stroke onset,[78–80] suggesting inadequate pial collaterals or particularly severe CPP reductions in the affected people (see Figure 6-3). Although in most instances the CBF is as profoundly reduced as the $CMRO_2$, moderately reduced or nearly normal CBF is occasionally encountered (notably in small, deep infarcts), reflecting spontaneous partial reperfusion.[81]

Marchal et al. found that the volume of the core as assessed within 5–18 hours postonset was linearly correlated to final infarct volume, as measured by computed tomography (CT) scanning approximately one month later.[72] The former underestimated the latter by a factor of two, however, because of subsequent metabolic deterioration of the penumbra (see the section Mapping the Penumbra). Thus, mapping the ischemic core in the acute stage of stroke helps predict the volume of final infarction. As expected, the volume of irreversible damage also positively correlates with the severity of admission neurologic deficit.[72]

Mapping the Penumbra

Acute-stroke PET often demonstrates critical ischemia, exhibiting features consistent with penumbra (see Figure 6-3).[9,78–82] In most instances, this involves the entire MCA cortical territory, with the striatocapsular area exhibiting early irreversible damage (see the section Mapping the Core and Figure 6-3). In some instances, however, the penumbra surrounds a limited cortical area with already irreversible damage. This tissue displays severely reduced CBF below the penumbral threshold of approximately 20 ml/100 ml per minute, strikingly increased OEF often above 0.80, and $CMRO_2$ above the threshold for viability. In a detailed voxel-based analysis of 11 patients studied within 5–18 hours after clinical onset of stroke, Furlan et al.[83] found that the range of CBF that characterized this tissue was 7–17 ml/100 ml per minute, close to the values reported in monkeys.[73] With a different approach to data analysis of the same patient sample, Marchal et al.[80] found a penumbra threshold of 22 ml/100 ml per minute, which is again very close to classic experimental data. From a study of 10 patients investigated within 12 hours of onset, Heiss et al.[74] reported a penumbra threshold of 14.5 ml/100 ml per minute, which lies on the low side presumably for methodologic reasons detailed elsewhere.[75] Another important feature of the penumbra is its expected alleviation with increases in arterial pressure. Although these are extremely difficult studies to perform, Ackerman et al.[71] reported in abstract form a patient in whom induced systemic hypertension resulted in reduced CBF and $CMRO_2$.

Both the incidence and the extent of the penumbra tend to decrease with elapsing interval since stroke onset. Thus, substantial cortical penumbra has been reported in 90% of patients studied within 6 hours of onset, in over 50% of those studied within 9 hours, and in about one-third of those studied between 5 and 18 hours.[74,78,84,85] These data suggest that the window for therapeutic opportunity may be protracted in at least a subset of patients. One study found that as late as 16 hours after symptom onset, up to 52% (range, 10–52%; mean, 32%) of the ultimately infarcted tissue still exhibited physiologic characteristics compatible with penumbra.[80] Based on semiquantitative CBF data, Heiss et al.[86] reported a smaller penumbral compartment (accounting for 18% of the finally infarcted volume) even though their patients were studied paradoxically within 3 hours. However, they used an unconventional classification of tissue subtypes evolving to infarction that considered a mildly hypoperfused component as distinct from penumbra, despite being clearly at risk of infarction. If this compartment is merged with the penumbra, then the findings are consistent with those of Marchal et al.[80] In a more recent report from a group of 10 patients studied within 12 hours from onset and using a similar tissue classification, Heiss et al.[74] reported a penumbra comprising approximately 20% of the final infarct. However, if the mildly hypoperfused compartment was also considered, then the at-risk compartment in this work was actually 45% across patients and up to 85% individually; again, the findings are consistent with Marchal et al.[80] Interestingly, in that study, large fractions of at-risk tissue were found in those patients studied within 12 hours of onset, confirming earlier findings[80] that in some patients with MCA territory stroke, a sizeable cortical penumbra may linger for hours. Using ^{18}F-MISO in acute stroke, Read et al.[7] also reported the frequent occurrence of hypoxic brain tissue, with the volume of the latter exhibiting the expected decline with elapsing time, but with hypoxic tissue still being found as late as 43 hours after onset in one case. However, because hypoxic tissue may represent penumbral as well as simply oligemic tissue, the relevance of this observation remains to be clarified.

Fate of the Penumbra

The penumbra can either progress to or escape from infarction, depending on subsequent events such as the occurrence of reperfusion. The transition from penumbra to core is signaled by a decline in $CMRO_2$, whereas the CBF further declines or remains stable.[78,80,82] With elapsing days, perfusion progressively increases in the necrotic tissue, representing improved collateral flow.[9,87] This whole process is epitomized by a dramatic fall in the OEF from initially very high to sometimes exceedingly low values (i.e., luxury perfusion), signaling the exhaustion of the tissue's oxygen needs. Of note, a marked gradual increase in ^{11}C-PK binding both within and surrounding the infarcted area has been reported, peaking around the second week and reflecting the microglial and macrophagic infiltration characteristic of the subacute stage of the infarction process.[5,6]

All or part of the penumbra may escape infarction.[82,83,84] Events such as partial or complete reperfusion—either spontaneous or therapeutic—and dampening of glutamate release from the core, may account for such favorable outcome. PET studies in baboons have documented that early reperfusion is capable of affecting the fate of the penumbra.[88,89] In humans, Heiss et al.[84] have reported that large volumes of tissue with CBF below approximately 12 ml/100 ml per minute (thus, likely penumbral) escape necrosis in patients successfully recanalized by intravenous thrombolysis administered within 3 hours of onset.

Oligemia

As stated above, the oligemic tissue is by definition hypoperfused but, in principle, not at risk for infarction. In other words, it displays a mild degree of misery perfusion with high OEF, but its CBF stands above the penumbra threshold. In distinguishing the penumbra from the oligemic tissue, Furlan et al.[83] documented that in some patients, the high OEF area was largely penumbral, whereas in others, it virtually was only oligemic, emphasizing the notion that acute stroke misery perfusion should not be equated with penumbra. As mentioned above, Heiss et al.[74,84] found that, according to their tissue classification scheme, a substantial portion (≥45% in three patients) of the ultimate infarction was only mildly hypoperfused (i.e., oligemic). This observation serves to stress the point that, because its perfusion is pressure dependent, the oligemic compartment, though not at risk of infarction in uncomplicated circumstances, may become incorporated in the penumbra and, hence, be incorporated into the core as a result of secondary events that tend to reduce the local CPP such as vasogenic edema and systemic hypotension. It is also possible that cells in the oligemic tissue are sensitive to systemic factors that aggravate the flow-to-metabolism mismatch such as hyperglycemia and pyrexia. These considerations are important because they explain the benefits of avoiding such complications in the clinic.

Early Spontaneous Hyperperfusion

In the 5- to 18-hour poststroke interval, hyperperfusion has been observed in approximately one-third of cases (see Figure 6-3).[79,89] It affects the MCA cortical ribbon either extensively or in a patchy fashion and sometimes the basal ganglia as well. Hyperperfusion is associated with reduced OEF and increased CBV, indicating luxury perfusion with abnormal vasodilatation. In most instances, the hyperperfused tissue does not exhibit reduced $CMRO_2$ but a mildly increased $CMRO_2$, suggesting postischemic rebound of cellular energy-dependent processes.[81] Importantly, in these studies, hyperperfused areas consistently exhibited intact morphology at late structural imaging,[81] suggesting early hyperperfusion is a marker of good tissue prognosis. Interpretation of these findings posits that recanalization spontaneously occurred before PET and resulted in efficient reperfusion of the penumbra. These findings are consistent with the well-established notion that infarct size is reduced by early recanalization[73] and suggest that the experimental concept of sudden tissue reoxygenation might exacerbate ischemic brain damage and may not apply to humans (see Marchal et al. for review).[90] The implications of hyperperfusion may, however, somewhat differ when it comes to therapeutic thrombolysis, as some reports suggest that postrecanalization hyperperfusion may herald poor tissue outcome.[91] It is conceivable that thrombolysis may, in certain circumstances, force reperfusion into an already irreversibly damaged vascular tree—an event that would otherwise rarely take place.

Clinical Correlates

In 30 patients investigated in the 5- to 18-hour poststroke interval, Marchal et al.[79,85] prospectively assessed the relationships between acute-stage PET findings and clinical outcome. Each patient was reproducibly classified into one of three visually defined patterns of PET changes (see Figure 6-3), namely (1) extensive subcortico-cortical core (pattern 1); (2) presence of penumbra without extensive core (pattern 2; this pattern is the equivalent of the mismatch pattern observed with diffusion-weighted and perfusion MRI, although formal cross-validation for the latter is still lacking); and (3) hyperperfusion without extensive core (pattern 3). There was a highly significant relationship between these patterns and subsequent neurologic course. Thus, all pattern-1 patients did poorly (malignant infarction with early death or poor outcome), whereas all patients classified as pattern 3 did well (complete or nearly complete recovery in all). Consistent with the penumbra concept, pattern-2 patients had an unpredictable course, ranging from death to full recovery. Importantly, the predictive value for final outcome was independent of admission neurologic scores (i.e., the PET patterns had significant independent predictive value over and above that of clinical scores alone).[85] Consistent findings regarding hyperperfusion have been reported by Heiss et al.,[91] who showed in a few cases that in both pre– and post–early intravenous thrombolysis, the occurrence of hyperperfusion was associated with good clinical and tissular outcome, unlike severe and persisting hypoperfusion. As noted above, however, massive post-thrombolysis hyperperfusion may occasionally develop in the already necrotic core.

Alleviation of Penumbra: Its Role in Clinical Recovery

Although pathophysiologic models have long predicted that survival of the penumbra should be one major determinant of recovery after ischemic stroke, it is only recently that this has been documented in humans. In a study of 11 patients with acute-stage misery perfusion, Furlan et al.[83] reported that the volume of penumbra that eventually escaped infarction was highly correlated with the extent of subsequent neurologic recovery. Less predictably, however, the best correlation was observed with 2-month recovery scores, which suggests that survival of the penumbra influences not only early but also late recovery (i.e., it provides an opportunity for subsequent peri-infarct neuronal reorganization). Heiss et al.[84] subsequently confirmed the findings of Furlan et al. These authors observed a significant correlation between the volume of critically hypoperfused tissue saved by thrombolysis and the change in neurologic scores between admission and 3 weeks. Likewise, using ^{18}F-MISO, Read et al.[92] reported that the degree of neurologic deterioration or improvement after MCA territory stroke was significantly related to the volume of initially hypoxic tissue that went on to infarct at subsequent structural imaging.

In the chronic stage, decreases in cortical uptake of ^{11}C-FMZ (or its single-photon emission CT analog, iodine-123–iomazenil) have been reported, occasionally affecting areas not showing frank infarction at structural imaging.[93] This finding has been taken as evidence for selective neuronal loss in the surviving penumbra, which might underlie neuropsychological deficits after subcortical infarction; thus, benzodiazepine-receptor imaging may allow us to differentiate cortical dysfunction induced by diaschisis (see the section Thalamo-Cortical Diaschisis) from that due to occult damage. However, reduced tracer uptake in the hypometabolic cortex after striatocapsular infarction is not a universal finding,[94] and in addition, histopathologic confirmation of neuronal loss in areas with reduced in vivo binding has been lacking thus far. The significance of these findings remains unclear to this date.

Implications for Therapy

Implications for General Management

Demonstration of high OEF in the setting of acute stroke implies that the autoregulation is overridden in the affected territory. This point is especially important in view of the frequent occurrence of reactive hypertension in this clinical setting. Thus, any lowering of the systemic arterial pressure (SAP) is likely to further reduce the CPP and in turn the CBF in the affected tissue, which can be harmful not only for the penumbra but also for the oligemia (see the section Oligemia). This may in turn explain why reductions in SAP in acute stroke have frequently been associated with worse outcome.[95] If, conversely, hyperperfusion and low OEF are present, then management of arterial hypertension may be possible and perhaps even advisable, particularly if early edema is demonstrated by CT or MRI, because some experimental studies suggest that hyperperfusion in necrotic tissue may promote the development of malignant brain swelling.

Implications for Specific Therapy and Trials

Based on the data reviewed in the section Clinical Correlates, physiologic imaging is helpful in depicting in each patient the pathophysiologic condition of the brain before aggressive therapy is considered. The following framework is proposed: (1) if pattern 3 (early spontaneous recanalization) is documented, outcome is invariably good, and no aggressive therapy should be considered; (2) if pattern 1 (early extensive necrosis) is documented, outcome is invariably poor with considerable risk of massive brain swelling and early death, and any treatment is likely to fail apart from those directed against vasogenic edema, such as surgical brain decompression; and (3) if pattern 2 (substantial penumbra [i.e., mismatch]) is documented, management should be directed at saving as much penumbra as possible; thus, this pattern characterizes the best candidates for urgent therapy. Specific trials should test whether incorporating physiologic imaging into the management flowchart of acute stroke has significantly added value despite the additional time required to perform the procedure. Likewise, although the above data suggest that pathophysiologically blind inclusion of acute stroke patients into trials may blur any beneficial effects of the agent being tested because of underlying pathophysiologic heterogeneity, the practice of adding physiologic imaging to improve sensitivity of therapeutic trials needs to be tested in its own right.

A final point is the observation that, whereas in some patients there is extensive tissue necrosis or, conversely, complete reperfusion only hours after stroke onset, in others, penumbra is seen up to 16 hours, suggesting that the individual therapeutic window should be considered in each case.[96] The positive results from the PRO-ACT II trial of intra-arterial thrombolysis performed up to 6 hours after onset in a selected sample of patients with documented MCA stem occlusion[97] further strengthen the notion that, in a subset of patients at least, some at-risk tissue is still present many hours into the pathologic process. Apart from thrombolysis, however, patients with extensive penumbra might also benefit from neuroprotective agents, provided they are devoid of SAP reduction effects.

REMOTE METABOLIC EFFECTS OF STROKE

Remote metabolic depression is characterized by coupled reductions in perfusion and metabolism in brain structures remote from, but connected with, the area damaged by the stroke. This effect is widely explained as depressed synaptic activity as a result of disconnection (either direct or transneural). Thus, mapping remote effects allows the identification of disrupted networks as a sequel of focal infarction. Although these effects are often referred to collectively as *diaschisis*,[98] this term conceals a variety of cellular derangements, from reversible hypofunction to evolving wallerian or trans-synaptic degeneration, which have the same PET expression. Importantly, some of these effects reflect purely functional, potentially recoverable synaptic derangement, which therefore may participate in both the acute clinical expression of stroke and subsequent recovery.

Crossed Cerebellar Diaschisis

Crossed cerebellar diaschisis (CCD)[9,99] affects the cerebellar hemisphere contralateral to supratentorial stroke (Figure 6-4). It occurs in approximately 50% of cortical or subcortical strokes but is more frequent and severe with large hemispheric or capsular strokes.[100] It generally results from damage to the glutamatergic cortico-ponto-cerebellar system (CPCS), inducing transneuronal functional depression, further documented by observations of CCD after unilateral brain stem lesion at the level of the crus cerebri or basis pontis. Although it is often associated with hemiparesis,[100] this association is not systematic and presumably results from strokes encroaching both the pyramidal and the CPCS fibers. The fact that CCD may develop within the first hours of stroke and subsequently disappear[101] indicates that it can be a transient manifestation of deafferentation. Accordingly, CCD can also tran-

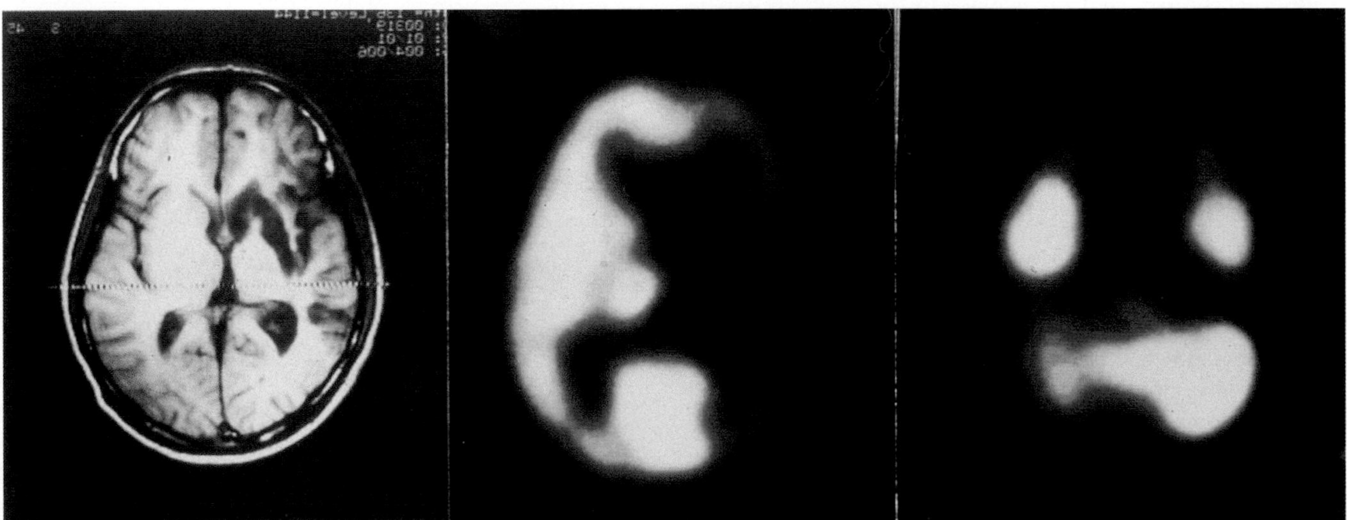

FIGURE 6-4. Remote metabolic effects of stroke. In this example of incomplete patchy cortico-subcortical middle cerebral artery territory infarction as depicted by chronic-stage magnetic resonance imaging (**left**), the positron emission tomography study of the cerebral metabolic rate of oxygen performed in the subacute stage revealed striking remote metabolic depression affecting the contralateral cerebellum (**right**) as well as the ipsilateral thalamus, striatum, and cortical ribbon (**middle**).

siently manifest in instances of reversible functional depression of the cerebral cortex, such as TIAs or balloon occlusion of the ICA.[102] In the majority of stroke patients, however, CCD tends to persist,[86,100] which suggests it might evolve into transneuronal degeneration in the long run. Yet, even in long-standing CCD, standard MRI rarely demonstrates atrophy, even though ipsilateral atrophy of the cerebral peduncle is occasionally seen, consistent with CPCS damage.[103]

The lack of CCD in acute MCA territory stroke predicts a good outcome, whereas its presence has little predictive value individually.[101] Although a relationship between CCD and ipsilateral ataxia has been anecdotally reported,[104] other studies indicate a lack of one-to-one association,[105] such that only ataxia due to CPCS damage will be translated into CCD. A relationship with ipsilateral flaccidity has also been reported,[106] but again, this was not a one-to-one association.

Contralateral Cerebral Effects

Although contralateral cerebral effects have long been thought to underlie some symptoms, such as agitation and confusion, and exacerbate the focal deficit, they have been elusive because of confounding factors, such as the lack of adequate controls and the use of CBF that has intrinsic physiologic variability. Recently, a lack of association between changes in contralateral hemisphere $CMRO_2$ and early changes in neurologic deficits was reported.[107] However, contralateral hemisphere hypometabolism develops in the subacute stage of MCA stroke, dissociated from the clinical recovery that takes place at this stage, presumably as a result of degeneration of severed transcallosal fibers.[107,108] It may be that the progressive alleviation of contralateral hemisphere hypometabolism that takes place in the long run partly underlies late improvements in cognitive deficits.[108–110]

Subcortico-Cortical Effects

Subcortical Aphasia

Reduced cortical CMRglc has been reported in small, deep left-sided infarcts such as thalamic or thalamocapsular stroke with language impairment,[109,111,112] suggesting that subcortical aphasia could be in part related to this remote functional effect. This idea is supported by the finding of a positive correlation between the impairment in distinct aphasia items (i.e., oral and written comprehension, naming, and repetition) and the severity of left parietotemporal hypometabolism.[113,114]

Subcortical Neglect

Marked ipsilateral cortical hypometabolism has been consistently reported after right-sided subcortical infarcts with left hemineglect.[109,115,116] Predominance of these effects over the frontal and parietal cortices suggests involvement of the subcortico-cortical network for directed attention. Consistent with this interpretation, motor neglect is characterized by sparing of the primary motor circuit (striatum, cerebellum, and motor strip) and hypometabolism of the "supra-motor" circuit (i.e., premotor, prefrontal, cingulate, and parietal cortices).[117,118]

Hemianopia

Damage to the optic radiations induces a significant reduction in glucose utilization in the disconnected part of the ipsilateral primary visual cortex,[119] sometimes spreading to the visual association areas and even to the contralateral visual cortex.[120]

Thalamo-Cortical Diaschisis

Infarcts in the anterior, medial, or lateral thalamus almost invariably induce a metabolic depression of the entire ipsilateral cortical mantle (maximal in the projection areas of the affected nuclei),[109,121,122] presumably as a result of involvement of the excitatory thalamo-cortical projections (Figure 6-5). As just noted, there are also significant relationships between the pattern of cortical hypometabolism and the aphasia profile or hemineglect after thalamic stroke.[109] A correlation between the degree of cognitive impairment after ventrolateral thalamotomy and the extent of thalamo-cortical diaschisis (TCD) has been reported,[109] whereas TCD is absent in pure sensorimotor stroke from posterolateral thalamic stroke.[123] Also, preferential frontal cortex hypometabolism has been associated with frontal-like syndromes and global amnesia after right- or left-sided thalamic infarction.[121,122] In patients with severe permanent amnesia and apathy from bilateral paramedian thalamic infarction ("thalamic dementia" from "strategic infarcts"), marked neocortical hypometabolism has been reported.[124,125]

Other Ipsilateral Effects

Striatal and thalamic hypometabolism is frequently found ipsilateral to cortico-subcortical stroke (see Figure 6-4).[9,103,111] As thalamic hypometabolism develops a few days after the stroke, it presumably represents active retrograde degeneration of the damaged thalamo-cortical neurons. This progression is further suggested by the finding of increased ^{11}C-PK binding in the thalamus ipsilateral to subacute cortical stroke,[126] whereas striatal hypometabolism probably reflects loss of glutamatergic input from the cortex. Left caudate and thalamic hypometabolism is significantly associated with Broca's (i.e., nonfluent) aphasia, as compared with Wernicke's or the conduction aphasias.[127] Thalamic hypometabolism has been associated with poor recovery of hand function after ischemic stroke.[128]

Iglesias et al.[129] recently assessed the issue of hypometabolism of the cortical ribbon ipsilateral to the

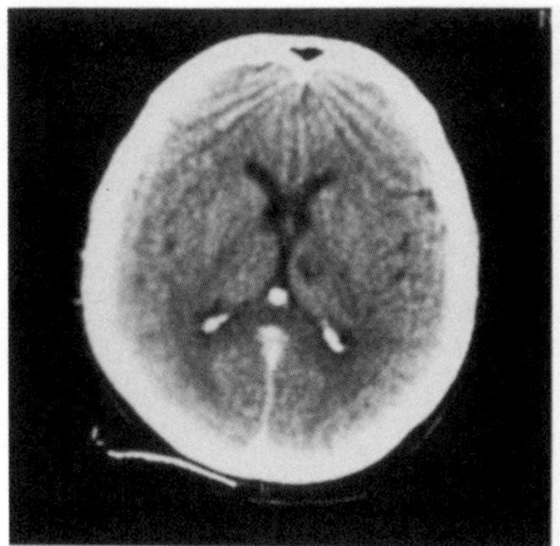
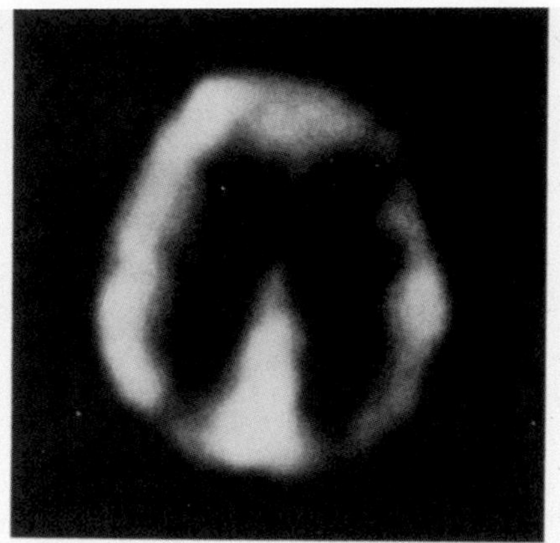
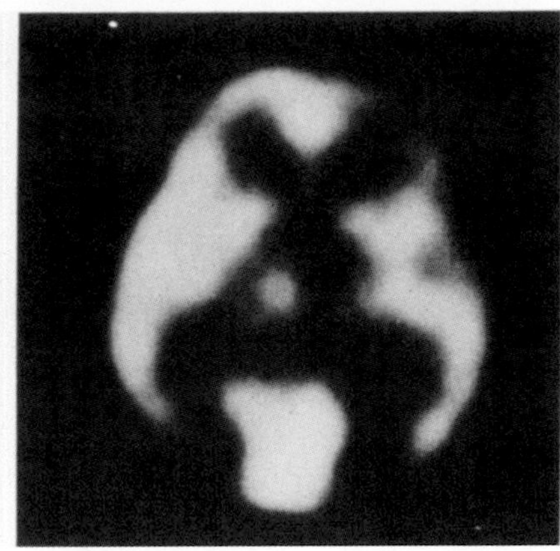

FIGURE 6-5. Thalamo-cortical diaschisis. Computed tomography scan (**left**) of a 57-year-old patient with small left lateral-ventral thalamic infarct inducing impaired verbal memory and verbal fluency with some general mental slowing. The positron emission tomography study of the cerebral metabolic rate of oxygen performed 2 months after onset (**middle, right**) revealed a metabolic depression affecting the entire cortical ribbon ipsilateral to the thalamic infarct, maximal over the frontal and parietotemporal association cortices with relative sparing of the primary cortices.

infarction in MCA territory stroke. They documented the effect develops over several days in spite of concomitant neurologic recovery. As in the case of contralateral cerebral hypometabolism, the hypothesis, proposed to explain these paradoxic findings, invokes the degeneration of terminals of neurons damaged by the infarct, a notion supported by the finding of a significant correlation between the severity of ipsilateral cortical $CMRO_2$ reduction and the size of the infarct in Iglesias et al.'s study. This, however, does not detract from the observation that there is a progressive improvement of this effect in the long run that may participate in the process of clinical recovery (see the section Role of Cortical Hypometabolism in Behavioral Recovery from Stroke).[108–110,130]

Role of Cortical Hypometabolism in Behavioral Recovery from Stroke

After subcortical stroke, the cortical metabolic depression tends to recover over the ensuing months in parallel with cognitive recovery.[109,130,131] Some mechanism of synaptic reorganization must, therefore, slowly creep in after the early trans-synaptic effect and underlie cognitive recovery. The lesser the subacute-stage defect in CMRglc around Wernicke's and Broca's areas, the better the outcome in terms of language comprehension and verbal fluency, respectively.[132] The observations that the peri-infarct area may be crucial for early recovery in aphasia are consistent with the previously described findings regarding the fate of the penumbra.[83] Thus, although language recovery within the first year appears to be linked primarily to metabolic recovery in the dominant hemisphere,[110] long-term language improvements seem to be related to slow metabolic recovery in the contralateral hemisphere, specifically in the homotopic frontal and thalamic areas.[133] Taken together, the available evidence suggests that recovery of cortical metabolism, both ipsilateral and contralateral, is associated with functional recovery after stroke and is one expression of neuronal reorganization after network damage.

REFERENCES

1. Baron JC, Frackowiak RSJ, Herholz K, et al. Use of positron emission tomography in the investigation of cerebral hemodynamics and energy metabolism in cerebrovascular disease. J Cereb Blood Flow Metab 1989;9:723–742.

2. Gibbs JM, Wise RJS, Leenders KL, et al. Evaluation of cerebral perfusion reserve in patients with carotid-artery occlusion. Lancet 1984;1:310–314.

3. Sette G, Baron JC, Mazoyer B, et al. Local brain hemodynamics and oxygen metabolism in cerebro-vascular disease: positron emission tomography. Brain 1989;112:931–951.

4. Schumann P, Touzani O, Young AR, et al. Evaluation of the ratio of cerebral blood flow to cerebral blood volume as an index of local cerebral perfusion pressure. Brain 1998;121:1369–1379.

5. Sette G, Baron JC, Young AR, et al. In vivo mapping of brain benzodiazepine receptor changes by positron emission tomography after focal ischemia in the anesthetized baboon. Stroke 1993;24:2046–2058.

6. Ramsay SC, Weiller C, Myers R, et al. Monitoring by PET of macrophage accumulation in brain after ischaemic stroke. Lancet 1992;239:1054–1055.

7. Read SJ, Hirano T, Abbott DF, et al. Identifying hypoxic tissue after acute ischemic stroke using PET and ^{18}F-fluoromisonidazole. Neurology 1998;51:1617–1621.

8. Baron JC, Rougemont D, Soussaline F, et al.

Local interrelationship of cerebral oxygen consumption and glucose utilization in normal subjects and in ischemic stroke patients: a positron tomography study. J Cereb Blood Flow Metab 1984;4:140–149.

9. Baron JC, Bousser MG, Comar D, et al. Noninvasive tomographic study of cerebral blood flow and oxygen metabolism in vivo: potentials, limitations and clinical applications in cerebral ischemic disorders. Eur Neurol 1981;20:273–284.

10. Frackowiak RSJ. The pathophysiology of human cerebral ischaemia: a new perspective obtained with positron tomography. QJM 1985;223:713–727.

11. Derdeyn CP, Grubb RL, Powers WJ. Cerebral hemodynamic impairment. Method of measurement and association with stroke risk. Neurology 1999;53: 251–259.

12. Baron JC, Bousser MG, Rey A, et al. Reversal of focal "misery-perfusion syndrome" by extra-intracranial arterial bypass in hemodynamic cerebral ischemia: a case study with ^{15}O positron tomography. Stroke 1981;12:454–459.

13. Lassen NA. The luxury perfusion syndrome and its possible relation to acute metabolic acidosis localised within the brain. Lancet 1966;2:1113–1115.

14. Samson Y, Baron JC, Bousser MG, et al. Effects of extra-intracranial arterial bypass on cerebral blood flow and oxygen metabolism in humans. Stroke 1985;16:609–616.

15. Derlon JM, Bouvard G, Viader F, et al. Impaired cerebral hemodynamics in internal carotid occlusion. Cerebrovasc Dis 1992;2:72–81.

16. Herold S, Brown MM, Frackowiak RSJ, et al. Assessment of cerebral haemodynamic reserve: correlation between PET parameters and CO_2 reactivity measured by the intravenous ^{133}xenon injection technique. J Neurol Neurosurg Psychiatry 1988;51:1045–1050.

17. Leblanc R, Yamamoto YL, Tyler JL, et al. Borderzone ischemia. Ann Neurol 1987;22:707–713.

18. Levine RL, Dobkin JA, Rozental JM, et al. Blood flow reactivity to hypercapnia in strictly unilateral carotid disease: preliminary results. J Neurol Neurosurg Psychiatry 1991;54:204–209.

19. Powers WJ, Press GA, Grubb RL, et al. The effect of hemodynamically significant carotid artery disease on the hemodynamic status of the cerebral circulation. Ann Intern Med 1987;106:27–35.

20. Yamauchi H, Fukuyama H, Kimura J, et al. Hemodynamics in internal carotid artery occlusion examined by positron emission tomography. Stroke 1990;21:1400–1406.

21. Derdeyn CP, Shaibani A, Moran CJ, et al. Lack of correlation between pattern of collateralization and misery perfusion in patients with carotid occlusion. Stroke 1999;30:1025–1032.

22. Sgouropoulos P, Baron JC, Samson Y, et al. Sténoses et occlusions persistantes de l'artère cérébrale moyenne: conséquences hémodynamiques et métaboliques étudiées par tomographie à positons. Rev Neurol (Paris) 1985;141:698–705.

23. Derdeyn CP, Powers WJ, Grubb RL. Hemodynamic effects of middle cerebral artery stenosis and occlusion. AJNR Am J Neuroradiol 1998;19:1463–1469.

24. Yamauchi H, Fukuyama H, Nagahama Y, et al. Significance of increased oxygen extraction fraction in five-year prognosis of major cerebral arterial occlusive diseases. J Nucl Med 1999;40:1992–1998.

25. Vorstrup S, Engell HC, Lindewald H, et al. Hemodynamically significant stenosis of the internal carotid artery treated with endarterectomy. J Neurosurg 1984;60:1070–1075.

26. Vorstrup S, Lassen NA, Henriksen L, et al. CBF before and after extracranial-intracranial bypass surgery in patients with ischemic cerebrovascular disease studied with ^{133}Xe-inhalation tomography. Stroke 1985;16:616–626.

27. Vorstrup S, Brun B, Lassen NA. Evaluation of the cerebral vasodilatory capacity by the acetazolamide test before EC-IC bypass surgery in patients with occlusion of the internal carotid artery. Stroke 1986;17: 1291–1298.

28. Carpenter DA, Grubb RL, Powers WJ. Borderzone hemodynamics in cerebrovascular disease. Neurology 1990;40:1587–1592.

29. Itoh M, Hatazawa J, Pozzilli C, et al. Positron CT imaging of an impending stroke. Neuroradiology 1988;30:276–279.

30. Yamauchi H, Fukuyama H, Fujimoto N, et al. Significance of low perfusion with increased oxygen extraction fraction in a case of internal carotid artery stenosis. Stroke 1992;23:431–432.

31. Kuwabara Y, Ichiya Y, Otsuka M, et al. Cerebral hemodynamic change in the child and the adult with moya-moya disease. Stroke 1990;21:272–277.

32. Kuwabara Y, Ichiya Y, Sasaki M, et al. Response to hypercapnia in moya-moya disease. Stroke 1997;28:701–707.

33. Taki W, Yonekawa Y, Kobayashi A, et al. Cerebral circulation and oxygen metabolism in Moyamoya disease of ischemic type in children. Child Nerv Syst 1988;4:259–262.

34. Taki W, Yonekawa Y, Kobayashi A, et al. Cerebral circulation and metabolism in adult's moyamoya disease: PET study. Acta Neurochir (Wien) 1989;100:150–154.

35. Ogawa A, Kameyama M, Muraishi K, et al. Cerebral blood flow and metabolism following superficial temporal artery to superior cerebellar artery bypass for vertebrobasilar occlusive disease. J Neurosurg 1992;76:955–960.

36. Mase M, Yamada K, Matsumoto T, et al. Cerebral blood flow and metabolism of steal syndrome evaluated by PET. Neurology 1999;52:1515–1516.

37. Delecluse F, Vooredecker P, Raftopoulos C. Vertebrobasilar insufficiency revealed by xenon-133 inhalation SPECT. Stroke 1989;20:952–956.

38. Derdeyn CP, Yundt KD, Videen TO, et al. Increased oxygen extraction fraction is associated with prior ischemic events in patients with carotid occlusion. Stroke 1998;29:754–758.

39. Powers WJ, Derdeyn CP, Fritsch SM, et al. Benign prognosis of never-symptomatic carotid occlusion. Neurology 2000;54:878–882.

40. Gibbs JM, Wise RJS, Thomas DJ, et al. Cerebral haemodynamic changes after extracranial-intracranial bypass surgery. J Neurol Neurosurg Psychiatry 1987;50:140–150.

41. Leblanc R, Tyler JL, Mohr G, et al. Hemodynamic and metabolic effects of cerebral revascularization. J Neurosurg 1987;66:529–535.

42. Muraishi K, Kameyama M, Sato K, et al. Cerebral circulatory and metabolic changes following EC/IC bypass surgery in cerebral occlusive diseases. Neurol Res 1993;15:97–103.

43. Powers WJ, Martin WRW, Herscovitch P, et al. Extracranial-intracranial bypass surgery: hemodynamic and metabolic effects. Neurology 1984;34:1168–1174.

44. Nariai T, Suzuki R, Matsushima Y, et al. Surgically induced angiogenesis to compensate for hemodynamic cerebral ischemia. Stroke 1994;25:1014–1021.

45. Kuwabara Y, Ichiya Y, Sasaki M, et al. PET evaluation of cerebral hemodynamics in occlusive cerebrovascular disease pre- and post-surgery. J Nucl Med 1998;39:760–765.

46. Ikezaki K, Matsushima T, Suzuki SO, et al. Cerebral circulation and oxygen metabolism in childhood moyamoya disease: a perioperative positron emission tomography study. J Neurosurg 1994;81:843–850.

47. Okada Y, Shima T, Nishida M, et al. Effectiveness of superficial temporal-artery-middle cerebral artery anastomosis in adult moya-moya disease. Stroke 1998;29:625–630.

48. The EC/IC bypass study group: failure of extracranial-intracranial arterial bypass to reduce the risk of ischemic stroke. N Engl J Med 1985;313:1191–1200.

49. Powers WJ, Grubb RL, Raichle M. Clinical results of extracranial-intracranial bypass surgery in patients with hemodynamic cerebrovascular disease. J Neurosurg 1989;70:61–67.

50. Powers WJ, Templel LW, Grubb RL. Influence of cerebral hemodynamics on stroke risk: one-year follow-up of 30 medically treated patients. Ann Neurol 1989;25:325–330.

51. Kleiser B, Widder B. Course of carotid artery occlusions with impaired cerebrovascular reactivity. Stroke 1992;23:171–174.

52. Kuroda S, Kamiyama H, Abe H, et al. Acetazolamide test in detecting reduced cerebral perfusion reserve and predicting long-term prognosis in patients with internal carotid artery occlusion. Neurosurgery 1993;32:912–919.

53. Webster MW, Makaroun MS, Steed DL, et al. Compromised cerebral blood flow reactivity is a predictor of stroke in patients with symptomatic carotid artery occlusive disease. J Vasc Surg 1995;21:338–345.

54. Yamauchi H, Fukuyama H, Nagahama Y, et al. Evidence of misery perfusion and risk for recurrent stroke in major cerebral arterial occlusive diseases from PET. J Neurol Neurosurg Psychiatry 1996;61:18–25.

55. Yonas H, Smith HA, Durham SR, et al. Increased stroke risk predicted by compromised cerebral blood flow reactivity. J Neurosurg 1993;79:483–489.

56. Gur AY, Bova I, Bornstein NM. Is impaired cerebral vasomotor reactivity a predictive factor of stroke in asymptomatic patients? Stroke 1996;27:2188–2190.

57. Grubb RL, Derdeyn CP, Fritsch SM, et al. Importance of hemodynamic factors in the prognosis of symptomatic carotid occlusion. JAMA 1998;280:1055–1060.

58. Klijn CJM, Kappelle LJ, Tulleken CAF, et al. Symptomatic carotid artery occlusion. Stroke 1997; 28:2084–2093.

59. Haisa T, Kondo T, Shimpo T, et al. Post-carotid endarterectomy cerebral hyperperfusion leading to intracerebral haemorrhage. J Neurol Neurosurg Psychiatry 1999;67:546.

60. Hosoda K, Kawaguchi T, Shibata Y, et al. Cerebral vasoreactivity and internal carotid artery flow help to identify patients at risk for hyperperfusion after carotid endarterectomy. Stroke 2001;32:1567–1573.

61. Derdeyn CP, Videen TO, Fritsch SM, et al. Compensatory mechanisms for chronic cerebral hypoperfusion in patients with carotid occlusion. Stroke 1999;30:1019–1024.

62. Yamauchi H, Fukuyama H, Nagahama Y, et al. Long-term changes of hemodynamics and metabolism after carotid artery occlusion. Neurology 2000;54:2095–2102.

63. Brown AP, Spetzler RF. Intracranial Arteriovenous Malformation: Cerebrovascular Hemodynamics. In HH Batjer (ed), Cerebrovascular Disease. Philadelphia: Lippincott–Raven, 1997;833–842.

64. Batjer HH, Devous MD. The use of acetazolamide-enhanced regional cerebral blood flow measurement to predict risk to arteriovenous malformation patients. Neurosurgery 1992;31:213–218.

65. Tyler JL, Leblanc R, Meyer E, et al. Hemodynamics and metabolic effects of cerebral arteriovenous malformations studied by positron emission tomography. Stroke 1989;20:890–898.

66. De Reuck J, Van Aken J, Van Landegem W, et al. Positron emission tomography studies of changes in

cerebral blood flow and oxygen metabolism in arteriovenous malformation of the brain. Eur Neurol 1989;29:294–297.

67. Fink GR. Effects of cerebral angiomas on perifocal and remote tissue: a multivariate positron emission tomography study. Stroke 1992;23:1099–1105.

68. Baron JC. Positron Emission Tomography. In HJM Barnett, JP Mohr, BM Stein, FM Yatsu (eds), Stroke: Pathophysiology, Diagnosis, and Management (3rd ed). London: Churchill Livingstone, 1998;101–119.

69. Baron JC. Mapping the ischaemic penumbra with PET: implications for acute stroke treatment. Cerebrovasc Dis 1999;9:193–201.

70. Powers WJ, Grubb RL Jr, Darriet D, et al. Cerebral blood flow and cerebral metabolic rate of oxygen requirements for cerebral function and viability in humans. J Cereb Blood Flow Metab 1985;5:600–608.

71. Ackerman RH, Lev MH, Mackay BC, et al. PET studies in acute stroke: findings and relevance to therapy. J Cereb Blood Flow Metab 1989;9[Suppl 1]:S359.

72. Marchal G, Benali K, Iglesias S, et al. Voxel-based mapping of irreversible tissue damage by PET in the acute stage of ischaemic stroke. Brain 1999;123: 2387–2400.

73. Jones TH, Morawetz RE, Crowell RM, et al. Thresholds of focal cerebral ischaemia in awake monkeys. J Neurosurg 1981;54:773–782.

74. Heiss WD, Kracht LW, Thiel A, et al. Penumbral probability thresholds of cortical flumazenil binding and blood flow predicting tissue outcome in patients with cerebral ischaemia. Brain 2001;124:20–29.

75. Baron JC. Mapping the ischaemic penumbra with PET: a new approach. Brain 2001;124:2–4.

76. Heiss WD, Grond M, Thiel A, et al. Permanent cortical damage detected by flumazenil positron emission tomography in acute stroke. Stroke 1998;29: 454–461.

77. Heiss WD, Kracht L, Grond M, et al. Early 11C-flumazenil/H_2O positron emission tomography predicts irreversible ischemic cortical damage in stroke patients receiving acute thrombolytic therapy. Stroke 2000:31:366–369.

78. Wise RJS, Bernardi S, Frackowiak RSJ, et al. Serial observations on the pathophysiology of acute stroke. The transition from ischaemia to infarction as reflected in regional oxygen extraction. Brain 1983;106:197–222.

79. Marchal G, Serrati C, Rioux P, et al. PET imaging of cerebral perfusion and oxygen consumption in acute ischaemic stroke: relation to outcome. Lancet 1993;341:925–927.

80. Marchal G, Beaudouin V, Rioux P, et al. Prolonged persistence of substantial volumes of potentially viable brain tissue after stroke: a correlative PET-CT study with voxel-based data analysis. Stroke 1996; 27:599–606.

81. Marchal G, Furlan M, Beaudouin V, et al. Early spontaneous hyperperfusion after stroke: a marker of favorable tissue outcome. Brain 1996;119:409–419.

82. Heiss WD, Huber M, Fink GR, et al. Progressive derangement of periinfarct viable tissue in ischemic stroke. J Cereb Blood Flow Metab 1992;12:193–203.

83. Furlan M, Marchal G, Viader F, et al. Spontaneous neurological recovery after stroke and the fate of the ischemic penumbra. Ann Neurol 1996;40:216–226.

84. Heiss WD, Grond M, Thiel A, et al. Tissue at risk of infarction rescued by early reperfusion: a positron emission tomography study in systemic recombinant tissue plasminogen activator thrombolysis of acute stroke. J Cereb Blood Flow Metab 1998;18:1298–1307.

85. Marchal G, Rioux P, Serrati C, et al. Value of acute-stage PET in predicting neurological outcome after ischemic stroke: further assessment. Stroke 1995;26:524–525.

86. Heiss WD, Thiel A, Grond M, et al. Which targets are relevant for therapy of acute ischemic stroke? Stroke 1999;30:1486–1489.

87. Lenzi GL, Frackowiak RSJ, Jones T. Cerebral oxygen metabolism and blood flow in human cerebral ischemic infarction. J Cereb Blood Flow Metab 1982;2:231–235.

88. Touzani O, Young AR, Derlon JM, et al. Progressive impairment of brain oxidative metabolism reversed by reperfusion following middle cerebral artery occlusion in anaesthetized baboons. Brain Res 1997;767:17–25.

89. Young AR, Sette G, Touzani O, et al. Relationships between high oxygen extraction fraction in the acute stage and final infarction in reversible middle cerebral artery occlusion. An investigation in anaesthetized baboons with positron emission tomography. J Cereb Blood Flow Metab 1996;16:1176–1188.

90. Marchal G, Young AR, Baron JC. Early post-ischaemic hyperperfusion: pathophysiological insights from positron emission tomography. J Cereb Blood Flow Metab 1999;19:467–482.

91. Heiss WD, Graf R, Löttgen J, et al. Repeat positron emission tomographic studies in transient middle cerebral artery occlusion in cats: residual perfusion and efficacy of postischemic reperfusion. J Cereb Blood Flow Metab 1997;17:388–400.

92. Read SJ, Hirano T, Abbott DF, et al. The fate of hypoxic tissue on ^{18}F-fluoromisonidazole positron emission tomography after ischemic stroke. Ann Neurol 2000;48:228–235.

93. Nakagawara J, Sperling B, Lassen NA. Incomplete brain infarction of reperfused cortex may be quantitated with iomazenil. Stroke 1997;28:124–132.

94. Takahashi W, Ohnuki Y, Ohta T, et al. Mechanism of reduction of cortical blood flow in striatocapsular infarction: studies using [123I]iomazenil SPECT. Neuroimage 1997;6:75–80.

95. Ahmed N, Nasman P, Wahlgren NG. Effects of intravenous nimodipine on blood pressure and outcome after stroke. Stroke 2000;31:1250–1255.

96. Baron JC, von Kummer R, Del Zoppo GJ. Treatment of acute ischemic stroke: challenging the concept of a rigid and universal time window. Stroke 1995;26:2219–2221.

97. Furlan A, Higashida R, Wechsler L, et al. Intra-arterial prourokinase for acute ischemic stroke. The PROACT II study: a randomized controlled trial. JAMA 1999;282:2003–2011.

98. Feeney D, Baron JC. Diaschisis. Stroke 1986;17:817–830.

99. Baron JC, Bousser MG, Comar D, et al. Crossed cerebellar diaschisis in human supratentorial brain infarction. Trans Am Neurol Assoc 1980;105:459–461.

100. Pantano P, Baron JC, Samson Y, et al. Crossed cerebellar diaschisis: further studies. Brain 1986;109: 677–694.

101. Serrati C, Marchal G, Rioux P, et al. Contralateral cerebellar hypometabolism: a predictor for stroke outcome? J Neurol Neurosurg Psychiatry 1994;57:174–179.

102. Brunberg JA, Frey KA, Horton JA, et al. $[^{15}O]H_2O$ positron emission tomography determination of cerebral blood flow during balloon test occlusion of the internal carotid artery. AJNR Am J Neuroradiol 1994;15:725–732.

103. Pappata S, Tran Dinh S, Baron JC, et al. Remote metabolic effects of cerebrovascular lesions: magnetic resonance and positron tomography imaging. Neuroradiology 1987;29:1–6.

104. Tanaka M, Kondo S, Hirai S, et al. Crossed cerebellar diaschisis accompanied by hemiataxia: a PET study. J Neurol Neurosurgery Psychiatry 1992;55:121–125.

105. Pappata S, Mazoyer B, Tran-Dinh S, et al. Cortical and cerebellar hypometabolic effects of capsular, thalamo-capsular, and thalamic stroke: a positron tomography study. Stroke 1990;21:519–524.

106. Pantano P, Formisano R, Ricci M, et al. Prolonged muscular flaccidity after stroke. Morphological and functional brain alterations. Brain 1995;118:1329–1338.

107. Iglesias S, Marchal G, Rioux P, et al. Do changes in oxygen metabolism in the unaffected cerebral hemisphere underlie early neurological recovery after stroke? A positron emission tomography study. Stroke 1996;27:1192–1199.

108. Heiss WD, Kessler J, Karbe H, et al. Cerebral glucose metabolism as a predictor of recovery from aphasia in ischemic stroke. Arch Neurol 1993;50:958–964.

109. Baron JC, D'Antona R, Pantano P, et al. Effects of thalamic stroke on energy metabolism of the cerebral cortex. Brain 1986;109:1243–1259.

110. Mimura M, Kato M, Kato M, et al. Prospective and retrospective studies of recovery in aphasia. Changes in cerebral blood flow and language functions. Brain 1998;121:2083–2094.

111. Kuhl DE, Phelps ME, Kowell AP, et al. Effects of stroke on local cerebral metabolism and perfusion. Mapping by emission computed tomography of ^{18}FDG and ^{13}NH3. Ann Neurol 1980;8:47–60.

112. Metter EJ, Wasterlain CG, Kuhl DE, et al. FDG positron emission computed tomography in a study of aphasia. Ann Neurol 1981;10:173–183.

113. Metter EJ, Riege WH, Hanson WR, et al. Subcortical structures in aphasia. Arch Neurol 1988;45: 1229–1134.

114. Karbe H, Szelies B, Herholz K, et al. Impairment of language is related to left parieto-temporal glucose metabolism in aphasic stroke patients. J Neurol 1990;237:19–23.

115. Perani D, Vallar G, Cappa S, et al. Aphasia and neglect after subcortical stroke. A clinical/cerebral perfusion correlation study. Brain 1987;110:1211–1229.

116. Bogousslavsky J, Miklossy J, Regli F, et al. Subcortical neglect neuropsychological, SPECT, and neuropathological correlations with anterior choroidal artery territory infarction. Ann Neurol 1988;23:448–452.

117. Fiorelli M, Blin J, Bakchine S, et al. PET studies of cortical diaschisis in patients with motor hemineglect. J Neurol Sci 1991;104:135–142.

118. Von Giesen HJ, Schlaug G, Steinmetz H, et al. Cerebral network underlying unilateral motor neglect: evidence from positron emission tomography. J Neurol Sci 1994;125:29–38.

119. Bosley T, Rosenquist AC, Kushner M, et al. Ischemic lesions of the occipital cortex and optic radiations: positron emission tomography. Neurology 1985;35:470–484.

120. Kiyosawa M, Bosley TM, Kushner M, et al. Middle cerebral artery strokes causing homonymous hemianopia: positron emission tomography. Ann Neurol 1990;28:180–183.

121. Kuwert T, Hennerici M, Langen KL, et al. Regional cerebral glucose consumption measured by positron emission tomography in patients with unilateral thalamic infarction. Cerebrovasc Dis 1991;1:327–336.

122. Szelies B, Herholz K, Pawlik G, et al. Widespread functional effects of discrete thalamic infarction. Arch Neurol 1991;48:178–182.

123. Chabriat H, Levasseur M, Pappata S, et al. Cortical metabolism in postero-lateral thalamic stroke: a PET study. Acta Neurol Scand 1992;86:285–290.

124. Levasseur M, Baron JC, Sette G, et al. Brain energy metabolism in bilateral paramedian thalamic infarcts: a positron emission tomography study. Brain 1992;115:795–807.

125. Bogousslavsky J, Regli F, Delaloye G, et al. Loss of psychic self-activation with bithalamic infarction. Acta Neurol Scand 1991;83:309–316.

126. Pappata S, Levasseur M, Gunn RN, et al. Thalamic microglial activation in ischemic stroke detected in vivo by PET and [^{11}C]PK11195. Neurology 2000; 55:1052–1054.

127. Metter EJ, Kempler D, Jackson C, et al. Cerebral glucose metabolism in Wernicke's Broca's, and conduction aphasia. Arch Neurol 1989;46:27–34.

128. Binkofski F, Seitz RJ, Arnold S, et al. Thalamic metabolism and corticospinal tract integrity determine motor recovery in stroke. Ann Neurol 1996;39:460–470.

129. Iglesias S, Marchal G, Viader F, Baron JC. Delayed intra-hemispheric remote metabolic depression after stroke: a PET study of its role in early recovery. Cerebrovasc Dis 2000;10:391–402.

130. Baron JC, Levasseur M, Mazoyer B, et al. Thalamo-cortical diaschisis: PET study in humans. J Neurol Neurosurg Psychiatry 1992;55:935–942.

131. Metter EJ, Jackson CA, Kempler D, et al. Temporoparietal cortex and the recovery of language comprehension in aphasia. Aphasiology 1992;6:349–358.

132. Karbe H, Kessler J, Herholz K, et al. Long-term prognosis of poststroke aphasia studied with positron emission tomography. Arch Neurol 1995;52:186–190.

133. Cappa SF, Perani D, Grassi F, et al. A PET follow-up study of recovery after stroke in acute aphasics. Brain Lang 1997;56:55–67.

CHAPTER 7

Imaging of Stroke with Single-Photon Emission Computed Tomography

José C. Masdeu

Single-photon emission computed tomography (SPECT), introduced to clinical medicine in the early 1980s, may be used to study regional cerebral perfusion or the regional density of various compounds in the brain. We first consider the applications of perfusion SPECT to cerebrovascular disease and, second, review the scant literature dealing with receptor imaging or markers of hypoxia in stroke.[1]

SINGLE-PHOTON EMISSION COMPUTED TOMOGRAPHY PERFUSION IMAGING

With the increasing availability of perfusion computed tomography (CT), including xenon-enhanced CT and diffusion-perfusion magnetic resonance imaging (MRI), is SPECT still a useful tool to study perfusion, an obviously important variable in stroke and stroke-prone patients? As interesting as this question may be, we only answer it partially in this review. Leaving aside for a moment the real-life availability of these techniques, there are no controlled studies comparing their usefulness and cost in the different settings relevant to clinical cerebrovascular disease, namely, (1) stroke prediction in the presymptomatic subject, (2) stroke prediction in the patient at risk, (3) diagnosis of an acute ischemic event, and (4) prognosis of the acute event.[2] Moreover, it is likely that such studies will never be carried out because the field of stroke imaging is evolving quickly, and the real applicability of the different modalities used to study stroke depends on the availability of each modality in the clinical setting. For this reason, this discussion focuses on the potential of SPECT to answer clinically the following relevant questions: (1) In the patient at risk of stroke, what are the mechanism and likelihood of suffering a stroke? (2) In the patient with a stroke-like syndrome, what is the mechanism, how should it be treated, and what is the prognosis for recovery?[3,4] A brief introduction to perfusion SPECT is first in order.

Technical Aspects

For the performance of SPECT, a flow tracer is first tagged with a radionuclide and injected into the patient (Figure 7-1). Using a gamma camera and the techniques of CT, a three-dimensional image of the distribution of a radionuclide in the brain is then obtained (Figure 7-2).[5–7] State-of-the-art SPECT systems can be expected to provide high-resolution (6–9 mm) imaging of statically distributed brain radiopharmaceuticals with patient imaging times of 10–20 minutes. Most systems are also capable of sequential image acquisitions; that is, they can produce multiple short studies back-to-back and, subsequently, to discard segments degraded by patient motion.

Risk of Stroke in Subjects at Risk

SPECT has been used to assess cerebral perfusion in subjects with large-vessel stenosis and perfusion change after a number of potentially therapeutic interventions. It has also been used to study perfusion reserve in patients with watershed infarcts and to predict which

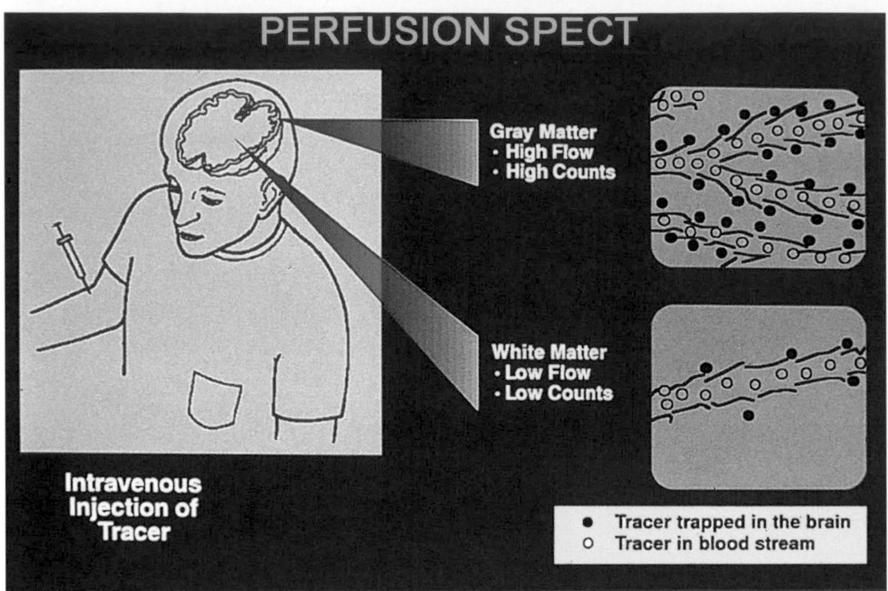

FIGURE 7-1. Injection of a single-photon emission computed tomography (SPECT) perfusion agent. These agents, highly lipid-soluble, tend to penetrate the blood-brain barrier and remain trapped in the perivascular space for several hours, enough to allow for imaging. Brain areas with high perfusion, such as the cerebral cortex, have higher counts than those with lower perfusion, such as the white matter.

patients with vasospasm secondary to subarachnoid hemorrhage are likely to develop cerebral infarction.

Assessment of Cerebral Perfusion with Large-Vessel Stenosis

Although SPECT, producing a qualitative measure of regional brain perfusion, cannot assess cerebrovascular reserve as well as positron emission tomography or xenon-enhanced CT,[8] it has been used to assess the changes in perfusion that occur after balloon angioplasty or stenting of cerebral vessels.[9,10] Suh et al. included a large area of hypoperfusion on SPECT as a criterion for the performance of middle cerebral artery (MCA) angioplasty in patients with a mild neurologic deficit.[11] In a small number of patients, they documented perfusion improvement after the procedure.

Vasodilation caused by hypercapnia (inhalation of 5% CO_2) or by acetazolamide injection (1 g i.v., 15 minutes before radionuclide injection) can be used to assess the vascular reserve of brain regions supplied by a stenotic or occluded artery. The two methods do not produce the same results. Hypercapnia, not acetazolamide, tends to increase systemic blood pressure.[12] Hypercapnia consistently increases regional perfusion in the affected arterial territory, whereas acetazolamide does so in only approximately one-half of patients. In some cases, it actually reduces perfusion in the affected area,

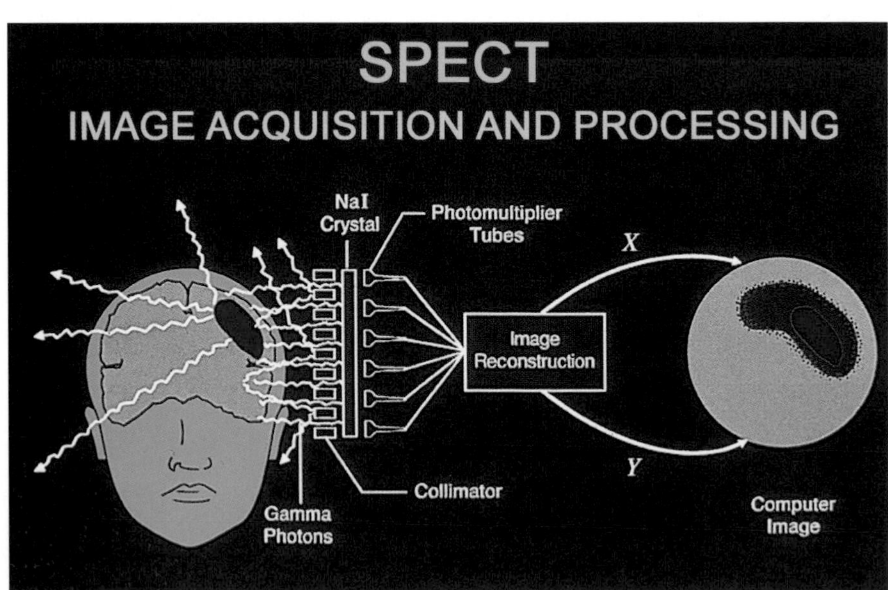

FIGURE 7-2. The distribution of a radionuclide in the brain is imaged by quantification of the photons that interact with sodium iodine (NaI) detectors. Careful collimation is essential for image quality. Mathematic algorithms similar to the ones used by other computed tomographic techniques, including Fourier transform, are used to reconstruct the distribution of the isotope in the brain. (SPECT = single-photon emission computed tomography.)

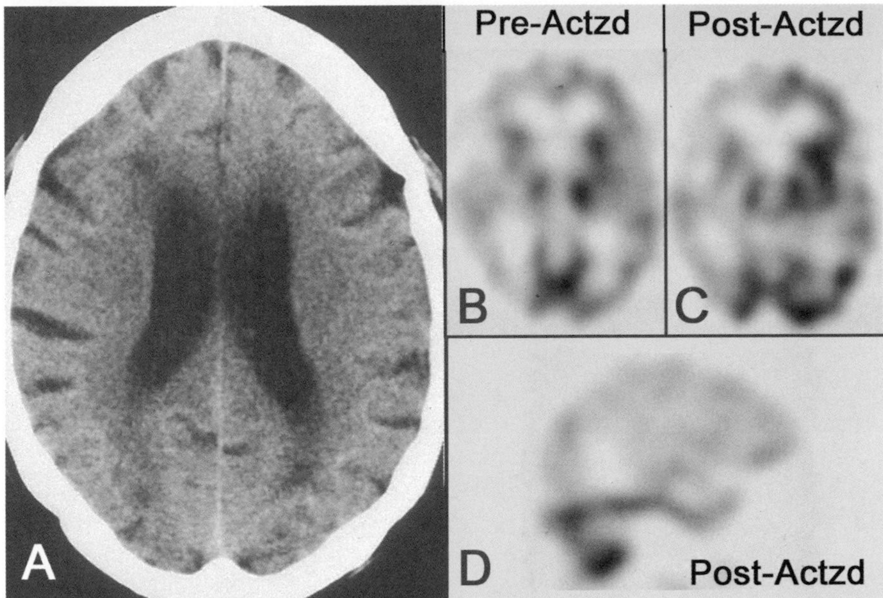

FIGURE 7-3. Use of acetazolamide (Actzd) challenge to assess vascular reserve and differentiate ischemia from diaschisis. A 51-year-old patient had transient left-arm weakness. A computed tomography scan (**A**) showed hypodense areas in the watershed of the left hemispheric white matter. Duplex ultrasound revealed occlusion of the right internal carotid artery at the bifurcation. Technetium-99m–hexamethyl propyleneamine oxime single-photon emission computed tomography before acetazolamide (**B**) showed hypoperfusion of the right middle cerebral artery (MCA) territory and the thalamus (usually supplied by the posterior circulation). Two days later, single-photon emission computed tomography was repeated after oral loading with acetazolamide (**C,D**). The difference between the hemispheres became more obvious. Perfusion of the previously hypoperfused right thalamus became normal (diaschisis), but not in the cortical distribution of the right MCA (**C**). Note the sharp difference between the ischemic territory of the MCA and the normal cortex supplied by the posterior cerebral artery from the posterior circulation (**D**).

likely because blood is being stolen by the normal circulation, vasodilated by acetazolamide administration (Figure 7-3).[12]

By using two isotopes, a technetium agent for a baseline blood flow measurement and an iodine agent for a post-acetazolamide blood flow measurement, the separate distributions can be measured using two windows on some of the modern three-headed scanners.[13] This greatly simplifies reactivity testing with SPECT and eliminates the need for multiple injections and subtraction techniques.[14,15]

Acetazolamide stress brain-perfusion SPECT has been found to be useful as a complementary method in determining selective carotid shunting during carotid endarterectomy. Eight of eight patients with a severely reduced vascular reserve needed shunts, as compared to four of 67 who had a less severe reduction.[16] The use of SPECT perfusion studies to predict the need for surgery in patients with asymptomatic stenosis of cerebral arteries is less well substantiated.[17,18]

Patients who have had cerebral infarction are also at risk for additional ischemic lesions. In a group of patients with watershed hemispheric infarcts ipsilateral to a stenotic artery, Moriwaki et al.[19] determined that those with white matter infarcts (see Figure 7-3) had less reserve than those with cortical infarcts. The second group may have compensated between the time of the infarction and the time of the SPECT or suffered infarction not on a hemodynamic, but on an embolic basis.

Subarachnoid Hemorrhage

Ischemia from vasospasm is a major cause of morbidity and mortality after subarachnoid hemorrhage (SAH).[20] In this setting, regional hypoperfusion on SPECT correlates with the presence and severity of delayed neurologic deficits.[21] SPECT facilitates the early diagnosis of cerebral hypoperfusion due to vasospasm and may help in differentiating hypoperfusion from other causes of deterioration after SAH (Figure 7-4). Because therapies exist for reducing the effects of vasospasm, the application of techniques for early and accurate diagnosis is of obvious importance.[22,23] Given the ability of SPECT to detect surface ischemia, this technique, when combined with transcranial Doppler, may prove a sensitive screen for the early detection of vasospasm and delayed ischemic deficits in an entire hemisphere or an isolated cortical branch.[21,24,25] Acetazolamide SPECT has been used within the first 18 days after SAH to predict which

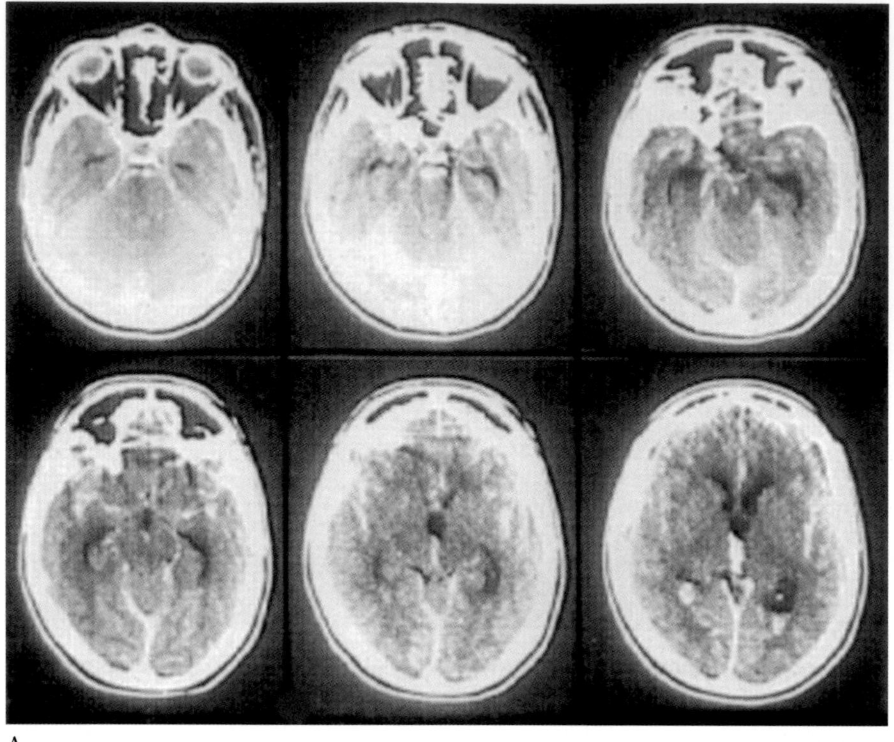

A

B

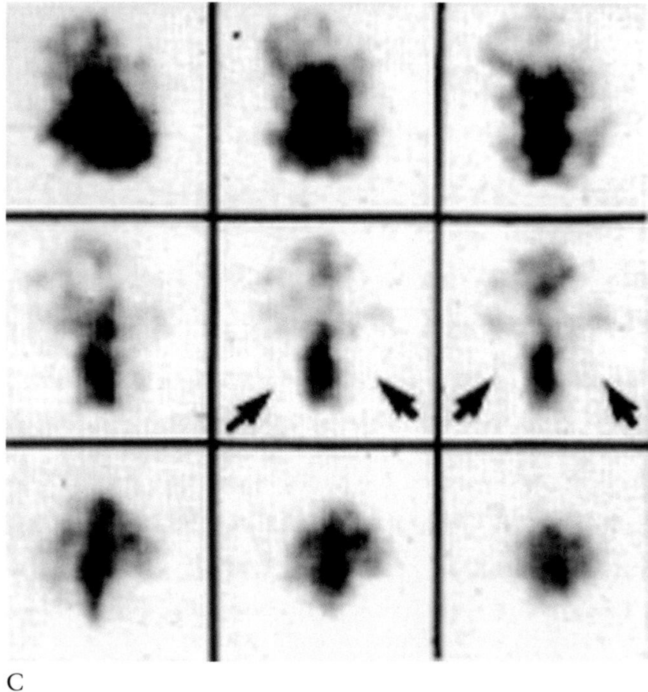

C

FIGURE 7-4. Vasospasm after subarachnoid hemorrhage. After massive subarachnoid hemorrhage on computed tomography (**A**), single-photon emission computed tomography obtained on day 2 was normal (**B**), but single-photon emission computed tomography on day 12 shows multiple perfusion defects in the hemispheres, particularly in the parietal watershed areas (*arrows*) and in the right cerebellar hemisphere (**C**). (Courtesy of Dr. Robert S. Hellman and Dr. Ronald S. Tikofsky, Section of Nuclear Medicine, Medical College of Wisconsin.)

patients are likely to develop cerebral infarction.[26,27] Early and extensive reduction in cerebral vasodilatory capacity correlated with the development of cerebral infarction due to vasospasm after SAH.

SPECT imaging has also been applied to the evaluation of arteriovenous malformations (AVMs). Blood steal from healthy tissue can be documented both at rest and after acetazolamide administration.[28] The presence of severe steal has prompted staging of the surgical resection and encouraged embolization as a preliminary treatment.[29] Awad and coworkers used SPECT to study cerebral perfusion before AVM resection as a means to predict which patients would develop malignant intracranial hypertension after resection.[30] Hypoperfusion was observed in seven of seven AVMs greater than 6 cm that were studied by this modality, and intractable intracranial pressure was observed postoperatively in five of these cases, despite preoperative staged embolization. Additional work is needed to define the role of preoperative hypoperfusion in the outcome of these patients. Cerebral ischemia due to blood shunting with carotid-cavernous fistulas can be also monitored with SPECT.[31]

Acute Stroke-Like Syndrome

For the diagnosis of stroke, time is of the essence. As evidence mounts that the therapeutic time window for acute stroke is narrow and that delaying effective therapy results in more tissue damage, the need to diagnose the cause of stroke as quickly as possible becomes more urgent. Because thrombolysis is effective in acute stroke and intracerebral hemorrhage is its main contraindication, CT has become the standard initial imaging modality for acute stroke. Spiral CT allows for the performance of CT angiography and perfusion CT; although, for perfusion, SPECT is an easier procedure and avoids the complications of iodinated contrast administration.[32] MRI with echoplanar imaging is replacing CT at some institutions, because it adds information on tissue damage and potentially reversible perfusion defects. It also provides vessel visualization.[33] Many see SPECT as an interesting technique, but one in which potential benefits are offset by the attendant delay in diagnosis and treatment.[34] Although SPECT was first approved by the U.S. Food and Drug Administration for the study of cerebral ischemia, this technique is not being used for acute stroke in the majority of U.S. hospitals.[35–37] However, a number of active stroke centers around the world are using perfusion SPECT for the evaluation of acute stroke.[4,38–40]

For it to be even potentially useful, SPECT must be performed quickly so that it does not delay thrombolysis.[39,41] In many hospitals, brain SPECT perfusion agents are only available during regular working hours, roughly one-third of the day. Lack of availability is one of the factors preventing SPECT from being included in many acute stroke protocols. Of the agents used for perfusion SPECT imaging, there is one that needs to be prepared shortly before injection (regular technetium-99m–hexamethyl propyleneamine oxime [^{99m}Tc-HMPAO]), but two others have a shelf life of approximately 6 hours (technetium-99m–ethyl-cysteinate-dimer [^{99m}Tc-ECD] and stable ^{99m}Tc-HMPAO). Thus, a syringe conveniently shielded can be left in the acute stroke care area or in the CT scan room, and the patient injected once a hemorrhage has been ruled out. Each compound requires at least 20–30 minutes to clear nonbrain tissue uptake, so that this process and getting the SPECT scanning unit ready can take place while the patient is finishing the CT scan. Intravenous thrombolysis can be started as soon as the CT information is available and stopped if the SPECT indicates that it will not be beneficial, either because the infarct is likely to improve spontaneously or because it is large with a high risk of hemorrhagic transformation.

Of the two compounds with a longer shelf life, stable ^{99m}Tc-HMPAO more closely matches true perfusion values and remains more stable in the brain for a longer period than ^{99m}Tc-ECD.[42,43] The uptake after ^{99m}Tc-ECD seems more dependent on tissue viability, and perhaps for this reason it has been found by some studies to be a better predictor of stroke evolution when given shortly after the acute event.[38,39] In addition, it has a better clearance from nonbrain tissues. Dynamic ^{99m}Tc-ECD SPECT correlates more closely than static images with true regional cerebral blood flow.[44] Some studies have also accurately predicted final infarct size by using ^{99m}Tc-HMPAO.[45–47]

For the evaluation of SPECT images, visual inspection may suffice and produce highly predictive results.[39] For semiquantitative evaluation, some studies have used the value of the region of interest relative to cerebellar perfusion, and other studies have used the value relative to the perfusion of the contralateral hemisphere.[46,48] The increasing interhemispheric difference observed in some studies with aging may reduce the usefulness of the interhemispheric measurement.[49]

Practical considerations are important, but we should examine the yield of the technique in an ideal situation, when it can be promptly performed on the stroke patient. SPECT may have a role in helping diagnose nonischemic neurologic deficits and in predicting the need for thrombolysis, separating the patients who would not benefit from it either because by the time the procedure is ready there is no perfusion deficit to be corrected by thrombolysis, or because the infarct is large and the ischemia profound, with attendant capillary necrosis and a high risk for bleeding. In patients with large infarcts, SPECT may

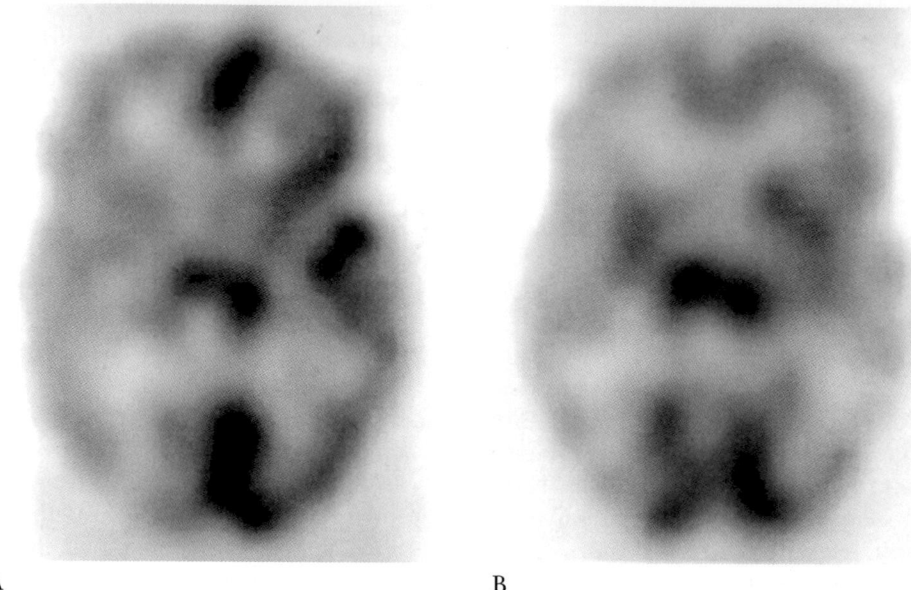

FIGURE 7-5. Postictal hemiplegia. **A.** Axial single-photon emission computed tomography (SPECT) showing increased perfusion of the left hemisphere obtained in a 58-year-old woman 26 hours after she was found in the street with a right-sided hemiplegia, global aphasia, and a gaze deviation to the left. Clinical findings persisted at the time of SPECT. Computed tomography was negative. Electroencephalogram obtained 12 hours before the SPECT had shown marked slowing over the left hemisphere but no epileptiform activity. Improvement ensued over a 1-week period, when the patient could give a history of having had a seizure disorder since her teens. Follow-up SPECT after the patient had improved showed symmetric perfusion of the hemispheres (**B**).

help determine which patients may benefit from holohemispheric decompression.

Nonischemic Neurologic Deficits

Occasionally, the clinical problem arises of differentiating ischemia from epilepsy as the cause of a sudden neurologic deficit, particularly in cases with a prolonged focal discharge, when the onset was not witnessed and the patient is unable to give a reliable account. Ischemia causes an area of hypoperfusion on SPECT, whereas epileptic phenomena are often manifested by hyperperfusion, although postictally there is hypoperfusion (Figure 7-5). Differentiating ischemia from focal epileptic phenomena is critical, as thrombolysis and other techniques to treat acute stroke are now available. Increased perfusion of the hemisphere contralateral to the affected limbs has also been reported in some cases of infantile alternating hemiplegia,[50] in cases of transient aphasia,[51] and with neurosarcoidosis.[52]

Prediction of Transient or Mild Ischemic Attack

Using ^{99m}Tc-ECD SPECT, Berrouschot et al.[53] studied 82 patients within 6 hours of stroke onset. By visual inspection, 23 had no perfusion deficit despite clinical symptoms. None of these patients had neurologic symptoms after 7 days. In the semiquantitative SPECT analysis, these patients had abnormal count densities in the affected region (activity <90%, but >70% compared with the contralateral side). All patients with subsequent infarction (n = 59) had values less than 70%.[53] Performance of the procedure in the first few hours seems critical for the usefulness of the test, both from the patient-management point of view and because the findings are less clear when the study is delayed (Figure 7-6).[54,55] Barber has called the apparently normal perfusion of a necrotic area *non-nutritional reperfusion.* This pattern on serial SPECT (hypoperfusion, normal perfusion, hypoperfusion) results most likely from perfusion being restored after neuronal damage has already occurred. Inflammatory tissue at the site of infarction causes arteriolar dilation in the days and weeks after the infarct, with the resultant normal perfusion pattern.[56,57] As the necrosed tissue is reabsorbed and inflammation abates, regional perfusion decreases, and the area becomes abnormal again on SPECT. This mechanism would also explain why failing to show an area of necrosis may happen more readily with ^{99m}Tc-HMPAO, a better marker of perfusion, than with ^{99m}Tc-ECD, which is poorly retained by areas of necrosis.[38,39]

Lesions in the cortex or deep gray nuclei are more likely to cause SPECT defects than purely white matter

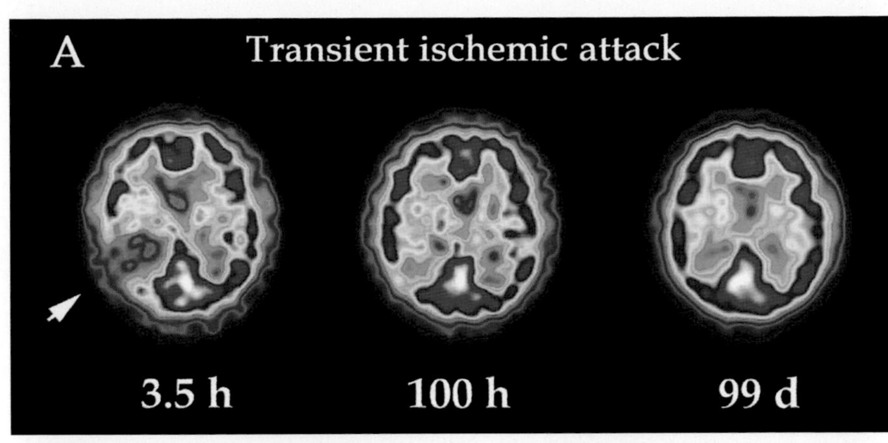

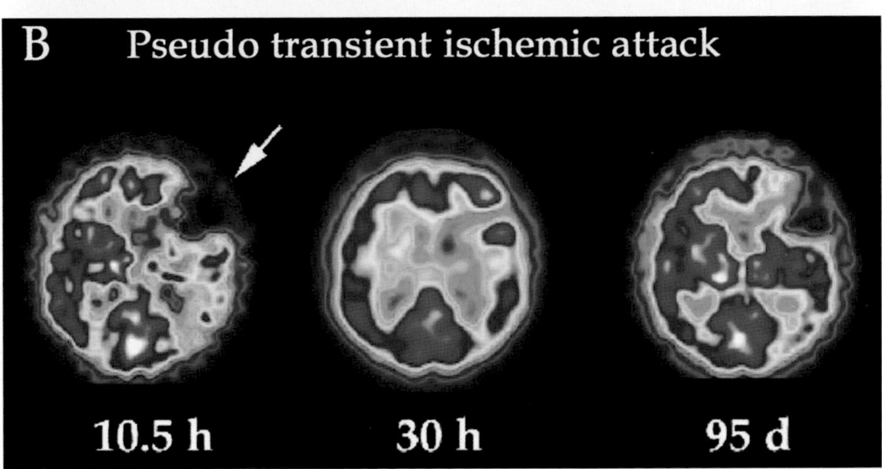

FIGURE 7-6. Serial technetium-99m–hexamethyl propyleneamine oxime single-photon emission computed tomography (SPECT) studies. **A.** SPECT study at 3.5 hours showing right middle cerebral artery territory hypoperfusion (*arrow*). At 100 hours, the deficit has largely resolved, which is consistent with early reperfusion. At 99 days, the early reperfusion has been maintained. **B.** SPECT study at 10.5 hours of stroke onset, showing left frontal hypoperfusion (*arrow*). At 30 hours, the deficit has largely resolved, which is consistent with early reperfusion. At 95 days, the hypoperfusion deficit has reappeared at the site of an infarct. Had the first SPECT been done at 30 hours, the deficit would have passed unnoticed. See text for explanation of the second (**B**) SPECT pattern. (Reprinted with permission from PA Barber, SM Davis, B Infeld, et al. Spontaneous reperfusion after ischemic stroke is associated with improved outcome. Stroke 1998;29:2522–2528.)

lesions, so that a normal SPECT study may also predict a lacunar stroke.[35,58]

Acute Ischemic Neurologic Deficit

After answering the critical question of whether the stroke is ischemic or hemorrhagic by the use of CT or gradient-echo MRI, the next step is to predict the likely usefulness of intravenous or, where permitted by protocol, intra-arterial thrombolysis. In some centers, decompression of a massively swollen hemisphere due to a large MCA infarct has been found to have a positive outcome if the procedure is performed before additional pressure damage occurs. It is, therefore, important to predict early who will develop severe hemispheric swelling (Figure 7-7).[59] Perfusion SPECT has been used to try to address these issues.

Earlier SPECT studies failed to show any advantage of SPECT over structured clinical evaluation (e.g., National Institutes of Health, Canadian, and Scandinavian stroke scales) to predict the evolution of acute stroke.[60] However, using ^{99m}Tc-ECD SPECT in the first 6 hours after stroke, Barthel and coworkers were able to determine which patients would develop massive MCA-territory necrosis with hemispheric herniation.[39] These patients have a high risk of hemorrhage following thrombolysis and could be helped by early decompressive hemicraniectomy.[59] Complete MCA infarctions were predicted with significantly higher accuracy with early SPECT (area under receiver operating characteristic curve [AUC] index 0.91) compared with early CT (AUC index 0.77) and clinical parameters (AUC index 0.73; $p < .05$). Furthermore, the predictive value increased when the findings on CT, clinical examination, and SPECT were considered.[39] Other studies have found SPECT to add predictive value to the clinical score on admission.[38,45,46] In summary, a patient with a normal ^{99m}Tc-ECD SPECT study performed within 3 hours of stroke onset, will most likely recover spontaneously and does not require thrombolysis. A patient with a dense deficit in the entire MCA distribution has a high risk of hemorrhage with thrombolysis and, depending on age and other factors, should be considered for decompressive hemicraniectomy. The patients most likely to benefit from thrombolysis are the ones with less-massive lesions.[39,41,45]

A mismatch in the area acutely affected, as seen on diffusion-weighted imaging and an MRI or SPECT perfusion studies, performed shortly after the acute event, predicts which infarcts become larger in the hours and days after the stroke. The infarct grows to match the

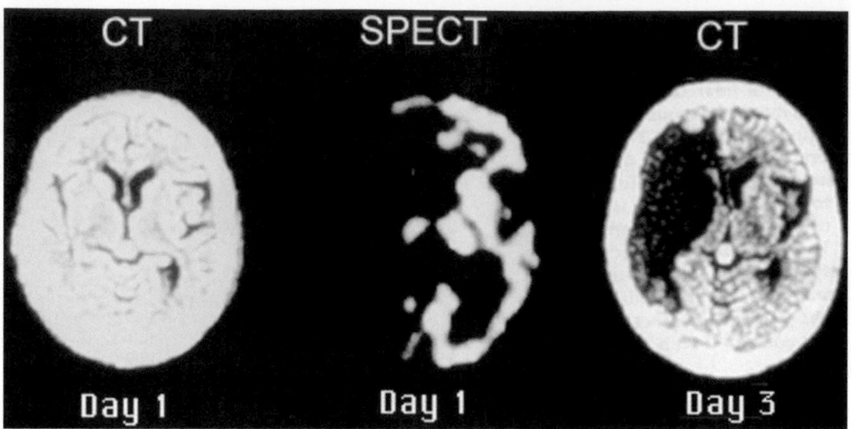

FIGURE 7-7. Acute stroke. Initial computed tomography (CT) did not show the lesion, clearly depicted by single-photon emission CT (SPECT). CT 3 days after stroke showing a large hemispheric infarction. (Courtesy of Dr. Ronald S. Tikofsky from the Section of Nuclear Medicine, Medical College of Wisconsin.)

area of severely decreased perfusion (between 12 and 20 ml/100 g per minute).[61–63] The area of mismatch is the ischemic penumbra that often becomes necrotic as the process evolves.[1] Using only ^{99m}Tc-ECD SPECT, the dynamic study approximates a perfusion map of the region, whereas decreased uptake in the static study shows the nonviable area of the brain, albeit with somewhat poor spatial resolution.[44] This information is important because patients with a mismatch may be most likely to benefit from acute stroke therapies. Clinical trials of acute stroke focusing on this subgroup might demonstrate a larger treatment effect and require fewer patients to show a significant benefit.

Because serial SPECT studies can be repeated after approximately 30 minutes using an initial smaller dose of the radioisotope and then a larger dose, or after a few minutes using two different isotopes (^{99m}Tc and iodine-123 [^{123}I]), or after approximately 24 hours using the same isotope and dose, SPECT has been used to evaluate the effect of different therapeutic strategies on brain perfusion (Figure 7-8). Among them are intra-arterial urokinase,[43,64,65] intravenous recombinant tissue plasminogen activator,[66–70] streptokinase,[71] and rheopheresis.[72,73] Strategies that seek to open an occluded vessel can be particularly well evaluated by perfusion SPECT, a much less invasive procedure than arterial angiography or iodine-contrast CT and a less costly procedure than perfusion MRI. For intra-arterial thrombolysis, Ueda et al.[65] found that ischemic tissue with perfusion greater than 55% of cerebellar flow still may be salvageable, even with treatment initiated 6 hours after onset of symptoms. Ischemic tissue with perfusion greater than 35% of cerebellar flow still may be salvageable with early treatment (<5 hours). Ischemic tissue with perfusion less than 35% of cerebellar flow may be at risk for hemorrhage with thrombolysis.[65]

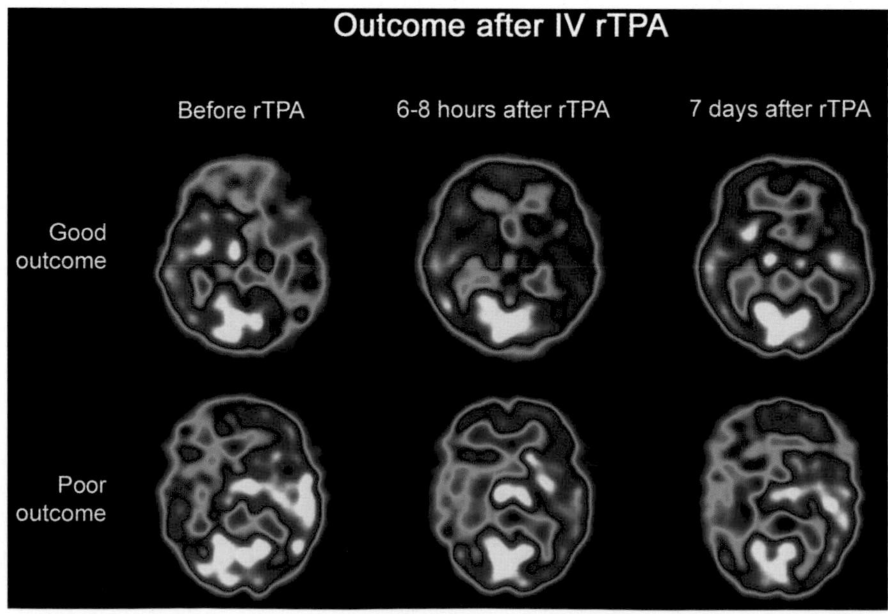

FIGURE 7-8. Repeated single-photon emission computed tomography with technetium-99m–ethyl-cysteinate-dimer in two patients (*top and bottom row*, respectively) at baseline before intravenous recombinant tissue plasminogen activator (rTPA) (*left column*), 6–8 hours after intravenous rTPA (*middle column*), and 7 days after intravenous rTPA (*right column*). The patient whose single-photon emission computed tomography is displayed at the top row had a good outcome, unlike the one at the bottom. (Reprinted with permission from J Berrouschot, H Barthel, S Hesse, et al. Reperfusion and metabolic recovery of brain tissue and clinical outcome after ischemic stroke and thrombolytic therapy. Stroke 2000;31:1545–1551.)

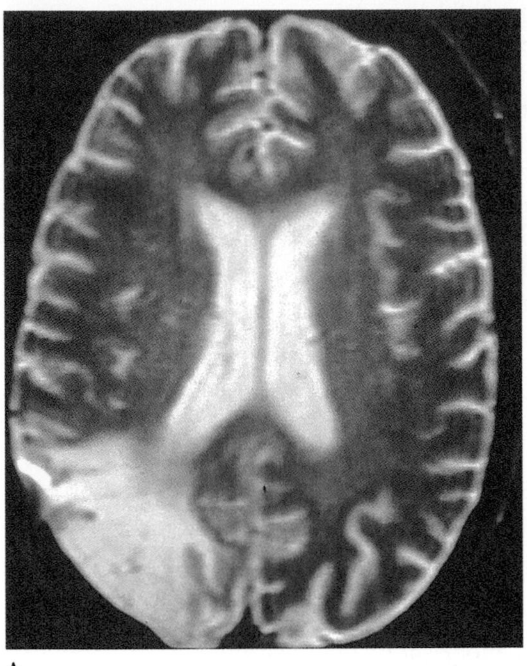
A

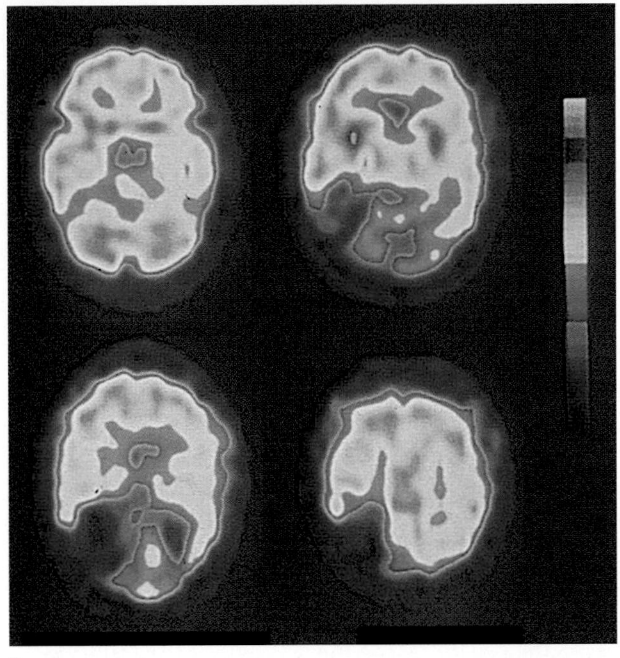
B

FIGURE 7-9. Mitochondrial encephalomyopathy with lactic acidosis and stroke-like episodes in a 41-year-old man who had impaired vision. **A.** Magnetic resonance image showing a right parieto-occipital infarct. **B.** Technetium-99m–ethyl-cysteinate-dimer single-photon emission computed tomography showing bilateral parieto-occipital hypoperfusion, better explaining the clinical symptoms. (Courtesy of DuPont Pharma and Johns Hopkins Department of Nuclear Medicine.)

SPECT has also been used to evaluate the effect on cerebral perfusion of a number of vasodilators, including pentoxifylline,[74] olprinone,[75] and nimodipine,[76] and vasoconstrictors, including cocaine.[77] In this regard, xenon-enhanced CT allows for the quantitative determination of regional cerebral blood flow, which can also be obtained with xenon-enhanced SPECT,[78] whereas SPECT with the more widely available radionuclides only provides a relative estimate.[8]

Other Cerebrovascular Disorders

Vascular Dementia

Compared with patients with Alzheimer's disease, those with vascular dementia, including *c*erebral *a*utosomal *d*ominant *a*rteriopathy with *s*ubcortical *i*nfarcts and *l*eukoencephalopathy (CADASIL), tend to have decreased perfusion in the basal ganglia and frontal lobes.[79,80] However, the "classical" pattern of Alzheimer's in SPECT, namely biparietal hypoperfusion, may be found in a small proportion of patients with vascular dementia.[81]

Mitochondrial Encephalomyopathy with Lactic Acidosis and Stroke-Like Episodes

In mitochondrial encephalopathies, SPECT may show a characteristic pattern of occipitoparietal hypoperfusion, even when the CT or MRI are normal or show only atrophy (Figure 7-9).[82,83] Some of the studies may show increased blood flow, which in some cases could be related to focal seizure activity.[83,84]

Takayasu's Arteritis

SPECT was abnormal in patients with a normal neurologic examination.[85]

Migraine

In migraine, decreased perfusion during the prodromal ischemic phase followed by hyperperfusion during the headache has been documented with xenon-enhanced SPECT.[86] SPECT has also been used to document decreased perfusion during the symptomatic phase of basilar migraine[87] and in the medial temporal region in some patients with acute confusional migraine.[88]

EXPERIMENTAL TRACERS FOR ISCHEMIC TISSUE

Tracers for ischemic tissue are still in the experimental stages, but their potential usefulness is exciting because, unlike purely perfusion agents, they could depict the ischemic tissue and, depending on the nature of the tracer, shed light on pathophysiologic mechanisms.

Cobalt 57 is taken up by ischemic tissue, possibly because of the similarity of this isotope to calcium.[89,90] ^{123}I-iomazenil binds to a central benzodiazepine receptor that is purely neuronal.[91,92] Partial ischemia may damage neurons while sparing astrocytes, and in this case the MRI may be normal. ^{123}I-iomazenil SPECT could be used in this case to detect the area of incomplete brain infarction.[93]

REFERENCES

1. Heiss WD. Ischemic penumbra: evidence from functional imaging in man. J Cereb Blood Flow Metab 2000;20:1276–1293.
2. Barber PA, Consolo HK, Yang Q, et al. Comparison of MRI perfusion imaging and SPECT in chronic stroke. Cerebrovasc Dis 2001;11:128–136.
3. Caplan LR. Question-driven technology assessment: SPECT as an example. Neurology 1991;41:187–191.
4. Ueda T, Yuh WT, Maley JE, et al. Current and future imaging of acute cerebral ischemia: assessment of tissue viability by perfusion imaging. J Comput Assist Tomogr 1999;23[suppl 1]:S3–S7.
5. Piez CW, Holman BL. Single photon emission computed tomography. Comput Radiol 1985;9:201–211.
6. English RJ, Brown SE. SPECT: Single Photon Emission Computed Tomography. A Primer (2nd ed). New York: Society of Nuclear Medicine, 1990.
7. Holman BL, Devous M Sr. Functional brain SPECT: the emergence of a powerful clinical method. J Nucl Med 1992;33:1888–1904.
8. Yonas H, Pindzola RR, Meltzer CC, Sasser H. Qualitative versus quantitative assessment of cerebrovascular reserves. Neurosurgery 1998;42:1005–1010; discussion 1011–1012.
9. Fessler RD, Lanzino G, Guterman LR, et al. Improved cerebral perfusion after stenting of a petrous carotid stenosis: technical case report. Neurosurgery 1999;45:638–642.
10. Laloux P, Richelle F, Meurice H, De-Coster P. Cerebral blood flow and perfusion reserve capacity in hemodynamic carotid transient ischemic attacks due to innominate artery stenosis. J Nucl Med 1995;36:1268–1271.
11. Suh DC, Sung KB, Cho YS, et al. Transluminal angioplasty for middle cerebral artery stenosis in patients with acute ischemic stroke. AJNR Am J Neuroradiol 1999;20:553–558.
12. Kazumata K, Tanaka N, Ishikawa T, et al. Dissociation of vasoreactivity to acetazolamide and hypercapnia. Comparative study in patients with chronic occlusive major cerebral artery disease. Stroke 1996;27:2052–2058.
13. Devous M Sr, Payne JK, Lowe JL. Dual-isotope brain SPECT imaging with technetium-99m and iodine-123: clinical validation using xenon-133 SPECT. J Nucl Med 1992;33:1919–1924.
14. Devous MD, Gassaway SK. Simultaneous SPECT imaging of Tc-99m- and I-123 labeled brain agents in patients using the PRISM scanner. J Nucl Med 1990;31:877.
15. Devous MD. Principles of Perfusion Imaging. In Neurology AAo, editor. AAN Annual Courses. 51st Annual Meeting of the American Academy of Neurology; 1999:9–28.
16. Kim JS, Moon DH, Kim GE, et al. Acetazolamide stress brain-perfusion SPECT predicts the need for carotid shunting during carotid endarterectomy. J Nucl Med 2000;41:1836–1841.
17. Takeuchi K, Maida K, Yoshida S, et al. Preoperative cerebrovascular screening before cardiovascular surgery in a high risk area of cerebrovascular events in Japan. J Cardiovasc Surg (Torino) 2000;41:911–914.
18. Ramsay SC, Yeates MG, Lord RS, et al. Use of technetium-HMPAO to demonstrate changes in cerebral blood flow reserve following carotid endarterectomy. J Nucl Med 1991;32:1382–1386.
19. Moriwaki H, Matsumoto M, Hashikawa K, et al. Hemodynamic aspect of cerebral watershed infarction: assessment of perfusion reserve using iodine-123-iodoamphetamine SPECT. J Nucl Med 1997;38:1556–1562.
20. Biller J, Godersky JC, Adams HP. Management of aneurysmal subarachnoid hemorrhage. Stroke 1988;19:1300–1305.
21. Davis SM, Andrews JT, Lichtenstein M, et al. Correlations between cerebral arterial velocities, blood flow, and delayed ischemia after subarachnoid hemorrhage. Stroke 1992;23:492–497.
22. Lewis DH, Eskridge JM, Newell DW, et al. Brain SPECT and the effect of cerebral angioplasty in delayed ischemia due to vasospasm. J Nucl Med 1992;33:1789–1796.
23. Le Roux PD, Newell DW, Eskridge J, et al. Severe symptomatic vasospasm: the role of immediate postoperative angioplasty. J Neurosurg 1994;80:224–229.
24. Caplan LR, Brass LM, DeWitt LD, et al. Transcranial Doppler ultrasound: present status. Neurology 1990;40:696–700.
25. Tranquart F, Ades PE, Groussin P, et al. Postoperative assessment of cerebral blood flow in subarachnoid haemorrhage by means of 99mTc-HMPAO tomography. Eur J Nucl Med 1993;20:53–58.
26. Kimura T, Shinoda J, Funakoshi T. Prediction of cerebral infarction due to vasospasm following aneurysmal subarachnoid haemorrhage using acetazolamide-activated 123I-IMP SPECT. Acta Neurochir 1993;123:125–128.
27. Tran Dinh YR, Lot G, Benrabah R, et al. Abnormal cerebral vasodilation in aneurysmal sub-

arachnoid hemorrhage: use of serial 133Xe cerebral blood flow measurement plus acetazolamide to assess cerebral vasospasm. J Neurosurg 1993;79:490–493.

28. Batjer HH, Devous MDS. The use of acetazolamide-enhanced regional cerebral blood flow measurement to predict risk to arteriovenous malformation patients. Neurosurgery 1992;31:213–217.

29. Batjer HH, Devous MD, Seibert GB, et al. Intracranial arteriovenous malformation: relationships between clinical factors and surgical complications. Neurosurgery 1989;24:75–79.

30. Awad IA, Magdinec M, Schubert A. Intracranial hypertension after resection of cerebral arteriovenous malformations. Predisposing factors and management strategy. Stroke 1994;25:611–620.

31. Chung TS, Lee JD, Suh JH, et al. Increased cerebral perfusion after detachable balloon embolization of carotid cavernous fistula on technetium-99m-HMPAO brain SPECT. J Nucl Med 1993;34:1987–1989.

32. Koenig M, Klotz E, Luka B, et al. Perfusion CT of the brain: diagnostic approach for early detection of ischemic stroke. Radiology 1998;209:85–93.

33. Hoggard N, Wilkinson ID, Griffiths PD. The imaging of ischaemic stroke. Clin Radiol 2001;56:171–183.

34. Cheung RT. Single-photon emission computed tomography-derived relative hypoperfusion volume after ischemic stroke. Stroke 1999;30:1733–1734.

35. Brass LM, Walovitch RC, Joseph JL, et al. The role of single photon emission computed tomography brain imaging with 99mTc-bicisate in the localization and definition of mechanism of ischemic stroke. J Cereb Blood Flow Metab 1994;14:S91–S98.

36. Masdeu J, Brass L, Holman L, Kushner M. Brain single-photon emission computed tomography. Neurology 1994;44:1970–1977.

37. Culebras A, Kase CS, Masdeu JC, et al. Practice guidelines for the use of imaging in transient ischemic attacks and acute stroke. A report of the Stroke Council, American Heart Association. Stroke 1997;28:1480–1497.

38. Mahagne MH, Darcourt J, Migneco O, et al. Early (99m)Tc-ethylcysteinate dimer brain SPECT patterns in the acute phase of stroke as predictors of neurological recovery. Cerebrovasc Dis 2000;10:364–373.

39. Barthel H, Hesse S, Dannenberg C, et al. Prospective value of perfusion and x-ray attenuation imaging with single-photon emission and transmission computed tomography in acute cerebral ischemia. Stroke 2001;32:1588–1597.

40. Karonen JO, Nuutinen J, Kuikka JT, et al. Combined SPECT and diffusion-weighted MRI as a predictor of infarct growth in acute ischemic stroke. J Nucl Med 2000;41:788–794.

41. Alexandrov AV, Masdeu JC, Devous M Sr, et al. Brain single-photon emission CT with HMPAO and safety of thrombolytic therapy in acute ischemic stroke. Proceedings of the meeting of the SPECT Safe Thrombolysis Study Collaborators and the members of the Brain Imaging Council of the Society of Nuclear Medicine. Stroke 1997;28:1830–1834.

42. Asenbaum S, Brucke T, Pirker W, et al. Imaging of cerebral blood flow with technetium-99m-HMPAO and technetium-99m-ECD: a comparison. J Nucl Med 1998;39:613–618.

43. Ogasawara K, Ogawa A, Ezura M, et al. Brain single-photon emission CT studies using 99mTc-HMPAO and 99mTc-ECD early after recanalization by local intraarterial thrombolysis in patients with acute embolic middle cerebral artery occlusion. AJNR Am J Neuroradiol 2001;22:48–53.

44. Ogasawara K, Ogawa A, Ezura M, et al. Dynamic and static 99mTc-ECD SPECT imaging of subacute cerebral infarction: comparison with 133Xe SPECT. J Nucl Med 2001;42:543–547.

45. Alexandrov AV, Black SE, Ehrlich LE, et al. Simple visual analysis of brain perfusion on HMPAO SPECT predicts early outcome in acute stroke. Stroke 1996;27:1537–1542.

46. Hirano T, Read SJ, Abbott DF, et al. Prediction of the final infarct volume within 6 h of stroke using single photon emission computed tomography with technetium-99m hexamethylpropylene amine oxime. Cerebrovasc Dis 2001;11:119–127.

47. Marchal G, Bouvard G, Iglesias S, et al. Predictive value of (99m)Tc-HMPAO-SPECT for neurological outcome/recovery at the acute stage of stroke. Cerebrovasc Dis 2000;10:8–17.

48. Baird AE, Austin MC, O'Keefe GJ, et al. Semiautomated analysis of the extent and severity of perfusion defects on brain SPECT images: validation studies. J Clin Neurosci 1999;6:121–127.

49. Baird AE, Donnan GA, Austin MC, et al. Asymmetries of cerebral perfusion in a stroke-age population. J Clin Neurosci 1999;6:113–120.

50. Aminian A, Strashun A, Rose A. Alternating hemiplegia of childhood: studies of regional cerebral blood flow using 99mTc-hexamethylpropylene amine oxime single-photon emission computed tomography. Ann Neurol 1993;33:43–47.

51. Lewis DH, Longstreth W Jr, Wilkus R, Copass M. Hyperemic receptive aphasia on neuroSPECT. Clin Nucl Med 1993;18:409–412.

52. Matsumoto K, Awata S, Matsuoka H, et al. Chronological changes in brain MRI, SPECT, and EEG in neurosarcoidosis with stroke-like episodes. Psychiatry Clin Neurosci 1998;52:629–633.

53. Berrouschot J, Barthel H, Hesse S, et al. Differentiation between transient ischemic attack and ischemic stroke within the first six hours after onset of symptoms by using 99mTc-ECD-SPECT. J Cereb Blood Flow Metab 1998;18:921–929.

54. Laloux P, Jamart J, Meurisse H, et al. Persisting perfusion defect in transient ischemic attacks: a new clinically useful subgroup? Stroke 1996;27:425–430.

55. Nuutinen J, Kuikka J, Roivainen R, et al. Early serial SPECT in acute middle cerebral artery infarction. Nucl Med Commun 2000;21:425–429.

56. Masdeu JC, Fine M. Cerebrovascular Disorders. In CF Gonzalez, CB Grossman, JC Masdeu (eds), Head and Spine Imaging. New York: Wiley, 1985;283–356.

57. Masdeu JC. Enhancing mass on CT: neoplasm or recent infarction? Neurology 1983;33:836–840.

58. Baird AE, Austin MC, McKay WJ, Donnan GA. Sensitivity and specificity of 99mTc-HMPAO SPECT cerebral perfusion measurements during the first 48 hours for the localization of cerebral infarction. Stroke 1997;28:976–980.

59. Berrouschot J, Barthel H, von Kummer R, et al. 99m technetium-ethyl-cysteinate-dimer single-photon emission CT can predict fatal ischemic brain edema. Stroke 1998;29:2556–2562.

60. Bowler JV, Wade JP, Jones BE, et al. Single-photon emission computed tomography using hexamethylpropyleneamine oxime in the prognosis of acute cerebral infarction. Stroke 1996;27:82–86.

61. Baron JC. Perfusion thresholds in human cerebral ischemia: historical perspective and therapeutic implications. Cerebrovasc Dis 2001;11:2–8.

62. Karonen JO, Vanninen RL, Liu Y, et al. Combined diffusion and perfusion MRI with correlation to single-photon emission CT in acute ischemic stroke. Ischemic penumbra predicts infarct growth. Stroke 1999;30:1583–1590.

63. Liu Y, Karonen JO, Vanninen RL, Ostergaard L, et al. Cerebral hemodynamics in human acute ischemic stroke: a study with diffusion- and perfusion-weighted magnetic resonance imaging and SPECT. J Cereb Blood Flow Metab 2000;20:910–920.

64. Ryu YH, Chung TS, Yoon PH, et al. Evaluation of reperfusion and recovery of brain function before and after intracarotid arterial urokinase therapy in acute cerebral infarction with brain SPECT. Clin Nucl Med 1999;24:566–571.

65. Ueda T, Sakaki S, Yuh WT, et al. Outcome in acute stroke with successful intra-arterial thrombolysis and predictive value of initial single-photon emission-computed tomography. J Cereb Blood Flow Metab 1999;19:99–108.

66. Sasaki O, Takeuchi S, Koizumi T, et al. Complete recanalization via fibrinolytic therapy can reduce the number of ischemic territories that progress to infarction. AJNR Am J Neuroradiol 1996;17:1661–1668.

67. Grotta JC, Alexandrov AV. tPA-associated reperfusion after acute stroke demonstrated by SPECT. Stroke 1998;29:429–432.

68. Berrouschot J, Barthel H, Hesse S, et al. Reperfusion and metabolic recovery of brain tissue and clinical outcome after ischemic stroke and thrombolytic therapy. Stroke 2000;31:1545–1551.

69. Nakano S, Iseda T, Ikeda T, et al. Thresholds of ischemia salvageable with intravenous tissue plasminogen activator therapy: evaluation with cerebral blood flow single-photon emission computed tomographic measurements. Neurosurgery 2000;47:68–71; discussion 71–73.

70. Umemura A, Suzuka T, Yamada K. Quantitative measurement of cerebral blood flow by (99m)Tc-HMPAO SPECT in acute ischaemic stroke: usefulness in determining therapeutic options. J Neurol Neurosurg Psychiatry 2000;69:472–478.

71. Yasaka M, O'Keefe GJ, Chambers BR, et al. Streptokinase in acute stroke: effect on reperfusion and recanalization. Australian Streptokinase Trial Study Group. Neurology 1998;50:626–632.

72. Rossler A, Berrouschot J, Barthel H, et al. Potential of rheopheresis for the treatment of acute ischemic stroke when initiated between 6 and 12 hours. Ther Apher 2000;4:358–362.

73. Berrouschot J, Barthel H, Koster J, et al. Extracorporeal rheopheresis in the treatment of acute ischemic stroke: a randomized pilot study. Stroke 1999;30:787–792.

74. Kruuse C, Jacobsen TB, Thomsen LL, et al. Effects of the non-selective phosphodiesterase inhibitor pentoxifylline on regional cerebral blood flow and large arteries in healthy subjects. Eur J Neurol 2000;7:629–638.

75. Yu Y, Mizushige K, Ueda T, et al. Effect of olprinone, phosphodiesterase III inhibitor, on cerebral blood flow assessed with technetium-99m-ECD SPECT. J Cardiovasc Pharmacol 2000;35:422–426.

76. Infeld B, Davis SM, Donnan GA, et al. Nimodipine and perfusion changes after stroke. Stroke 1999;30:1417–1423.

77. Wallace EA, Wisniewski G, Zubal G, et al. Acute cocaine effects on absolute cerebral blood flow. Psychopharmacology (Berl) 1996;128:17–20.

78. Matsuda M, Lee H, Kuribayashi K, et al. Comparative study of regional cerebral blood flow values measured by Xe CT and Xe SPECT. Acta Neurol Scand Suppl 1996;166:13–16.

79. Starkstein SE, Sabe L, Vazquez S, et al. Neuropsychological, psychiatric, and cerebral blood flow findings in vascular dementia and Alzheimer's disease. Stroke 1996;27:408–414.

80. Mellies JK, Baumer T, Muller JA, et al. SPECT study of a German CADASIL family: a phenotype with migraine and progressive dementia only. Neurology 1998;50:1715–1721.

81. Kuwabara Y, Ichiya Y, Otsuka M, et al. Differential diagnosis of bilateral parietal abnormalities in I-

123 IMP SPECT imaging. Clin Nucl Med 1990;15: 893–899.

82. Lien LM, Lee HC, Wang KL, et al. Involvement of nervous system in maternally inherited diabetes and deafness (MIDD) with the A3243G mutation of mitochondrial DNA. Acta Neurol Scand 2001;103: 159–165.

83. Miyamoto A, Oki J, Takahashi S, et al. Serial imaging in MELAS. Neuroradiology 1997;39:427–430.

84. Peng NJ, Liu RS, Li JY, et al. Increased cerebral blood flow in MELAS shown by Tc-99m HMPAO brain SPECT. Neuroradiology 2000;42:26–29.

85. Hoffmann M, Corr P, Robbs J. Cerebrovascular findings in Takayasu disease. J Neuroimaging 2000;10:84–90.

86. Andersen AR, Friberg L, Olsen TS, Olesen J. Delayed hyperemia following hypoperfusion in classic migraine. Single photon emission computed tomographic demonstration. Arch Neurol 1988;45:154–159.

87. La-Spina I, Vignati A, Porazzi D. Basilar artery migraine: transcranial Doppler EEG and SPECT from the aura phase to the end. Headache 1997;37:43–47.

88. Nezu A, Kimura S, Ohtsuki N, et al. Acute confusional migraine and migrainous infarction in childhood. Brain Dev 1997;19:148–151.

89. Stevens H, Van de Wiele C, Santens P, et al. Cobalt-57 and technetium-99m-HMPAO-labeled leukocytes for visualization of ischemic infarcts. J Nucl Med 1998;39:495–498.

90. Stevens H, Knollema S, Piers DA, et al. Cobalt-57 as a SPECT tracer in the visualization of ischaemic brain damage in patients with middle cerebral artery stroke. Nucl Med Commun 1998;19:573–580.

91. Hatazawa J, Satoh T, Shimosegawa E, et al. Evaluation of cerebral infarction with iodine 123-iomazenil SPECT. J Nucl Med 1995;36:2154–2161.

92. Sasaki M, Ichiya Y, Kuwabara Y, et al. Benzodiazepine receptors in chronic cerebrovascular disease: comparison with blood flow and metabolism. J Nucl Med 1997;38:1693–1698.

93. Nakagawara J, Sperling B, Lassen NA. Incomplete brain infarction of reperfused cortex may be quantitated with iomazenil. Stroke 1997;28:124–132.

CHAPTER

8

Xenon-Enhanced Computed Tomography Cerebral Blood Flow

Howard Yonas and Elad I. Levy

HISTORICAL PERSPECTIVE

The measurement of cerebral blood flow (CBF) with the xenon-enhanced computed tomography (XeCT) CBF method is built on the extensive work of the pioneers in CBF that utilized xenon-133 as a diffusible tracer of CBF. With decades of experience in measuring CBF with radioactive xenon, the observation by Haughton and Winkler[1–4] that xenon was radiodense led investigators to attempt to measure CBF by combining stable xenon with CT imaging.[5,6] The breakthrough work in the field was accomplished by Gur et al.,[7] who not only provided a means of measurement of CBF by integrating the measurement of the end tidal concentration of stable xenon with the progressive enhancement of CT imaging during a relatively short inhalation period, but also provided the means to do this for every voxel of the CT image, thereby providing a tomographic, high-resolution image of CBF.

PROBLEMS AND SOLUTIONS

The clinical application of this potentially useful technology had to overcome a number of real and potential obstacles before it could fulfill its clinical potential. The fact that xenon, although a noble gas, was biologically active and at 80% was an anesthetic agent presented an initial hurdle for the clinical use of xenon as a contrast agent. Although the safety record of even high concentrations of xenon inhalation was excellent, with a rapid clearance and no allergic or other adverse reactions, the fact that even low levels of xenon altered the sensorium in some patients did present a problem. The report by Winkler in 1985 that 100% xenon inhalation was associated with apnea also raised concerns about the safety of a radiologic study that utilized a potentially anesthetic agent.[8] Concern was further raised by the observation that xenon inhalation tended to raise CBF and thereby violated the Frick principle that a tracer of CBF not alter CBF.

The initial efforts with CBF measurement were directed toward obtaining enough enhancement for deriving reliable quantitative information, combined with the need to minimize the concentration and duration of inhalation. Early clinical studies demonstrated an unacceptable incidence of side effects at concentrations above 35%, especially when inhaled for more than 5 minutes. Even the relatively primitive CT scanners of the late 1970s, however, provided an adequate signal to noise ratio below that concentration. Novel approaches to the calculation of CBF were used to generate quantitative CBF maps with only a 4.3-minute xenon inhalation period combined with eight CT images at each CT level of study.[7] With this configuration, sensory side effects were infrequent, mild, and rapidly reversible (<3%).[9] Subsequent improvements in CT technology have made it possible to maintain the same high signal to noise ratio while lowering the xenon concentration into the mid-20% range associated with a significant reduction in flow activation and xenon-related symptomatology.

Early studies of the effect of xenon inhalation on CBF confirmed that xenon did raise CBF, but to a moderate degree and in a delayed manner. Despite this tendency, confidence in the reliability of the technique was gained with a series of cross-correlation studies that showed the ability of this noninvasive technology to provide information similar to that provided by microspheres[10,11] and iodoantipyrine.[12] Statistical correlation was found with these standard laboratory technologies at high, low, and normal flow levels of CBF. Normative patient studies demonstrated that CBF values obtained with the XeCT method were within the published normative ranges for gray, white, and mixed cortical flow.[13] The reason for the stability and apparent accuracy of the technology was explained by a number of authors who used mathematic simulation approaches to explore the effect of the time course of flow activation on the calculation of flow.[14] These studies consistently concluded that the effect of the 15–30% flow activation is less than a 5% effect on calculated flow compared with real flow. The disparity was explained by the observation that flow activation does not become significant until 2.5 minutes of xenon inhalation, which is after the essential early data for flow measurement are recorded. Although flow within white matter is affected to a greater degree than gray matter, even white matter flow values are not altered greater than 5% due to xenon-related flow activation.

The potential for blood flow activation to elevate intracranial pressure (ICP) in patients with head injury was another early concern. A report by an early investigator that did not compensate for the ventilation effects of the xenon as a heavy gas did report an elevation of ICP.[15] Subsequent studies have demonstrated that if the CO_2 is kept constant, with the use of a volume priority ventilator that automatically increases ventilator pressure to maintain the volume of exchanged gas, no significant increase of ICP occurs.[16] In patients with elevated ICP, the use of moderate hyperventilation also negates any tendency for ICP elevation during xenon inhalation.

Although Winkler[8] raised concerns that xenon could cause apnea, from tens of thousands of clinical studies at 33% xenon and 67% oxygen, it has been learned that respiratory pauses for more than 20 seconds are rare.[9] On closer examination, the respiratory difficulties were most often due to respiratory obstruction similar to sleep apnea. Attention to neck positioning and further lowering the concentration of xenon has made respiratory irregularities even less frequent and rarely significant. Simply coaching the patient to take a deep breath often terminates a brief respiratory pause. No significant clinical injury associated with xenon inhalation has been reported.

Despite resolution of many of the technical issues related to the efficacy and safety of XeCT CBF, an early effort to commercialize the XeCT CBF technology was a failure for many reasons. Those early systems were simply too unreliable and too slow to deliver clinically relevant information. Studies required the CT scan computer not be used for imaging for at least 1 hour while three flow images were calculated. With the evolution of modern CT scanners, more levels could be studied with lower xenon concentrations.[17] With faster computers, not only could the calculation of flow be accomplished within 5 seconds per level, but a far superior "numeric" integration methodology could be used that provided a more stable solution for the measurement of CBF. The ability to fast-transfer images via network systems also meant that air curve and CT information could be merged within a dedicated computer within seconds of study completion, while freeing the scanner to proceed with other imaging tasks. Thus, today a six-level flow study that takes 4.5 minutes to acquire can be transferred, calculated, and displayed in less than a total time of 10 minutes. Last, the availability of technology that can blend xenon/oxygen mixtures and maintain a steady delivery with a closed loop system has also reduced the cost of xenon per study by 80% to levels costing less than those currently associated with iodinated contrast agents (Figure 8-1). These improvements in the technologies on which XeCT CBF are directly dependent have made this a very different technology from what was brought to the market in 1985.[17]

The last problem related to XeCT has been the inability to obtain xenon gas due to U.S. Food and Drug Administration (FDA)–related issues. Because the approval for xenon/oxygen was originally by the "grandfather" process, in that it was used before current regulations, the gas mix was made available by the one manufacturer that had demonstrated "prior use." In February of 2001, that manufacturer decided to withdraw from this market and with that action removed the only approved source of medical-grade xenon in the United States. Currently, work with this technology is on hold while other manufacturers are seeking to complete the FDA process.

TECHNIQUE

Xenon is a radiodense, highly lipid-soluble inert (noble) gas with a molecular number adjacent to iodine, so that its tissue concentration can be accurately measured by CT imaging. The concentration of xenon in the blood flowing to the brain is dependent on several factors: CBF, arterial concentration, the relative distribution of xenon between the blood and each tissue compartment (brain-blood partition coefficient, or λ, which is 0.7 for gray matter and 1.4 for white matter), and duration of xenon exposure. Using the Kety-Schmidt equations, these variables are integrated to produce a quantitative CBF image with a flow calculation for each of the 24,000 voxels per CT level of study.[11]

The above variables are related mathematically by the following modifications of the Kety-Schmidt equations:

$$C_{XcBr}(t) = \lambda k \int_0^t C_{XeArt}(u) e^{-k(t-u)} du$$

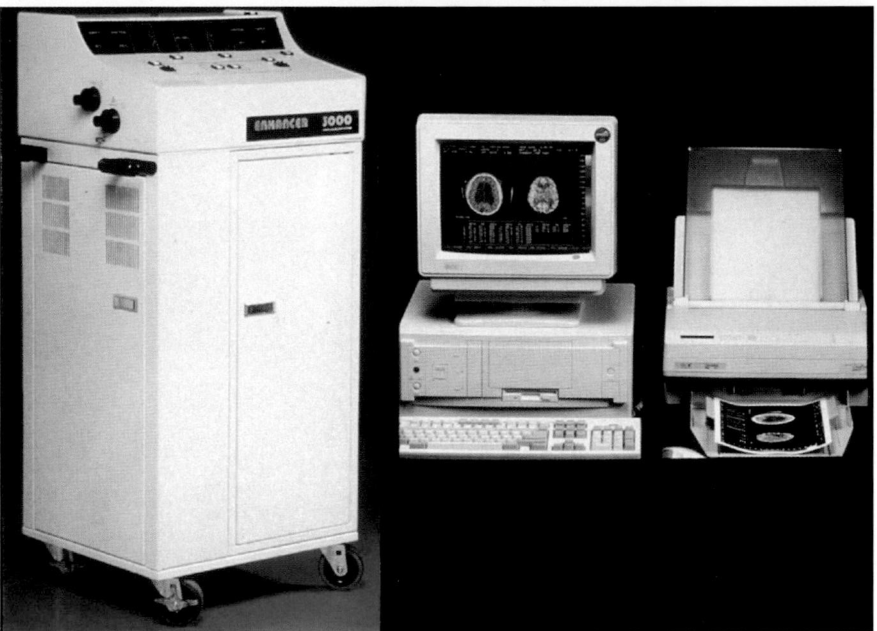

FIGURE 8-1. The xenon-enhanced computed tomography cerebral blood flow system involves a semi- and then closed-loop delivery device that blends 80% xenon and 20% oxygen to deliver the desired xenon concentration, which can range from 26% to 35% within 1%. This device minimizes the amount of xenon needed per study while delivering a constant level of contrast. The system works equally well with spontaneously breathing patients as well as ventilated patients.

$$F = \lambda k$$

where $C_{XeBr}(t)$ is the time-dependent concentration of xenon in the blood supplying the brain, λ is the blood-brain partition coefficient, k is the uptake flow rate constant, $C_{XeArt}(u)$ is the time-dependent arterial concentration of xenon, and F is the CBF.[9]

The time-dependent arterial concentration of xenon accumulation is related by the following equation:

$$C_{XeArt}(u) = C_{Xemax}(1 - e^{-bu})$$

$$C_{Xemax} = C(\%)_{max}\,(5.15)\,(S_{Xe})\,(0.01)$$

where C_{Xemax} is the maximum arterial xenon concentration, u is the elapsed time, b is the rate uptake constant, $C\,(\%)_{max}$ is the maximum percent uptake of xenon, 5.15 is the density of xenon (mg/ml) at 37°C and at 1 atmosphere of pressure, and S_{Xe} is the solubility of xenon in blood. The validity of these equations assumes that arterial xenon uptake is instantaneously in equilibrium with the end-tidal pulmonary xenon concentration (which is true for most patients without severe lung disease or right to left cardiopulmonary shunting).[11]

The Ostwald solubility of xenon in blood is related to the hematocrit of the patient by the following equation:

$$S_{Xe} = 0.1 + 0.0011\ (\%\ \text{hematocrit})$$

To generate graphic representation of CBF, the Hounsfield enhancement is calculated from the following equation:

$$HE = C_{XeBr} / \,(U_p^{w} / U_p^{Xe})$$

where U_p^{w} and U_p^{Xe} are the mass attenuation coefficients of water and xenon.

Although there are many approaches to calculate CBF with stable xenon, the strategy using only the "wash-in" information minimizes the effects of flow activation due to xenon inhalation. In this format, two baseline CT scans are obtained before administering xenon. These images are averaged for numeric advantage and then subtracted from each of the six xenon-enhanced images obtained at each CT level of study during or following 4.3 minutes of xenon administration (providing C_{XeBr} [t]).[11] Because only eight images are needed at each CT level of study, programmed table movements allow for the study of six to ten 10-mm thick levels during each examination.

Before entering the solution of the Kety-Schmidt equation, the database is cleared of voxels that have a buildup curve not characteristic of a diffusible tracer within brain tissue. Voxels with a rapid buildup typical of an artery are deleted from the database, and surrounding "good" voxels are averaged and substituted. This maneuver guarantees that the XeCT CBF map is an image of flow within tissue and not within the arterial bed.

The CBF image is displayed in reference to or with a fixed color scale (Figure 8-2). Due to a relatively high noise level, a single voxel ($1 \times 1 \times 10$ mm^3), error is reduced to relatively low levels (12%) with the grouping of more than 100 adjacent voxels.[18] Acceptable mean normative flows for XeCT CBF are 80 + 20 ml/100 g per

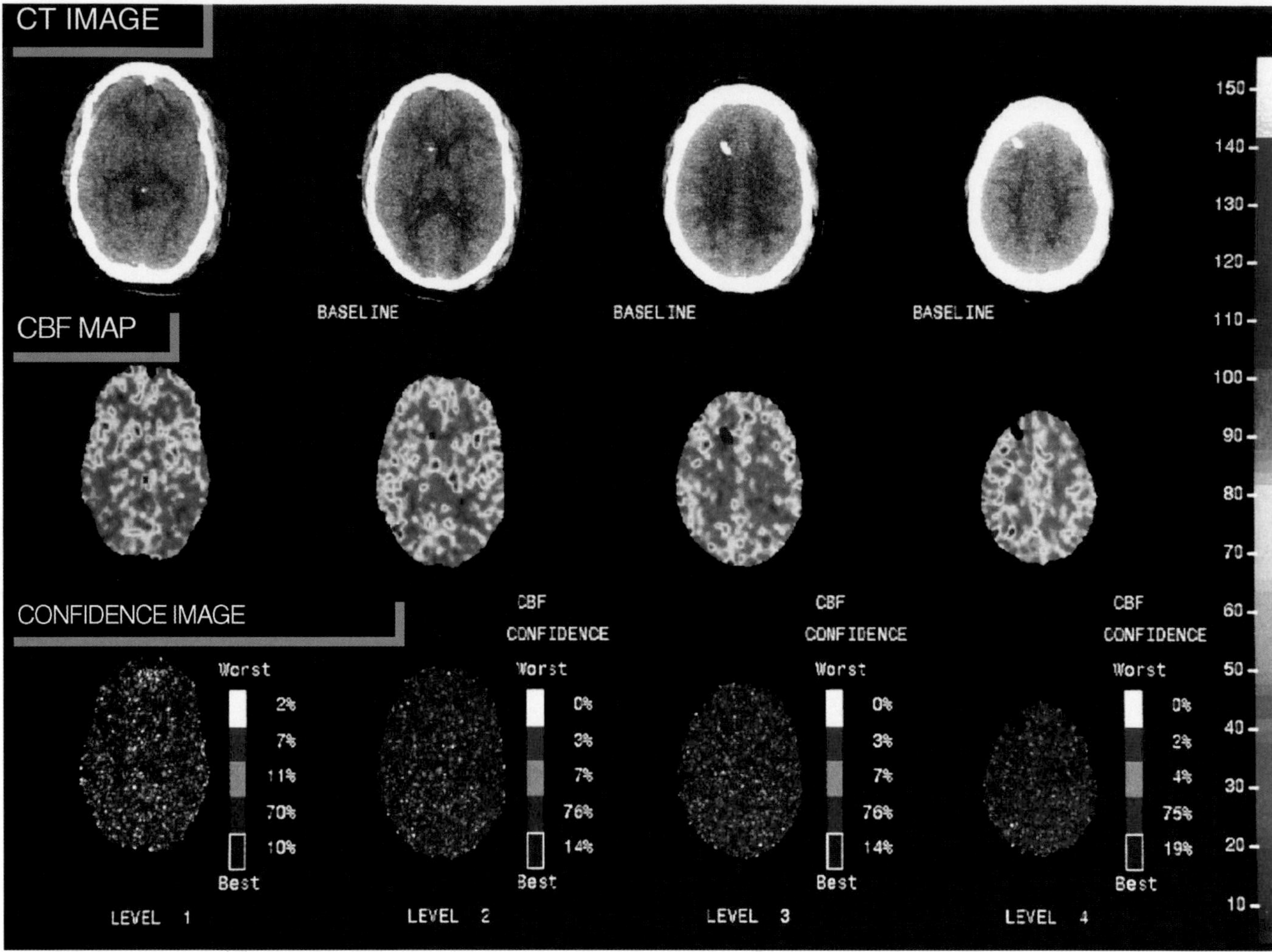

FIGURE 8-2. A normal four-level, xenon-enhanced computed tomography cerebral blood flow (CBF) study is displayed, showing the computed tomographic scan of each level of study (**top**), the CBF study (**middle**), and the confidence image (**bottom**). The scale on the far right is fixed for the technology, with a color change with every 20 cc/100 g per minute and with flow values below 8 cc/100 g per minute highlighted in lavender. The color scale with the confidence image indicates a scale that provides an assessment of the quality of the information.

minute for healthy gray matter, 20 + 2 ml/100 g per minute for white matter, and mixed cortical flows are 50 + 10 ml/100 g per minute.[13] Gray matter flows and mixed cortical flow values are somewhat age dependent, with values decreasing in the elderly.

LIMITATIONS AND ADVANTAGES

The major clinical limitation of XeCT CBF is an intolerance to head motion. Because the tissue curve for each voxel is acquired by directly subtracting each of six xenon-enhanced images from the baseline images, any motion between images significantly degrades this high-resolution (FWHM <4 mm) technology. Although later images can be deleted from the calculation with a relatively small loss of accuracy, the first three images are critical to obtaining a quantitative image. Head fixation, including a specially designed head holder, together with good patient cooperation aided by the occasional (10–20%) use of mild sedation have lessened the frequency of deterioration of studies due to motion and has generated useful studies in 87% of acute stroke patients (M. Kilpatrick, *personal communication*, 2000). Computational strategies for motion correction before entering the calculation of flow should minimize this problem in the future.

Bone-induced artifacts are a second limitation. Scatter artifacts created by bone ridges and extremely high densities, such as the petrous apex, make the calculation of flow within regions of scatter artifact impossible with this technique. By aligning images along the orbital meatal line, artifact-free images are obtained for 90% of the supratentorial compartment. The highest level of cortical imaging is limited by "beam hardening" artifacts due to the extreme curvature of the skull. The posterior fossa can for the most part be imaged by using an extreme gan-

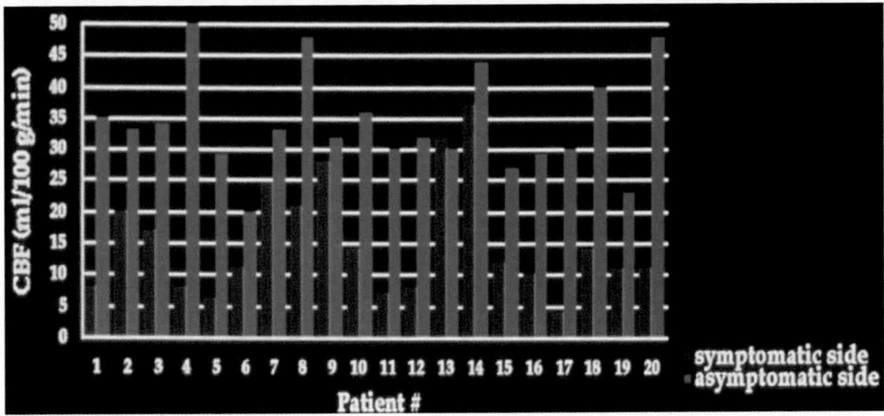

FIGURE 8-3. Mean cerebral blood flow (CBF) values for the middle cerebral artery territory on the ipsilateral and contralateral hemispheres to a major ischemic stroke display great heterogeneity between and within patients. Whereas the mean flow for the "symptomatic" side was 15 cc/100 g per minute, flow on the asymptomatic side was 34 cc/100 g per minute and not the "norm" of 50 cc/100 g per minute. Although all patients had a similar neurologic deficit, flow within the symptomatic side varied from 4 to 48 cc/100 g per minute. The wide spectrum clearly indicates the need to differentiate a group of patients with major vascular territories that are irreversibly ischemic from those within the penumbra and, in turn, from those that are no longer ischemic due to reperfusion.

try angle and neck flexion. Imaging of the lower pons and medulla can only be obtained by using a gantry angle perpendicular to the clivus with the mouth open to minimize scatter artifact due to dentition. A higher-photon energy can be used (100 or 120 vs. 80 kilovolt [peak]) to lessen bone artifact. This approach lessens the CT scanner sensitivity to xenon and requires an alteration of the flow constant for the calculation of CBF.

Another limitation of XeCT is the inability to directly measure multiple variables. Although XeCT CBF is able to accurately measure a broad range of flow values, a single study cannot determine whether a regional reduction of flow is due to reduced demand or supply. Because of the relatively rapid washout of xenon, a second study can, however, be performed within 20 minutes, providing adequate time for altering a physiologic variable, thereby providing two data points. By altering the blood pressure or the acid–base balance between studies, the integrity of autoregulation or the vascular reserve status can be assessed.[19] This type of approach does provide access to information about cerebral blood volume, vasoregulation, and vascular reserve without the cost and limitations of positron emission tomography.

The importance of the ability of XeCT to measure flow on a real, quantitative scale should be stressed. XeCT-generated numbers can be directly referenced to the laboratory studies that have provided an understanding about the relationship between the time and depth of flow values below 20 cc/100 g per minute, and reversible and irreversible ischemia. Studies that provide only qualitative CBF examine only a ratio, assuming an ability to identify a known normal region of CBF for comparison. As described by Rubin et al.[20] and Firlik et al.,[21] transhemispheric and cerebellar diaschisis may result or does occur in the first few hours after large hemispheric thromboembolic strokes. Firlik et al. reported that whereas ipsilateral flow values to a hemispheric ischemic stroke were approximately 15, contralateral flow values were 35 cc/100 g per minute. In the same paper, Firlik et al. demonstrated that the actual flow values both ipsilateral as well as contralateral to an ischemic insult varied significantly between patients (Figure 8-3), further demonstrating that no prediction can be made concerning flow values either ipsi- or contralateral. This unpredictable degree of metabolic suppression throughout all regions of the brain means that any strategy built on calculating a ratio between the injured region and a "known normal reference region" is frequently in error.

An important feature of the current XeCT CBF system is the minimal additional time required to collect and process data.[17] Because quantitative data can be obtained on the same scanner bed used to obtain a conventional CT scan, patients are not subjected to the risks of additional delays due to the necessity of transport to another scanner. The rapid integration into patient-specific management is aided by the fact that the CBF image can be directly correlated with CT-defined anatomy.

Three additional advantages of XeCT CBF are due to technical issues that make the study increasingly reliable and potentially useful. First, XeCT is the only CBF technology that solves for and integrates information concerning the partition coefficient.[22] By solving for a tissue-specific coefficient (λ), XeCT-generated flow values should be more accurate, even in disease states. Because the partition coefficient is linearly related to CBF, by not solving for this variable, flow values in diseased tissue can easily be in error by 50%. Second, XeCT is the only technology that attempts to quantitatively assess the quality of the flow data that are being provided for clinical assessment. The confidence image integrates a "best fit analysis" of the tissue data points together with the number of enhanced scans used in the map creation as well as the degree of enhancement due to the concentration of xenon actually achieved from end-tidal sampling.[17] Thus, this technology provides the reader a means of rapidly assessing the quantitative status of the study, helping to avoid the error of over-relying on the values generated from a poor-quality study due to excessive motion or inadequate xenon concentration. Third, the availability of a flow phantom allows for the standardization of flow values generated by all centers irrespective of the CT manufacturer. Potential alterations of flow values, due to vagaries within and between scanners, are compensated for by the integration of a correction constant generated with the aid of the phantom. Thus, a value of 20 cc/100 g per minute generated at one site should be the same and have the same vital implications of this number obtained elsewhere.

CLINICAL APPLICATIONS

Cerebral Blood Flow–Guided Management of Thromboembolic Stroke

XeCT CBF is capable of answering many of the critical questions inherent in the management of acute ischemic stroke victims and specifically for the selection of stroke patients most and least likely to benefit from thrombolytic therapy. The goal of thrombolytic therapies is to re-establish perfusion to potentially viable brain tissue. Concurrent with that goal is the need to know when tissue is not amenable to reperfusion therapy, either because it is no longer ischemic or because it is already irreversibly ischemic. The former does not require reperfusion therapy, and the latter may be additionally injured by causing a potentially harmful hemorrhagic complication. The goal is to find a patient with a significant volume of tissue in the 8–20 cc/100 g per minute range, commonly referred to as the *ischemic penumbra* (Figure 8-4). This is the prime target of therapy because without reperfusion this tissue progresses from a reversible to an irreversible injury. Such differentiation is readily attainable with XeCT CBF studies.

The importance of a single flow measurement has been questioned because it is only a "snapshot" of a complex and evolving process. Animal modeling of hemispheric infarction has demonstrated that regions with very low flow levels from the onset are very stable.[23–26] A similar observation has been made with positron emission tomography using another model of hemispheric ischemia.[27] Thus, the observation of near-zero flow at any time in the first 6 hours after stroke onset is highly predictive that flow had been near zero from the onset of the ischemic insult. This consistency of very low flow values explains why they do predict the volume of dead tissue[28] and the likelihood of progression to life-threatening herniation.[29,30]

It has also been argued that only technologies that measure metabolism can determine if an infarction has occurred, with this question being most relevant in the set-

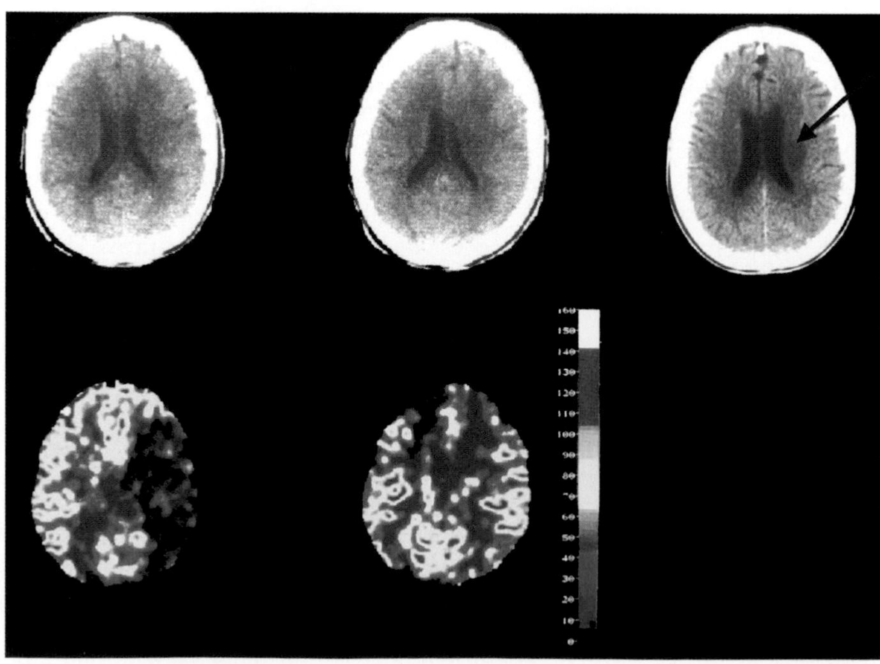

FIGURE 8-4. The computed tomographic scan (**top**) and the xenon-enhanced computed tomography cerebral blood flow study (**bottom**) were obtained in a patient with middle cerebral artery occlusion 3 hours after onset of a right-sided deficit. Middle cerebral artery territorial flow on the left was a mean of 15 cc/100 g per minute. Emergent angiography confirmed middle cerebral artery occlusion, after which intra-arterial urokinase was infused with rapid clot lysis. The next day, flow within the territory was normal, and only on late follow-up films was a small infarction within the distribution of the striate arteries identified (*arrow*).

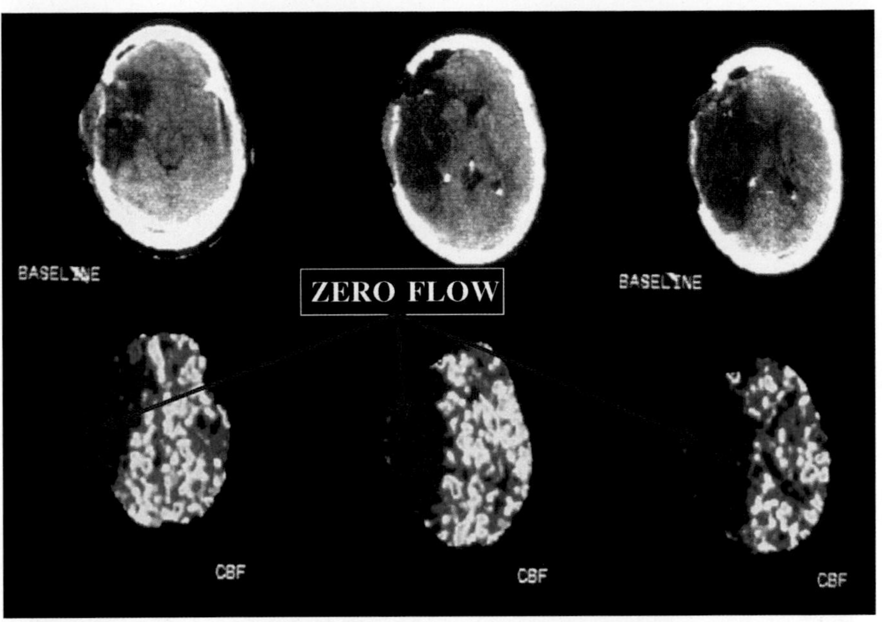

FIGURE 8-5. This three-level xenon-enhanced computed tomography cerebral blood flow (CBF) study was obtained the day after a decompressive craniotomy for massive brain swelling, following carotid and middle cerebral artery occlusion 3 days prior. Despite the decompression, there is still significant midline shift, and it is evident that nearly all of the tissue that is "infarcted" on computed tomography has no effective flow remaining. Availability of this type of information before surgery has been the basis for making the decision in some patients for performing a "strokectomy."

ting of reperfusion after ischemic infarction. In the world of acute stroke therapy, however, the only question that needs to be answered is whether a region of the brain is persistently ischemic and potentially recoverable if reperfusion can be accomplished. Firlik et al.[31] identified 12 stroke victims who had normal flow levels when initially studied within the first 6 hours poststroke onset; nine fully recovered without therapeutic intervention. The other three presumably achieved reperfusion after developing an irreversible injury. Thus, with the finding of low but not ischemic levels of flow, there was no indication for reperfusion therapy, and 9 out of 12 patients subsequently resolved their deficits without any intervention. If reperfusion takes place after an irreversible injury has occurred, the rapid appearance of low densities and evidence of mass effect is also useful in understanding the nature of the injury. Thus, even without a measurement of metabolism, the finding of flows in the 20 cc/100 g per minute range in association with well-defined CT evidence of infarction 3 hours after stroke onset clearly provides the insight that there is a large stroke with reperfusion and accelerated edema due to reperfusion of the injured tissues. Thus, integration of the anatomic information provided by CT imaging with quantitative flow information does provide vital insights needed to help guide acute stroke management even if reperfusion occurs.[26,31]

The importance of being able to define the "core" or region with irreversible ischemic injury cannot be overstressed (Figure 8-5). Reperfusion of tissue that is already dead is a waste of valuable resources and only increases the risk of hemorrhagic complications. Goldstein et al.[32] demonstrated that when the flow level of the entire middle cerebral artery (MCA) territory was less than 13 cc/100 g per minute, and two adjacent standard cortical regions of interest were below 9 cc/100 g per minute, the risk of hemorrhage was significantly increased. A similar threshold for irreversibility was observed in a case report involving basilar artery occlusion by Levy et al.[33] Similarly, Firlik et al.[31] reported that if the MCA average flows were 9 cc/100 g per minute, the patients were at significantly increased risk of developing malignant edema or hemorrhage, or both, thereby progressing to the clinical picture of life-threatening brain herniation. These patients in a separate report were reasonable candidates for aggressive stroke volume reduction (strokectomy) after CBF studies had defined irreversible ischemic injuries from the onset (see Figure 8-5).[29]

In an examination of the ischemic penumbra, Kaufmann et al.[28] reported that the volume of hemispheric tissue with flow values between 7 and 20 cc/100 g per minute after middle cerebral occlusion was not significantly increased on the side of occlusion. They thereby questioned where the penumbra constituted a significant target for therapy. A recent re-evaluation of the penumbra in patients with acute M1 occlusion was reported by Jovin et al.[23] When they examined flow within only the middle cerebral territory, they did find a significant and relatively constant penumbra of approximately 20–30%. The remarkable finding in this report is that the outcome and risk of complication did not correlate with the volume of penumbra but instead with the volume of the core.

CBF studies are useful for prediction of patient outcomes after stroke as well as for guiding clinical management with therapeutic interventions. Kilpatrick et al.[34] reported that rather than the time from onset, the persistent level of perfusion, and therefore the quality of persistent collateral supply was a significantly better prognostic indicator of the incidence of infarction. Rubin et al.[35] demonstrated, from a study of the intake National Institutes of Health stroke scale and MCA flow

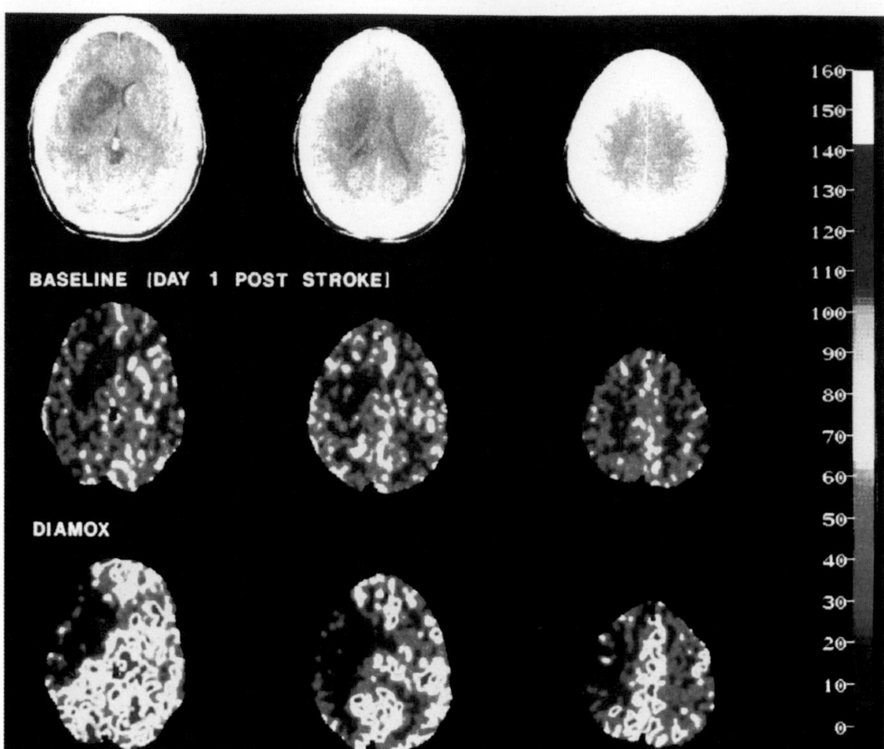

FIGURE 8-6. This 60-year-old woman presented with a left hemiplegia and was found to have occlusion of her middle cerebral artery. The computed tomographic scan (**top**) for this three-level study shows infarction of the basal ganglia. The baseline study (**middle**) demonstrates symmetrically low but nonischemic level of perfusion to the lateral cortex. After Diamox (**bottom**), flow within the entire brain, except for the right middle cerebral artery territory, increased by 50%, whereas flow within the middle cerebral artery territory fell by 50%. Study demonstrates that while the patient has re-established adequate collateral flow to right cortex at rest, the region remained at risk for further ischemic injuries with physiologic stress.

values compared with the outcome, that the levels of flow could discriminate groups of patients who had a good outcome, a poor outcome, and a group with a less predictable course depending on therapy used.

The ability and utility of integrating the observations based on CT with XeCT CBF and CT angiography were reported by Kilpatrick et al.[36] By integrating the information gained with all three technologies in 51 patients studied within 24 hours of stroke onset, it was possible to identify subgroups who were good candidates for reperfusion therapy well past the 3-hour window for tissue plasminogen activator. A patient without CT evidence of infarction with penumbral levels of perfusion (8–30 cc/100 g per minute) with major vessel occlusion should be an ideal candidate for reperfusion therapy. Conversely, a patient with a normal CT, no definable vessel occlusion on CT angiography, and normal flow would not be a candidate for thrombolytic therapy.[28] The fact that flow values strongly predicted the clinical outcome as well as the likelihood of CT conversion provided support that this type of paradigm is valid and worthy of further study.

Assessing Stroke Risk and the Need for Surgical Revascularization

After the pioneering efforts of Yasargil in the 1970s that showed the feasibility of bypass surgery to the arteries of the brain, the superficial temporal artery–MCA bypass procedure became a standard of care for patients with symptomatic carotid occlusion or inoperable stenosis, or both. With the conclusions of the International Cooperative Study of Extracranial-Intracranial Arterial Anastomosis that there was no significant benefit of this operation, this procedure almost ceased to be performed.[37] Because bypass surgery is a purely hemodynamic procedure, many have contended that the study failed to show utility because it failed to identify a group of patients who were hemodynamically compromised.

Early efforts to study compromised physiology involved the measurement of CBF combined with a "stress" test. Most efforts involved an examination of the response to a challenge that should increase CBF, presuming that normally there should be the ability to vasodilate further. Although many combinations of stress induction and flow measurement have been reported, the combination of a quantitative CBF study and acetazolamide has won wide acceptance. Acetazolamide normally increases CBF by greater than 20%, with a mean increase of 35%, and patients with a degree of activation of flow less than 20% have a "compromise of reserve."[38]

With the most severe levels of compromise, primary collateral channels are lost, and territorial blood supply shifts to secondary collateral routes (i.e., ophthalmic and pial).[39] With a severe compromise of blood supply, maximum vasodilation and a loss of autoregulation of blood pressure occur in conjunction with a paradoxic decrease of CBF in response to acetazolamide. In this setting, the acid–base shift induced by acetazolamide maximally dilates adjacent vessel beds and produces a "steal phenomenon" (Figure 8-6). When this happens, the maximal ischemic challenge is most evident within the deep white matter at a borderzone between the vessels arising from the ependymal surface of the ventricle and the penetrating vessels from the surface.[40] This type of deep white matter injury has been directly related to the symptoms of ischemic claudication, which is a hallmark clinical sign of a severe compromise of cerebrovascular reserve.

The critical question is whether any study paradigm can predict future events and specifically if they could identify a high-risk group for subsequent stroke. A natural history study demonstrated that a "steal phenomenon" (regional decrease in CBF greater than 5% and a baseline flow below 45 cc/100 g per minute) was highly predictive of patients at increased ischemic rise (12.6 times greater chance of stroke with $p = .0007$).[41] History of stroke or transient ischemic attacks, baseline CBF, or degree of stenosis did not correlate with an increased stroke rate. Webster et al.[42] added 32 additional patients to the series and analyzed the results with or on a reactivity threshold of minus 5%. This study also demonstrated the highly significant ability of a study of flow reserve to identify a high-risk subset, although with less power than the prior report.[41] Although many of the new strokes in the additional group were contralateral to the side with the greatest negative reactivity, it is important to understand that in this study of patients with bilateral occlusive disease, 89% of new strokes were still in territories with negative reactivity.

A seemingly contradictory result was reported by Yokota et al.,[43] who performed CBF studies with a qualitative technology, hexametazime single-photon emission CT and observed no increase of stroke incidence in the group with compromised reserve. An explanation for the negative results of Yokota et al. was supplied by Yonas et al.,[44] who demonstrated that a qualitative assessment was unable to identify the high-risk patients 50% of the time. The subsequent prospective natural history study by Kuroda et al.[45] provided validation of the ability of a quantitative CBF study combined with an acetazolamide challenge to identify a high-risk subgroup. They observed that a "steal phenomenon" did identify an equally high-risk subgroup as reported by Grubb et al.,[46] who used a raised oxygen extraction fraction measurement to identify a high-risk subgroup. A surgical trial randomizing patients based on oxygen extraction fraction is under way in the United States, with a secondary goal being to also obtain enough concurrent cerebrovascular reserve data to be able to use either technology in the future to help identify high-risk patients.

One series of surgical cases in which flow reserve was used to select a group at exceptionally high risk was reported by Przybylski et al.[47] All 12 of their patients had bilateral carotid occlusive disease, recurrent blood pressure–related ischemic symptoms, and a negative reactivity within both hemispheres. Within 27 days, all 12 developed strokes in borderzone regions. After extracranial-intracranial bypass procedures, all 12 stabilized clinically and had improved hemodynamic parameters. This study demonstrated that a group at very high stroke risk can be identified and safely operated on with clinical and physiologic benefit.

Management of Severe Traumatic Brain Injury

Several investigators have described a role for the measurement of CBF in the acute and subacute management of patients post head trauma. From the perspective of triage and prognostication, multiple reports have noted that the lowest flow values after head injury are observed or obtained on entry to the hospital, and that these initial flow values were predictive of outcome.[48–50] These studies have indicated the potential harm of hyperventilation initially post trauma as well as the observation that when the global flow value was below 20 cc/100 g per minute that the most likely outcome was either a vegetative state or death.

ICP measurements have become the standard by which head trauma patients are managed, presuming that it is a useful index of intracranial mass effect and cerebral perfusion. The studies of Marion et al.[16] and Darby et al.[51] have shown that CBF changes, just like the underlying process, are commonly heterogeneous, with one area of the brain being ischemic and another hyperemic. Thus, directing care toward only the ICP can easily result in the aggressive use of hyperventilation therapy, with the result being inducing ischemia in normal regions while shifting even more blood into irreversibly injured, contused brain tissue.[52] Therapy should ideally be focused on the protection of the retained normal tissue, and this type of patient-specific and injury-specific therapy requires the type of tomographic quantitative CBF information provided by XeCT CBF.

Although focal flow and metabolic information is becoming increasingly available, providing access to continuous information, there remains the need to reference the focal data to tomographic information. Only with a global "look" at physiologic changes will the focal data be useful for guiding clinical management. Acting on focal information can obviously be misleading if the probe is within the only ischemic area, and the rest of the brain is normal or hyperemic.

CBF normally falls as $P\text{CO}_2$ is lowered. This response is lost only with a severe and probably irreversible brain injury. The utility of repeat XeCT CBF studies was demonstrated by Marion and Bouma[16] and by Adelson et al.,[50] showing that the variability of CBF reactivity was extreme and unpredictable (1.3–8.5% per mm Hg change in $P\text{CO}_2$). These authors concluded that awareness of the changes of CBF to changes in CO_2 is imperative for proper management of ICP in critically injured patients.

The role of CBF studies in the trauma population is not limited to patients with severe traumatic brain injury. Other uses include assessing the hemodynamic significance of vascular injuries resulting from skull base injuries.[53] The hemodynamic significance of a carotid-cavernous fistula is readily assessed with a XeCT CBF study with or without a challenge study depending on the level of CBF seen with the baseline study.

Management Dilemmas Involving Brain Death

Decisions regarding the withdrawal of life support are often difficult for physicians as well as the patient's family. XeCT CBF studies in this setting provide a graphic demonstration of the damage that has occurred. The diagnosis of brain death is not complicated when the clinical examination, electroencephalogram (EEG), and anatomic injury are consistent with the diagnosis of brain death. When a patient has received sedative medications, the diagnosis can be more complex, and in that setting, the finding of essentially no blood flow is of clinical utility.[54–56]

The value of the ability to accurately measure CBF has been evident when all of the diagnostic studies are not in agreement. The measurement of no flow within the posterior circulation with retained anterior circulation flow helps explain the presence of EEG activity despite an examination consistent with brain death.[55] These findings provided the necessary insight in a woman with a ruptured posterior circulation aneurysm to help guide the family to withdraw ventilatory support due to the bleak prognosis despite the persistent EEG activity.

Planned Vessel Sacrifice

Surgical treatment of large aneurysms and some tumors of the skull base often involves decision making that could require carotid artery sacrifice. Some believe that balloon test occlusion (BTO) coupled with blood flow data and neurologic examinations are insufficient to predict stroke risk, thus necessitating revascularization procedures in all these patients.[57] Others evaluate stroke risk using intraarterial BTO in combination with either a qualitative or quantitative measure of CBF. In one study,[58] 156 patients who passed the initial clinical BTO underwent a XeCT CBF study in combination with a second balloon test. Fourteen patients exhibited reduced flow values between 20 and 30 cc/100 g per minute on the side of test occlusion. Such patients fall into a category of elevated stroke risk for whom bypass surgery before vessel sacrifice is indicated. By using a "qualitative" strategy, the number of candidates for surgical revascularization would have been at least twice as large.[59] The safety of this strategy was provided by Mathis et al.,[60] who reported the results of BTO studies with CBF acquisition in 500 patients. Complications related to this procedure occurred in 3.2% of the patients, and 0.4% of the complications were symptomatic and permanent. Thus, BTO coupled with a quantitative CBF measurement and neurologic examinations is a relatively safe strategy for identifying that relatively small subgroup of patients who would benefit from a bypass despite clinically passing BTO.

Linskey et al.[59] demonstrated a 3% incidence of delayed deficit and a 9% incidence of imaging-defined borderzone-defined deficits; all of the injuries in that series occurred in patients with combined intracranial tumors that underwent carotid sacrifice during skull base procedures.

Vasospasm

Despite angiographic narrowing being present in 50% of patients after subarachnoid hemorrhage, delayed symptoms due to ischemia probably occur in no more than 5–10% of patients. The delayed appearance of a region with flow below 20 cc/100 g per minute has correlated with delayed clinical deterioration and the finding of severe vasospasm on angiography.[61,62] If not rapidly elevated, flow regions with flow values below 15 cc/100 g per minute went on to infarction. Thus, it is apparent that a physiologic study capable of defining patients at ischemic risk deserves to be integrated into the care of aneurysm patients if unnecessary "therapies" are to be minimized, and if necessary ones are to be instituted in a timely manner.

Although transcranial Doppler sonography is widely used for monitoring large vessel vasospasm, correlative CBF studies have demonstrated an unacceptably high false-positive rate. Elevated transcranial Doppler recordings that are supposed to identify a patient at high risk of ischemia, in fact, correspond with hyperemia more often than with ischemia.[63]

XeCT CBF studies have been effectively used to identify patients with delayed ischemic neurologic deficits as well as to assess the efficacy of interventions. Repeat CBF studies either before or after starting hypertensive therapy serve as a useful tool for identifying those patients at increased stroke risk.[64] At our institution, we have used the CBF information to identify patients with a failure of autoregulation who are dependent on hypertensive therapy to be free of a neurologic deficit. Of 14 patients who met flow criteria,[65] all had severe angiographic vasospasm, and, after angioplasty was accomplished in 13 of 14 patients, 12 were clinically improved. CBF levels after treatment were also elevated to nonischemic levels in all regions. In a parallel study of 15 patients[66] who met the same selection criteria, papaverine was the primary treating agent because of the location of the spasm (primarily anterior cerebral). Though all patients selected by clinical and blood flow criteria had severe angiographic narrowing, and vasospasm was at least partially resolved in every patient, significant clinical improvement was demonstrated in only six patients. Post-treatment CBF was assessed in 13 cases and showed improvement in six. Thus, CBF studies were effective in identifying individuals at very high stroke risk due to vasospasm as well as for guiding and evaluating treatment decisions.

SUMMARY

Since the 1980s, XeCT-derived CBF information has demonstrated the capacity to play an integral role in the diagnosis and management of several clinical conditions relevant to a number of clinical specialties. The ability to efficiently obtain quantitative information regarding CBF physiology has proven to be a useful paradigm for guiding therapeutic interventions. Although the absence of flow is a powerful finding for guiding against reperfusion therapy, many technologies can identify this phenomenon. CBF information should also be able to distinguish tissue still at risk and tissue no longer at ischemic risk. Quantitative flow values combined with a physiologic challenge provide a useful paradigm for distinguishing when low flow is due to low supply or low demand. Similarly, measuring the response to a vasodilatory or autoregulatory challenge provides insights into whether the patient is at increased risk of subsequently developing an ischemic injury. As the cost for this technology is modest, and the implementation relatively simple, it is reasonable to expect that XeCT CBF will be able to play an increasing role in patient management, assuming current FDA regulatory problems are overcome.

REFERENCES

1. Haughton V, Schmidt J, Syvertsen A, et al. Detection of demyelinated plaques with xenon-enhanced computed tomography. Neuroradiology 1980;20:181–183.

2. Haughton V, Donegan J, Walsh P, et al. Clinical cerebral blood flow measurement with inhaled xenon and CT. AJR Am J Roentgenol 1980;134:281–283.

3. Winkler S, Spira J. Radiopacity of xenon under hyperbaric conditions. AJR Am J Roentgenol, Radium Ther Nucl Med 2001;96:1035–1040.

4. Winkler S, Sackett J, Holden J, et al. Xenon inhalation as an adjunct to computerized tomography of the brain: preliminary study. Invest Radiol 1977;12:15–18.

5. Drayer BP, Wolfson S, Reinmuth OM, et al. Xenon enhanced CT for analysis of cerebral integrity, perfusion, and blood flow. Stroke 1978;9:123–130.

6. Drayer BP, Friedman A, Osborne D, et al. Anatomic applications of xenon-enhanced CT scanning: visual image analysis and brain-blood partition coefficient studies in man. AJNR Am J Neuroradiol 1983;4:577–582.

7. Gur D, Good WF, Wolfson SKJ, et al. In vivo mapping of local cerebral blood flow by xenon-enhanced computed tomography. Science 1982;215: 1267–1268.

8. Winkler S, Turski P. Potential hazards of xenon inhalation. AJNR Am J Neuroradiol 1985;6: 974–975.

9. Latchaw R, Yonas H, Pentheny S, et al. Adverse reactions to xenon-enhanced CT cerebral blood flow determination. Radiology 1987;163:251–254.

10. Gur D, Yonas H, Jackson DL, et al. Measurements of cerebral blood flow during xenon inhalation as measured by the microspheres method. Stroke 1985;16:871–874.

11. DeWitt DS, Fatouros PP, Wist AO, et al. Stable xenon versus radiolabeled microsphere cerebral blood flow measurements in baboons. Stroke 1989;20:1716–1723.

12. Wolfson SK, Clark J, Greenberg JH, et al. Xenon-enhanced computed tomography compared with [^{14}C] iodoantipyrine for normal and low cerebral blood flow states in baboons. Stroke 1990;21:751–757.

13. Yonas H, Darby JM, Marks EC, et al. CBF measured by Xe-CT: approach to analysis and normal values. J Cereb Blood Flow Metab 1991;11:716–725.

14. Obrist WD, Zhang Z, Yonas H. Effect of xenon-induced flow activation on xenon-enhanced computed tomography cerebral blood flow calculations. J Cereb Blood Flow Metab 1998;18:1192–1195.

15. Harrington TR, Manwaring K, Hodak J. Local Basal Ganglion and Brain Stem Blood Flow in the Head-Injured Patient Using Stable Xenon-Enhanced CT Scanning. Berlin: Springer-Verlag, 1986;680–686.

16. Marion DW, Bouma GJ. The use of stable xenon-enhanced computed tomographic studies of cerebral blood flow to define changes in cerebral carbon dioxide vaso-responsivity caused by a severe head injury. Neurosurgery 1991;29:869–873.

17. Pindzola RR, Yonas H. The xenon-enhanced computed tomography cerebral blood flow method. Neurosurgery 1998;43:1488–1492.

18. Good WF, Gur D. The effect of computed tomography noise and tissue heterogeneity on cerebral blood flow determination by xenon-enhanced computed tomography. Med Phys 1987;14:557–561.

19. Yonas H, Pindzola RR, Johnson DW. Xenon/computed tomography cerebral blood flow and its use in clinical management [review]. Neurosurg Clin N Am 1996;7:605–616.

20. Rubin G, Levy EI, Scarrow AM, et al. Remote effects of acute ischemic stroke: a xenon CT cerebral blood flow study. Cerebrovasc Dis 1000;10:221–228.

21. Firlik AD, Kaufmann AM, Wechsler LR, et al. Quantitative cerebral blood flow determinations in acute ischemic stroke. Relationship to computed tomography and angiography [published erratum appears in Stroke 1998 Apr;29(4):873]. Stroke 1997;28:2208–2213.

22. Johnson DW, Stringer WA, Marks MP, et al. Stable xenon CT cerebral blood flow imaging: rationale for and role in clinical decision making [review]. AJNR Am J Neuroradiol 1991;12:201–213.

23. Jovin T, Goldstein S, Gebel J, et al. Patterns of core and penumbra in acute MCA occlusion and their clinical correlates. Stroke 2001;32(1):51.

24. Brenowitz G, Yonas H. Selective occlusion of blood supply to the anterior perforated substance of the dog: a highly reproducible stroke model. Surg Neurol 1990;33:247–252.

25. Yonas H, Wolfson SKJ, Dujovny M, et al. Selective lenticulostriate occlusion in the primate. A highly focal cerebral ischemia model. Stroke 1981; 12:567–572.

26. Yonas H, Gur D, Claassen D, et al. Stable xenon-enhanced CT measurement of cerebral blood flow in reversible focal ischemia in baboons. J Neurosurg 1990;73:266–273.

27. Sakoh M, Ostergaard L, Rohl L, et al. Relationship between residual cerebral blood flow and oxygen metabolism as predictive of ischemic tissue viability: sequential multitracer positron emission tomography scanning of middle cerebral artery occlusion during the critical first 6 hours after stroke in pigs. J Neurosurg 2000;93:647–657.

28. Kaufmann AM, Firlik AD, Fukui MB, et al. Ischemic core and penumbra in human stroke [see comments]. Stroke 1999;30:93–99.

29. Kalia KK, Yonas H. An aggressive approach to massive middle cerebral artery infarction. Arch Neurol 1993;50:1293–1297.

30. Firlik AD, Yonas H, Kaufmann AM, et al. Relationship between cerebral blood flow and the development of swelling and life threatening herniation in acute ischemic stroke. J Neurosurg 1998;89:243–249.

31. Firlik AD, Rubin G, Yonas H, et al. Relation between cerebral blood flow and neurologic deficit resolution in acute ischemic stroke. Neurology 1998;51: 177–182.

32. Goldstein S, Yonas H, Gebel J, et al. Acute cerebral blood flow as a predictive physiologic marker for symptomatic hemorrhagic conversion and clinical herniation after thrombolytic therapy. Stroke 2000;31:275.

33. Levy EI, Scarrow A, Kanal E, et al. Reversible ischemia determined by xenon-enhanced CT after 90 minutes of complete basilar artery occlusion. AJNR Am J Neuroradiol 1998;19:1943–1946.

34. Kilpatrick M, Goldstein S, Yonas H, et al. Sensitivity and specificity of quantitative cerebral blood flow vs. time from symptom onset as a predictor of cerebral infarction. Stroke 2000;32:348.

35. Rubin G, Firlik AD, Levy EI, et al. Relationship between cerebral blood flow and clinical outcome in acute stroke. Cerebrovasc Dis 2000;10:298–306.

36. Kilpatrick MM, Yonas H, Goldstein S, et al. CT-based assessment of acute stroke: CT, CT angiography, and xenon-enhanced CT cerebral blood flow. Stroke 2001;32:2543–2549.

37. EC/IC Bypass Study Group. Failure of extracranial-intracranial arterial bypass to reduce the risk of ischemic stroke. N Engl J Med 1985;313:1191–1200.

38. Okazawa H, Yamauchi H, Sugimoto K, et al. Effects of acetazolamide on cerebral blood flow, blood volume, and oxygen metabolism: a positron emission tomography study with healthy volunteers. J Cereb Blood Flow Metab 2001;21:1472–1479.

39. Smith HA, Thompson-Dobkin J, Yonas H, et al. Correlation of xenon-enhanced computed tomography-defined cerebral blood flow reactivity and collateral flow patterns. Stroke 1994;25:1784–1787.

40. Firlik AD, Firlik KS, Yonas H. Physiological diagnosis and surgical treatment of recurrent limb shaking: case report. Neurosurgery 1996;39:607–611.

41. Yonas H, Smith HA, Durham SR, et al. Increased stroke risk predicted by compromised cerebral blood flow reactivity. J Neurosurg 1993;79:483–489.

42. Webster MW, Makaroun MS, Steed DL, et al. Compromised cerebral blood flow reactivity is a predictor of stroke in patients with symptomatic carotid artery occlusive disease. J Vasc Surg 1995;21:338–344.

43. Yokota C, Hasegawa Y, Minematsu K, et al. Effect of acetazolamide reactivity on long-term outcome in patients with major cerebral artery occlusive diseases. Stroke 1998;29:640–644.

44. Yonas H, Pindzola RR, Meltzer CC, et al. Qualitative versus quantitative assessment of cerebrovascular reserves. Neurosurgery 1998;42:1005–1012.

45. Kuroda S, Houkin K, Kamiyama H, et al. Long-term prognosis of medically treated patients with internal carotid or middle cerebral artery occlusion: can acetazolamide test predict it? Stroke 2001;32:2110–2116.

46. Grubb RL, Derdeyn CP, Fritsch SM, et al. Importance of hemodynamic factors in the prognosis of symptomatic carotid occlusion. JAMA 1998;280:1055–1060.

47. Przybylski GJ, Yonas H, Smith HA. Reduced stroke risk in patients with compromised cerebral blood flow reactivity treated with superficial temporal artery to distal middle cerebral artery bypass surgery. J Stroke Cerebrovasc Dis 1998;7:302–309.

48. Bouma GJ, Muizelaar JP, Stringer WA, et al. Ultra-early evaluation of regional cerebral blood flow in severely head-injured patients using xenon-enhanced computerized tomography. J Neurosurg 1992;77:360–368.

49. Marion DW, Darby J, Yonas H. Acute regional cerebral blood flow changes caused by severe head injuries. J Neurosurg 1991;74:407–414.

50. Adelson PD, Clyde B, Kochanek PM, et al. Cerebrovascular response in infants and young children following severe traumatic brain injury: a preliminary report. Pediatr Neurosurg 1997;26:200–207.

51. Darby JM, Yonas H, Marion DW, et al. Local "inverse steal" induced by hyperventilation in head injury. Neurosurgery 1988;23:84–88.

52. Resnick DK, Subach B, Marion DW. The significance of carotid canal involvement in basilar cranial fracture. Neurosurgery 1997;40:1177–1181.

53. Wahlig JB, McLaughlin MR, Burke JP, et al. The role of xenon-enhanced computed tomography in the management of a traumatic carotid-cavernous fistula: case report. J Trauma-Inj Infection Crit Care 1999;46:181–185.

54. Darby J, Yonas H, Brenner RP. Brainstem death with persistent EEG activity: evaluation by xenon-enhanced computed tomography. Crit Care Med 1987;15:519–521.

55. Darby JM, Yonas H, Gur D, et al. Xenon-enhanced computed tomography in brain death. Arch Neurol 1987;44:551–554.

56. Pistoia F, Johnson DW, Darby JM, et al. The role of xenon CT measurements of cerebral blood flow in the clinical determination of brain death. AJNR Am J Neuroradiol 1991;12:97–103.

57. Lawton M, Hamilton M, Morcos J, et al. Revascularization and aneurysm surgery: current techniques, indications, and outcome. Neurosurgery 1996;38:83–92.

58. Witt JP, Yonas H, Jungreis C. Cerebral blood flow response pattern during balloon test occlusion of the internal carotid artery. AJNR Am J Neuroradiol 1994;15:847–856.

59. Linskey ME, Jungreis CA, Yonas H, et al. Stroke risk after abrupt internal carotid artery sacrifice: accuracy of preoperative assessment with balloon test occlusion and stable xenon-enhanced CT [see comments]. AJNR Am J Neuroradiol 1994;15:829–843.

60. Mathis JM, Barr JD, Jungreis CA, et al. Temporary balloon test occlusion of the internal carotid artery: experience in 500 cases. AJNR Am J Neuroradiol 1995;16:749–754.

61. Yonas H, Sekhar L, Johnson DW, et al. Determination of irreversible ischemia by xenon-enhanced computed tomographic monitoring of cerebral blood flow in patients with symptomatic vasospasm. Neurosurgery 1989;24:368–372.

62. Fukui MB, Johnson DW, Yonas H, et al. XeCT cerebral blood flow evaluation of delayed symptomatic cerebral ischemia after subarachnoid hemorrhage. AJNR Am J Neuroradiol 1992;13:265–270.

63. Clyde BL, Resnick DK, Yonas H, et al. The relationship of blood velocity as measured by transcranial doppler ultrasonography to cerebral blood flow as determined by stable xenon computed tomographic studies after aneurysmal subarachnoid hemorrhage. Neurosurgery 1996;38:896–904.

64. Darby JM, Yonas H, Marks EC, et al. Acute cerebral blood flow response to dopamine induced hypertension after subarachnoid hemorrhage. J Neurosurg 1994;80:857–864.

65. Firlik AD, Kaufmann AM, Jungreis CA, et al. Effect of transluminal angioplasty on cerebral blood flow in the management of symptomatic vasospasm following aneurysmal subarachnoid hemorrhage. J Neurosurg 1997;86:830–839.

66. Firlik KS, Kaufmann AM, Firlik AD, et al. Intra-arterial papaverine for the treatment of cerebral vasospasm following aneurysmal subarachnoid hemorrhage. Surg Neurol 1999;51:66–74.

CHAPTER

9

Magnetic Resonance Imaging

Heidi C. Roberts, Timothy P. L. Roberts, and Randall T. Higashida

Cerebrovascular diseases encompass disturbances of blood flow in the major blood vessels such as the carotid and intracranial arteries and abnormalities of perfusion of brain tissue. Thus, both blood flow assessment of the feeding vessels and the evaluation of tissue perfusion are of interest in neuroradiologic imaging techniques when used in conjunction with other developing neuroimaging techniques such as diffusion-weighted imaging, which is sensitive to distinct physiologic aspects of tissue viability.[1–5] Magnetic resonance imaging (MRI) can provide a composite picture of the origin, severity, and tissue impact of an ischemic event, the intactness of compensatory mechanisms, and the etiology of the pathophysiologic cascade. A full and physiologically specific characterization of ischemic and neighboring tissue should serve to stratify patients for the various developing treatment regimens, monitor the efficacy of such interventions, and predict risk of unfavorable outcomes associated with therapy.

Imaging options available for the study of cerebrovascular diseases center on invasive catheter angiography, the gold standard for ultimate verification of the site of vascular stenosis or occlusion and an indicator of the extent of collateral blood supply. However, noninvasive imaging methods that focus on the qualitative and quantitative assessment of regional cerebral blood flow (CBF), perfusion, and the consequences of tissue viability are the subject of much development, not only for the reduction in radiation exposure they provide, but also for a more thorough tissue characterization and, thus, selection of appropriate treatment strategies. Beyond lumenography (yielded by x-ray angiography), methods such as MRI offer approaches to assessment of large vessel flow and tissue perfusion as well as indicators of tissue functional integrity at cellular and metabolic levels. Through "perfusion" MRI and its analog, "perfusion" computed tomography (CT), we are also able to study the nature of the blood supply to a tissue, to assess delays of such perfusion in terms of stenotic effects or collateral pathways, and to assess vascular reactivity via hemodynamic challenges. This chapter addresses the use of MRI to study CBF and perfusion, highlighting both qualitative and quantitative methodologic approaches.

An intrinsic feature of MRI that is primarily responsible for the widespread and wide-ranging development of the technology is the potential sensitivity of the magnetic resonance (MR) signal to a variety of factors that may be related to physiologically relevant feature of the physicochemical microenvironment. By appropriate selection of MR pulse sequence and parameter options, sensitivity can be biased in favor of particular tissue features, and this image contrast can be interpreted (by inference) in terms of underlying physiology. Of critical importance to the study of CBF and vascular physiology in ischemic disease is exploitation of the flowing nature of blood. Three distinct approaches derive image contrast from this phenomenon and thus generate images that are sensitized to, and consequently reflect, blood flow:

- Quantitative large vessel flow assessment using the phase-contrast approach[6,7] in which the pixelwise velocity of blood is reflected by the phase part of the complex MR image.

- The dynamic imaging (or tracking) of an intravenously injected "bolus" of exogenous contrast agent (gadolinium-based) via its intravascular retention (in the presence of an intact blood-brain barrier) and the influence of the tracer on local image signal intensity. Subsequent kinetic modeling allows estimation of perfusion-related parameters.[8–11]
- Assessment of tissue perfusion by the magnetic "labeling" or "tagging" of inflowing arterial blood (arterial spin labeling methods). Blood that has been subjected to such tagging contributes a different signal intensity compared to untagged, or stationary, water.[12–14]

LARGE VESSEL FLOW WITH PHASE-CONTRAST VELOCITY ENCODING

Phase-contrast methods are a class of MRI sequences with the incorporation of velocity-encoding gradient pulses—equal and opposite gradient pulses. Stationary water molecules remain unencoded (i.e., acquire no accumulated phase), but moving molecules are imperfectly refocused due to their change of location between encoding and decoding gradient pulses and thus acquire a phase angle proportional to their velocity. Using the complex (i.e., magnitude *and* phase) information inherent to the MR signal (but mostly ignored in favor of the simpler magnitude-only data), it is possible to infer pixel-by-pixel velocity maps.[6,7]

By such instantaneous measuring of velocity at a variety of discrete time points within the cardiac cycle, it is possible to create a velocity-time profile that can be integrated to determine volume flux per cardiac cycle (ml/R-R interval) or *vascular stroke volume*.[7,15] This can then be interpreted quantitatively to assess the impact of vascular stenosis (Figure 9-1), which might only be amenable to morphometric assessment using x-ray or MR angiographic approaches. Furthermore, quantitative assessment of vessel flow before and after interventional treatment (e.g., with balloon angioplasty or intra-arterial stent placement) allows an objective index of the treatment efficacy. Recent developments in integrated MRI and x-ray angiography suites are facilitating the near real-time availability of such efficacy assessment.[16]

Phase-contrast velocity-encoding methods are limited by the assumption that all water molecules within the pixel are moving with a constant (and equal) velocity; consequently, interpretation is degraded by accelerating or turbulent flow or by partial volume effects (particularly at pixels partly overlapping the vessel wall). Partial volume errors are somewhat mitigated in the construction of vascular flow rates rather than velocities, wherein the bulk flow through a pixel is estimated as the product of its area and its velocity. If velocity is underestimated by the inclusion of vessel wall, lumen area will be commensurately overestimated, and the product will be robust. However, the nature of fluid flow is not necessarily uniform across the vessel (plug flow). In areas close to the vessel wall (even neglecting partial volume effects), there will be a gradient of velocities across a pixel, thus contaminating phase-based effective velocity estimates.[17]

Primarily as a result of these factors, velocity-encoded phase-contrast flow quantification is limited to application in larger vessels such as the carotid arteries[7,15] and major segments of the middle cerebral arteries. Nonetheless, it is invaluable in quantitatively documenting the degree of flow reduction associated with stenosis and allows the assessment of the extent of flow restoration after angioplasty or stent placement.[16]

PERFUSION IMAGING WITH DYNAMIC SUSCEPTIBILITY CONTRAST

In addition to flow in large arteries, MRI can assess the adequacy of the blood supply beyond an atherosclerotic artery itself. Indeed, distal tissue perfusion has become the focus of much effort in the noninvasive characterization of acute and chronic ischemic disease.

Certain ions, including gadolinium, are termed *paramagnetic*. That is, in the presence of an external magnetic field (e.g., in an MR scanner), they become magnetized. If the gadolinium ions are compartmentalized (i.e., not uniformly distributed or mixed), this magnetization will lead to a spatial nonuniformity of magnetic field. Such variations in magnetic field homogeneity (magnetic susceptibility effects) lead to attenuated nuclear MR signal and, consequently, regional signal loss on appropriately weighted MR images. The degree of field inhomogeneity can be characterized by an exponential time constant, T2*, which relates to the rate at which nuclear MR signal is lost from such a region over time. A long T2* value implies persistent signal, which must be a consequence of a locally homogeneous external magnetic field. A short T2* is a hallmark of field inhomogeneity, such as that associated with compartmentalized paramagnetic moieties. T2*-sensitive imaging is performed using a simple gradient-recalled echo approach (remember that spin-echo imaging was developed specifically to mitigate the effects of local field inhomogeneity and is thus relatively insensitive to the presence of such magnetic field disruptions), or, in a majority of applications, gradient-recalled echo-planar imaging (which shares the T2* sensitivity of the gradient-recalled echo approach but combines it with ultrafast image acquisition). Using gradient-recalled echo-planar imaging allows multiple two-dimensional slices covering the entire head to be acquired in a dynamic mode with a temporal resolution of 1–3 seconds, each with appropriate T2* sensitivity. In practice, such negative contrast associated with paramagnetic contrast media is exploited as follows (Table 9-1)[11]:

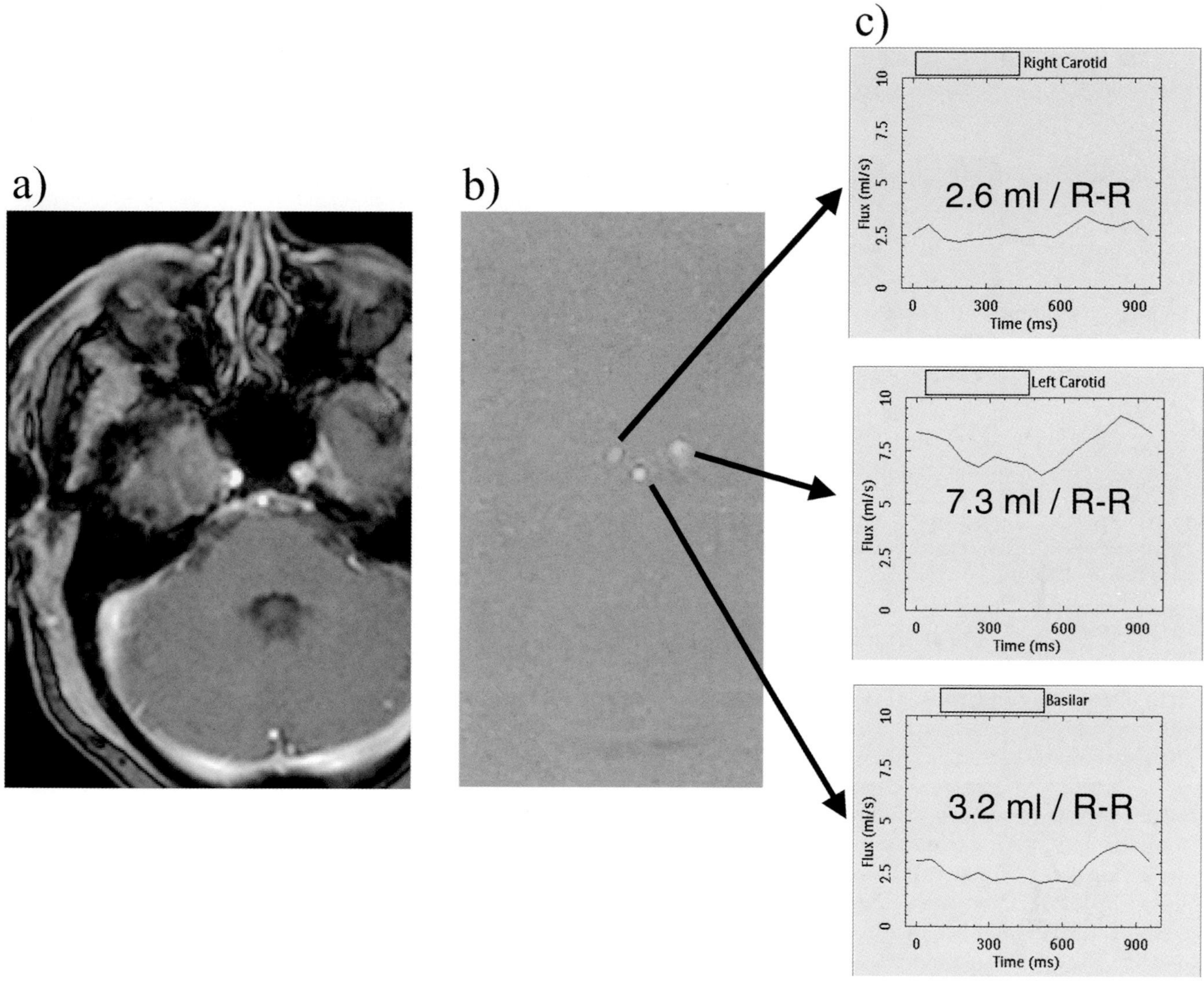

FIGURE 9-1. Two-dimensional Q-flow of carotid artery stenosis. Magnitude (**A**) and phase (**B**) magnetic resonance images at an axial level through the carotid and basilar arteries using a velocity-encoded phase-contrast sequence in a patient with stenosis of the right carotid artery. Velocity profiles through each of the vessels can be integrated over a single cardiac cycle to yield vessel stroke volumes for each vessel, reflecting the volume flux of blood through the vessel per cardiac cycle. **C.** Right carotid (*top*), left carotid (*middle*), basilar artery (*bottom*). Flow in the stenotic carotid is markedly reduced (2.6 ml/R-R cycle) compared to the contralateral vessel (7.3 ml/R-R cycle).

Dynamic T2*-weighted imaging is performed repeatedly on a multislice set at temporal resolutions of 1–3 seconds over a period of approximately 2 minutes. As such, approximately 60 multislice volumes are typically acquired. After the acquisition of a few baseline or precontrast scans, an intravenous bolus administration of gadolinium-diethylenetriaminepentaacetic acid (GdDTPA) is commenced. The site of injection varies but is typically the antecubital vein. Standard clinically approved GdDTPA may be used at a routine dose (0.1 mmol gadolinium per kg body weight). For added sensitivity, a double dose may be selected (0.2 mmol/kg body weight). To maintain a tight bolus profile, injection rates are generally fast (2–5 ml per second) and are commonly performed using a power injector. At 5 ml per second, a 15-ml injection volume (standard dose for a 75-kg man) represents a 3-second bolus duration. Although the bolus becomes somewhat dispersed as it mixes in the intravascular space, it is an assumption that it maintains its bolus characteristic during first pass through the brain. Furthermore, because the intact blood-brain barrier retains such contrast media in the intravascular space, signal loss associated with the transit of the contrast media bolus through the brain is a regional marker of perfusion; conversely, absence of such signal loss is evidence of hypoperfusion—"where blood is not flowing, gad is not going" (Figure 9-2). Additional sensitivity is obtained using negative contrast associated with such

TABLE 9-1. Typical Data Acquisition Parameters of a Magnetic Resonance Bolus Tracking Experiment*

		Comments
Sequence	Gradient-recalled echo-planar imaging	If not an echo-planar imaging facility, a single-slice fast-gradient echo sequence (e.g., SPGR/FLASH, TR = 35 ms, TE = 25 ms, flip = 30 degrees) has been used.
TE	Long (50–70 ms)	To allow imaging of contrast agent–related susceptibility (negative-enhancing) effects.
Number of slices	6–7 (or more if scanner permits without compromising temporal resolution)	Usually focused supratentorially; infratentorial impairment of image quality due to susceptibility artifacts from bone.
Temporal resolution	1–3 secs	—
Number of phases (time points)	Approximately 40 with 2 secs/multislice image set (imaging time of 80 secs)	To ensure coverage of the entire contrast agent transit.
Contrast agent	0.1–0.2 mmol/kg body weight	Gradient-recalled echo-planar imaging sequence is sensitive to contrast agent, so double dose is rarely required.
Injection rate	4–5 ml/sec	To approximate ideal bolus.

FLASH = fast low-angle shot; SPGR = spoiled gradient-recalled acquisition in the steady state; TE = echo time; TR = repetition time.
*Many variations exist, with different sensitivities, advantages, and disadvantages. This table represents a commonly used implementation and a basis for clinical adoption.

agents by exploiting the spatial extent of the magnetic field disruptions and, thus, also generating signal loss in the surrounding parenchymal tissue as well as in the microvasculature itself.

It is the kinetics of such signal loss that offer the most promise for clinical studies of the cerebrovasculature. A variety of information can be derived from observing the regional variations in the time course of signal loss associated with contrast agent bolus transit (Figure 9-3). A number of physiologic models can be used to allow inferences into tissue perfusion from such dynamic data.[18] However, a first step in all of these is to establish the concentration-time curve of the tracer (contrast agent) itself. Although the signal loss associated with the passage of the contrast media bolus does indeed relate to contrast agent concentration, this relationship is not linear. As stated previously, the signal loss arises from heterogeneity in magnetic field associated with compartmentalization of the contrast agent. This compartmentalization is occurring within the capillary bed; thus, the degree of signal loss is somewhat dependent on the microvascular architecture. Furthermore, the signal loss associated with magnetic susceptibility field variations is additionally mediated by water molecule diffusion through these field disturbances, which relates to water mobility in tissue and hindrances in the form of cell membranes and vascular walls. Finally, the total signal loss within a region or voxel is also a composite mix of T2-type signal loss within the intravascular spaces as well as the previously described T2*-type signal loss in areas of heterogeneous field. Despite these limitations, the definition of a single effective transverse relaxation time constant, T2*, and its associated relaxation rate, R2* (= 1/T2*), allows an assumption to be made that change in effective transverse relaxation rate is approximately proportional to tracer concentration.[8] The change in relaxation rate (ΔR2*) can be obtained simply by constructing the ratio of instantaneous to precontrast signal intensity, taking its natural logarithm, reversing its sign, and dividing by the echo time in milliseconds (see Figure 9-2).

Regional analysis of the time-series dynamic images acquired during bolus contrast administration followed by such mathematic manipulation allows the construction of concentration-time curves for every pixel in the image. Such curves typically are characterized by a period of little change (before bolus arrival), followed by a period of very rapid increase in tracer concentration (as the bolus enters the microvasculature of the tissue being imaged), followed by a slower decay (as the tracer washes out). Recirculation of the tracer generally prevents the concentration-time curve from fully recovering to baseline. (Note: If the integrity of the blood-brain barrier is compromised such that the contrast agent extravasates into the extravascular space during its passage, the concentration-time curve will appear to decay much more slowly and will tend not to recover toward baseline in a typical imaging period.) Some characteristic features of these concentration-time curves can be identified and form the basis of the most straightforward (and widespread) analysis strategies (Figure 9-4)[10]:

1. Every curve has a peak. This peak can be readily identified and measured. Its amplitude reflects the peak local concentration of tracer and is thus highly dependent on vascular volume within the pixel and lack

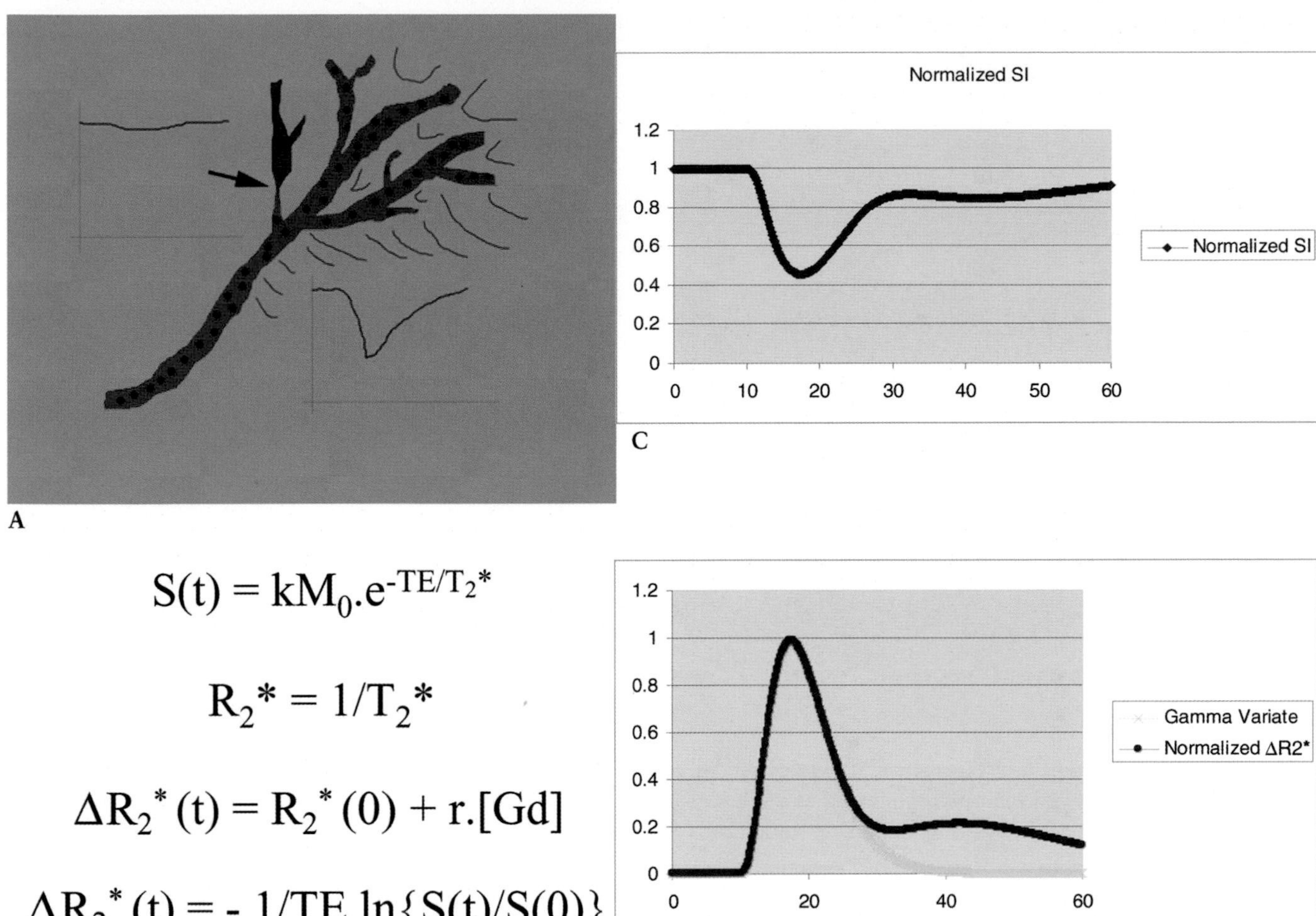

FIGURE 9-2. Dynamic susceptibility contrast. **A.** Schematically, contrast agents (*black dots*) remain intravascular and disturb the local field homogeneity during their passage, leading to transient signal loss. Distal to a vessel occlusion (*arrow*), no contrast agent arrives, so there is no commensurate signal loss. **B.** Equations to relate signal intensity on dynamic susceptibility-weighted magnetic resonance imaging to changes in transverse relaxation rate (ΔR_2^*), which is generally taken to be proportional to instantaneous contrast agent concentration. **C.** Schematic signal intensity (SI)–versus-time curve during contrast passage. **D.** Corresponding $\Delta R2^*$-versus-time (*brown line*) derived from the equations (**B**). To correct for recirculation of contrast agent, a curve fit (gamma variate) is often applied (*blue line*).

of bolus dispersion by the time of arrival in the pixel. Consequently, unambiguous physiologic interpretation of peak maps remains complex, but a pronounced signal change can be considered to reflect a relatively large vascular fractional volume and a relatively intact bolus profile. Because bolus dispersion occurs over time, an intact bolus profile might be considered indicative of relatively direct, likely antegrade flow.

2. The peak occurs at a certain time after injection, or at a certain time after the first elevation of tracer levels above baseline. The time of arrival of the bolus peak (either relative to time of injection or time of onset of arrival) is indicative of the wash-in component of bolus transit. Consequently, it is highly sensitive to obstructions or path deviations, which might cause a delay in the delivery of the contrast agent bolus to the tissue. Areas of delayed perfusion are sensitively depicted on time-of-arrival maps and may be considered to represent tissue at risk. The question of how much delay constitutes serious risk remains unresolved, as it is certainly influenced by other parameters of cerebral perfusion.

3. The curve has a width. Given the definition of a baseline and a peak, any curve allows definition of a width relating wash-in to wash-out phases of bolus transit. Commonly practiced is the estimation of full width at half maximum (FWHM), which may be constructed by measuring the time taken to achieve 50% of the peak contrast tracer concentration during wash-in to the time taken for contrast agent levels to decrease to

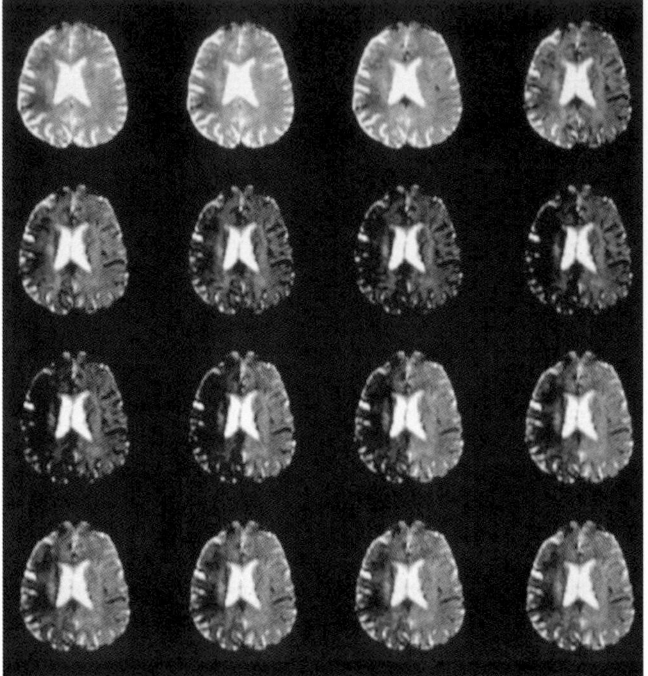

A

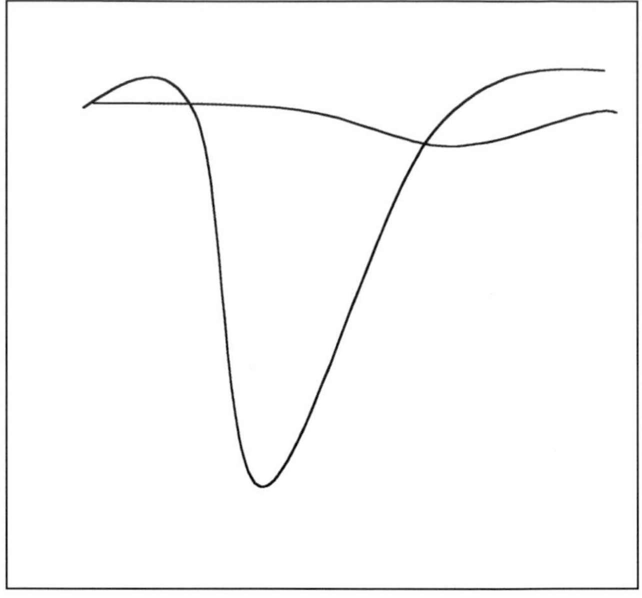

B

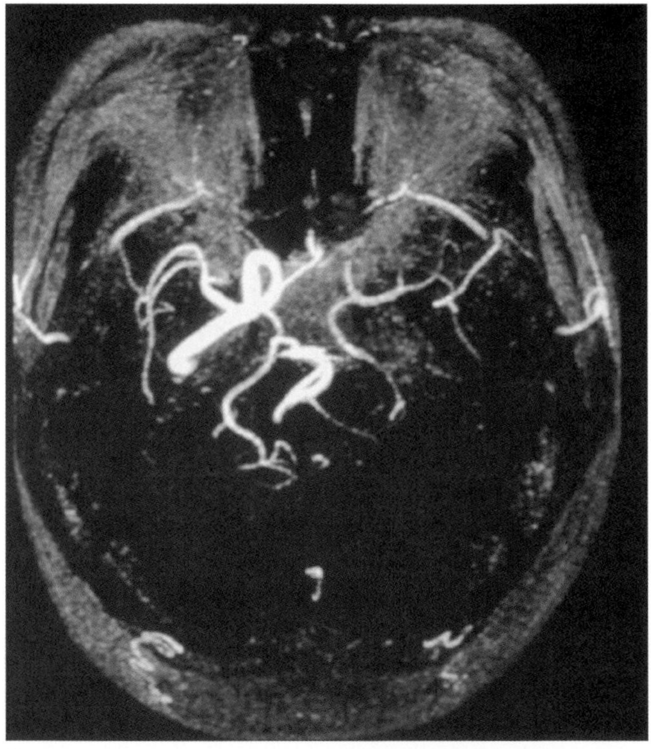

C

FIGURE 9-3. **A.** Sixteen of a series of dynamic susceptibility-weighted (gradient-recalled echo-planar) images at a single level (from a multislice acquisition) in a patient with left carotid artery occlusion. Contrast agent–induced signal loss is severely limited ipsilateral to the occlusion. **B.** Schematic signal intensity curves from left and right hemispheres. **C.** Magnetic resonance angiogram confirms major vessel occlusion on left side.

50% of their peak value (on their wash-out progression toward baseline). In practice, the width of the contrast bolus peak depends not only on the tissue-related dispersion of the contrast bolus (indicative of the microcirculation), but also on the inherent duration and profile of the contrast agent bolus itself. It is worth keeping in mind that a typical single dose of 14 cc of contrast media (to a 70-kg patient) requires a 7-second injection at a rate of 2 ml per second. Thus, an inherent width of 7 seconds should be expected, even without the additional injection site–to–feeding artery bolus dispersion in the vascular system. This prompts measurement of the arterial form of the bolus before its arrival in tissue. The FWHM of a contrast agent bolus, however, can be seen to reflect, in part, the nature of the transit of the bolus through the tissue, so it is commonly approxi-

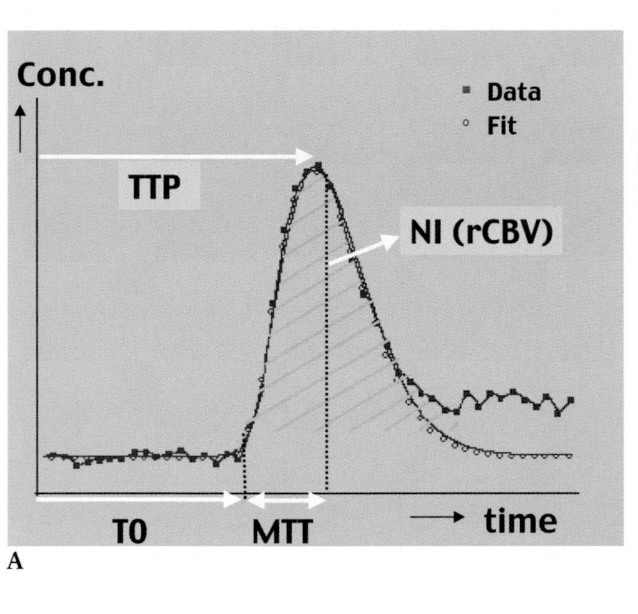

A

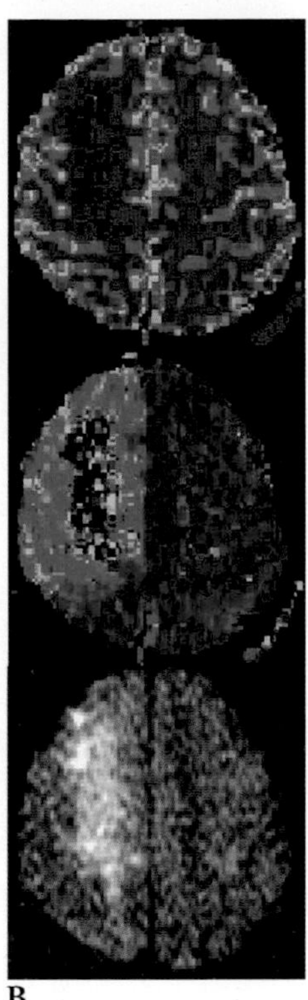
B

FIGURE 9-4. **A.** Transverse relaxation rate–versus-time curve can yield perfusion parameters, time of first arrival of contrast (T0), time to peak (TTP), mean transit time (MTT; first moment of contrast agent–versus-time curve—often approximated by width of transit curve, but see text for limits to this approximation), and negative integral (NI; area under the curve, proportional to cerebral blood volume). Again, a gamma-variate fit (*smooth line*) corrects for recirculation effects. **B.** Pixel-by-pixel map of relative cerebral blood volume (rCBV) clearly depicting an infarct as area of hypoperfusion (absent) in right deep white matter (*top*). Corresponding TTP map indicating infarct surrounded by a large area (*green*) of delayed perfusion (*middle*). It may be speculated that this represents tissue at risk. Corresponding diffusion-weighted image shows hyperintensity corresponding to the severely hypoperfused zone but not (yet) the peripheral area of delayed perfusion (*bottom*). (Conc. = concentration.)

mately related to the physiologically relevant descriptor, the mean transit time of the tissue.

4. The curve has an area. Again, given definition of a baseline and a peak, any curve must have an "integral" or "area under it." Because any change in signal intensity is related to the instantaneous tracer concentration, the integrated signal changes or area under the tracer concentration–time curve can be interpreted as relating to the total amount of tracer that passes through the voxel over time. As such, it is interpreted as proportional to the cerebral blood volume of the voxel. The proportionality constant, however, cannot be obtained without measurement of a vascular reference, and so it is commonplace to consider maps of the area under the curve as indicative of relative cerebral blood volume (rCBV). Furthermore, because recirculation of the contrast agent after the first pass typically prevents complete return of signal intensity to baseline, precontrast levels, and integration thereof, would thus lead to overestimation of the first-pass bolus area, essentially counting the contrast agent more than once. Thus, truncation or curve fitting of the data (often using the gamma-variate function) is usually performed (see Figure 9-4).

Interpretation of these perfusion parameters in the context of underlying pathology forms the basis of the clinical use of cerebrovascular perfusion imaging. However, to extend these perfusion parameters toward more absolute, quantitative, and reproducible use makes some assumptions, primarily about the nature (duration) of the bolus. Furthermore, to generate absolute cerebral blood volume maps from relative cerebral blood volume maps or to determine tissue transit time appropriately[19] requires knowledge of the arterial input function (i.e., the concentration-time curve of tracer in the feeding vessel). This poses both the methodologic question of how to measure concentration of the tracer in the feeding vessel and the philosophical questions of which is the best reference vessel to use in ischemia and whether the same reference vessel should be used in the analysis of all tissue regions. Complete answers to both types of questions remain under investigation (Figure 9-5).

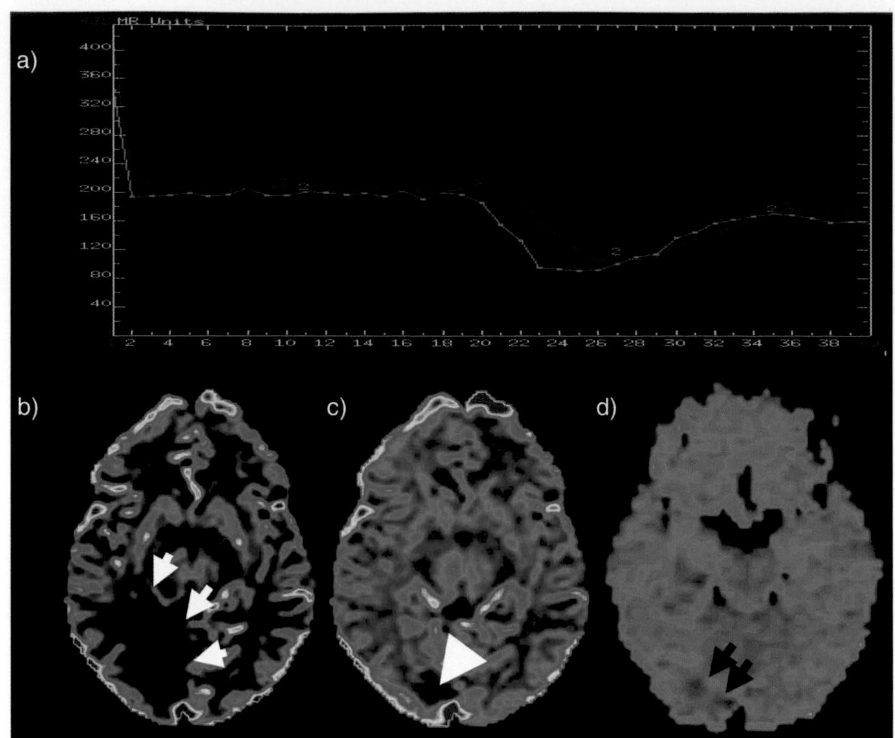

FIGURE 9-5. For the process of deconvolution, knowledge of the arterial input function is critical. **A.** In this example of a patient with a posterior cerebral artery insult, arterial input functions in the posterior cerebellar artery itself (*pink*) and in the more readily visualized ipsilateral middle cerebral artery (*green*) were drawn. **B–D.** Cerebral blood flow (CBF) maps derived from deconvolution using the two putative arterial input functions reveal markedly different results. **B.** Using the middle cerebral artery as an arterial input function suggests an extensive region of low CBF (*white arrows*). **C.** Using the posterior cerebral artery curve suggests only a focal posterior region of low CBF (*white arrowhead*). **D.** Corresponding apparent diffusion coefficient map (*lower right*) suggests only a small focal area (*black arrows*) of injury (at this time point), in agreement with the CBF map derived using the posterior cerebral artery as an arterial reference. (Images courtesy of Prof. J. Provenzale, Duke University Medical Center, Durham, North Carolina.)

The leading approach in the pursuit of more quantitative physiologic modeling of bolus contrast media transit through cerebral tissues is described as *arterial deconvolution*.[20,21] By simultaneously measuring signal intensity in a major artery (such as the internal carotid artery or the middle cerebral artery), an estimate of contrast agent concentration in the feeding vessels can similarly be obtained. In practice, arterial imaging may be practically limited by confounding effects of rapid and pulsatile flow. Furthermore, the relationship between signal change and tracer concentration may be somewhat different in pixels entirely contained within a vascular structure (in which field homogeneity is, in fact, locally good, the field strength simply being shifted relative to the bulk surrounding tissue). In such structures, signal loss is primarily associated with contrast agent–mediated T2-type dephasing, rather than with field heterogeneity or T2*-type signal loss. This introduces a different proportionality constant in the relationship between tracer concentration and effective change in relaxation rate derived from dynamic T2*-sensitive MRI. Assuming, however, that the concentration-time curve in a feeding artery can, in fact, be estimated, the tracer kinetic model of Zierler[22] can be applied (formally known as *the model of a nondiffusible tracer*). The impact of the tissue transit on the entering bolus can be described mathematically by the operation of convolution of a tissue residue function on the arterial input function. What is observed by dynamic imaging is this convolved product. Given knowledge of the arterial input function [a(t)], the mathematic operation of deconvolution permits extraction of the tissue residue function [h(t)] from the tissue concentration–time curve [T(t)] (Figure 9-6). The tissue residue function can then be used to extract the mean transit time from the first moment of h(t). Absolute CBF is then obtained by applying the central volume theorem: CBF = CBV/mean transit time, in which absolute CBV is obtained by computing the ratio of rCBV in tissue (described previously) to the similarly derived rCBV (area under the curve) in the (100% blood) arterial input. As such, arterial deconvolution offers the promise of more quantitative estimation of cerebral perfusion parameters: absolute CBV, quantitative CBF, and bolus-independent timing parameters, suggesting widespread application and comparability across patients.[23] As discussed above, choice of the appropriate arterial input

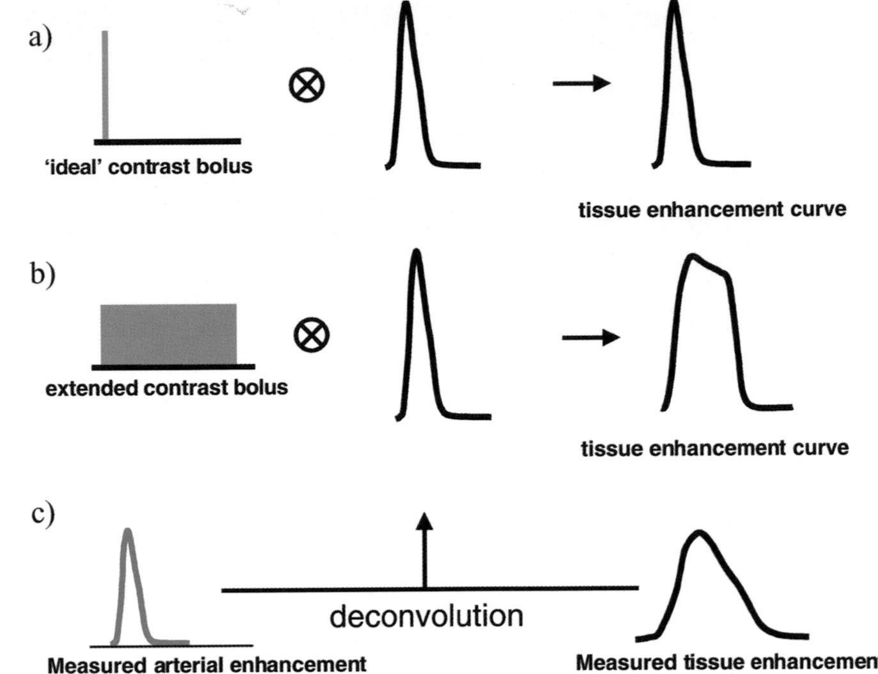

FIGURE 9-6. Convolution. **A.** An ideal "spike" or delta function arterial input is convolved with the intrinsic tissue residue function (*center*) to yield the tissue enhancement curve (*right*). In practice, this is not realizable. **B.** An extended rectangular bolus would be similarly convolved to yield a broader tissue enhancement curve. **C.** In reality, knowledge of the geometry of the arterial input (*left*) and measurement of the tissue enhancement curve (*right*) allows deconvolution of the desired tissue residue function (*center*) from which transit time can be derived.

remains contentious, and the nonlinearity between MR-derived estimates of relaxation rate and local tracer concentration remains a theoretic concern, the magnitude of which is yet to be fully established.

It is interesting that, in the context of the above limitations, bolus-tracking perfusion imaging can be performed with dynamic CT. Indeed, primarily because of imminent availability and easier accessibility of the patient, CT has emerged as the imaging technique of choice for suspected acute ischemic stroke in many institutions. Just as in MR perfusion, the transit of a tracer, which in this case is the iodinated contrast agent, is observed using dynamic imaging and described with similar perfusion parameter maps (Figure 9-7).[24] Indeed, because the density change observed with CT relates to the concentration of tracer itself (and not via an indirect reporting mechanism as in MRI), many of the above linearity concerns are mitigated. Arterial input deconvolution methods can be straightforwardly applied (arterial signal estimation is not confounded by flow effects in CT), and quantitative parameters of perfusion can be extracted with high spatial resolution (without anatomic/geometric distortion effects associated with echo-planar imaging in MRI, especially near the brain stem).[25,26] These advantages are offset by the larger volume of contrast media needed for CT imaging (typically at least 40 cc), leading to a longer bolus duration, although this can be mathematically accounted for in the deconvolution analysis. Dynamic CT is also limited in anatomic coverage. Despite the advent of multidetector arrays and faster gantry revolution times, typical anatomic coverage is limited to a few centimeters of extent if high temporal resolution is required (using a multidetector array, these few centimeters may be split into several contiguous thinner slices or sections). The *toggling table* approach[24] compromises temporal resolution for the opportunity of imaging at multiple distinct anatomic levels by the rapid toggling of the table between two or more positions, allowing interleaved imaging. More generally, disadvantages of CT include the necessity of ionizing radiation (of particular impact in the pediatric population) and the possible adverse reactions associated with iodinated contrast media. Finally, in comparison to MRI, perfusion CT is limited by the lack of availability of other types of physiologic imaging (primarily the sensitivity to cytotoxic edema, with diffusion-weighted imaging or the metabolic information available from MR spectroscopy).

ARTERIAL SPIN LABELING

An entirely different MRI strategy for the measurement of CBF, without the use of exogenous tracers, has also been proposed. Using the principle of magnetic tagging, it is possible to label arterial blood proximal to a tissue of interest.[12,13] If the selected artery ultimately feeds the imaged tissue, the effects of such tagging are manifest as signal variations in the tissue image (when compared to a similar image acquired in the absence of arterial tagging) (Figure 9-8). Such approaches are known collectively as *arterial spin labeling* and exist in several different forms, reflecting primarily whether the arterial blood is magnetically tagged before its perfusion into a tissue or whether the tissue itself is tagged; thus untagged blood subsequently perfuses into it.[12–14,27–29] An extensive review of

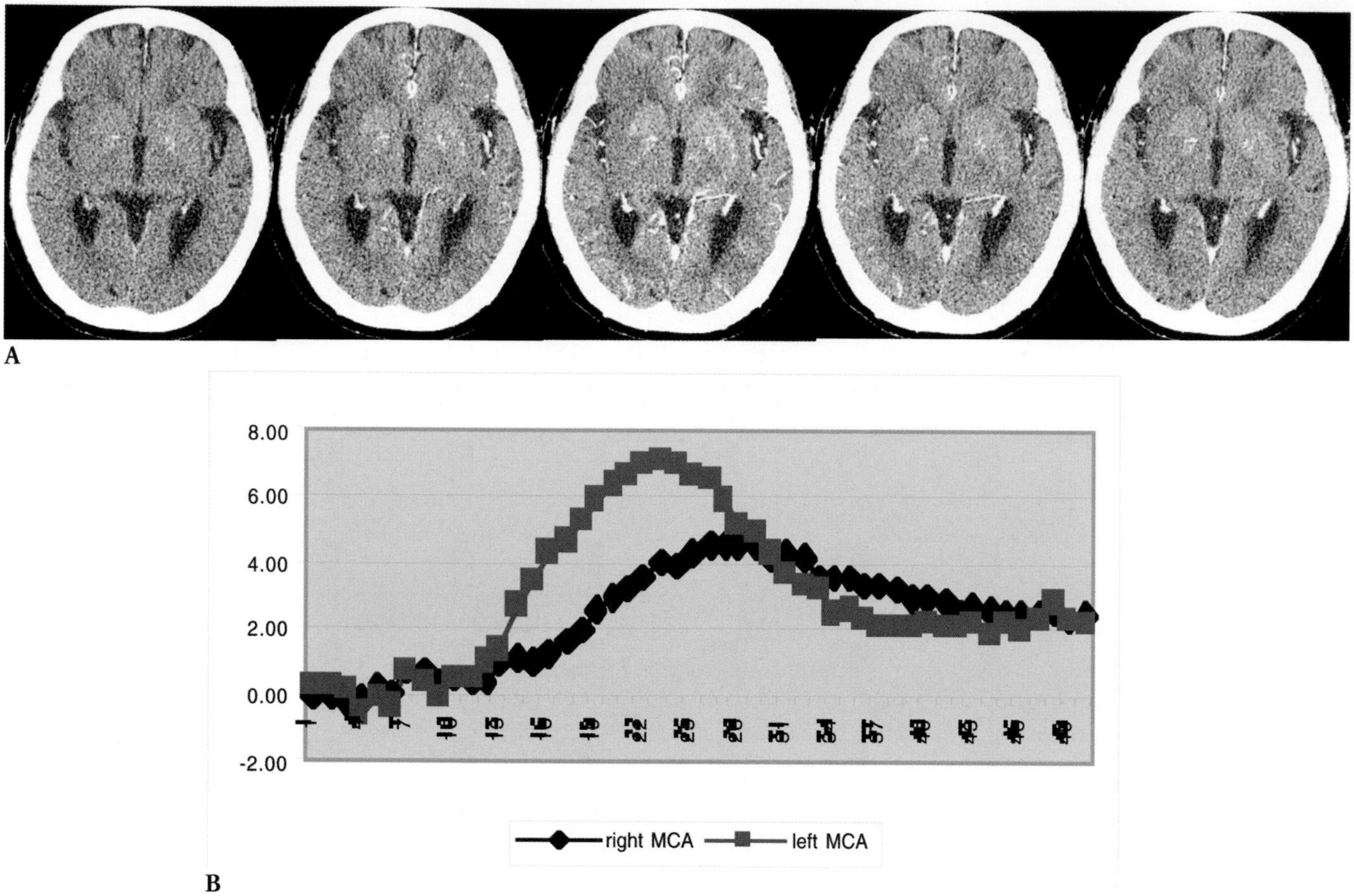

FIGURE 9-7. **A.** Dynamic computed tomography images during contrast agent injection. Image density variations over time correspond more directly to contrast concentration (there is no need to perform the algebraic manipulations and concentration approximations used in magnetic resonance imaging). **B.** Whereas the left middle cerebral artery (MCA) territory demonstrates sharp contrast agent–induced enhancement (*pink*), the ischemic right MCA territory shows delayed and attenuated contrast agent effects (*blue*).

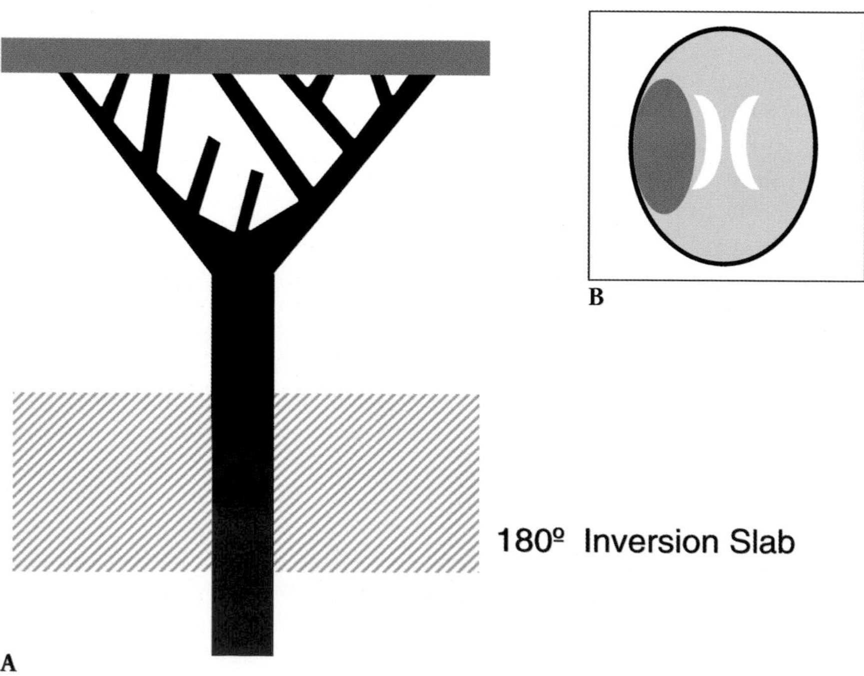

FIGURE 9-8. Schematic of arterial spin labeling. **A.** Upstream blood has its magnetization inverted via a slab selective 180 degrees inversion radiofrequency pulse in this example. Subsequently, inverted or tagged blood flows and perfuses into the imaging plane (*gray*). Correspondingly, the perfused zone can be identified on the resulting image (**B**). Generally two images are acquired (with and without tagging); subtraction reveals the perfused zone and can lead to quantitation of perfusion in physiologic units.

the idiosyncrasies and technical considerations of arterial spin labeling methods is beyond the scope of this chapter; indeed, these methods are the subject of considerable evolution and development. Nonetheless, arterial spin labeling methodologies have a number of intrinsic features that set them apart from bolus tracking with exogenous contrast agents. By using magnetic manipulation rather than exogenous contrast injection, it is possible to perform repeated arterial spin labeling experiments within a short period, either for the improvement of signal to noise ratio or for the monitoring of dynamic changes in blood flow and perfusion. Because it is water that is being tagged to form our tracer, we can use the kinetic models of freely diffusible tracers, which allow quantitative estimation of CBF (Figure 9-9).[12,30] Because the image signal to noise ratio and blood flow estimation precision is limited by the rapid fading of the tags or longitudinal relaxation of the labeled water molecules, it is likely that higher magnetic field strengths (e.g., 3T and above) will be fertile ground for the further investigation of arterial spin labeling methods (because the longitudinal relaxation time constant, T1, of blood increases with increasing field strength, leading to improved tag persistence).

Although it was a goal (perhaps the "holy grail") of the development of noninvasive cerebral perfusion methodologies to achieve a pixelwise mapping of CBF in quantitative and physiologically relevant terms (ml/100 g per minute), it has become increasingly appreciated that other facets of cerebral perfusion, such as the time of arrival or peak,[31] might play a role in the diagnostic and prognostic use of cerebral perfusion methods in study of cerebrovascular disease. Consequently, a combination of perfusion-related parameters might, in fact, offer a more complete and prognostically useful description of the state of cerebral perfusion, the integrity of the microvasculature, and the viability of the tissue it serves. Indeed, extending this concept to repeated assessment of cerebral perfusion parameters after hemodynamic challenges, such as administration of acetazolamide (Diamox)[32] or changes in partial pressure of blood gases O_2 and CO_2,[33–35] seems likely to allow increased insight into the functional integrity of the vascular system as an index of autoregulatory capacity.

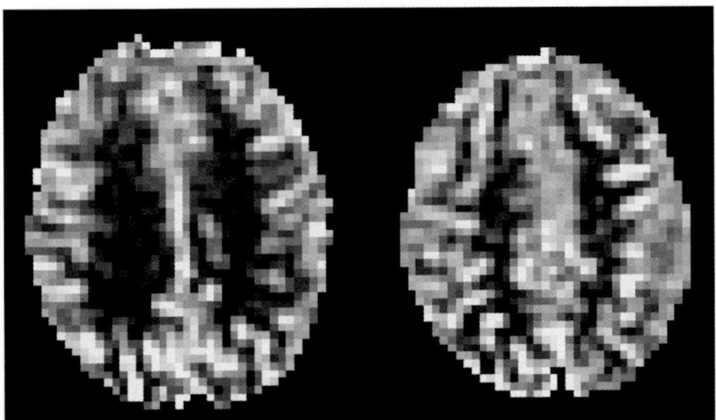

FIGURE 9-9. Example of pixel-by-pixel cerebral blood flow maps from a healthy volunteer derived using arterial spin labeling and clearly identifying gray and white matter perfusion differences. (Images courtesy of Mr. J. Poublanc, Dr. A. Crawley, and Prof. D. Mikulis, University of Toronto, Canada.)

Thus, ongoing and future developments of cerebral perfusion imaging methodologies will target the robust and quantitative estimation of CBF itself, the evaluation of the role of parameters beyond flow (including, but not limited to, timing parameters), and the sensitivity of these parameters to tissue responses to hemodynamic challenges. Future applications include further stratification of tissue at risk defined by abnormality on one or more cerebral perfusion parameter maps and the quantitative estimation of the collateral versus antegrade contributions to tissue perfusion, because these factors are of significant consideration in the selection of patient management strategies and interventional therapies. As these issues become addressed, use of cerebral perfusion methods is becoming increasingly widespread and of increasing diagnostic and prognostic value in the study of cerebrovascular disease. Whereas the initial target appears to be in the observation and delineation of hypoperfusion in acute cerebral ischemia, further application to vasculitis, chronic occlusive vascular disease, vasospasm, and a host of other vascular compromises is promising.

REFERENCES

1. Moseley ME, Kucharczyk J, Mintorovitch J, et al. Diffusion-weighted MR imaging of acute stroke: correlation with T2-weighted and magnetic susceptibility-enhanced MR imaging in cats. AJNR Am J Neuroradiol 1990;11:423–429.
2. Wendland MF, White DL, Aicher KP, et al. Detection with echo-planar MR imaging of transit of susceptibility contrast medium in a rat model of regional brain ischemia. J Magn Reson Imaging 1991; 1:285–292.
3. Kucharczyk J, Mintorovitch J, Asgari HS, Moseley M. Diffusion/perfusion MR imaging of acute cerebral ischemia. Magn Reson Med 1991:19:311–315.
4. Warach S, Chien D, Li W, et al. Fast magnetic resonance diffusion-weighted imaging of acute human stroke. Neurology 1992;42(9):1717–1723.
5. Sorensen AG, Buonanno FS, Gonzalez RG, et al. Hyperacute stroke: evaluation with combined multisection diffusion-weighted and hemodynamically weighted echo-planar MR imaging. Radiology 1996; 199(2):391–401.
6. Underwood SR, Firmin DN, Rees RS, Longmore DB. Magnetic resonance velocity mapping. Clin Phys Physiol Meas 1990;11[suppl A]:37–43.
7. Furst G, Sitzer M, Hofer M, et al. Quantifica-

tion of carotid blood flow velocity using MR phase mapping. J Comput Assist Tomogr 1994;18(5):688–696.

8. Villringer A, Rosen BR, Belliveau JW, et al. Dynamic imaging with lanthanide chelates in normal brain: contrast due to magnetic-susceptibility effects. Magn Reson Med 1988;6:164–174.

9. Rosen BR, Belliveau JW, Vevea JM, Brady TJ. Perfusion imaging with NMR contrast agents. Magn Reson Med 1990;14(2):249–265.

10. Kucharczyk J, Roberts T, Moseley ME, Watson A. Contrast-enhanced perfusion-sensitive MR imaging in the diagnosis of cerebrovascular disorders. J Magn Reson Imaging 1993(1):241–245.

11. Kucharczyk J, Vexler ZS, Roberts TP, et al. Echo-planar perfusion-sensitive MR imaging of acute cerebral ischemia. Radiology 1993;188(3):711–717.

12. Detre JA, Leigh JS, Williams DS, Koretsky AP. Perfusion imaging. Magn Reson Med 1992;23(1):37–45.

13. Edelman RR, Siewert B, Darby DG, et al. Qualitative mapping of cerebral blood-flow and functional localization with echo-planar MR imaging and signal targeting with alternating radio-frequency. Radiology 1994;192:513–520.

14. Kwong KK, Chesler DA, Weisskoff RM, et al. MR perfusion studies with T1-weighted echo planar imaging. Magn Reson Med 1995;34(6):878–887.

15. Bendel P, Buonocore E, Bockisch A, Besozzi MC. Blood flow in the carotid arteries: quantification by using phase-sensitive MR imaging. AJR Am J Roentgenol 1989;152(6):1307–1310.

16. Roberts TPL, Roberts HC, Martin AJ, et al. Using a combined MRI/X-ray angiography suite for the quantitative online evaluation of carotid stent placement. Proc Am Soc Neuroradiol 2002:167.

17. Wolf RL, Ehman RL, Riederer SJ, Rossman PJ. Analysis of systematic and random error in MR volumetric flow measurements. Magn Reson Med 1993;30(1):82–91.

18. Perkiö J, Aronen HJ, Kangasmäki A, et al. Evaluation of four post-processing methods for determination of cerebral blood volume and mean transit time by dynamic susceptibility contrast imaging. Magn Reson Med 2002;47:973–981.

19. Weisskoff RM, Chesler D, Boxerman JL, Rosen BR. Pitfalls in MR measurement of tissue blood flow with intravascular tracers: which mean transit-time? Magn Reson Med 1993;29:553–559.

20. Lythgoe MF, Thomas DL, Calamante F. Acute changes in MRI diffusion, perfusion, T1 and T2 in a rat model of oligemia produced by partial occlusion of the middle cerebral artery. Magn Reson Med 2000;44:706–712.

21. Østergaard L, Weisskoff RM, Chesler DA, et al. High resolution measurement of cerebral blood flow using intravascular tracer bolus passages. Part I. Mathematical approach and statistical analysis. Magn Reson Med 1996;36:715–725.

22. Zierler KL. Equations for measuring blood flow by external monitoring of radioisotopes. Circ Res 1965;16:309–321.

23. Sorensen AG, Copen WA, Ostergaard L, et al. Hyperacute stroke: simultaneous measurement of relative cerebral blood volume, relative cerebral blood flow, and mean tissue transit time. Radiology 1999;210(2):519–527.

24. Roberts HC, Roberts TPL, Smith WS, et al. Multisection dynamic CT perfusion for acute cerebral ischemia: the "toggling-table" technique. AJNR Am J Neuroradiol 2001;22:1077–1080.

25. Eastwood JD, Lev MH, Azhari T, et al. CT perfusion scanning with deconvolution analysis: pilot study in patients with acute middle cerebral artery stroke. Radiology 2002;222(1):227–236.

26. Cenic A, Nabavi DG, Craen RA, et al. Dynamic CT measurement of cerebral blood flow: a validation study. AJNR Am J Neuroradiol 1999;20:63–73.

27. Edelman RR, Chen Q. EPISTAR MRI: multislice mapping of cerebral blood flow. Magn Reson Med 1998:40:800–805.

28. Kim SG. Quantification of relative cerebral blood flow change by flow-sensitive alternating inversion recovery (FAIR) technique: application to functional mapping. Magn Reson Med 1995;34:293–301.

29. Dixon WT, Du LN, Faul DD, et al. Projection angiograms of blood labeled by adiabatic fast passage. Magn Reson Med 1986;3:454–462.

30. Calamante F, Williams SR, van Bruggen N, et al. A model for quantification of perfusion in pulsed labelling techniques. NMR Biomed 1996;9(2):79–83.

31. Grandin CB, Duprez TP, Oppenheim C, et al. Which MR-derived perfusion parameters are the best predictors of infarct growth in hyperacute stroke? Comparative study between relative and quantitative measurements. Radiology 2002;223:361–370.

32. Gückel FJ, Brix G, Schmiedek P, et al. Cerebrovascular reserve capacity in patients with occlusive cerebrovascular disease: assessment with dynamic susceptibility contrast-enhanced MR imaging and the acetazolamide stimulation test. Radiology 1996;201:405–412.

33. Zaharchuk G, Bogdanov AA, Marota JJ, et al. Continuous assessment of perfusion by tagging including volume and water extraction (CAPTIVE): a steady-state contrast agent technique for measuring blood flow, relative blood volume fraction, and the water extraction fraction. Magn Reson Med 1998;40:666–678.

34. Zaharchuk G, Mandeville JB, Bogdanov AA, et al. Cerebrovascular dynamics of autoregulation and hypoperfusion. An MRI study of CBF and changes in total and microvascular cerebral blood volume during hemorrhagic hypotension. Stroke 1999;30:2197–2204.

35. Zaharchuk G, Yamada M, Sasamata M, et al. Is all perfusion-weighted magnetic resonance imaging for stroke equal? The temporal evolution of multiple hemodynamic parameters after focal ischemia in rats correlated with evidence of infarction. J Cereb Blood Flow Metab 2000;20:1341–1351.

SECTION

III

Ischemic Cerebrovascular Disease

CHAPTER

10

Acute Stroke

Tudor G. Jovin and Lawrence R. Wechsler

The National Institute of Neurological Disorders and Stroke trial demonstrated that intravenous (i.v.) tissue plasminogen activator (t-PA) administered within 3 hours of symptom onset is efficacious in acute ischemic stroke.[1] This resulted in approval of i.v. t-PA for acute ischemic stroke by the U.S. Food and Drug Administration (FDA), marking the beginning of a new era in acute stroke therapy. More recently, the Prolyse in Acute Cerebral Thromboembolism (PROACT) II investigators reported improved outcomes in patients with middle cerebral artery (MCA) occlusion treated with intra-arterial prourokinase within 6 hours of symptom onset, extending the window for thrombolytic therapy.[2] Numerous reports indicating that recanalization therapy with intra-arterial thrombolytic agents dramatically improved outcomes in a condition with an otherwise dire natural history, such as basilar artery thrombosis, even as late as 24 hours after symptom onset,[3] add to the mounting evidence that intra-arterial recanalization therapy can be beneficial for selected patients with acute ischemic stroke.

Despite these advances, 5 years after FDA approval of i.v. t-PA, thrombolytic therapy continues to be underused. Post-marketing studies have estimated nationwide rates of i.v. t-PA use as low as 1.5%.[4] The comparable rates of intra-arterial thrombolysis use are not known, but are likely to be even lower. Even the most active stroke centers in the country have only been able to report a modest 5–10% i.v. t-PA use.[5] One of the reasons for these observed modest use rates is the strict adherence to the 3-hour therapeutic window in the case of intravenous thrombolysis and to the 6-hour window in the case of intra-arterial therapy. Due to deficiencies in the nationwide infrastructure for timely triage and evaluation of patients eligible for thrombolytic therapy, and due to lack of public education regarding the signs and symptoms of stroke and the need for urgent medical attention they require, the majority of patients with acute ischemic stroke are not evaluated within 3 hours of symptom onset. Further contributing to the low use rate of thrombolytic therapy is the fact that in patients who are unable to provide an adequate history, the time of stroke onset is often unknown, thus excluding potentially eligible patients from treatment.

Even in patients who receive intra-arterial or intravenous thrombolysis therapy, favorable outcomes occur in only approximately 40% of patients,[1,2] and the risk of symptomatic intracerebral hemorrhage is increased several-fold. Nevertheless, despite all the imperfections associated with its current use, thrombolytic therapy represents an important step forward in acute stroke management. Ideally, however, a much larger number of patients should receive the most appropriate form of therapy, resulting in better outcomes and less symptomatic hemorrhages. Imaging provides the possibilities of selecting patients based on physiology rather than time, potentially leading to improved outcomes, reduced complications, and increased proportion of patients eligible for treatment.

There is evidence that i.v. t-PA is not as effective for strokes caused by occlusion of large caliber arteries, such as the internal carotid artery (ICA) and main stem MCA, and that the desired therapeutic effect of i.v. t-PA (i.e., vessel recanalization) is related to the size of the affected vessel. Wolpert et al.[6] reported recanalization rates ranging from 20% for ICA occlusion to 50% for MCA distal branch occlusion. The Thrombolytic Therapy of Acute

Thrombotic/Thromboembolic Stroke Study[7] suggested a recanalization rate of no more than 30% for large vessel occlusion with i.v. t-PA doses of 0.8 mg/kg or 1.0 mg/kg. Tomsick et al.[8] reported a less favorable outcome of i.v. t-PA therapy in patients with hyperdense MCA sign on computed tomography (CT) and a National Institutes of Health Stroke Scale (NIHSS) score of greater than 10, compared to patients without this sign, suggesting a poor therapeutic response to i.v. t-PA in MCA mainstem occlusion. Schneweis et al.,[9] in a case series of 20 patients with proximal MCA occlusion treated with i.v. t-PA, reported favorable outcomes (modified Rankin score, 0–2) in only 30% of these patients. In contrast, a higher rate of favorable outcomes compared to intravenous thrombolysis alone has been reported in MCA occlusion patients treated with either intra-arterial therapy or with a combination of both intra-arterial and intravenous therapy.[2,10] This suggests that imaging modalities capable of identifying the vascular occlusion site in the acute setting might provide important information for guiding specific therapy in individual patients with acute stroke.

Neuroprotectant drugs constitute another category of potentially beneficial treatments for acute stroke. Although a plethora of compounds have been shown to have neuroprotectant effects in the laboratory animal, none of the drugs tested to date in phase III trials has been proved to positively affect outcomes in humans.[11] Flaws in the design of the drug trials, which based patient selection on chronologic rather than physiologic criteria, contributed to the negative results encountered. The clinical outcome measures used in these trials have been deemed not sufficiently reliable given the relatively low number of patients enrolled. Therefore, a need for surrogate markers of drug efficacy has been recognized.[12] New imaging modalities have the potential of addressing some of the deficiencies encountered in the design of neuroprotectant drug trials, and use of neuroimaging techniques in patient selection or as surrogate markers for outcome, or both, may provide evidence of drug efficacy in selected patients with acute stroke.

WHY IMAGING?

At present, with the exception of head CT to rule out intracerebral hemorrhage, selection criteria for thrombolytic therapy are entirely clinical and are based in part on a rigid time limit. This may not be the best selection method, as the wide spectrum of outcomes after thrombolytic therapy suggests that the amount of salvageable brain tissue in acute stroke varies from individual to individual. The concept of a fixed therapeutic time window in acute stroke has been questioned by many authors,[13] and, increasingly, selection of patients undergoing thrombolytic therapy based on physiologic criteria and on knowledge of the vascular occlusion site has been deemed more appropriate. In contrast to clinical assessment alone, some of the current imaging modalities used in conjunction with clinical assessment are able to provide this type of information.

The ideal imaging modality for acute stroke should be fast and safe. It should be able to detect acute hemorrhage, allow assessment of the large extra- and intracranial arteries, and provide information regarding the proportion of tissue irreversibly damaged in relationship to the tissue at risk.

Although improvement in technology has greatly decreased scan time, all imaging techniques require time, and "time is brain." The information obtained must be sufficiently valuable to offset the possibility of increasing the area of irreversible damage during the time needed to perform the scan. Assessment of the tissue infarcted in relationship to the tissue at risk would require knowledge of the extent of the ischemic core in relationship to the ischemic penumbra and to the tissue perfused beyond penumbral thresholds.

The ischemic penumbra represents tissue that is functionally impaired but structurally intact. According to various authors, beyond certain time limits, it corresponds to cerebral blood flow values from 17 to 22 ml/100 g per minute upper limit to 7–12 lower limit.[4–6,14–17] Salvaging this tissue by restoring its normal blood flow is the aim of reperfusion therapy. The ischemic core represents tissue that is irreversibly damaged. It corresponds to blood flow values of less than 7–12 ml/100 g per minute. By definition, reperfusing this tissue should not yield any therapeutic benefit. In fact, evidence suggests that in patients with large ischemic cores, thrombolytic therapy may be detrimental by significantly increasing the risk of symptomatic intracerebral hemorrhage and the development of malignant edema and herniation.[18,19]

Several imaging modalities have been used in the setting of acute stroke. Some are easier to apply than others. Positron emission tomography (PET) imaging provides considerable physiologic information, but requires a sophisticated and time-consuming infrastructure for its administration as well as a significant degree of cooperation on the part of the patient, making it ill suited for studying acute stroke patients. CT- and magnetic resonance imaging (MRI)–derived technologies are the most likely candidates for imaging of acute stroke. Both have the potential for providing information about the presence of hemorrhage, extent of infarcted brain, tissue perfusion, and vascular anatomy. Ultrasound allows detection of vascular occlusions in the major extra- or intracranial arteries, but cannot yet measure perfusion or allow assessment of extent of infarction. Single-photon emission CT (SPECT) may be used to image cerebral blood flow, but cannot be used to exclude hemorrhage, and thus requires a CT or MRI in addition to the SPECT study, adding significant time to the imaging protocol.

In summary, in the future, neuroimaging is expected to overcome some of the deficiencies associated with the current use of thrombolytic therapy as well as with selection of patients eligible for neuroprotectant treatment. In particular, it is hoped that in addition to reliably excluding the presence of intracerebral hemorrhage, neuroimaging will be able to identify the vascular occlusion site and will be capable of discerning between reversible and irreversible ischemia, making possible patient selection based on physiologic rather than chronologic criteria. CT and MRI technologies used individually or in combination are the imaging modalities best suited for these purposes.

COMPUTED TOMOGRAPHY IMAGING IN ACUTE STROKE

The routine, noncontrasted head CT together with CT-derived technologies such as xenon-enhanced computed tomography (XeCT), CT angiography (CTA), and CT perfusion can provide extremely useful information regarding presence of hemorrhage, presence and extent of irreversibly damaged tissue, quantitative data regarding tissue perfusion, and a highly accurate assessment of the large extra- and intracranial arteries. All CT-derived imaging modalities are fast, noninvasive, and have the potential of wide availability as they only require addition of equipment or software to already existing CT scanners that are in wide use throughout the country. A noncontrasted head CT is still the modality of choice for exclusion of intracerebral hemorrhage. Because most of the patients evaluated for acute stroke symptoms undergo CT scanning immediately on arrival to the hospital, the addition of other scanning sequences adds minimal time.

Noncontrast Head Computed Tomography Evaluation of Acute Stroke

Noncontrast head CT represents the only imaging modality used for evaluation of acute stroke patients in the vast majority of U.S. hospitals. Its main utility resides in its ability to exclude the presence of hemorrhage in a fast and reliable manner. In many instances, it can also detect other causes of acute neurologic deficit mimicking a stroke, such as tumor, subdural hematoma, vascular malformation, or sinus thrombosis. In acute ischemic stroke, it can provide important additional information with respect to the vascular occlusion site and extent and location of ischemic tissue.

As early as 1983, Gacs et al.[20] suggested that hyperdensity of a major extra- or intracranial artery in a patient with acute stroke reflects the presence of thrombus in that vessel. Since then, this finding has been confirmed by other reports,[21] although false-positive hyperdensity has also been described, mainly due to high hematocrit or vessel wall calcification.[22] The hyperdense MCA artery sign, highly suggestive of thrombus in the MCA or its major branches, has been extensively described in the literature. It is defined as an MCA that is denser than its counterpart and denser than any vessel of similar size.[23] Tomsick et al.[24] reported a sensitivity of 78% and a specificity of 93% of this sign for detection of MCA thrombus. A hyperdense basilar artery has been described as a sign of basilar artery thrombosis.[25,26] In a case series reported by Castillo et al.,[27] a hyperdense basilar artery was present in 7 of 11 patients with angiographically proven basilar artery thrombosis. Overall, data regarding the accuracy of the hyperdense basilar artery sign as a predictive factor for basilar artery thrombosis are lacking.

Hyperdensity of an arterial structure (seen as a dot) in the sylvian fissure relative to the contralateral side or to other vessels within the sylvian fissure was defined as the "MCA dot sign."[28] This sign, described in 16% of patients who received i.v. t-PA in a recent case series, is believed to represent thromboembolic occlusion of the distal MCA branches, but no angiographic data are available to confirm this contention.

Parenchymal changes on the acutely performed noncontrasted head CT can also provide useful information for the treating physician. In severe ischemia involving large areas of the brain, these changes can appear as early as 1 hour after onset.[23] The presence or absence of these changes, which usually reflect ischemic edema or tissue necrosis, or both, depends on the duration, location, and size of the tissue affected.

There is increasing evidence that parenchymal hypodensity on CT represents tissue perfused at under tissue viability thresholds.[29–31] Reperfusing this tissue is therefore not only unlikely to result in any benefit, but it may lead to worse outcomes by increasing the risk of intracerebral hemorrhage and development of malignant edema. Data from the European-Australasian Acute Stroke Study I (ECASS I)[32] and ECASS II[33] suggest that patients with hypoattenuation on pretreatment head CT exceeding one-third of the MCA territory are at high risk for developing symptomatic intracerebral hemorrhage. Although this has not been confirmed in all thrombolytic trials, there is a growing consensus among treating physicians that these patients should not undergo thrombolytic therapy. Considerable differences exist between physicians involved in acute stroke care and even between neuroradiologists in grading the extent of MCA involvement as greater or less than one-third MCA territory,[34–36] with interobserver agreement rates ranging from 45%[36] to 77%, the latter with a κ of 0.39, indicating only a fair degree of agreement.[34] According to the ATLANTIS criteria, involvement of greater than one-third MCA territory is defined as substantial involvement of two or more of the following four areas: frontal, parietal, temporal, or both basal ganglia and insula.[34]

Other early CT changes in acute stroke include lentiform nucleus obscuration, caused by cellular edema in the basal ganglia[37] that is closely correlated to proximal MCA occlusion; loss of insular ribbon signifying ischemia in the area supplied by the insular segment of the MCA and its claustral branches, which represents a watershed area between the anterior and posterior circulation;[38] and loss of gray-white matter differentiation and sulcal effacement most likely representing ischemic cortical edema.[30] The significance of these findings as predictors of worse outcomes and development of intracerebral hemorrhage is still unclear. Patel et al.[39] analyzed 616 out of 624 baseline CT scans of patients enrolled in the National Institute of Neurological Disorders and Stroke trial and concluded that although these changes are prevalent in acute stroke patients, they are not independently associated with increased risk of adverse outcome after i.v. t-PA treatment. However, both among patients who received t-PA and among those who did not receive thrombolysis, the percentage of patients with good outcomes (modified Rankin score, 0 or 1) was highest in the group of patients without early changes and higher in the group of patients with changes comprising less than one-third MCA territory than in those patients with changes involving more than one-third MCA territory (48% vs. 33% vs. 21%, respectively, in the t-PA–treated group; 29% vs. 28% vs. 15%, respectively, in the placebo group). Roberts et al.,[40] in an analysis of baseline CT scans of patients enrolled in the PROACT II trial, correlated the volume of early CT changes with clinical outcomes and reported that regardless of the baseline CT abnormality volume, there was a better outcome in recombinant prourokinase patients compared with control patients. However, similar to the findings reported by Patel et al., the percentage of patients with favorable outcomes at 90 days decreased with increasing baseline CT abnormality volume in both treatment groups. There seems to be considerable disagreement even between experienced stroke neurologists in recognizing these changes,[35,36] with observed agreement rates ranging from 68% to 85% (κ of 0.35 to 0.2, respectively) in one study[35] to 65% in another study.[36] Currently, most clinicians do not base their treatment decisions on the presence or absence of these findings.

More recently, the CT-based Alberta Stroke Programme Early CT Score (ASPECTS) has been shown to predict outcome and development of intracerebral hemorrhage with reasonable accuracy in thrombolysis-treated stroke patients.[41] The score divides the MCA territory into 10 regions of interest. The territory of the MCA is allotted 10 points. One point is subtracted for an area of early ischemic change, such as focal swelling or parenchymal hypoattenuation, for each of the defined regions. A normal CT scan has an ASPECTS value of 10 points. A score of 0 indicates diffuse ischemia throughout the territory of the MCA. In a study conducted on 203 patients who received intravenous thrombolysis, using a cutoff baseline ASPECTS score of 7, the sensitivity of ASPECTS for functional outcome was 0.78, and specificity was 0.96; the values for symptomatic intracerebral hemorrhage were 0.90 and 0.62, respectively. Agreement between observers for ASPECTS, with knowledge of the affected hemisphere, was better than that described in other studies looking at interobserver agreement for early CT changes in acute stroke.

Computed Tomography Angiographic Evaluation of Acute Stroke

With the advent of helical CT technology, a CT angiogram added to the noncontrast head CT in the acute stroke patient can be performed in 5–10 minutes, providing fast and reliable information about the patency of the extra- and intracranial and anterior and posterior cerebral circulation. It has the disadvantage of using iodinated contrast medium, which carries a small risk of adverse reactions such as allergic reactions and renal impairment. In the acute stroke patient who is agitated and not cooperating, motion artifacts can also be problematic. The technique is prone to the usual CT artifacts caused by bony structures. Nevertheless, a high diagnostic accuracy of CTA in detection of intracranial high-grade stenoses or occlusion could be demonstrated by several authors,[42–46] making it, in conjunction with CT-based perfusion studies, an extremely useful tool for triaging patients to the appropriate form of thrombolytic therapy (i.e., intravenous, combined intravenous/intra-arterial, or intra-arterial thrombolysis versus no thrombolytic therapy), depending on the time of onset of symptoms, stroke severity, and arterial territory affected (Figure 10-1). For stroke centers without intra-arterial thrombolysis capabilities, CTA may provide a rapid means for selection of patients who could benefit from transfer to a center where intra-arterial thrombolysis can be performed. CTA can also provide useful information regarding the presence of occlusion or high-grade stenoses within the extracranial circulation, as well as regarding the presence and extent of collaterals, which can guide blood pressure management, improve prognostication, and shed light on the etiology of the stroke, important for further management beyond the hyperacute phase.

Xenon-Enhanced Computed Tomography Cerebral Blood Flow Evaluation in Acute Stroke

XeCT cerebral blood flow (CBF) can be easily obtained in acute stroke patients by adding another approximately 10–20 minutes of scanning time to the noncontrasted head CT. Thus, the entire CT scanning sequence

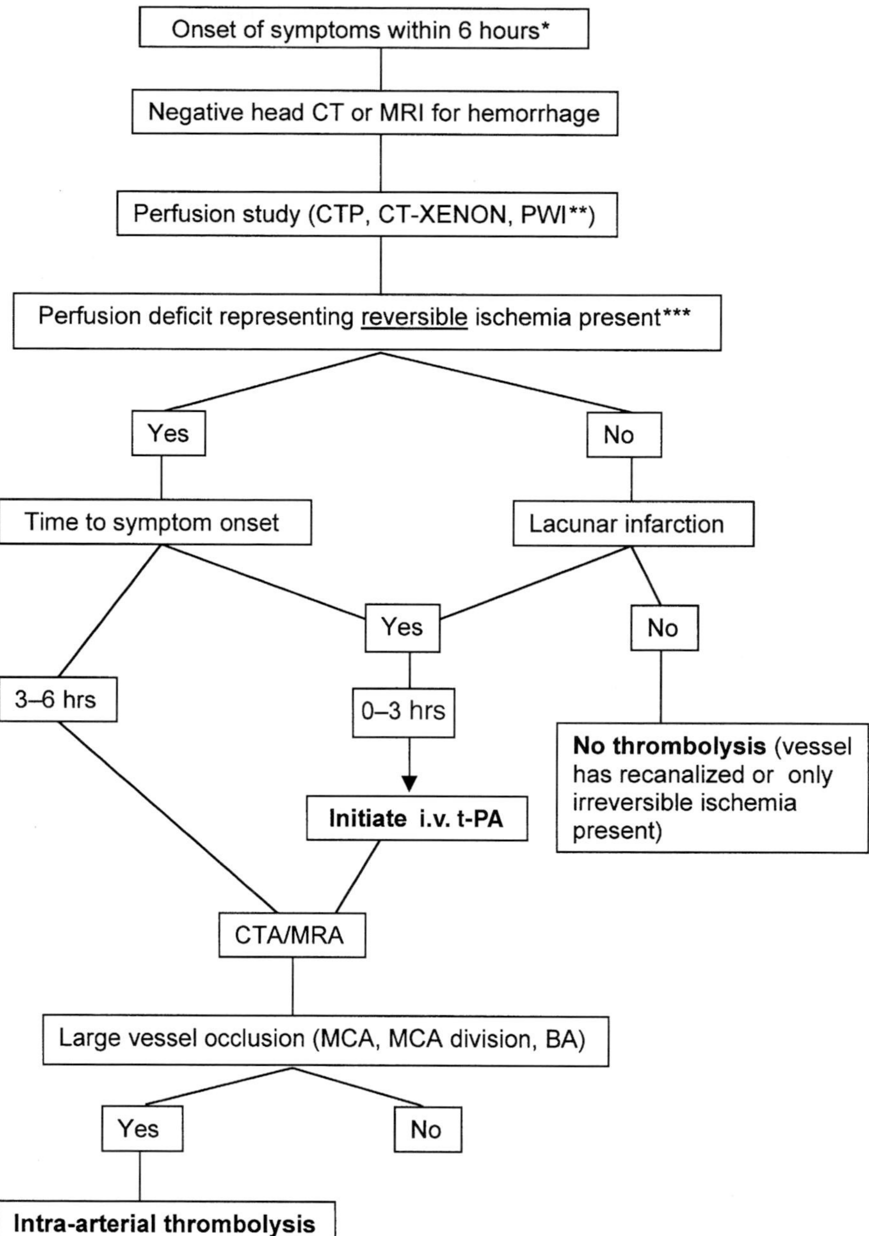

FIGURE 10-1. Proposed algorithm for neuroimaging-guided thrombolytic therapy. (BA = basilar artery; CT = computed tomography; CTA = computed tomography angiography; CTP = computed tomography perfusion; MCA = middle cerebral artery; MRA = magnetic resonance angiography; MRI = magnetic resonance imaging; PWI = perfusion-weighted imaging; t-PA = tissue plasminogen activator.) *It is hoped that in the future, thrombolytic therapy will be guided by factors other than time. Currently, however, one major determinant of eligibility for thrombolytic therapy remains time to symptom onset. **May be combined with diffusion-weighted imaging (DWI). ***Reversible ischemia may be determined by quantitative cerebral blood flow (CBF) measurements (penumbral values of regional CBF) or by DWI/PWI mismatch.

of CT and XeCT CBF followed, if necessary, by CTA requires only 20–30 minutes. The technique is safe,[47] and its major limitations are sensitivity to motion artifacts and, like any other CT-based technology, poor visualization of structures within the posterior fossa. The major advantage of the XeCT CBF technology is that it provides quantitative blood flow data with excellent anatomic resolution. Using previously established[14–16,48–50] flow definitions for ischemic penumbra and ischemic core, it is possible to appreciate the amount of brain tissue that is at risk versus tissue that is already infarcted. This is especially important because, as found in 28 patients with main-stem MCA occlusion studied within 6 hours of symptom onset,[51] the same vascular occlusion site can lead to a great variability in the amount of core versus penumbra even when the patients are studied at the same points in time relative to their symptom onset. Although the concept of one measurement in time has been encountered with skepticism because it represents a "snapshot" of a dynamic process, primate models of MCA occlusion have demonstrated with continuous vessel occlusion that flows in the irreversible ischemia range have a predictable time course.[52]

Knowledge of the extent of the tissue that is already infarcted is important because it may lead to a better selection of patients who might benefit from recanalization therapy. Goldstein et al.[19] demonstrated that the risk of symptomatic intracerebral hemorrhage after i.v. t-PA administration is significantly increased if large areas of the MCA territory are perfused at blood flow values that correspond to ischemic core. Firlik et al.[18] showed that perfusion of the entire cortical MCA territory at under tissue viability thresholds is associated with the development of malignant cerebral edema. Conversely, normal cerebral blood flow in a presumed symptomatic territory indicates that spontaneous recanalization has already occurred, and thrombolytic therapy may unnecessarily expose the patient to the risk of intracerebral hemorrhage. In one series of 12 acute stroke patients with normal flows in the symptomatic arterial territory studied within 6 hours of stroke onset, Firlik et al.[53] demonstrated that nine patients recovered without any therapeutic intervention. The other three patients presumably achieved vessel recanalization after irreversible damage had already occurred.

Kilpatrick et al.[54] analyzed the predictive value for subsequent development of infarction by CT and for good outcome as determined by discharge-to-home disposition in 31 acute stroke patients studied within 6 hours of symptom onset with CT, CTA, and XeCT CBF. Patients with no infarction on initial CT and normal XeCT CBF had significantly fewer new infarctions and were discharged home more often than those with compromised CBF. The same held true for patients with an open ICA and MCA by CTA and normal CT compared to those with an occluded ICA or MCA, or both, by CTA. Either was superior to baseline CT and NIHSS in prediction of outcome. Both enabled the selection of a group of patients not identifiable by CT alone that would have done well without being exposed to the risks of thrombolytic therapy. The study included too few patients to statistically assess the role of combining CTA and XeCT CBF information.

These retrospective studies addressing the value of quantitative CBF measurement in hyperacute stroke await validation from prospective studies that will ideally define flow thresholds in relationship to extent of affected MCA territory, which will guide patient selection for recanalization therapy.

Computed Tomography Perfusion Evaluation in Acute Stroke

CT perfusion has been recently added to the diagnostic armamentarium of acute stroke. It can provide quantitative blood flow data, currently limited to only a few contiguous levels within the brain, resulting in a relatively small sampling volume, which represents one of the major drawbacks of this technique. Its applicability is theoretically similar to that of XeCT or any other quantitative perfusion imaging modality. Several reports using semi-quantitative CBF measurements have indicated that CT perfusion provides useful information for acute stroke management.[45,55–59] The presence and extent of perfusion deficits in acute stroke patients could be identified with high degrees of accuracy. Wintermark et al.[60] reported that in a small series of acute stroke patients with large vessel occlusion, a cerebral blood volume threshold of less than 2.5 ml/100 g was highly predictive of infarction irrespective of whether the patients received successful recanalization therapy. A highly predictive relationship between the whole-brain–perfused blood volume lesion and final infarct in patients who were successfully reperfused was reported by Lev et al.[61] However, a reliable differentiation between reversible and irreversible ischemia based on this technique has so far not been reported. In general, experience with this imaging modality is still limited, and the technique awaits validation in humans through comparison with more standard quantitative blood flow measurement techniques such as PET or XeCT.

MAGNETIC RESONANCE IMAGING IN ACUTE STROKE

Until the advent of the newer MRI sequences, especially diffusion and perfusion MRI, MRI had a limited role in the assessment of hyperacute stroke patients. The availability of these techniques as well as the significant reductions in the amount of time required to perform these scans have led to a rapid growth in the number of centers performing MRI in acute stroke patients, such that many authors regard MRI as the future imaging modality of choice in acute stroke.[62] One remaining problem that used to limit the use of MRI as a single imaging modality in acute stroke is its inability to reliably visualize hyperacute blood, making an additional head CT often necessary, which added additional scanning time. Newer MRI techniques, such as gradient echo sequences, that are highly sensitive to the presence of blood will likely obviate the need for additional CT scanning in the future.

Diffusion Magnetic Resonance Imaging in Acute Stroke

In acute ischemic brain lesions, diffusion MRI (DWI) detects areas of restricted diffusion of hydrogen ions caused by shift of water from the interstitial to the intracellular space. This coincides with ischemia-induced membrane depolarization due to sodium/potassium adenosine triphosphatase failure.[63] The restricted diffusion of water can be quantified by the apparent diffusion coefficient. In humans, DWI was reported to be able to detect ischemic lesions as early as 39 minutes after stroke onset.[64] These changes appear hours before the appearance of signal abnormalities on conventional

MRI sequences such as T2 or fluid-attenuated inversion recovery.[64–66] In a recent study in which DWI in acute stroke patients was compared to findings at autopsy, Kelly and coworkers[67] were able to report a sensitivity of 88.5% and a specificity of 96.6% for this imaging modality in the detection of ischemic lesions within the brain. The acute DWI lesion volume was reported by several investigators to correlate well with clinical outcome.[66,68,69] It was initially thought that the DWI lesion represented irreversible ischemia. However, evidence in the recent literature documenting reversal or regression of DWI lesions in acute stroke patients after recanalization therapy[66,68–71] led to a reappraisal of this concept. It is by now clear that DWI, although extremely useful in establishing the presence, location, and extent of the ischemic lesion, is currently not capable of differentiating between reversible and irreversible injury. Whether this will be possible by establishing apparent diffusion coefficient thresholds that will discern between reversible and irreversible ischemia remains to be established by future studies.

Perfusion Magnetic Resonance Imaging in Acute Stroke

Perfusion MRI (PWI) provides information about tissue perfusion at multiple levels within the brain. For most of its applications, the technique is based either on dynamic tracking of a bolus of a paramagnetic contrast agent (dynamic susceptibility contrast) or on arterial spin labeling. Relative cerebral blood volume, relative cerebral blood flow, and qualitative mean transit time can be obtained, but techniques that allow quantitative assessment of perfusion parameters, though described by various research units,[72] are still not available in routine clinical practice. PWI can be useful in determining whether vessel recanalization has occurred (in which case it is normal) and in determining the extent of the brain tissue at risk, which has been shown by some authors[66,69] to strongly correlate with clinical outcome. However, the lack of quantitative data makes PWI unable to reliably identify either the upper limit or the lower limit of the ischemic penumbra. Neumann-Haefelin and coworkers[73] suggested that using mean transit time and time to peak (TTP) might allow some quantification of the degree of ischemia. They reported that a TTP enhancement delay of longer than 6 seconds in regions with normal DWI findings was associated with a high risk of lesion enlargement. Because more moderate perfusion deficits (TTP delays ≥4 and <6 seconds) appear to also contribute to the acute clinical deficit, they suggested that TTP delay of approximately 4 seconds might be the threshold for functional impairment of brain tissue. Although several other authors have reported greater sensitivity of TTP maps compared to cerebral blood volume maps in detecting abnormalities in acute stroke, further studies will be necessary to clarify this approach.

Diffusion/Perfusion Magnetic Resonance Imaging in Acute Stroke

Perhaps the most useful application of MRI in acute stroke is the information derived from the combined DWI/PWI sequences. Because the diffusion abnormality is presumed to represent an approximation of the irreversible ischemic lesion, and the perfusion abnormality is thought to represent the brain territory at risk, the area of mismatch between DWI and PWI is considered still viable but at risk of undergoing infarction and corresponds theoretically to the concept of ischemic penumbra.

Several investigators who performed MRI in patients with acute stroke[69,74–78] reported that the final infarct size was significantly larger than the initial DWI lesion in patients in whom the initial PWI lesion was larger than the initial DWI lesion, whereas the final infarct size was equal to or decreased in size compared to the initial DWI lesion in patients in whom the initial PWI lesion was equal in size or smaller than the initial DWI lesion. This observation reinforces the concept that the PWI lesion that exceeds the DWI lesion represents tissue at risk, which, in the absence of vessel recanalization, will progress to infarction. Schellinger and coworkers,[75] on a prospective case series of 51 patients studied within 5 hours of symptom onset with PWI/DWI, reported that vessel occlusion was associated with a PWI/DWI mismatch on the initial MRI, whereas vessel patency was associated with PWI/DWI match. In this study, clinical outcome scores and lesion volumes on follow-up MRI differed significantly between the group of patients who achieved vessel recanalization compared with the group of patients who did not recanalize. The authors suggest that the presence of PWI/DWI mismatch should guide recanalization therapy within 6 hours of symptom onset according to the following algorithm: No thrombolysis is recommended in patients without PWI/DWI mismatch and without vessel occlusion and in patients with large infarctions exceeding 33–50% of the MCA territory according to DWI. Thrombolysis is strongly recommended in patients with MCA occlusions distal to the lenticulostriate branches and with presence of a PWI/DWI mismatch as well as in patients with distal ICA or proximal MCA occlusions and presence of a PWI/DWI mismatch. Careful and reluctant consideration for thrombolysis should be given to patients who have no PWI/DWI mismatch but have evidence of vessel occlusion; in patients with PWI/DWI mismatch, vessel occlusion, and DWI lesion volume between 33% and 50% of the MCA territory; and in patients with PWI/DWI mismatch but without vessel occlusion. Two prospective trials, DEFUSE in the United States and DIAS in

Germany, investigating the benefit of patient selection for i.v. thrombolytic therapy within 3–6 hours of symptom onset, based on the presence of PWI/DWI mismatch, are currently ongoing. Although PWI/DWI-guided thrombolytic therapy in acute stroke is a concept embraced by many investigators, one factor that makes standardization of such an approach problematic remains the lack of quantitative data regarding the degree of ischemia.

FIGURE 10-2. ▶ Case illustrations of functional imaging-guided clinical decision making in hyperacute stroke at our institution. **A–D.** *Case 1.* Vascular occlusion site identified. Tissue at risk is compromised but still salvageable. Thrombolytic therapy appropriate. A 64-year-old man presented with acute-onset expressive aphasia, left gaze deviation, right homonymous hemianopsia, and right hemiplegia. Admission National Institutes of Health Stroke Scale (NIHSS) was 19. A noncontrasted head computed tomography (CT) scan was normal. He received 0.6 mg/kg i.v. tissue plasminogen activator (t-PA) (0.09 mg/kg bolus) at 2 hours and 15 minutes after symptom onset and underwent a xenon-enhanced CT cerebral blood flow (XeCT CBF) at 2 hours and 30 minutes after symptom onset, which demonstrated diminished blood flow in the entire left middle cerebral artery (MCA) territory (mean MCA flow, 21 mg/100 ml per minute). However, left MCA cerebral blood flow values were in a range compatible with reversible ischemia. It was therefore thought that he failed to achieve vessel recanalization with i.v. t-PA, but there were still large areas of penumbral flow (i.e., hypoperfused areas at risk of undergoing infarction but potentially salvageable) in the left MCA territory. He underwent emergent cerebral angiography demonstrating occlusion of the left M1 MCA segment (*arrow*) and good filling of the distal MCA territory through leptomeningeal collaterals. Within 3 hours of symptom onset, he underwent intra-arterial thrombolysis with t-PA over approximately 2 hours, at the end of which a control angiogram revealed complete recanalization of the M1 and M2 segments with evidence of filling defects in some of the distal left MCA branches. The observed vessel recanalization correlated with a dramatic improvement in the patient's clinical deficits. Follow-up brain magnetic resonance imaging revealed infarcts in the left basal ganglia, corona radiata, frontal operculum, insular cortex, and parietal cortex. The patient's deficits resolved gradually over the ensuing days, such that at discharge from hospital his NIHSS was 0.

Emerging Magnetic Resonance Techniques: Magnetic Resonance Spectroscopy and Sodium Magnetic Resonance Imaging

The utility of magnetic resonance spectroscopy in hyperacute stroke is still under investigation, and magnetic resonance spectroscopy studies performed on patients within 3–6 hours of symptom onset are, to this date, lacking. A recent report in the literature[79] conducted on patients studied within 72 hours suggests that *N*-acetyl aspartate measurements in the area of infarction provide a useful measure of residual neuronal activity and, hence, indicate the severity of ischemia as well as the potential for recovery. Other authors have reported that lactate measurements in acute stroke may provide useful information for the clinician. Barker et al.[80] reported that tissue containing elevated lactate but no other spectroscopic or MRI abnormality can be identified in the early stages of stroke and suggested that such regions may represent an ischemic zone at risk of infarction.

Recent reports[81] have suggested that sodium MRI may be an imaging modality capable of identifying irreversibly ischemic tissue by measuring sodium concentration in the ischemic brain. It was suggested that a sodium concentration of greater than 70 mmol/L reliably predicts infarction. Experience with this imaging technique is limited, and the method awaits validation by future studies. At present, the long scanning sequences make this modality clinically impractical in the time frame needed for decision making.

Magnetic Resonance Angiography in Acute Stroke

The advantages derived from precise knowledge of the presence and site of vascular occlusion in hyperacute stroke have been alluded to earlier in this chapter (Figures 10-2 through 10-4). Magnetic resonance angiography (MRA) is capable of providing this type of information with minimal time added to the other scanning sequences used in hyperacute stroke. Time-of-flight (TOF) MRA and contrast MRA, the most commonly used MRA imaging techniques, allow visualization of the large arteries that form the extra- and intracranial circulation. In TOF, the degree of stenosis is often overestimated. Gadolinium-enhanced MRA is probably more accurate than TOF MRA[82,83] and requires less than 1 minute for completion. It is therefore likely to emerge as the MRA imaging modality of choice in hyperacute stroke patients. The utility of MRA in the diagnosis of extracranial cerebrovascular disease has been extensively studied, and a discussion on this topic is beyond the scope of this chapter. There are relatively little data available regarding the accuracy of MRA in the diagnosis of intracranial occlusive disease, and further studies are needed to address this issue.

POSITRON EMISSION TOMOGRAPHY IN ACUTE STROKE

In stroke, PET techniques are capable of providing the most accurate assessment of the brain tissue at risk in relationship to the tissue irreversibly damaged through

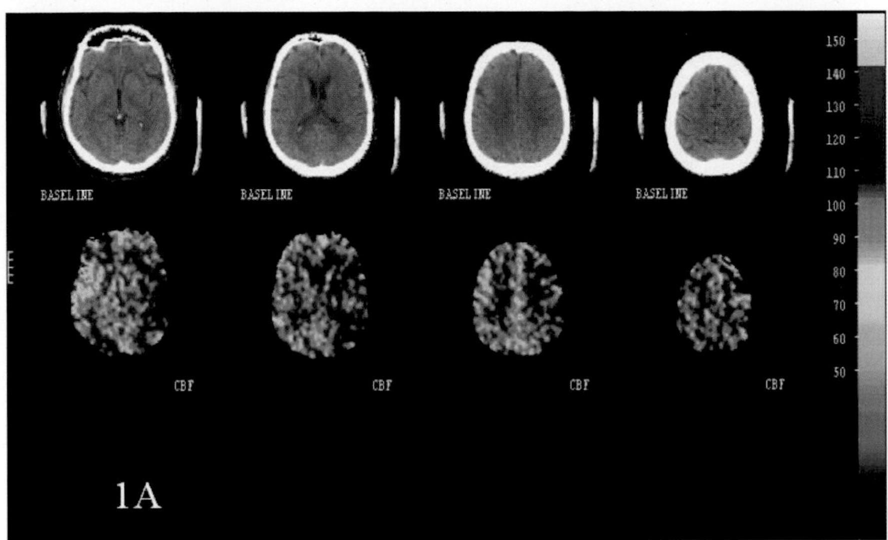
BASELINE
BASELINE
BASELINE
BASELINE
CBF
CBF
CBF
CBF
150
140
130
120
110
100
90
80
70
60
50
1A

A

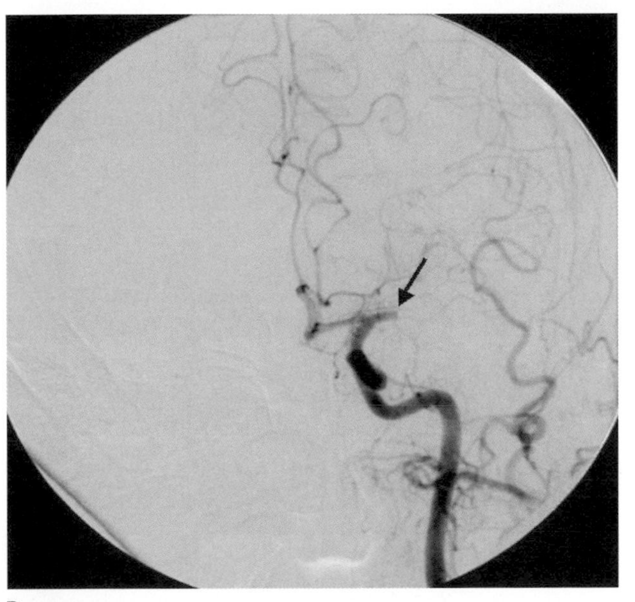

B

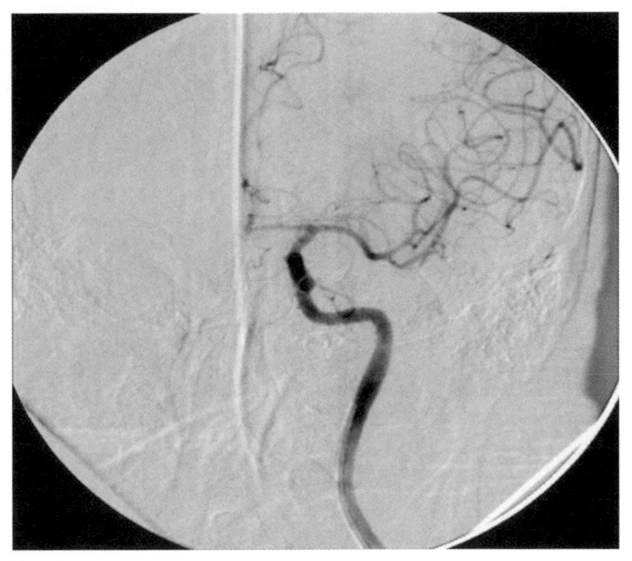

C

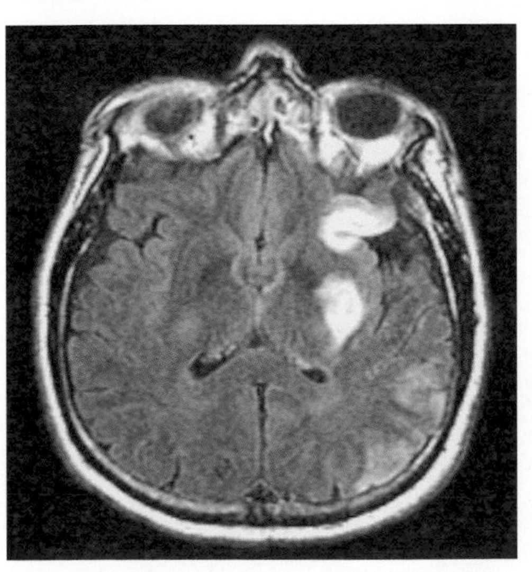

D

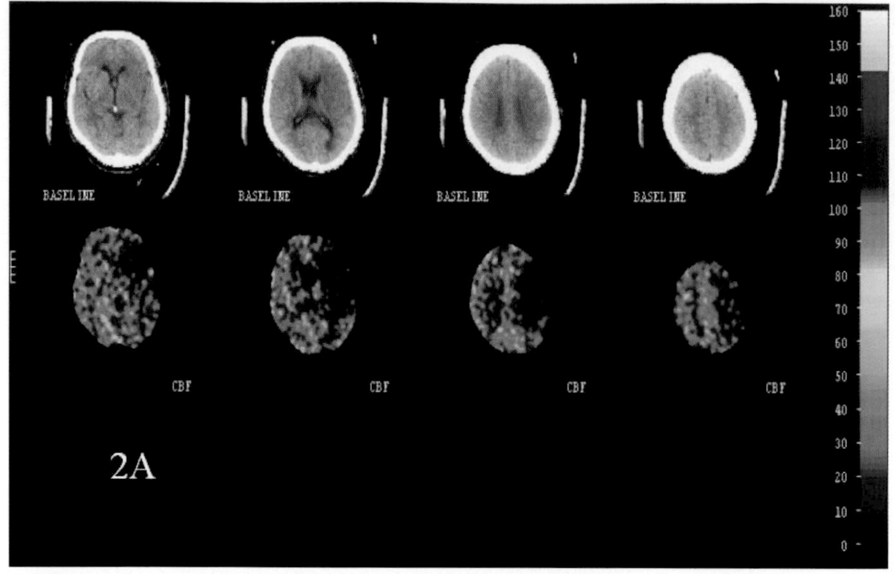
BASELINE
BASELINE
BASELINE
BASELINE
CBF
CBF
CBF
CBF
2A
160
150
140
130
120
110
100
90
80
70
60
50
40
30
20
10
0

A

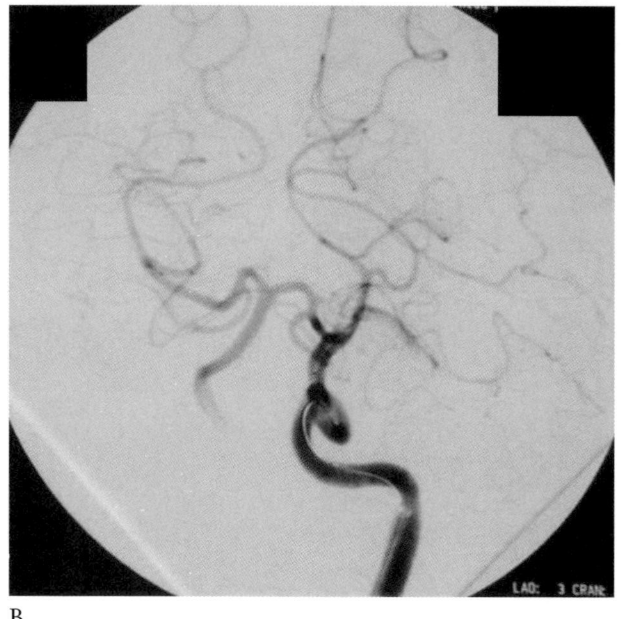
LAO: 3 CRAN

B

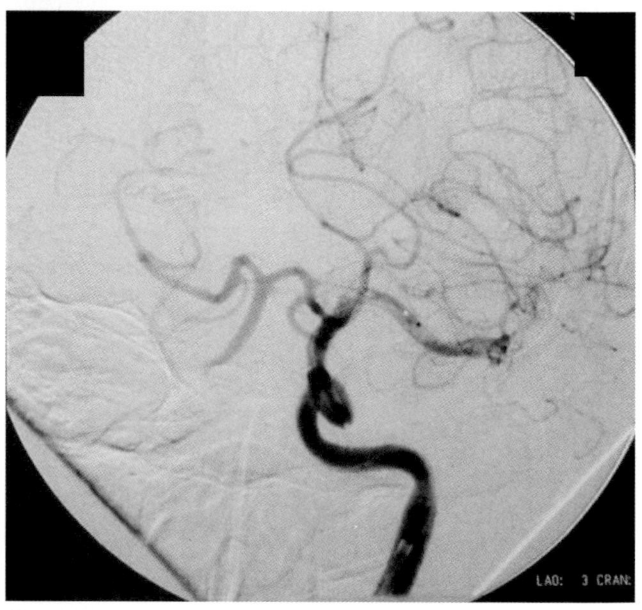
LAO: 3 CRAN

C

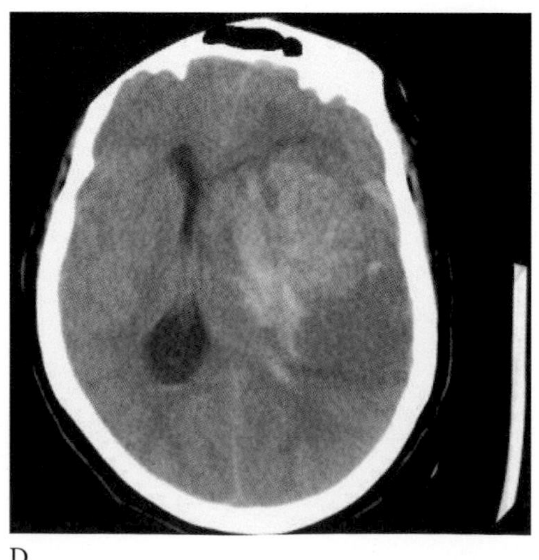

D

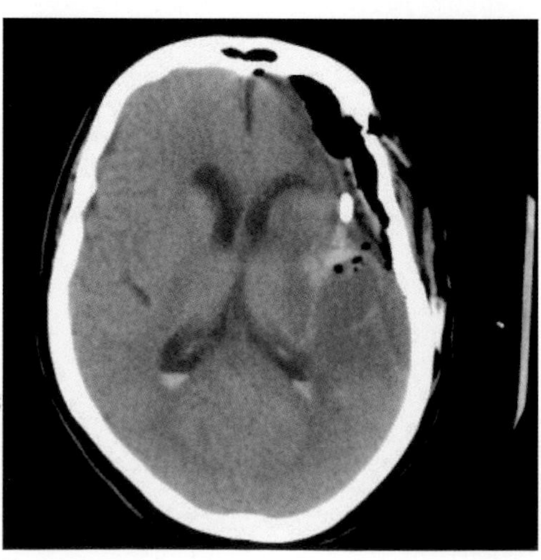

E

◀ FIGURE 10-3. **A–E.** *Case 2*. Vascular occlusion site identified. Tissue at risk is irreversibly compromised. Thrombolytic therapy is inappropriate. A 59-year-old woman developed sudden onset of aphasia and right hemiplegia. A head computed tomography revealed the presence of hypoattenuation involving greater than one-third left middle cerebral artery (MCA) territory as well as loss of cortical grey-white matter differentiation in the left MCA territory. Xenon-enhanced computed tomography cerebral blood flow obtained at the same time revealed reduced cerebral blood flow values in the MCA territory (mean cortical MCA flow, 13 mg/100 ml per minute), indicating irreversible ischemia involving large areas of the left MCA territory. An emergent left common carotid angiogram revealed the presence of critical left internal carotid artery (ICA) stenosis at its origin, for which angioplasty was performed (C), and distal ICA occlusion. For the terminal ICA occlusion, she underwent angioplasty followed by intra-arterial thrombolysis with 2 million units urokinase over 2 hours. The infusion was begun at 6 hours after onset of symptoms. A postinfusion angiogram revealed patent anterior cerebral artery, MCA (with multiple filling defects consistent with thrombi), and patent anterior division MCA. Within the ensuing 12 hours, the patient developed a clinical picture consistent with transtentorial herniation. Head computed tomography demonstrated the presence of hemorrhagic transformation of a large left MCA infarction with intraventricular extension, significant mass effect, and midline shift. She underwent surgical removal of the hemorrhage and strokectomy. One month after surgery, she still had significant language impairment and right hemiplegia.

its potential, depending on the tracer used, to concomitantly measure cerebral blood flow and metabolism. Additionally, new markers of permanent ischemic damage have been described recently.[16,84,85] PET studies on acute stroke patients have been performed in a handful of research centers around the world,[29,49,86] but due to the cumbersome infrastructure and patient cooperation required to perform the study, it is unlikely that PET will have a role in the routine clinical evaluation of hyperacute stroke in the near future.

SINGLE-PHOTON EMISSION COMPUTED TOMOGRAPHY IN ACUTE STROKE

Like many other methods that assess perfusion, SPECT has been shown to be accurate in predicting outcomes in acute stroke,[87] including in patients treated with thrombolytics.[88,89] Shimosegawa et al.[90] reported an infarction threshold uptake of 60% of contralateral value by SPECT. Ueda et al.[88] reported that tissue with a CBF below 35% of that in the cerebellum represents irreversible ischemia that cannot be salvaged by intra-arterial thrombolysis within 5 hours of symptom onset. In agreement with findings reported in acute stroke patients who underwent XeCT CBF studies before or during thrombolytic therapy,[19] this study suggested that the tissue perfused below reversible ischemia thresholds is at considerable risk of hemorrhagic transformation. In a study comprising 28 patients with acute stroke studied with technetium-99m–ethyl-cysteinate-dimer SPECT before undergoing successful intra-arterial thrombolysis within 6 hours of symptoms, Ogasawara et al.[89] demonstrated that brain SPECT can be used to differentiate patients with reversible ischemia from those with irreversible brain damage. In hyperacute stroke, SPECT is capable of providing reliable information if vessel recanalization has occurred (in which case, it is normal), but as it represents an essentially qualitative CBF assessment method, the degree of ischemia cannot be quantified. Despite its wide availability and relative ease of use, SPECT will be unlikely to play a major role in hyperacute stroke diagnostics in the future mainly due to the fact that it only provides information about tissue perfusion, making the addition of other imaging modalities (CT to exclude hemorrhage; CTA, transcranial Doppler [TCD], or MRA to assess the brain vasculature) often necessary.

TRANSCRANIAL DOPPLER ASSESSMENT IN ACUTE STROKE

TCD is an imaging method that is fast, inexpensive, noninvasive, widely available, feasible in almost any clinical setting, and relatively easy to use, characteristics that make it an excellent tool for the evaluation of hyperacute stroke patients in conjunction with other imaging modalities. One major limitation of this imaging method is that it is highly operator dependent, but in the hands of a skilled operator it has been shown to detect occlusion of the ICA and of the major arteries of the circle of Willis with high accuracy.[91] Another limitation of the method is that vessel insonation cannot be obtained in a significant proportion of patients.[92] However, the advent of ultrasound contrast substances, such as Levovist (currently not FDA approved) seems to largely eliminate this inconvenience.[93,94] In addition, emerging ultrasound techniques, such as power Doppler imaging, harmonic contrast imaging, and three-dimensional transcranial power Doppler ultrasound imaging, have potential for improved morphologic delineation of the extra- and intracranial vessels. One major additional advantage of TCD is that it allows continuous monitoring of the insonated vessel, which may provide important information regarding the timing and occurrence of vessel recanalization with potentially immediate therapeutic consequences.[95,96] Another possible advantage of this imaging technique is suggested by in vitro experiments

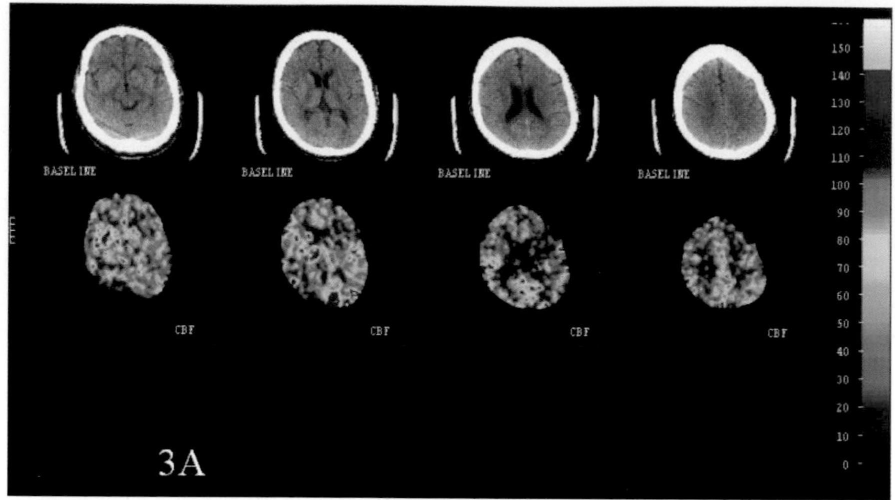
BASEL INE
BASEL INE
BASEL INE
BASEL INE
CBF
CBF
CBF
CBF
150
140
130
120
110
100
90
80
70
60
50
40
30
20
10
0
3A

A

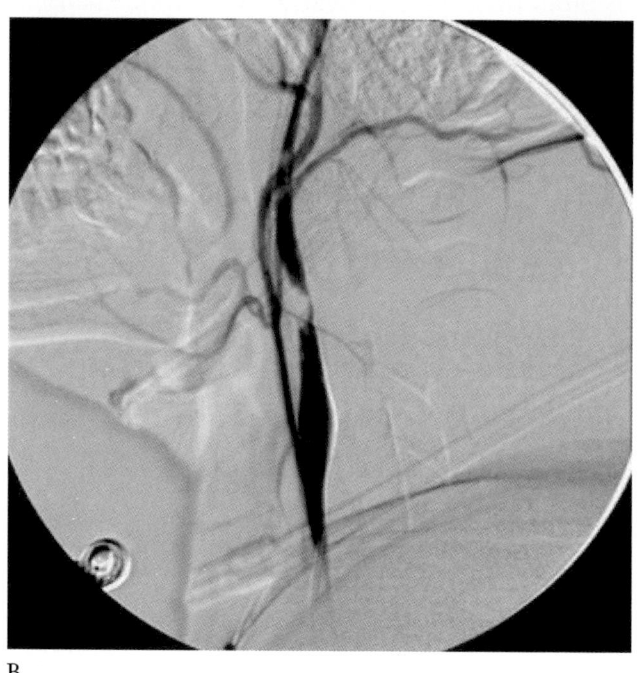

B

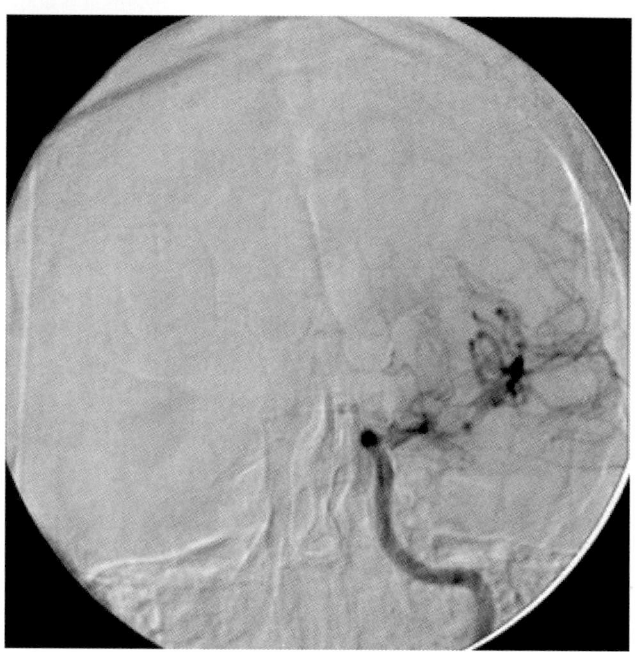

C

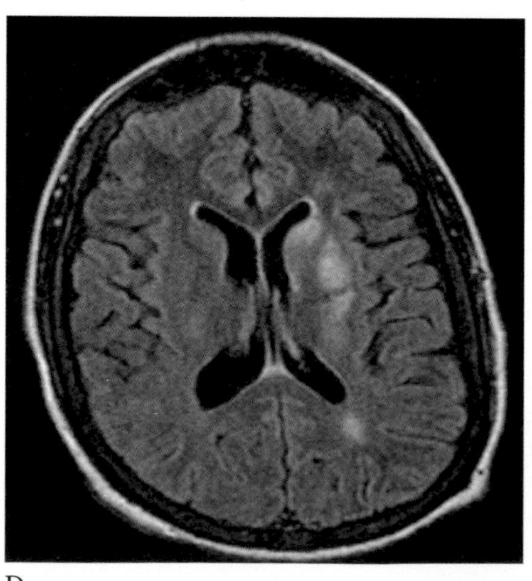

D

◀ FIGURE 10-4. **A–D.** *Case 3*. Vascular occlusion site identified. Tissue at risk is only minimally compromised due to abundant collaterals. Thrombolytic therapy withheld. A 23-year-old, right-handed man developed a severe right hemiparesis, global aphasia, and right homonymous hemianopsia 3 days after heart transplantation for idiopathic cardiomyopathy. An emergent noncontrasted head computed tomography at 1 hour after onset of his symptoms revealed no early computed tomography changes in the left middle cerebral artery (MCA) territory. This was followed immediately by a xenon-enhanced computed tomography cerebral blood flow study showing only minimally diminished flows in the left MCA distribution (mean cortical MCA flow, 45 ml/100 mg per minute). Emergent cerebral angiography demonstrated a left proximal ICA dissection and thrombus in the M1 segment of the left MCA with minimal contrast penetration. Good filling of the distal M2 branches was noted via collaterals. It was decided not to pursue thrombolytic therapy because the only mildly diminished flow in the left MCA territory by xenon-enhanced computed tomography and the presence of good leptomeningeal collaterals by angiography were considered to be predictive of good outcome even without thrombolysis. Over the ensuing hours, the patient's deficits resolved gradually and by the next day only a mild right arm paresis was present, which completely cleared subsequently. Follow-up brain magnetic resonance imaging revealed a small left basal ganglia infarct.

and preliminary studies of acute stroke patients,[97] showing that ultrasound may enhance the lytic action of thrombolytic agents. Further prospective data are necessary to clarify this issue.

CONCLUSION

The ideal imaging modality for the acute stroke patient should be available emergently with little setup time. There should be no contraindications to the test and little or no risk and discomfort to the patient. It should enable the clinician to exclude other causes for strokelike symptoms and must reliably identify hemorrhage. The test should be capable of differentiating between the tissue irreversibly affected in relationship to the tissue at risk. It should also be capable of assessing the brain vasculature such that patient selection would occur based on physiologic criteria rather than chronologic criteria. None of the available techniques yet meets these criteria for an ideal imaging method in acute stroke. The ability of CT- and magnetic resonance–based technologies to select patients with viable brain more likely to respond and less likely to hemorrhage has not been established. However, both techniques have the potential to fulfill the previously mentioned requirements and are likely to emerge as the two imaging modalities of choice for hyperacute stroke patients in the future.

REFERENCES

1. The National Institute of Neurological Disorders and Stroke rt-PA Stroke Study Group. Tissue plasminogen activator for acute ischemic stroke. N Engl J Med 1995;333(24):1581–1587.

2. Furlan A, Higashida R, Wechsler L, et al. Intra-arterial prourokinase for acute ischemic stroke. The PROACT II study: a randomized controlled trial. Prolyse in Acute Cerebral Thromboembolism. JAMA 1999;282(21):2003–2011.

3. Phan TG, Wijdicks EF. Intra-arterial thrombolysis for vertebrobasilar circulation ischemia. Crit Care Clin 1999;15(4):719–742.

4. Alberts MJ. tPA in acute ischemic stroke: United States experience and issues for the future. Neurology 1998;51(3 Suppl 3):S53–S55.

5. Chiu D, Krieger D, Villar-Cordova C, et al. Intravenous tissue plasminogen activator for acute ischemic stroke: feasibility, safety, and efficacy in the first year of clinical practice. Stroke 1998;29(1):18–22.

6. Wolpert SM, Bruckmann H, Greenlee R, et al. Neuroradiologic evaluation of patients with acute stroke treated with recombinant tissue plasminogen activator. The rt-PA Acute Stroke Study Group. AJNR Am J Neuroradiol 1993;14(1):3–13.

7. Genentech. Summary basis for approval: Activase TM for acute ischemic stroke. New Drug Application (PLA96-0350).

8. Tomsick T, Brott T, Barsan W, et al. Prognostic value of the hyperdense middle cerebral artery sign and stroke scale score before ultra-early thrombolytic therapy. AJNR Am J Neuroradiol 1996;17(1):79–85.

9. Schneweis S, Grond M, Neveling M, et al. Intravenous thrombolysis in proximal middle cerebral artery occlusion. Cerebrovasc Dis 2001;11(3):212–215.

10. Ernst R, Pancioli A, Tomsick T, et al. Combined intravenous and intra-arterial recombinant tissue plasminogen activator in acute ischemic stroke. Stroke 2000;31(11):2552–2557.

11. DeGraba TJ, Pettigrew LC. Why do neuroprotective drugs work in animals but not humans? Neurol Clin 2000;18(2):475–493.

12. Muir KW, Grosset DG. Neuroprotection for acute stroke: making clinical trials work. Stroke 1999;30(1):180–182.

13. Baron JC, von Kummer R, del Zoppo GJ. Treatment of acute ischemic stroke. Challenging the concept of a rigid and universal time window. Stroke 1995;26(12):2219–2221.

14. Baron JC. Perfusion thresholds in human cerebral ischemia: historical perspective and therapeutic implications. Cerebrovasc Dis 2001;11(Suppl 1):2–8.

15. Symon L, Branston NM, Strong AJ, Hope TD. The concepts of thresholds of ischaemia in relation to

brain structure and function. J Clin Pathol Suppl (R Coll Pathol) 1977;11:149–154.

16. Heiss WD, Kracht LW, Thiel A, et al. Penumbral probability thresholds of cortical flumazenil binding and blood flow predicting tissue outcome in patients with cerebral ischaemia. Brain 2001;124(Pt 1):20–29.

17. Heiss WD, Graf R. The ischemic penumbra. Curr Opin Neurol 1994;7(1):11–19.

18. Firlik AD, Yonas H, Kaufmann AM, et al. Relationship between cerebral blood flow and the development of swelling and life-threatening herniation in acute ischemic stroke. J Neurosurg 1998;89(2):243–249.

19. Goldstein S, Yonas H, Gebel JM. Acute cerebral blood flow as a predictive physiologic marker for symptomatic hemorrhagic conversion and clinical herniation after thrombolytic therapy. Stroke 2000; 31(1):275.

20. Gacs G, Fox AJ, Barnett HJ, Vinuela F. CT visualization of intracranial arterial thromboembolism. Stroke 1983;14(5):756–762.

21. Schuknecht B, Ratzka M, Hofmann E. The "dense artery sign"—major cerebral artery thromboembolism demonstrated by computed tomography. Neuroradiology 1990;32(2):98–103.

22. Rauch RA, Bazan C 3d, Larsson EM, Jinkins JR. Hyperdense middle cerebral arteries identified on CT as a false sign of vascular occlusion. AJNR Am J Neuroradiol 1993;14(3):669–673.

23. Gaskill-Shipley MF. Routine CT evaluation of acute stroke. Neuroimaging Clin North Am 1999;9(3): 411–422.

24. Tomsick TA, Brott TG, Chambers AA, et al. Hyperdense middle cerebral artery sign on CT: efficacy in detecting middle cerebral artery thrombosis. AJNR Am J Neuroradiol 1990;11(3):473–437.

25. Ehsan T, Hayat G, Malkoff MD, et al. Hyperdense basilar artery. An early computed tomography sign of thrombosis. J Neuroimag 1994;4(4):200–205.

26. Hankey GJ, Khangure MS, Stewart-Wynne EG. Detection of basilar artery thrombosis by computed tomography. Clin Radiol 1988;39(2):140–143.

27. Castillo M, Falcone S, Naidich TP, et al. Imaging in acute basilar artery thrombosis. Neuroradiology 1994;36(6):426–429.

28. Barber PA, Demchuk AM, Hudon ME, et al. Hyperdense sylvian fissure MCA "dot" sign: a CT marker of acute ischemia. Stroke 2001;32(1):84–88.

29. Grond M, von Kummer R, Sobesky J, et al. Early x-ray hypoattenuation of brain parenchyma indicates extended critical hypoperfusion in acute stroke. Stroke 2000;31(1):133–139.

30. von Kummer R, Weber J. Brain and vascular imaging in acute ischemic stroke: the potential of computed tomography. Neurology 1997;49(5 Suppl 4):S52–S55.

31. Firlik AD, Kaufmann AM, Wechsler LR, et al. Quantitative cerebral blood flow determinations in acute ischemic stroke. Relationship to computed tomography and angiography. Stroke 1997;28(11): 2208–2213.

32. von Kummer R, Allen KL, Holle R, et al. Acute stroke: usefulness of early CT findings before thrombolytic therapy. Radiology 1997;205(2):327–333.

33. Larrue V, von Kummer RR, Muller A, Bluhmki E. Risk factors for severe hemorrhagic transformation in ischemic stroke patients treated with recombinant tissue plasminogen activator: a secondary analysis of the European-Australasian Acute Stroke Study (ECASS II). Stroke 2001;32(2):438–441.

34. Kalafut MA, Schriger DL, Saver JL, Starkman S. Detection of early CT signs of >1/3 middle cerebral artery infarctions: interrater reliability and sensitivity of CT interpretation by physicians involved in acute stroke care. Stroke 2000;31(7):1667–1671.

35. Grotta JC, Chiu D, Lu M, et al. Agreement and variability in the interpretation of early CT changes in stroke patients qualifying for intravenous rtPA therapy. Stroke 1999;30(8):1528–1533.

36. Wardlaw JM, Dorman PJ, Lewis SC, Sandercock PA. Can stroke physicians and neuroradiologists identify signs of early cerebral infarction on CT? J Neurol Neurosurg Psychiatry 1999;67(5):651–653.

37. Tomura N, Uemura K, Inugami A, et al. Early CT finding in cerebral infarction: obscuration of the lentiform nucleus. Radiology 1988;168(2):463–467.

38. Truwit CL, Barkovich AJ, Gean-Marton A, et al. Loss of the insular ribbon: another early CT sign of acute middle cerebral artery infarction. Radiology 1990;176(3):801–806.

39. Patel SC, Levine SR, Tilley BC, et al. Lack of clinical significance of early ischemic changes on computed tomography in acute stroke. JAMA 2001;286: 2830–2838.

40. Roberts HC, Dillon WP, Furlan AJ, et al. Computed tomographic findings in patients undergoing intra-arterial thrombolysis for acute ischemic stroke due to middle cerebral artery occlusion: results from the PROACT II trial. Stroke 2002;33:1557–1565.

41. Barber PA, Demchuk AM, Zhang J, Buchan AM. Validity and reliability of a quantitative computed tomography score in predicting outcome of hyperacute stroke before thrombolytic therapy. ASPECTS Study Group. Alberta Stroke Programme Early CT Score. Lancet 2000;355:1670–1674.

42. Brandt T, Knauth M, Wildermuth S, et al. CT angiography and Doppler sonography for emergency assessment in acute basilar artery ischemia. Stroke 1999;30:606–612.

43. Wildermuth S, Knauth M, Brandt T, et al. Role of CT angiography in patient selection for thrombolytic

therapy in acute hemispheric stroke. Stroke 1998; 29(5):935–938.

44. Shrier DA, Tanaka H, Numaguchi Y, et al. CT angiography in the evaluation of acute stroke. AJNR Am J Neuroradiol 1997;18(6):1011–1020.

45. Lev MH, Nichols SJ. Computed tomographic angiography and computed tomographic perfusion imaging of hyperacute stroke. Top Magn Reson Imaging 2000;11(5):273–287.

46. Knauth M, von Kummer R, Jansen O, et al. Potential of CT angiography in acute ischemic stroke. AJNR Am J Neuroradiol 1997;18(6):1001–1010.

47. Latchaw RE, Yonas H, Pentheny SL, Gur D. Adverse reactions to xenon-enhanced CT cerebral blood flow determination. Radiology 1987;163(1):251–254.

48. Heiss WD, Graf R, Grond M, Rudolf J. Quantitative neuroimaging for the evaluation of the effect of stroke treatment. Cerebrovasc Dis 1998;8(Suppl 2):23–29.

49. Baron JC, Marchal G. Ischemic core and penumbra in human stroke. Stroke 1999;30:1150–1153.

50. Furlan M, Marchal G, Viader F, et al. Spontaneous neurological recovery after stroke and the fate of the ischemic penumbra. Ann Neurol 1996;40(2):216–226.

51. Jovin TG, Goldstein S, Gebel J, et al. Patterns of core and penumbra in acute MI occlusion and their clinical correlates. Stroke 2001;32(1):348.

52. Jovin T, Yonas H, Nemoto EM, et al. The ischemic core follows a predictable time course in acute middle cerebral artery infarction. Neurology 2001; 56(8)(Suppl 3):A369.

53. Firlik AD, Rubin G, Yonas H, Wechsler LR. Relation between cerebral blood flow and neurologic deficit resolution in acute ischemic stroke. Neurology 1998;51(1):177–182.

54. Kilpatrick MM, Yonas H, Goldstein S, et al. CT-based assessment of acute stroke: CT, CT angiography, and xenon-enhanced CT cerebral blood flow. Stroke 2001;32:2543–2549.

55. Hunter GJ, Hamberg LM, Ponzo JA, et al. Assessment of cerebral perfusion and arterial anatomy in hyperacute stroke with three-dimensional functional CT: early clinical results. AJNR Am J Neuroradiol 1998;19(1):29–37.

56. Lee KH, Lee SJ, Cho SJ, et al. Usefulness of triphasic perfusion computed tomography for intravenous thrombolysis with tissue-type plasminogen activator in acute ischemic stroke. Arch Neurol 2000; 57(7):1000–1008.

57. Lee KH, Cho SJ, Byun HS, et al. Triphasic perfusion computed tomography in acute middle cerebral artery stroke: a correlation with angiographic findings. Arch Neurol 2000;57(7):990–999.

58. Rother J, Jonetz-Mentzel L, Fiala A, et al. Hemodynamic assessment of acute stroke using dynamic single-slice computed tomographic perfusion imaging. Arch Neurol 2000;57(8):1161–1166.

59. Mayer TE, Hamann GF, Baranczyk J, et al. Dynamic CT perfusion imaging of acute stroke. AJNR Am J Neuroradiol 2000;21(8):1441–1449.

60. Wintermark M, Reichhart M, Thiran JP, et al. Prognostic accuracy of cerebral blood flow measurement by perfusion computed tomography, at the time of emergency room admission, in acute stroke patients. Ann Neurol 2002;51:417–432.

61. Lev MH, Segal AZ, Farkas J, et al. Utility of perfusion-weighted CT imaging in acute middle cerebral artery stroke treated with intra-arterial thrombolysis: prediction of final infarct volume and clinical outcome. Stroke 2001;32:2021–2028.

62. Fisher M, Albers GW. Applications of diffusion-perfusion magnetic resonance imaging in acute ischemic stroke. Neurology 1999;52(9):1750–1756.

63. Kohno K, Hoehn-Berlage M, Mies G, et al. Relationship between diffusion-weighted MR images, cerebral blood flow, and energy state in experimental brain infarction. Magn Reson Imaging 1995;13(1):73–80.

64. Yoneda Y, Tokui K, Hanihara T, et al. Diffusion-weighted magnetic resonance imaging: detection of ischemic injury 39 minutes after onset in a stroke patient. Ann Neurol 1999;45(6):794–797.

65. Schlaug G, Siewert B, Benfield A, et al. Time course of the apparent diffusion coefficient (ADC) abnormality in human stroke. Neurology 1997;49(1):113–119.

66. Tong DC, Yenari MA, Albers GW, et al. Correlation of perfusion- and diffusion-weighted MRI with NIHSS score in acute (6.5 hour) ischemic stroke. Neurology 1998;50(4):864–870.

67. Kelly PJ, Hedley-Whyte ET, Primavera J, et al. Diffusion MRI in ischemic stroke compared to pathologically verified infarction. Neurology 2001;56(7):914–920.

68. Lovblad KO, Baird AE, Schlaug G, et al. Ischemic lesion volumes in acute stroke by diffusion-weighted magnetic resonance imaging correlate with clinical outcome. Ann Neurol 1997;42:164–170.

69. Barber PA, Darby DG, Desmond PM, et al. Prediction of stroke outcome with echoplanar perfusion- and diffusion-weighted MRI. Neurology 1998;51: 418–426.

70. Kidwell CS, Saver JL, Mattiello J, et al. Thrombolytic reversal of acute human cerebral ischemic injury shown by diffusion/perfusion magnetic resonance imaging. Ann Neurol 2000;47:462–469.

71. Krueger K, Kugel H, Grond M, et al. Late resolution of diffusion-weighted MRI changes in a patient with prolonged reversible ischemic neurological deficit after thrombolytic therapy. Stroke 2000;31:2715–2718.

72. Calamante F, Thomas DL, Pell GS, et al. Measuring cerebral blood flow using magnetic resonance

imaging techniques. J Cereb Blood Flow Metab 1999;19:701–735.

73. Neumann-Haefelin T, Wittsack HJ, Wenserski F, et al. Diffusion- and perfusion-weighted MRI. The DWI/PWI mismatch region in acute stroke. Stroke 1999;30:1591–1597.

74. Schlaug G, Benfield A, Baird AE, et al. The ischemic penumbra: operationally defined by diffusion and perfusion MRI. Neurology 1999;53:1528–1537.

75. Schellinger PD, Fiebach JB, Jansen O, et al. Stroke magnetic resonance imaging within 6 hours after onset of hyperacute cerebral ischemia. Ann Neurol 2001;49:460–469.

76. Schellinger PD, Jansen O, Fiebach JB, et al. Feasibility and practicality of MR imaging of stroke in the management of hyperacute cerebral ischemia. AJNR Am J Neuroradiol 2000;21:1184–1189.

77. Schellinger PD, Jansen O, Fiebach JB, et al. A standardized MRI stroke protocol: comparison with CT in hyperacute intracerebral hemorrhage. Stroke 1999;30:765–768.

78. Baird AE, Benfield A, Schlaug G, et al. Enlargement of human cerebral ischemic lesion volumes measured by diffusion-weighted magnetic resonance imaging. Ann Neurol 1997;41:581–589.

79. Pereira AC, Saunders DE, Doyle VL, et al. Measurement of initial *N*-acetyl aspartate concentration by magnetic resonance spectroscopy and initial infarct volume by MRI predicts outcome in patients with middle cerebral artery territory infarction. Stroke 1999;30:1577–1582.

80. Barker PB, Gillard JH, van Zijl PC, et al. Acute stroke: evaluation with serial proton MR spectroscopic imaging. Radiology 1994;192:723–732.

81. Thulborn KR, Gindin TS, Davis D, Erb P. Comprehensive MR imaging protocol for stroke management: tissue sodium concentration as a measure of tissue viability in nonhuman primate studies and in clinical studies. Radiology 1999;213:156–166.

82. Remonda L, Heid O, Schroth G. Carotid artery stenosis, occlusion, and pseudo-occlusion: first-pass, gadolinium-enhanced, three-dimensional MR angiography—preliminary study. Radiology 1998;209:95–102.

83. Sardanelli F, Zandrino F, Parodi RC, De Caro G. MR angiography of internal carotid arteries: breath-hold Gd-enhanced 3D fast imaging with steady-state precession versus unenhanced 2D and 3D time-of-flight techniques. J Comput Assist Tomogr 1999;23:208–215.

84. Heiss WD, Kracht L, Grond M, et al. Early [(11)C]flumazenil/H(2)O positron emission tomography predicts irreversible ischemic cortical damage in stroke patients receiving acute thrombolytic therapy. Stroke 2000;31:366–369.

85. Heiss WD, Grond M, Thiel A, et al. Permanent cortical damage detected by flumazenil positron emission tomography in acute stroke. Stroke 1998; 29:454–461.

86. Heiss WD, Grond M, Thiel A, et al. Tissue at risk of infarction rescued by early reperfusion: a positron emission tomography study in systemic recombinant tissue plasminogen activator thrombolysis of acute stroke. J Cereb Blood Flow Metab 1998; 18:1298–1307.

87. Marchal G, Bouvard G, Iglesias S, et al. Predictive value of (99m)Tc-HMPAO-SPECT for neurological outcome/recovery at the acute stage of stroke. Cerebrovasc Dis 2000;10:8–17.

88. Ueda T, Sakaki S, Yuh WT, et al. Outcome in acute stroke with successful intra-arterial thrombolysis and predictive value of initial single-photon emission-computed tomography. J Cereb Blood Flow Metab 1999;19:99–108.

89. Ogasawara K, Ogawa A, Doi M, et al. Prediction of acute embolic stroke outcome after local intra-arterial thrombolysis: value of pretreatment and posttreatment 99mTc-ethyl cysteinate dimer single photon emission computed tomography. J Cereb Blood Flow Metab 2000;20:1579–1586.

90. Shimosegawa E, Hatazawa J, Inugami A, et al. Cerebral infarction within six hours of onset: prediction of completed infarction with technetium-99m-HMPAO SPECT. J Nucl Med 1994;35:1097–1103.

91. Demchuk AM, Christou I, Wein TH, et al. Accuracy and criteria for localizing arterial occlusion with transcranial Doppler. J Neuroimaging 2000;10:1–12.

92. Babikian VL, Feldmann E, Wechsler LR, et al. Transcranial Doppler ultrasonography: year 2000 update. J Neuroimaging 2000;10:101–115.

93. Nabavi DG, Droste DW, Schulte-Altedorneburg G, et al. Diagnostic benefit of echocontrast enhancement for the insufficient transtemporal bone window. J Neuroimaging 1999;9:102–107.

94. Postert T, Braun B, Meves S, et al. Contrast-enhanced transcranial color-coded sonography in acute hemispheric brain infarction. Stroke 1999;30:1819–1826.

95. Burgin WS, Malkoff M, Felberg RA, et al. Transcranial Doppler ultrasound criteria for recanalization after thrombolysis for middle cerebral artery stroke. Stroke 2000;31:1128–1132.

96. Alexandrov AV, Demchuk AM, Felberg RA, et al. Intracranial clot dissolution is associated with embolic signals on transcranial Doppler. J Neuroimaging 2000;10:27–32.

97. Alexandrov AV, Demchuk AM, Felberg RA, et al. High rate of complete recanalization and dramatic clinical recovery during tPA infusion when continuously monitored with 2-MHz transcranial doppler monitoring. Stroke 2000;31(3):610–614.

CHAPTER

11

Cerebral Infarction during Its Subacute Stage

David E. Thaler, Michael A. Sloan, and Viken L. Babikian

The overwhelming majority of stroke patients comes to medical attention within the first week from the onset of stroke symptoms but after the first 6 hours. Thrombolysis is not likely to be useful during this time except in unusual circumstances. These patients face predictable medical and neurologic complications. Imaging data in this setting are acquired to confirm the diagnosis, monitor the progression of tissue changes, understand the mechanism of ischemia, plan treatment, and assess prognosis.

DIAGNOSTIC CONFIRMATION

It is estimated that 5–15% of patients presenting to medical attention with a diagnosis of brain infarction have their original diagnosis changed after a complete evaluation. Intraparenchymal hemorrhage, brain tumor, subdural hematoma, or intracranial infection can present with symptoms mimicking those of brain ischemia. Neuroimaging studies are useful for discriminating between these etiologies and establishing a definitive diagnosis. Noncontrast-enhanced brain computed tomography (CT) or magnetic resonance imaging (MRI) studies are considered standard practice in the United States. A precise and early diagnosis is important for obvious therapeutic reasons.

In addition to their role in diagnosis, imaging studies help in monitoring the progression of brain parenchymal changes during the first week. Acute brain infarcts are dynamic lesions, and they evolve rapidly during the first 2–4 weeks. Radiographic studies are particularly useful during this period to monitor mass effect and hemorrhagic transformation.

Radiographic Signs of Acute Cerebral Infarction

A number of findings consistent with ischemia may be demonstrated on imaging studies performed during the acute stage that follows the first 6 hours. The ability of CT and MRI to show these ischemic lesions depends on several factors: the generation of the CT or MRI scanner; MRI sequences; lesion age, location, and size; severity of ischemia; and use of contrast enhancement. In general, the evolution of the appearance of ischemic lesions on CT or MRI studies reflects the neuropathologic processes occurring at the cellular level.

During the first 24 hours after the onset of a nonlacunar ischemic stroke, CT scanning may show a poorly demarcated area of subtle decrease in density of the gray or white matter. The gray matter may become isodense with white matter and lead to a blurring of the gray-white junction. This finding represents intracellular cytotoxic edema; its presence in a vascular distribution becomes more distinct in the first few days after stroke onset. By 8 hours after stroke onset, approximately 20% of CT scans are abnormal.[1,2] Specific signs of early infarction that have been reported include the hyperdense middle cerebral artery (MCA) sign suggesting acute MCA occlusion by an embolus (Figure 11-1); attenuation of the lentiform nucleus; loss of the insular ribbon; hemisphere sulcal effacement (Figure 11-2); and the hyperdense sylvian fissure "MCA dot" sign, a marker of occlusion of MCA branch(es) in the sylvian fissure.[3,4] In one study[3] of patients imaged during the 14 hours after stroke onset, the hyperdense MCA sign, when present, was usually accompanied by at least one of the other early signs of brain infarction. Intravenous contrast

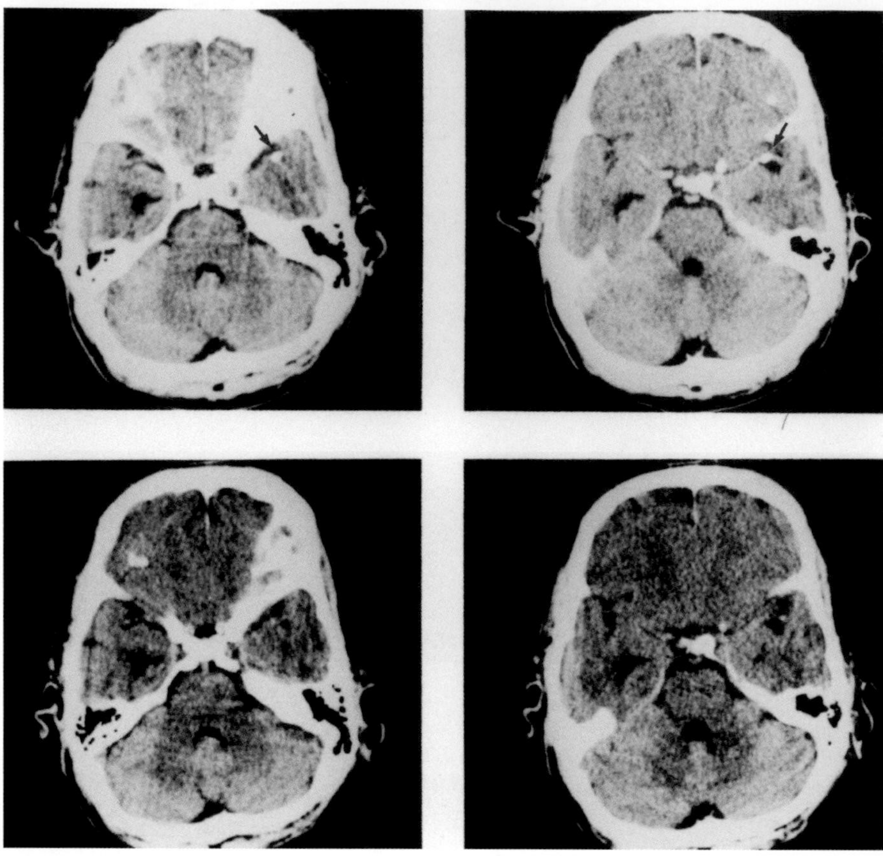

FIGURE 11-1. Embolus in the middle cerebral artery. A brain computed tomography scan obtained 2 hours after the onset of symptoms of brain infarction shows an embolus (*arrows*) caught in the left middle cerebral artery M1 segment (**top**). A repeat study 24 hours later (**bottom**) shows passage of the embolus. (Reprinted with permission from the American Roentgen Ray Society/Am J Roentgenol.)

agents used with CT and MRI scans can extravasate into the area of the infarction. This is thought to be due to a breakdown of the blood-brain barrier in those areas. It is more evident on T1-weighted MRI scans.[5]

In general, MRI is superior to CT for the detection of cerebral infarcts.[6] The earliest changes in the infarct region are low (dark) signal on T1-weighted images and high (bright) signal on T2-weighted images, reflecting prolongation of T1 and T2 relaxation times by an increase in tissue water content. Abnormal MRI findings may be present within 1–3 hours of stroke onset but are more reliably found after 8 hours, reaching a maximum at 24–48 hours.[7,8] Negative MRI studies may be observed in 7–20% of acute stroke patients and may relate to lesion size and location and strength of the magnet.[9] Diffusion-weighted MRI (DWI) is particularly useful in detecting areas of acute brain infarction,[10] and fluid-attenuated inversion recovery sequences produce a strong T2 signal and a suppressed cerebrospinal fluid signal, leading to improved detection of cortical or periventricular infarcts.[11] Diffusion-weighted images have a false-negative rate of approximately 6%. The detection rate is lower for lesions located in the posterior fossa and during the first 24 hours of brain infarction.[12]

In the absence of cerebral infarction, areas of poor perfusion may be detectable with MRI scanning. This is true even for MRI scanners, which are not capable of perfusion-weighted imaging (PWI). Vascular enhancement or the hyperintense artery sign may reflect the presence of slow flow associated with large vessel stenosis or occlusion and an inadequate collateral circulation.[13]

Mass Effect

Over the first 7 days after stroke onset, CT and MRI scans demonstrate the emergence of mass effect that reflects tissue necrosis and edema. Edema can be seen within hours from the onset of stroke, and edematous areas expand, causing mass effect. The greatest degree of mass effect occurs within 3–5 days.[14–17] Neuroimaging studies are particularly useful during this period because the clinical assessment of mass effect may be difficult in patients with severe deficits.

The neuroimaging appearance differs depending on the location of the infarct. Above the tentorium, there may be effacement of sulci, compression of the ipsilateral lateral ventricle, midline shift, displacement of the septum pellucidum, dilation of the contralateral temporal horn, and lateral displacement of the pineal gland. In the infratentorial compartment, the posterior fossa appears "tight" as the cerebrospinal fluid spaces, including cisterns and ventricles, become compressed. An especially ominous sign for the development of hydrocephalus is compression of the fourth ventricle. Another sign may also be torsion of the brain stem. The demonstration of secondary bleeding in the pons (Duret's hemorrhages) is rare. On occasion,

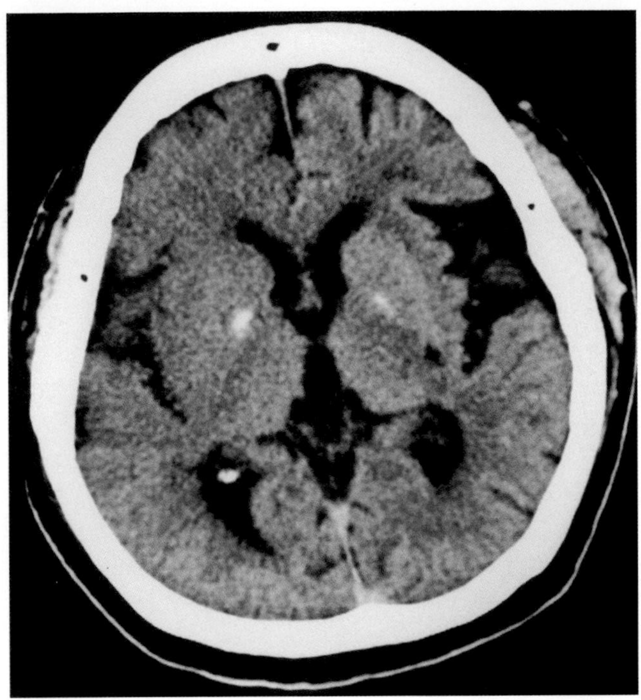
A

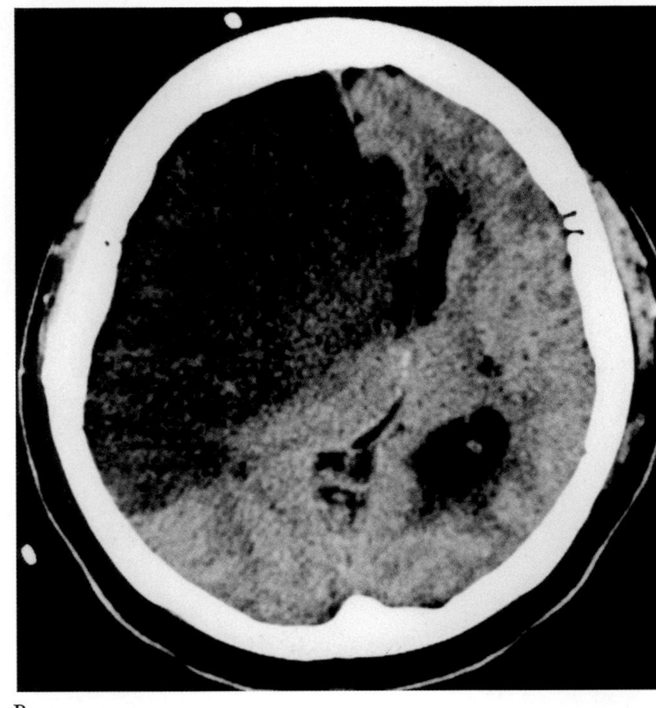
B

FIGURE 11-2. Early infarct signs and subacute cerebral edema. **A.** Computed tomography image of a patient presenting with a right middle cerebral artery syndrome taken several hours after symptom onset. There is asymmetry in the appearance of the cortex in the insula. There is a subtle loss of differentiation of the internal capsule from the basal ganglia on the right. Two days later (**B**), the patient was deeply comatose and developed a Babinski's sign on the right (Kernohan's notch phenomenon). There is severe edema of the right middle and anterior cerebral artery territories, with mass effect and midline shift to the left.

transtentorial herniation of the temporal lobe is accompanied by extrinsic compression of the posterior cerebral artery, causing a secondary infarction in that territory.

The amount of lateral brain displacement seen on CT scans correlates with the change in the level of consciousness.[18] Displacement of the septum pellucidum occurs before the lateral displacement of the pineal gland.[19] The degree of horizontal midline displacement of the latter correlates with the risk of early death.[20] A displacement of 4 mm or more, as measured by CT, identifies patients at a particularly increased risk.[20] In several studies,[19,21–25] age older than 45 years, persistent hypertension, presence of hyperdense MCA sign, early brain swelling, and CT hypodensity of more than 50% of the MCA territory have been associated with herniation, neurologic deterioration, and death. If there is a hypodense area that encompasses more than 50% of the MCA territory within 18 hours of stroke onset, malignant MCA infarction develops in 90% of cases.[26]

Hemorrhagic Transformation

Bleeding into an area of cerebral infarction is known as *hemorrhagic transformation*. This is often confused with a primary intracerebral hemorrhage. The subject has been extensively reviewed.[27–33] Hemorrhagic transformation may be diagnosed by the appearance of blood within the presumed ischemic infarct location if blood densities are not present on the initial CT image, or if blood densities on the first CT scan are surrounded by a larger hypodense area that appears consistent with an area of ischemic stroke[32] (Figure 11-3). Hemorrhagic transformation usually results from the restoration of blood flow into a recently ischemic area that contains abnormal blood vessels. Permeability changes in the blood-brain barrier occur between 2 and 6 hours after experimental focal ischemia and reperfusion. Mild to moderate bleeding is believed to result from diapedesis through ischemic endothelium. Severe bleeding, leading to confluent hematomas, occurs when vessel walls rupture (Figure 11-4). Significant acute hypertension may contribute to or produce hemorrhagic transformation in the setting of persistent vessel occlusion, presumably by accentuating retrograde flow into damaged blood vessels through leptomeningeal collaterals.

The frequency of hemorrhagic transformation is up to 71% in pathologic studies and 5–43% in CT-based studies of patients with cardioembolic stroke. DWI and perfusion-weighted MRI techniques may improve its early detection.[34] Hemorrhagic transformation usually develops within the first few days after stroke onset but may occur up to 2 weeks later. In rare patients with

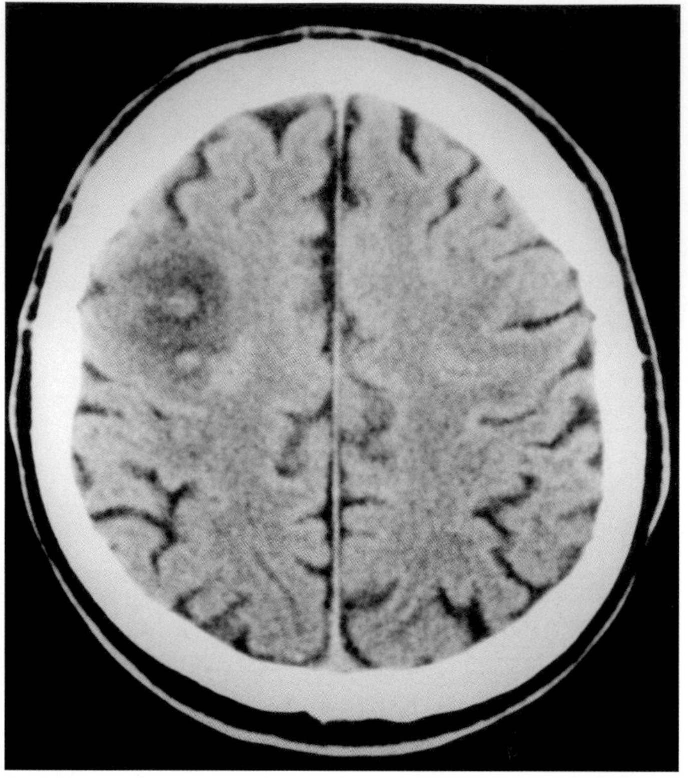

A

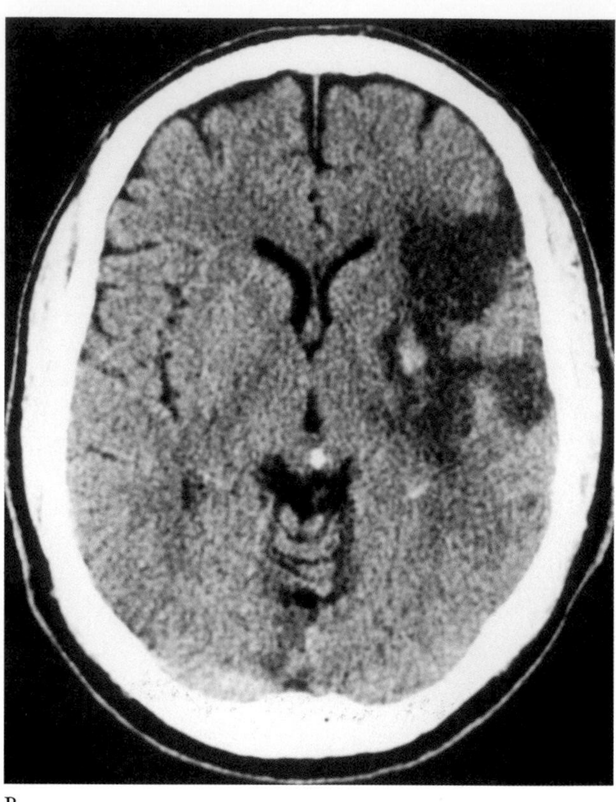

B

FIGURE 11-3. **A,B.** Spontaneous hemorrhagic transformation. Examples of hemorrhagic transformation seen on computed tomography scans several days after ischemic strokes. These patients were not treated with systemic anticoagulation.

ischemic infarction, the CT scan may show what appears to be a primary intracerebral hemorrhage a few days later.[35] Whether these constitute extreme cases of hemorrhagic transformation is not known, nor is the role of antithrombotic agents in the pathogenesis of hemorrhage in this setting clearly understood.

Risk factors for hemorrhagic transformation include severe neurologic deficit, depressed level of consciousness, large infarct size, early infarct signs on CT scan, significant reduction in apparent diffusion coefficient on DWI scan, mass effect, and brain shift across the midline.[29,31,32,36–38] The majority of hemorrhagic transformations are asymptomatic. This helps to distinguish them from primary intracerebral hemorrhages, which typically cause symptoms unless they are very small.

Radiographic Signs of Subacute and Chronic Cerebral Infarction

During the period from 8 to 21 days, mass effect and edema gradually subside and resolve. When the resolution of mass effect and edema leads to an isodense area on CT scan, the infarct may become less conspicuous due to the so-called fogging effect (Figure 11-5).[39,40] On MRI scanning, signal changes are similar to the earlier time phase, with hypointensity on T1-weighted images and hyperintensity on T2-weighted images. Contrast enhancement occurs on both CT and MRI.[41–43] The pattern of contrast enhancement is gyral with cortical infarction (see Figure 11-5) and ring-like in deep basal ganglia infarction. The gyral pattern may be diagnostically useful when there is a question of brain infarction versus tumor invasion. Subtle enhancement is detected more easily with MRI than with CT scanning.[5] Contrast enhancement of CT scans may be needed to visualize the infarction during the time in which the fogging effect may be present.

The chronic phase of infarction begins a few weeks after stroke onset. On CT and MRI images, the lesion appears as a distinct, well-marginated zone of cystic encephalomalacia. The density on CT or intensity on MRI is similar to cerebrospinal fluid. There is usually a surrounding area of gliosis that is seen best on MRI fluid-attenuated inversion recovery sequences. Calcification may be seen on some CT scans. For cortical infarctions, there is loss of brain tissue volume and the development of prominent cortical sulci. There is usually compensatory dilation of the adjacent lateral ventricle. Wallerian degeneration of motor fibers may produce atrophy along the course of a corticospinal tract, which is often seen as a marked asymmetry at the level of the

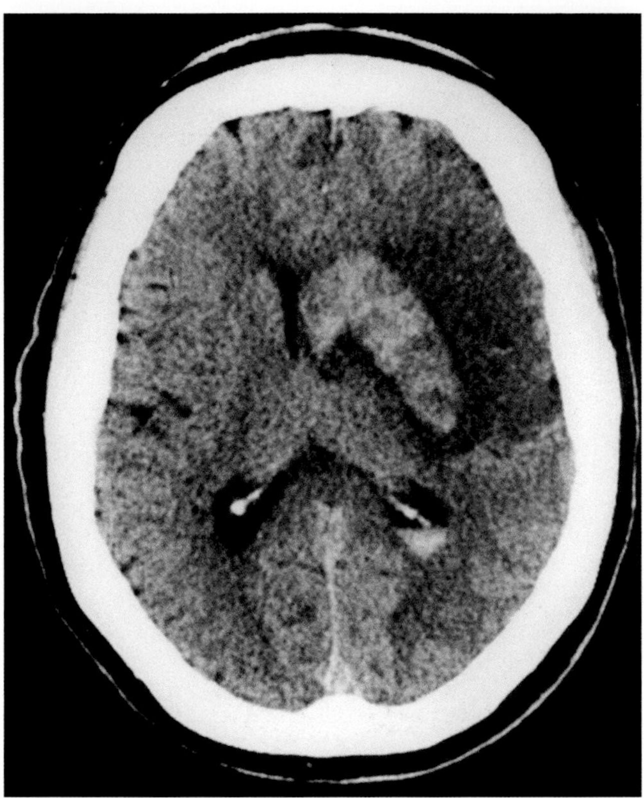

FIGURE 11-4. Hematoma after anticoagulation. Confluent hematoma in a subacute infarct. This patient was receiving intravenous heparin. The hematoma ruptured into the ventricular system, with pooling of blood visible in the occipital horn of the left lateral ventricle.

cerebral peduncles. Contrast enhancement subsides within 6–8 weeks. This suggests that the integrity of the blood-brain barrier has become reestablished.

UNDERSTANDING MECHANISM

Stroke diagnosis is inferential. This is subjective and error-prone because the clinician uses judgment to assign a mechanism to a particular brain infarct. The problem is complicated by the facts that stroke is a heterogeneous disease and that an individual patient often has more than one potential explanation for his or her infarct.[44] An adequate evaluation of a stroke patient is geared at detecting all potential causes of brain ischemia and identifying the ones pertinent to the infarct. Therapy is tailored to the most likely mechanism given all the circumstances of the case, including the patient's preference.

Knowledge of the clinical and radiologic characteristics of stroke subtypes can help in identifying mechanism. An exhaustive list of all stroke subtypes and their radiologic patterns is beyond the scope of this chapter. In the following section, we focus on the major stroke subtypes and their common radiologic patterns.

Small Deep Infarcts and Lacunes

Few terms have been more widely misused than *lacunar stroke*. A *lacune* can be defined as an ischemic brain lesion in the territory of a single penetrating artery. Many physicians use the term to describe infarcts that are small in volume. Others use it to describe patients with minor neurologic deficits. Given that strokes of small volume can be caused by small emboli and that lacunes can cause severe deficits, these are mistaken assumptions. The initial description of the lacunar syndromes was on the basis of careful clinical and pathologic observations,[45–49] and the classic lacunar syndromes are presented in Table 11-1.

Lesions corresponding to these syndromes are usually located in the territories of the small penetrating arteries (Figure 11-6). A correlation with hypertension and hypertensive arteriolopathy is recognized. The utility of the lacunar hypothesis rests, in part, in the suggestion that the underlying pathophysiology is predicted by the syndrome. Although there is little doubt that the clinical presentation strongly suggests a small lesion in the deep parts of the brain, the pathophysiologic mechanism is not always so clear.

In a patient with vascular risk factors who presents with a typical lacunar syndrome, if the MRI demonstrates a single lesion in the appropriate location, then the diagnosis is fairly secure. However, some caution against overconfidence when confronted with a clinical lacunar syndrome is in order. DWI scans done in patients with lacunar syndromes show multiple acute infarcts in up to one out of six patients,[50] and embolic sources can often be found in this setting. This argues for a thorough investigation of all patients even if they present with "just a lacune." Some radiologic and clinical characteristics may help to distinguish small vessel disease from embolism in patients with small deep strokes—namely, secondary hemorrhagic transformation, subinsular involvement, and better recovery of neurologic deficits.[51]

The presence of older, clinically silent lesions in typical lacunar locations is supporting evidence for small vessel disease. There may also be varying amounts of increased T2 signal present in the periventricular white matter. This is variably referred to as *periventricular white-matter disease*, *ischemic-gliotic change*, or *leukoariosis*. The hemispheric white matter is primarily supplied by long penetrating arteries originating at right angles from the cortical pial network. The subcortical U fibers receive their blood supply from shorter vessels supplying the cortex and white matter. The periventricular white matter receives its blood supply from ventriculofugal branches of subependymal arteries that also supply the basal ganglia, internal capsule, and part of the thalamus.

The term *leukoariosis* was coined to describe periventricular or subcortical areas of hypodensity on

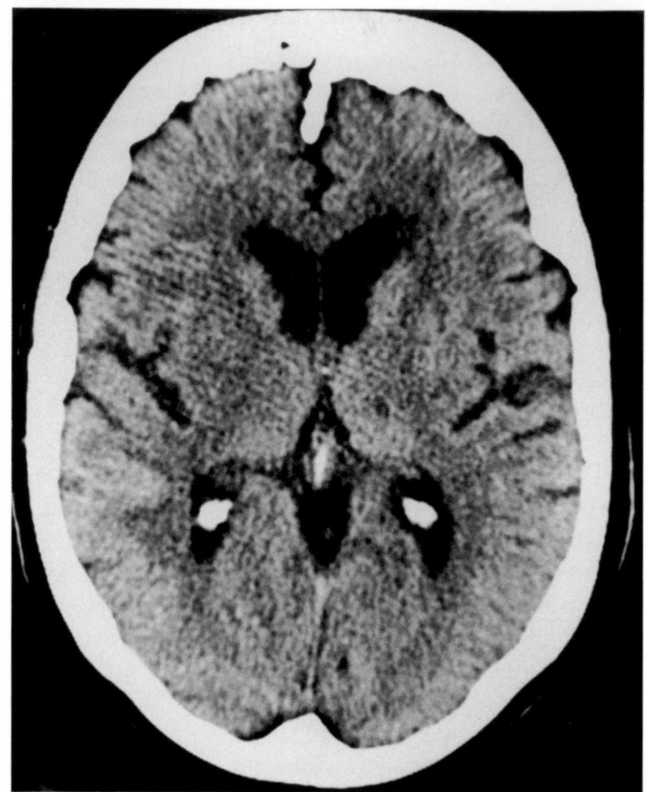

A

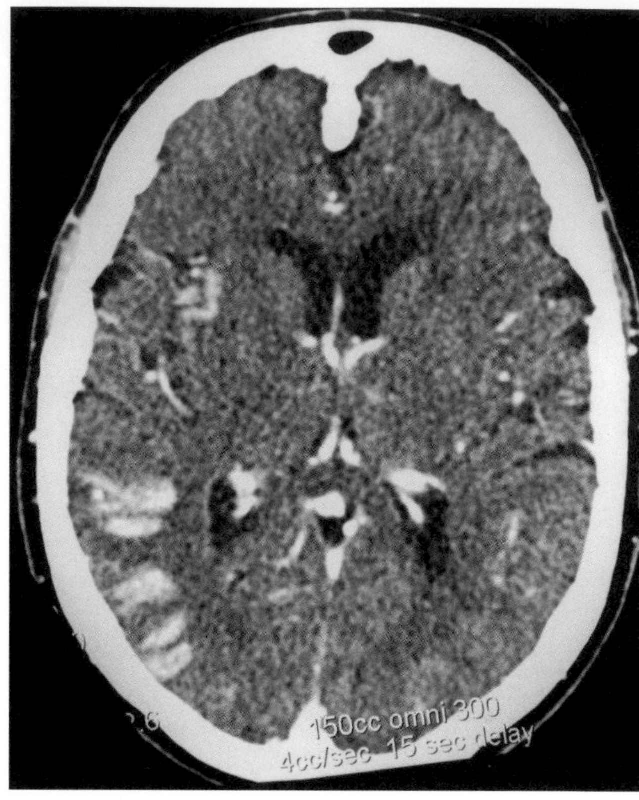

B

FIGURE 11-5. Subacute "fogging" effect and contrast enhancement. Computed tomography image of a patient seen 2 weeks after developing a right parietal syndrome. The unenhanced image (**A**) was read as normal. After the administration of intravenous contrast, the gyral enhancement clearly demonstrates the area of infarction (**B**). The patient's cardiac pacemaker precluded the use of magnetic resonance imaging.

CT or hyperintensity on MRI T2-weighted sequences.[52] The most common risk factor for leukoariosis is aging, but hypertension and cardiac disease are also associated with it.[53–61] The combined effects of aging (lengthening, tortuosity, and reduced lumen of long penetrating vessels) and hypertension (lipohyalinosis, arteriolosclerosis, and fibrinoid necrosis) may raise the minimum blood pressure needed to perfuse the distal aspects of the periventricular white matter. Thus, normal or relatively low blood pressure levels and several other hemodynamic variables may lead to deep white-matter hypoperfusion, particularly in the elderly.[56,58–60,62] Decreased vasomotor reactivity to carbon dioxide inhalation has been reported in elderly patients with periventricular white-matter lesions,[63] and it may be a marker of small vessel disease. Binswanger's disease may be a more extreme example of this phenomenon.[59,64,65] Despite all of these observations, histopathologic data on the subject are sparse.

TABLE 11-1. Localization of Typical Lacunar Syndromes

Syndrome	*Typical localization*
Pure motor stroke	Internal capsule, basis pontis
Pure sensory stroke	Lateral thalamus
Ataxic hemiparesis	Pons, internal capsule/thalamus, corona

Small Cortical Infarcts

Single and small cortical infarcts are often seen in the MCA territory.[66] Atherosclerotic narrowing of the ipsilateral internal carotid artery (ICA) and cardiac lesions associated with embolism are the most commonly identified pathologies in those patients. Together, they account for over half of all superficial anterior circulation strokes,[67] suggesting that embolic occlusion of distal pial MCA arterioles is the most likely mechanism for the stroke. Small vessel disease and in situ thrombosis are not common in pial vessels. Atherosclerotic debris and cardiogenic thrombi are not the only embolic particles, however. Infective endocarditis can produce friable vegetations; cardiac procedures can produce air embolism; and patent foramen ovale can allow the transit of venous thromboemboli into the

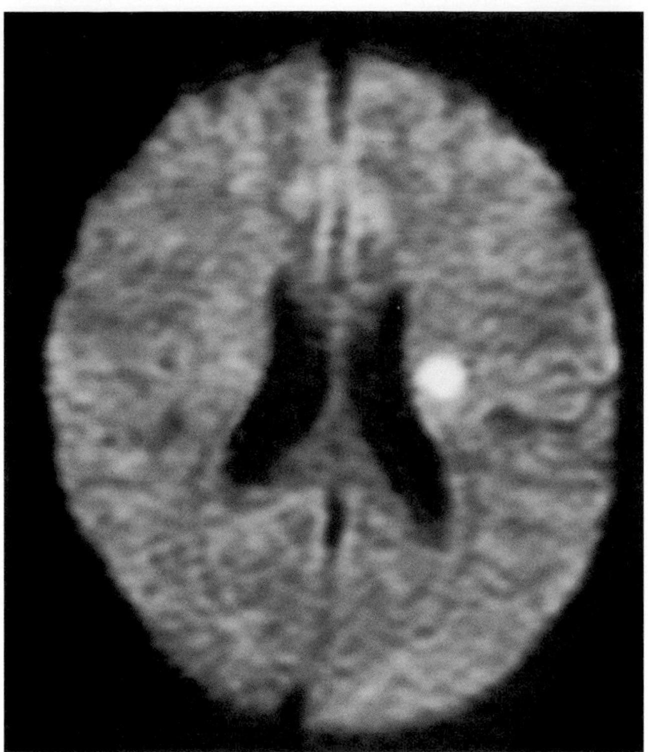

FIGURE 11-6. Lacunar infarction. Diffusion-weighted magnetic resonance image of a patient presenting with right hemiparesis. There is a lesion typical of a lacune in the left corona radiata.

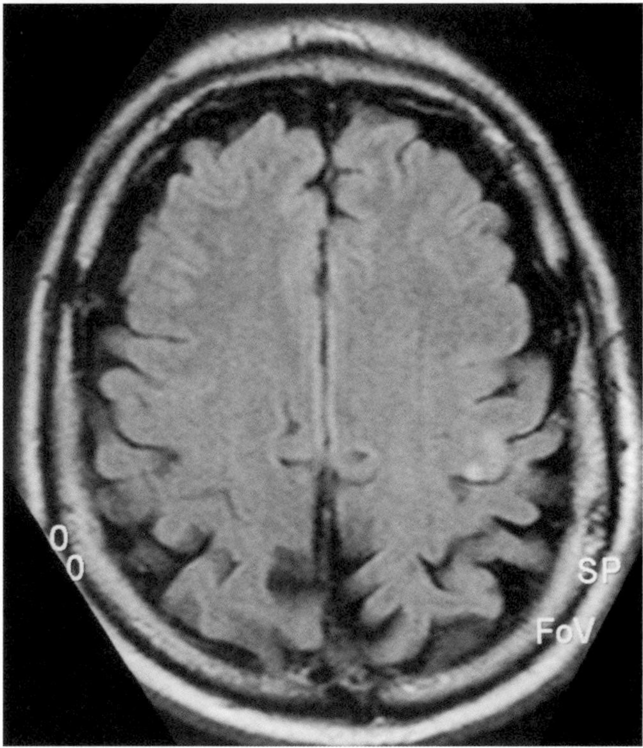

FIGURE 11-7. Small cortical infarction. Magnetic resonance image of a 46-year-old man who presented with right face and hand weakness. He had a patent foramen ovale. The fluid-attenuated inversion recovery image shows a bright signal in the left posterior frontal lobe. The finding was confirmed by the diffusion-weighted image and apparent diffusion coefficient map.

arterial side of the circulation, causing paradoxic embolization (Figure 11-7).

Similar mechanisms cause posterior cerebral circulation infarcts. Extracranial vertebral artery stenosis, usually in the V4 segment, plays a role analogous to that of extracranial ICA lesions. Vertebral artery stenoses are not detected regularly, in part because of the lack of noninvasive vascular imaging methods.[68] Contrast-enhanced CT and magnetic resonance angiography (MRA) are now permitting better visualization of the V1 and V4 segments without the need for conventional angiography. Stenotic lesions at the vertebral artery origin may be responsible for approximately one-third of all small pial infarcts in the posterior circulation. This is a proportion similar to that attributed to ICA origin stenosis in the anterior circulation.

Large Hemispheric Infarcts

Large hemispheric infarction is often due to a confluence of factors, such as poor collateral arterial supply, insufficient washout of embolic particles, and inadequate spontaneous thrombolysis and recanalization that conspire against a good outcome. Large MCA or posterior cerebral artery territory infarcts are usually a result of embolic occlusions. The ICA is again a frequent donor of emboli, but the pathologic lesions vary.[69] They include ICA stenosis or occlusion secondary to atherosclerosis, thromboembolism, and dissection (Figure 11-8). Patients without ICA disease are usually found to have a cardiac source of embolism such as atrial fibrillation, severe left ventricular wall motion abnormalities, and prosthetic valves or native valvular disease.

For the larger posterior cerebral artery territory strokes, if there is no cardiac source of embolus, then artery-to-artery embolization is commonly found.[70] As is the case for small infarcts, vertebral artery atherostenosis is a common source of these emboli. A persistent fetal origin of a posterior cerebral artery may implicate an ICA source for a posterior circulation embolus.

Multiple Acute Infarcts

When patients present with multiple acute brain infarcts, parsimony suggests that there should not be a different diagnosis for each lesion. For example, although it is possible that a patient with acute infarcts in the cerebellum and the frontal lobe has both ICA and vertebral artery atherosclerotic lesions that became symptomatic simulta-

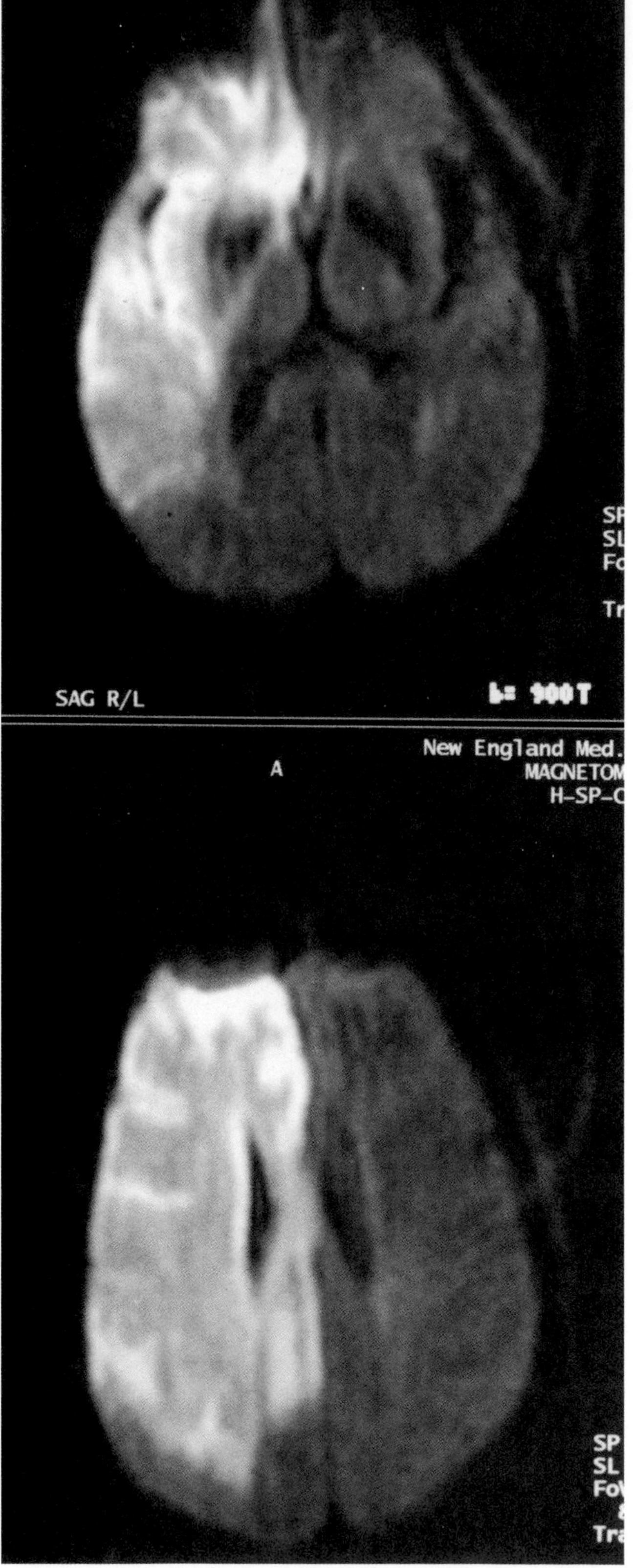

FIGURE 11-8. Large hemispheric infarction. Diffusion-weighted magnetic resonance image of a patient with an acute carotid occlusion. The entire right middle cerebral artery and anterior cerebral artery territories are infarcted.

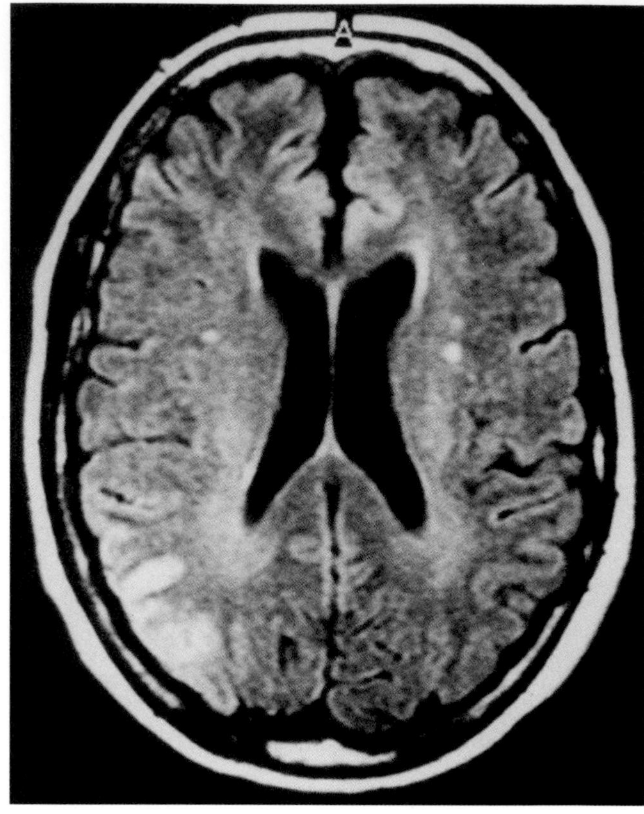

FIGURE 11-9. Multifocal brain embolism. The patient presented with a right parietal syndrome of sudden onset. The diffusion-weighted magnetic resonance image shows areas of restricted diffusion in the posterior right parietal lobe as well as the right and left periventricular white matter. This is consistent with embolism from a cardiac or aortic arch source. The patient was in atrial fibrillation. No other cerebrovascular lesions were detected.

neously, it would be more elegant to conclude that there was a proximal source, such as atrial fibrillation, that was responsible for both lesions. DWI is the most sensitive MRI sequence to detect multiple strokes[71] and enables detection of clinically unsuspected infarcts with regularity (Figure 11-9).[72] Unsuspected lesions are usually irrelevant in terms of neurologic impairment but may be critical for understanding the vascular etiology.

In a patient presenting with acute stroke, the discovery of one or more unsuspected areas of infarction in different vascular territories should prompt a search for a proximal source for embolism that might otherwise have been neglected. One study has examined the stroke etiology in patients with multiple acute strokes in different patterns.[73] Patients were divided into four groups based on the location of their infarcts: group A, one hemisphere, anterior circulation; group B, two hemispheres, anterior circulation; group C, posterior circulation; group D, anterior and posterior circulations. In groups A and C, the common etiology was large artery atherosclerosis because both ICA and vertebral artery disease were detected. In group B, many patients had an associated systemic abnormality such as a malignancy or hypercoagulable state. Group D included patients with cardiogenic embolism, isolated central nervous system angiitis, and other proximal sources of embolism such as catheter angiography. None of these groups had exclusive rights to a single etiologic category, implying that all patients deserve careful consideration of the etiology of their lesions. It should be noted that isolated central nervous system angiitis does not have a characteristic neuroradiologic picture and that single or multiple infarcts or intracranial hemorrhage can be present at the time of initial presentation.

Stroke between Vascular Territories: Borderzone Infarcts

Although physicians still use the term *insufficiency of arterial supply* to describe the cause of cerebral ischemia to colleagues and patients, true borderzone infarcts are relatively rare and account for less than 10% of all ischemic strokes.[74] They carry great etiologic significance because of therapeutic considerations. A key component of borderzone infarcts between the MCA and anterior cerebral artery is low perfusion pressure (Figure 11-10). Borderzone infarcts between the MCA and posterior cerebral artery territories are often associated with embolization.[75] Pathologic studies support the notion that capillaries in the borderzone territories may be particularly poor at clearing cerebral microemboli.[76] Unilateral borderzone strokes arise from a complex set of circumstances that includes large artery occlusive disease, decreased cerebral perfusion pressure, and the showering of microemboli that is usually of cholesterol. Bilateral borderzone strokes are more often associated with profound or prolonged decreases in blood pressure that might occur during cardiac bypass surgery or cardiac arrest.[75] They are more common in patients without any demonstrable large artery occlusive disease. PWI within 24 hours of symptom onset may be particularly helpful in determining stroke mechanism in this setting.[77]

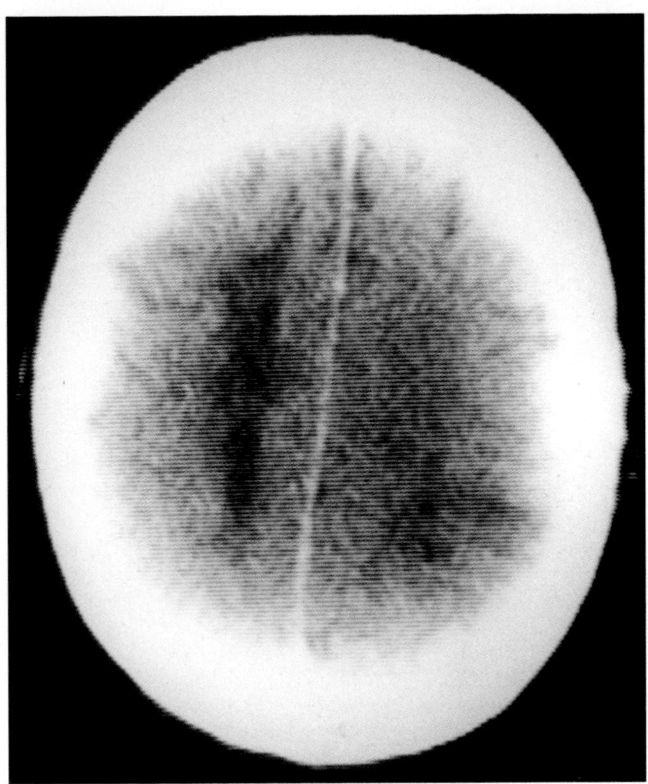

FIGURE 11-10. Borderzone infarct. This computed tomography scan shows evidence of borderzone infarction between the right middle and anterior cerebral artery territories in a patient with ipsilateral internal carotid artery stenosis. The scan also shows evidence of a previous infarct in the left posterior parietal region.

PLAN TREATMENT

Therapeutic Decisions in the Subacute Stage

As indicated at the beginning of this chapter, mass effect and hemorrhagic transformation are frequent complications after brain infarction. Initial treatment measures for brain edema and mass effect include relative dehydration of the brain with diuretics and hyperosmolar agents. When these measures fail, hyperventilation, barbiturates, and surgical decompression may be instituted. Of particular relevance in this context is the presence of mass effect in the posterior fossa (Figure 11-11). It can progress rapidly, leading to respiratory arrest and cardiac dysrhythmias. Decompression of the cerebellum can be lifesaving and is a generally accepted procedure.[78] Hemicraniectomy for patients with massive MCA infarction (see Figure 11-2) can be lifesaving, but it is not currently considered a standard procedure.[79] Neuroimaging studies are obtained to confirm the clinical impression and to rule out confounding complications such as intraparenchymal hemorrhage, infarct extension, or brain stem infarction.

Stroke in progression refers to the neurologic deterioration during the hours and days after the development of the initial symptoms of cerebral ischemia. Its frequency ranges between 10% and 30%.[80] In more than 50% of cases, progression occurs within the first 24 hours after presentation; in the remaining cases, progression usually occurs during the subsequent 3- or 4-day period.[80] The mechanism of progression has not been adequately studied, and it often remains undetermined in routine clinical practice. A high blood glucose level is an independent predictor of progression, and patients with brain hemorrhage and noncardioembolic infarction are at greater risk

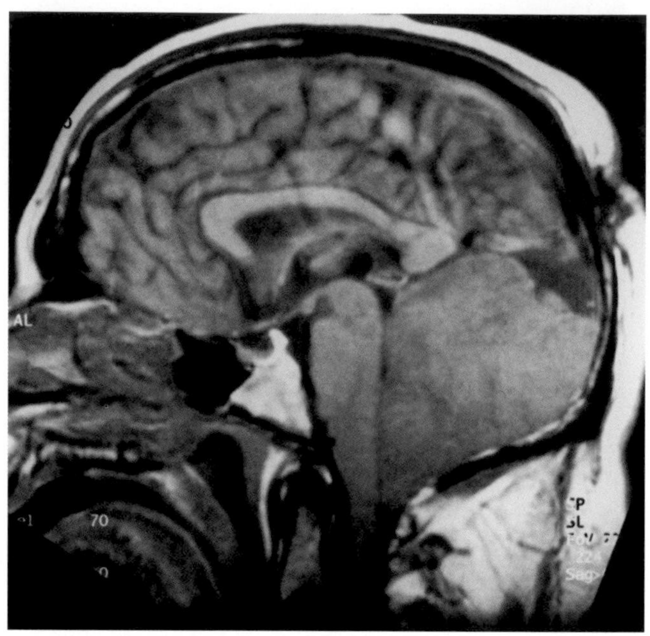

A

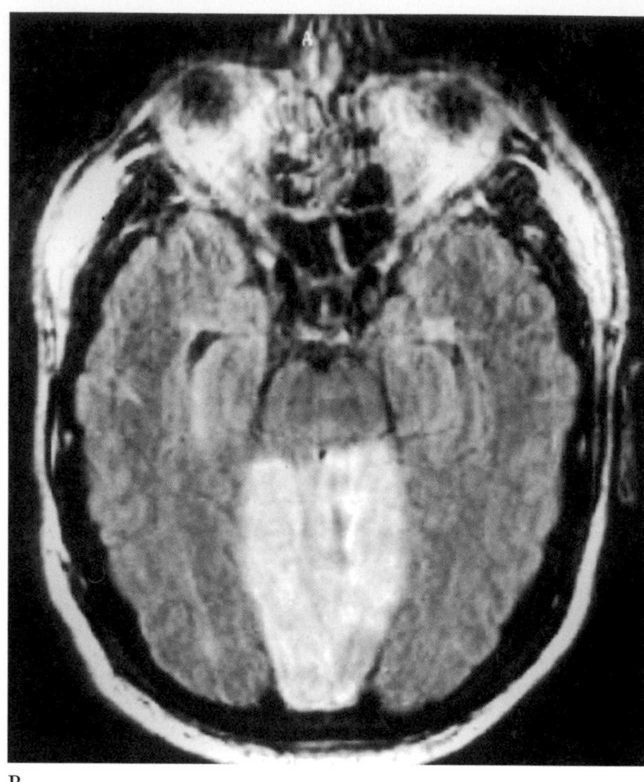

B

FIGURE 11-11. Massive posterior fossa swelling and herniation. **A.** Sagittal T1 magnetic resonance image of a patient with fatal expansion of the posterior fossa contents due to edema after a cerebellar infarct. Note the severe anterior, superior, and inferior herniation. The pons has been displaced anteriorly and is severely distorted. **B.** This axial fluid-attenuated inversion recovery magnetic resonance image is at the level of the pontomesencephalic junction. There is increased signal in the midline cerebellum that has herniated upward, obliterating the adjacent cerebrospinal fluid spaces.

for worsening.[81] Recurrent embolism is often suspected. Transcranial Doppler studies suggest that patients with carotid artery stenoses may have ongoing microembolization for a period of several days after the initial manifestations of cerebral ischemia.[82]

To prevent stroke progression or recurrence until the workup is completed, anticoagulation is occasionally prescribed to selected patients with a stroke that may be due to embolism. Patients with stenosis or occlusion of a large artery, such as the ICA, may benefit from early anticoagulation, but there are insufficient data from clinical trials to support this practice routinely.[83,84] The risks of causing or exacerbating a secondary intracranial hemorrhage must be weighed against the benefits of reducing recurrence and improving outcome. Conservative clinicians delay anticoagulation during the first few days after the onset of stroke symptoms. Some evidence suggests, however, that anticoagulants are acceptably safe even when hemorrhagic transformation has been demonstrated by imaging studies.[85,86] As indicated in the preceding paragraphs, hemorrhagic transformation is usually asymptomatic and does not require a specific treatment. Its detection often prompts tighter control of hypertension and frequent monitoring of the activated partial thromboplastin time and international normalized ratio. The relationship of hemorrhagic transformation to frank hemorrhage is not well understood.

Stroke in progression can also occur in hemodynamic or borderzone infarction. Inadequate collateral channels and severe stenosis or occlusion of the main artery may markedly limit brain blood flow. These relatively isolated brain regions are highly susceptible to absolute or relative hypotension. Treatment is aimed at optimizing perfusion pressure by keeping the head of the bed flat and allowing hypertension to be untreated. Induced hypertension may be useful and is the subject of ongoing study.[87]

The term *ischemic penumbra* was introduced to describe a region of hypoperfused but viable brain tissue surrounding an area of infarction. A penumbra is often detected in the hypoperfused brain regions described in the preceding paragraph. It was traditionally detected by positron emission tomography,[88] but DWI and PWI studies can also identify these areas (see Chapter 19). The penumbra can be detected in approximately one-third of acute stroke patients, and it can persist for many hours after the onset of symptoms.[88] Although it does not have any immediate treatment implications at the time of this writing, the finding of a penumbra theoretically expands the therapeutic window. In certain patients with a demonstrated region of uninfarcted but hypoperfused brain, thrombolytic or neuroprotective therapy could be effective long after time limits accepted today.

Although antithrombotic therapy is prescribed to most patients presenting with a stroke, not all embolic particles are composed of platelets and fibrin, and potentially helpful treatments are not provided when a correct diagnosis is missed. Neuroimaging studies can occasionally be helpful in determining the composition of emboli. Particles composed of calcium often originate at the mitral or aortic valves, and they can be detected by CT.[89] Antithrombotic therapy is unlikely to be helpful for these patients, and surgery has been recommended for some. In the fat embolism syndrome usually associated with long bone fractures, emboli are composed of fat globules and elements of bone marrow. Massive brain embolism can be detected,[90] but neuroimaging findings specific to the condition have not been described. Treatment is mainly directed at associated pulmonary complications. Air embolism, a condition traditionally associated with diving accidents,[91] is now increasingly recognized as a complication of cardiac procedures.[92] Trapped air emboli can be detected by CT.[93] Hyperbaric oxygen may be the best approach to treating this form of arterial occlusion.

Secondary Stroke Prevention

Several antiplatelet medications have been tested for efficacy in the subacute setting after stroke. There is a small but significant benefit to the early administration of aspirin after stroke. Recurrent strokes are prevented in significant numbers with only a marginal impact on hemorrhagic complications.[94,95]

In addition to addressing the immediate neurologic and medical complications associated with acute stroke, the clinician is faced with the task of identifying the cause of the event. The evaluation of stroke patients during this stage includes appropriate imaging of the extracranial and intracranial brain arteries, the ascending aortic arch, and the cardiac chambers. Blood tests are obtained to assess vascular risk factors and hypercoagulable states. Arteries are usually imaged with MRI, ultrasound, or CT techniques, and occasionally, with conventional angiography. Advantages and limitations of these technologies are reviewed in other chapters of the book. Transesophageal echocardiography is increasingly considered to be the technique of choice to evaluate the cardiac chambers and aortic arch.[96] As soon as arterial and cardiac evaluations are completed, therapy is adjusted to the specific mechanism of stroke. Stroke is clearly a heterogeneous condition, and treatment is aimed at specific identified pathologies.

Carotid Stenosis

Extracranial ICA atherosclerotic stenosis is detected in approximately 15–25% of stroke patients, even though it may be unrelated to the ischemic event in some.[97] Conclusive studies indicate that symptomatic ICA stenosis of more than 50% is best treated surgically.[98] For the benefit to be achieved, however, the endarterectomy must be accomplished with a complication rate that does not exceed 6%. This rate is often exceeded outside of clinical trials.[99] Endarterectomy is also performed as an emergency procedure for stenosis or occlusion,[100] but this practice is infrequent. Although contrast angiography remains the gold standard to determine the degree of stenosis, it is often replaced with a combination of ultrasound, MRA, or CT angiography, in an effort to avoid complications.[101] A single noninvasive test may misclassify a stenosis as potentially operable up to 25% of the time. A combination of noninvasive studies such as MRA and ultrasound can reduce the rate of misclassification to approximately 10%, suggesting that there is still a role for conventional angiography in the assessment of carotid artery disease. Carotid artery angioplasty and stenting are increasingly recommended for patients at high risk of perioperative complications, although data from randomized trials do not yet support this practice.[102]

The overwhelming majority of ICA stenoses are secondary to atherosclerosis, but intraluminal clot,[103] fibromuscular dysplasia, and spontaneous or traumatic dissection[104] are also occasionally detected. Similar pathologic changes, particularly dissection, are also seen in the extracranial vertebral artery. Each of these conditions has its particular treatment. Anticoagulation is often prescribed for intraluminal clot formation, and stenting has been used for patients with dissection.[105]

ICA stenosis is a recognized risk factor for cerebral infarction even in asymptomatic patients. The findings of the Asymptomatic Carotid Atherosclerosis Study[106] indicate that elective endarterectomy for patients with stenosis of 60% or more is statistically beneficial when compared with medical management. There are caveats from this study. The natural history of asymptomatic ICA stenosis is benign when compared with the clinical course of symptomatic patients. The annual risk of stroke is 1–2% rather than approximately 13% in patients with symptoms. The statistical benefit of surgery does not appear unless the patient lives for 5 years after the procedure. This means that the complications from the procedure—brain and myocardial infarction and death—must not exceed 3%. The safety of the surgery has been hard to replicate outside of clinical trials. Because of these factors, some centers are reluctant to recommend routine endarterectomy for patients without symptoms of ICA disease.

Because of the cautions mentioned previously, several studies have tried to identify subsets of patients with asymptomatic ICA stenosis who are at a particularly high risk for stroke. Some of these patients have reduced ipsilateral MCA vasomotor reactivity on transcranial Doppler testing.[107–113] One study showed a moderate but statistically significant correlation between carbon dioxide reactivity and the nitrogen acetyl-aspartate/choline ratio, the latter being an indicator of disordered cerebral metabolism in noninfarcted tissue with reduced blood flow.[114,115] These metabolic changes were most severe in patients with contralateral ICA occlusion. An exhausted vasomotor reactivity is also an independent predictor of the occurrence of transient ischemic attack or stroke.[116–118] The prognosis of a patient with ICA occlusion is significantly influenced by the number and effectiveness, but not the type, of intracranial collateral vessels.[119] Subjects with markedly reduced vasomotor reactivity may be particularly attractive candidates for a revascularization procedure while still asymptomatic.

The potential for surgery in people without symptoms has led to screening for carotid stenosis. Indications regarding whom should be screened have not been established. Color duplex imaging, and particularly Doppler-mode assessment, is most commonly used to detect extracranial carotid artery stenosis and to monitor its progression over time (Figure 11-12). Despite substantial limitations, ultrasound has acceptable accuracy when determining severity of stenosis. MRA is also used in this setting, but its cost prohibits repeat imaging. As is the case for symptomatic patients, concordant results from two or more noninvasive tests decrease the risk of misclassifying the severity of stenosis.[120]

Intracranial Stenosis

Intracranial arterial occlusion or stenosis is commonly detected by neuroimaging studies during the days after a new infarct (Figure 11-13). Many of these lesions are secondary to intraluminal brain embolism rather than atherosclerosis of the arterial wall, and they tend to be transient.[121] Currently available imaging techniques, including contrast angiography, do not reliably discriminate between embolism and atherosclerosis. The diagnosis is usually established on repeat imaging weeks or months later, when lysis of the embolic particle leads to recanalization.

Symptomatic intracranial arterial plaques causing more than 50% stenosis are associated with a high risk of recurrent stroke. Retrospective studies suggest that warfarin anticoagulation, with an international normalized ratio of 2 to 3, may be superior to aspirin in preventing stroke recurrence.[122] The Warfarin-Aspirin Symptomatic Intracranial Disease Study, a large prospective, multicenter investigation, is in progress at the time of this writing. Thus, both anticoagulation and antiplatelet agents are considered acceptable forms of treatment—anticoagulation being perhaps used more often in patients not randomized into clinical studies. Antithrombotic treatments fail in some patients with more than 50% stenosis.[123] Stenting without balloon angioplasty has recently been tested in patients with severe stenoses of the basilar or MCA.[124,125] Short-term results have been satisfactory, but experience with this technology remains limited.

Cardiogenic Embolus

It is now well established that chronic, nonvalvular, atrial fibrillation is associated with brain embolism and infarction.[126] At least five large atrial fibrillation trials have conclusively demonstrated that warfarin anticoagulation is effective in reducing the stroke risk. The reduction of risk is substantial and may be as high as 86%. The associated increased risk of systemic and intracranial hemorrhage is offset by the benefit of the treatment.[127,128] Aspirin is less effective but may be used in some patients.[129] It has been suggested that echocardiographic markers, such as left atrial appendage thrombi and spontaneous echo contrast, are predictors of recurrent embolism.[130] Brain infarcts in this condition tend to be large and are associated with high morbidity and mortality. Neuroimaging studies in atrial fibrillation show silent brain infarction in 10–20% of patients, but when compared to symptomatic infarcts, the latter are more often of the deep lacunar type.[131]

A severe stenosis of the extracranial ICA ipsilateral to the symptomatic side can be detected in some patients with atrial fibrillation, raising questions regarding the source of embolism. Analysis of the patient's symptoms may be helpful in some cases. For example, a history of multiple episodes of stereotypic transient ischemic attacks or of transient monocular blindness is consistent with symptomatic carotid disease, whereas embolism in several arterial territories indicates a cardiac source such as atrial fibrillation. A transcranial Doppler embolus detection study may be helpful in this setting, because microembolism is common in extracranial ICA stenosis but less frequent in atrial fibrillation. Thus, imaging of the ICA is indicated for patients with stroke and atrial fibrillation who are potential candidates for endarterectomy.

Whether warfarin anticoagulation should be routinely prescribed to patients with reduced left ventricular ejection fraction is a matter of debate. The ejection fraction can be measured by echocardiography and gated radionuclide scanning. It is not invariably associated with symptomatic heart failure, but when less than 30%, it is associated with recurrent stroke. In patients with heart failure, the yearly stroke rate is rel-

FIGURE 11-12. **A–D.** Progressive internal carotid artery stenosis. Consecutive Doppler studies show a progressive increase of flow velocities. The peak-systolic velocity (PSV) was 191 cm per second at baseline (**A**) and 315 cm per second 38 months later (**D**). The corresponding end-diastolic velocities (EDVs) were 54 cm per second and 104 cm per second. The patient remained asymptomatic during this period. (RI = resistance index.)

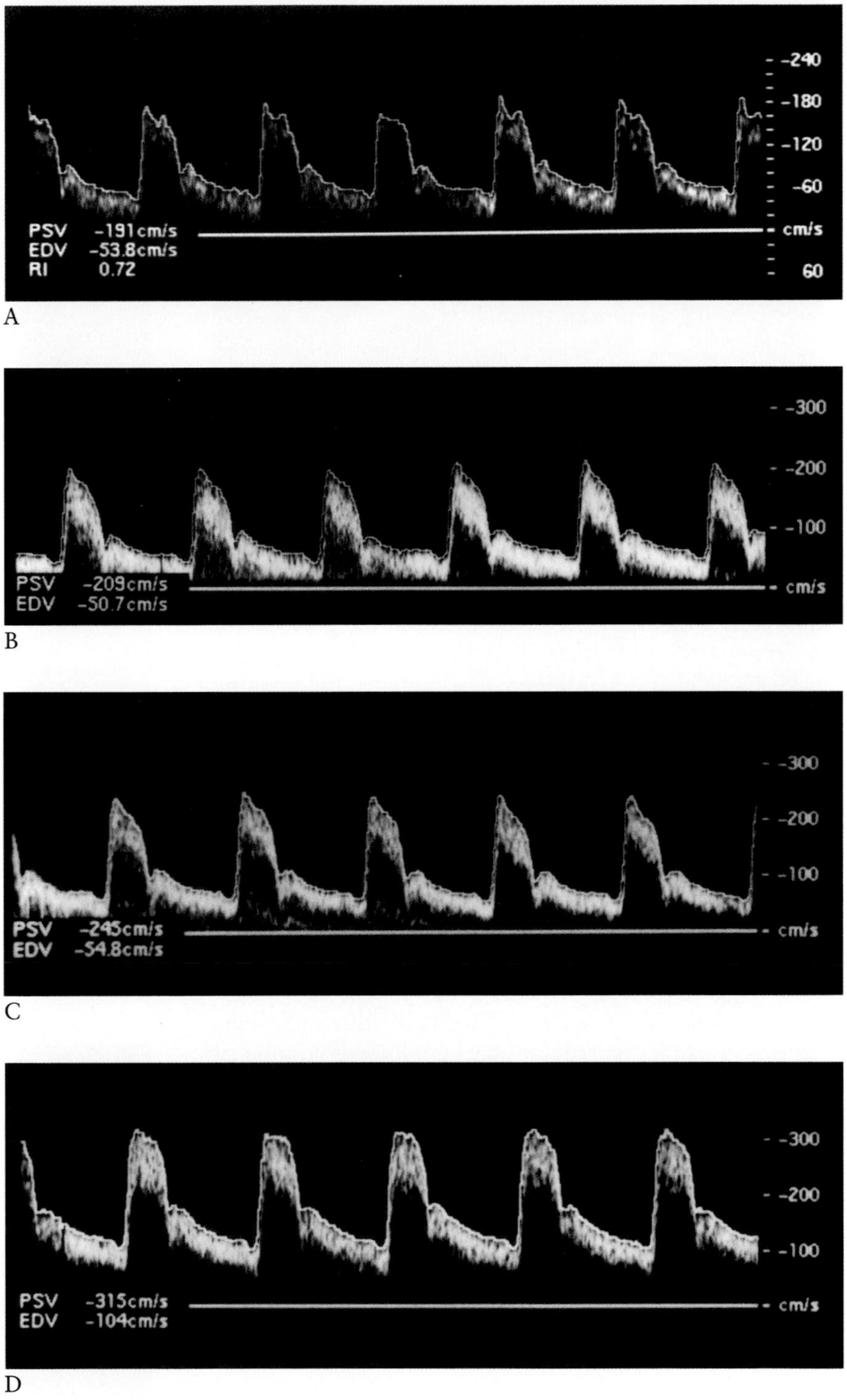

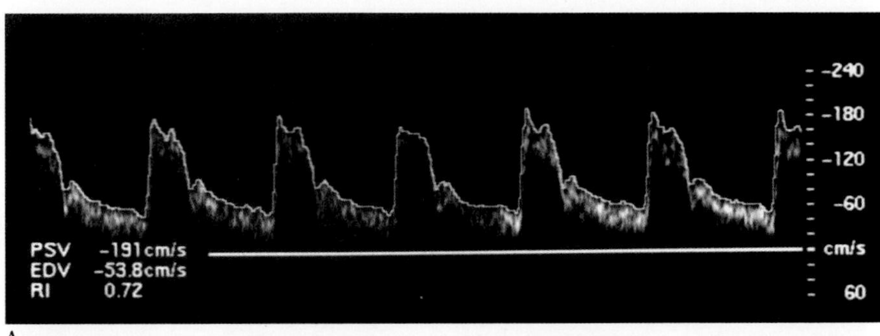

A

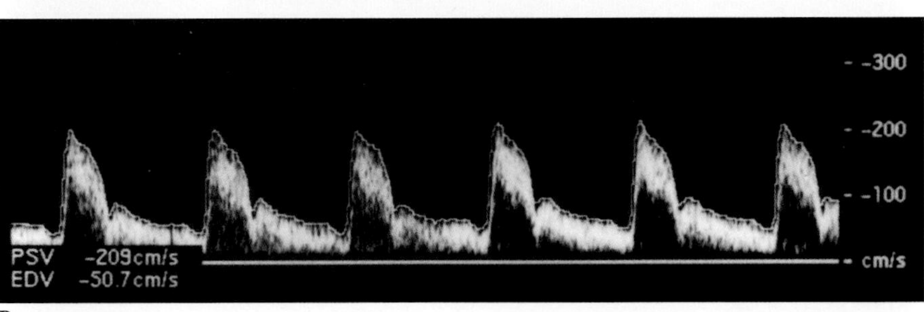

B

C

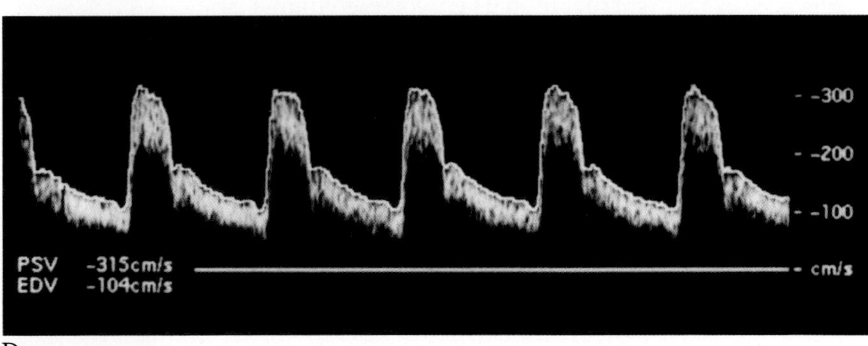

D

atively low, ranging between 1.3% and 3.5%,[132] but a decreased ejection fraction after myocardial infarction is an independent predictor of increased risk for stroke.[133] Warfarin is prescribed to selected high-risk patients.

The increased use of transesophageal echocardiography to evaluate stroke patients during recent years has identified aortic arch thick plaque formation as an independent risk factor for recurrent ischemic stroke (Figure 11-14).[96] Oral anticoagulants may have an added benefit in the treatment of these patients.[134]

ASSESS PROGNOSIS

The prognosis for functional recovery and for recurrent stroke depends greatly on the size and location of an

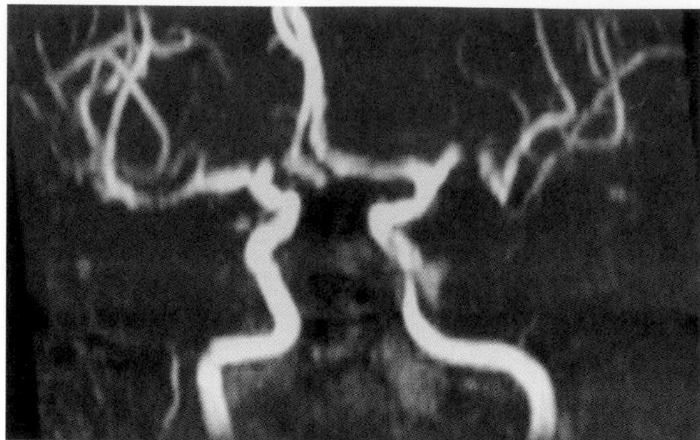

FIGURE 11-13. Intracranial atherosclerosis. Intracranial magnetic resonance angiogram showing bilateral middle cerebral artery stenoses (there is a flow gap on the left) and a stenosis in the precavernous left internal carotid artery.

infarct as well as its cause. In addition, the presence of previous infarcts further increases the likelihood of a persistent deficit. A number of techniques for imaging the brain and its blood supply have been applied to predict outcome after ischemic stroke. Observations made during the Randomized Trial of Tirilazad Mesylate in Patients with Acute Stroke reveal a definite but modest correlation between subacute CT infarct volume and clinical outcome.[135] The presence of two or three early CT infarct signs has been associated with large areas of MCA-territory infarct and poor neurologic outcome.[3] The presence of the sylvian fissure MCA dot sign by itself suggests that the patient is more likely to do well than if a dense MCA is seen.[4] These and other radiologic signs are, in fact, surrogate markers for the volume of infarcted tissue.

Studies using MRI with DWI and PWI sequences show a discrepancy between the volume of the DWI and PWI lesions (the DWI/PWI mismatch) during the hours to days after the onset of symptoms.[136–140] Although there is some controversy as to whether the DWI/PWI mismatch corresponds to the ischemic penumbra, these and other MRI variables, such as the apparent diffusion coefficient, identify the area at risk for infarction. When the DWI lesion is smaller than the PWI area of abnormality, the latter correlates with final infarct volume,[139,140] and there tends to be progressive enlargement of the DWI lesion.[136] The absence of flow in the affected MCA on MRA[137] and time-to-peak delays of more than 6 seconds[140] predict DWI lesion enlargement. The size of the DWI lesion, when measured within 48 hours after the onset of stroke, may be an independent risk factor for functional independence.[141] Greater age and higher scores on the National Institutes of Health Stroke Scale also contribute to a worse prognosis. With the addition of magnetic reso-

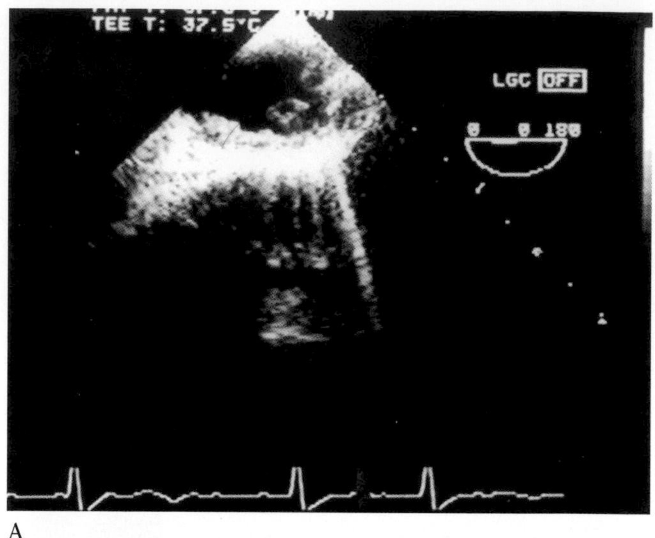

A

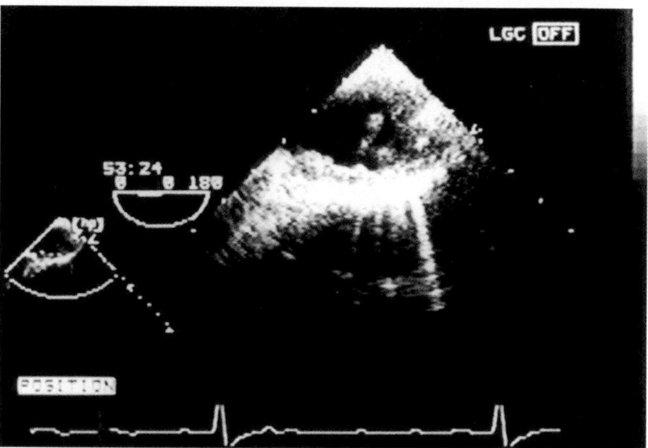

B

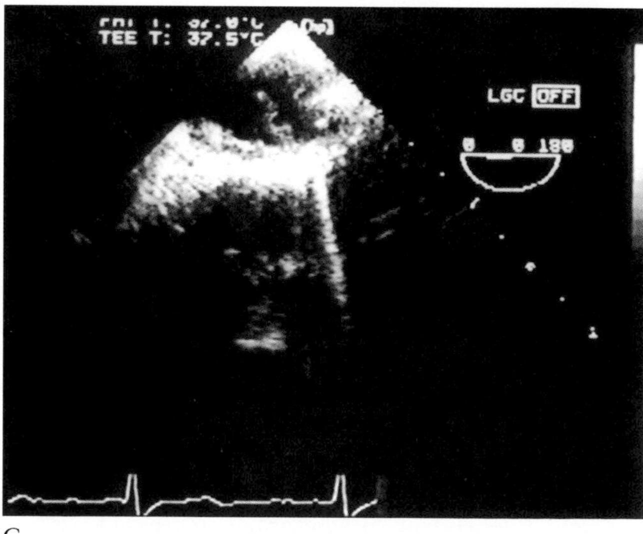

C

FIGURE 11-14. **A–C.** Atherosclerotic plaque in the aortic arch. Transesophageal echocardiogram (TEE) showing an atherosclerotic plaque with a mobile thrombus in the ascending aortic arch. The patient presented with symptoms of an acute brain infarct.

nance spectroscopy imaging, the extent and degree of the T2 hyperintensity may directly reflect the amount of neuronal damage.[142–144] Combining the lactate/choline ratio[143] or the nitrogen acetyl-aspartate concentration[144] with lesion volume might add prognostic information, although this method is not without its critics.[145,146]

Transcranial Doppler has also been used to evaluate the relationship between vascular patency, perfusion status or vasomotor reactivity, and ischemic stroke outcome. In patients with ICA territory stroke, clinical severity, CT lesion size, and transcranial Doppler findings are independent predictors of outcome at 30 days.[147] Not surprisingly, major intracranial arterial occlusions are associated with poor neurologic recovery,[147–150] whereas normal results are a predictor of early improvement.[151,152] One study[153] suggested that when transcranial Doppler is combined with carotid duplex sonography, the presence and total number of arteries with suspected occlusive lesions are associated with an increased risk of further vascular events and death within 6 months.

Transcranial color-coded sonography, particularly with contrast enhancement, has been used to evaluate brain parenchyma and vascular status in the setting of acute stroke. Transcranial color-coded sonography can demonstrate areas of hypoechogenicity in the MCA distribution, suggestive of brain infarction as shown on CT scan. This may be accompanied by abnormal blood flow velocity patterns.[154,155] In patients with severe, space-occupying MCA territory ischemic stroke, serial monitoring of midline shift may identify patients at risk of cerebral herniation and death.[156,157] Transcranial color-coded sonography measurements of the midline shift and the ventricular system are highly reproducible and highly specific for death caused by midline shift-associated cerebral herniation.[154,157–160] Experience in this setting remains limited.

Single-photon emission CT performed within 5 days after stroke onset can aid in stroke prognosis. The volume[161–165] and severity[161–163,166–170] of perfusion defects are directly and significantly associated with poor neurologic and functional outcome or mortality. It is unclear whether single-photon emission tomography adds much to the predictive power of the neurologic examination.[165,167,170]

These diverse techniques provide complementary anatomic and physiologic information that can be used to estimate ischemic stroke prognosis. Except for specific instances, such as the treatment of mass effect and herniation, their overall impact on the assessment of prognosis remains limited at present. Future research should evaluate the use of combined testing modalities to the extent possible to determine which technique(s) provide optimal, independent prognostic information in specific patient populations.

REFERENCES

1. Fieschi C, Argentino C, Lenzi GL, et al. Clinical and instrumental evaluation of patients with ischemic stroke within the first six hours. J Neurol Sci 1989;91:311–322.
2. Bose A, Pacia SV, Fayad P, et al. Cerebral blood flow (CBF) imaging compared to CT during the initial 24 hours of cerebral infarction. Neurology 1990;40[Suppl 1]:190.
3. Moulin T, Cattin F, Crepin-Leblond T, et al. Early CT signs in acute middle cerebral artery infarction: predictive value for subsequent infarct locations and outcome. Neurology 1996;47:366–375.
4. Barber PA, Demchuk AM, Hudson ME, et al. Hyperdense sylvian fissure MCA "dot sign": a CT marker of acute ischemia. Stroke 2001;32:84–88.
5. Sato A, Takahashi S, Soma Y, et al. Cerebral infarction: early detection by means of contrast-enhanced cerebral arteries CT MR imaging. Radiology 1991;178:433–439.
6. Bryan RN, Levy LM, Whitlow WD, et al. Diagnosis of acute cerebral infarction: comparison of CT and MR imaging. AJNR Am J Neuroradiol 1991;12:611–620.
7. Yuh WT, Crain MR. Magnetic resonance imaging of acute cerebral ischemia. Neuroimaging Clin N Am 1992;1:421–439.
8. Baird AE, Warach S. Magnetic resonance imaging of acute stroke. J Cereb Blood Flow Metab 1998;18:583–609.
9. Alberts MJ, Faulstich ME, Gray L. Stroke with negative brain magnetic resonance imaging. Stroke 1992;23:663–667.
10. Lansberg MG, Albers GW, Beaulieu C, et al. Comparison of diffusion-weighted MRI and CT in acute stroke. Neurology 2000;54:1557–1561.
11. Brant-Zawadzki M, Atkinson D, Detrick M, et al. Fluid-attenuated inversion recovery (FLAIR) for assessment of cerebral infarction: initial clinical inexperience in 50 patients. Stroke 1996;27:1187–1191.
12. Oppenheim C, Stanescu R, Dormont D, et al. False-negative diffusion-weighted MR findings in acute ischemic stroke. AJNR Am J Neuroradiol 2000;21: 1434–1440.
13. Kamran S, Bates V, Bakshi R, et al. Significance of hyperintense vessels on FLAIR MRI in acute stroke. Neurology 2000;55:265–269.
14. Houser OW, Campbell JK, Baker EL, et al. Radiologic evaluation of ischemic cerebrovascular syndromes with emphasis on computed tomography. Radiol Clin North Am 1982;20:123–142.
15. Grond M, von Kummer R, Sobesky J, et al. Early x-ray hypoattenuation of brain parenchyma indicates extended critical hypoperfusion in acute stroke. Stroke 2000;31:133–139.

16. Masdeu JC, Berhooz A-K, Rubino FA. Evaluation of recent cerebral infarction by computed tomography. Arch Neurol 1977;34:417–424.

17. Yock DH, Marshall WH. Recent ischemic brain infarcts at computed tomography: appearance pre and post contrast infusion. Radiology 1975;117: 599–600.

18. Ropper AH. Lateral displacement of the brain and level of consciousness in patients with an acute hemispheric mass. N Engl J Med 1986;314:953–958.

19. Wijdicks EFM, Diringer MN. Middle cerebral artery territory infarction and early brain swelling: progression and effect of age on outcome. Mayo Clin Proc 1998;73:829–836.

20. Pullicino PM, Alexandrov AV, Shelton JA, et al. Mass effect and death from severe acute stroke. Neurology 1997;49:1090–1095.

21. von Kummer R, Meyding-Lamade U, Forsting M, et al. Sensitivity and prognostic value of early CT in occlusion of the middle cerebral artery trunk. AJNR Am J Neuroradiol 1994;15:9–15.

22. Frank JI. Large hemisphere infarction, deterioration, and intracranial pressure. Neurology 1995;45: 1286–1290.

23. Hacke W, Schwab S, Horn M, et al. "Malignant" middle cerebral artery territory infarction: clinical course and prognostic signs. Arch Neurol 1996; 53:309–315.

24. Toni D, Fiorelli M, Bastianello S, et al. Acute strokes improving during the first 48 hours of onset: predictability, outcome, and possible mechanisms: a comparison with early deteriorating strokes. Stroke 1997;28:10–14.

25. Krieger DW, Demchuk AM, Kasner SE, et al. Early clinical and radiological predictors of fatal brain swelling in ischemic stroke. Stroke 1999;30:287–292.

26. Haring H-P, Dilitz E, Pallua A, et al. Attenuated corticomedullary contrast: an early cerebral computed tomography sign indicating malignant middle cerebral artery infarction. A case-control study. Stroke 1999;30:1076–1082.

27. Hart RG, Easton JD. Hemorrhagic infarcts. Stroke 1986;17:586–589.

28. Pessin M, del Zoppo GJ, Estol C. Thrombolytic agents in the treatment of stroke. Clin Neuropharmacol 1990;13:271–289.

29. Pessin MS, Teal PA, Caplan LR. Hemorrhagic infarction: guilt by association. AJNR Am J Neuroradiol 1991;12:1123–1126.

30. Moulin T, Crepin-Leblond T, Chopard JL, et al. Hemorrhagic infarcts. Eur Neurol 1993;34:64–77.

31. Lyden PD, Zivin JA. Hemorrhagic transformation after cerebral ischemia: mechanisms and incidence. Cerebrovasc Brain Metab Rev 1993;5:1–16.

32. Sloan MA. Neurologic Complications of Thrombolytic Therapy. In J Biller (ed), Iatrogenic Neurology. Woburn, MA: Butterworth–Heinemann, 1998: 335–378.

33. del Zoppo GJ, von Kummer R, Hamann GF. Ischaemic damage of brain microvessels: inherent risks for thrombolytic treatment in stroke. J Neurol Neurosurg Psychiatry 1998;63:1–9.

34. Nighoghossian N, Hermier M, Berthezene Y, et al. Early diagnosis of hemorrhagic transformation: diffusion/perfusion-weighted MRI versus CT scan. Cerebrovasc Dis 2001;11:151–156.

35. Bogousslavsky J, Regli F, Uske A, et al. Early spontaneous hematoma in cerebral infarct: is primary cerebral hemorrhage overdiagnosed? Neurology 1991;41:837.

36. Lodder J. CT-detected hemorrhagic infarction. Relation with the size of the infarct and the presence of midline shift. Acta Neurol Scand 1984;70:329–335.

37. Chamorro A, Vila N, Saiz A, et al. Early anticoagulation after large cerebral embolic infarction: a safety study. Neurology 1995;45:861–865.

38. Tong DC, Adami A, Moseley ME, et al. Relationship between apparent diffusion coefficient and subsequent hemorrhagic transformation following acute ischemic stroke. Stroke 2000;31:2378–2384.

39. Becker H, Desch H, Hacker H, et al. CT fogging effect with ischemic cerebral infarcts. J Neuroradiol 1979;18:185–192.

40. Skriver EB, Olsen TS. Transient disappearance of cerebral infarctions on CT scan, the so-called fogging effect. Neuroradiology 1981;22:61–65.

41. Pullicino P, Kendall BE. Contrast enhancement in ischemic lesions. J Neuroradiol 1980;19:235–239.

42. Weisberg LA. Computerized tomographic enhancement patterns in cerebral infarction. Arch Neurol 1980;37:21–24.

43. Crain MR, Yuh WT, Greene GM. Cerebral ischemia: evaluation with contrast-enhanced MR imaging. AJNR Am J Neuroradiol 1991;12:631–639.

44. Caplan L. Multiple potential risks for stroke. JAMA 2000;283:1479–1480.

45. Fisher CM. Pure sensory stroke involving the face, arm, and leg. Neurology 1965;15:76–80.

46. Fisher CM. A lacunar stroke: the dysarthria-clumsy hand syndrome. Neurology 1967;17:614–617.

47. Fisher CM. Thalamic pure sensory stroke: a pathological study. Neurology 1978;28:1141–1144.

48. Fisher CM. Ataxic hemiparesis: a pathological study. Arch Neurol 1978;35:126–128.

49. Fisher CM, Curry HB. Pure motor hemiplegia from vascular origin. Arch Neurol 1965;13:30–44.

50. Ay H, Oliveira-Filho J, Buonanno FS, et al. Diffusion-weighted imaging identifies a subset of lacunar infarction associated with embolic source. Stroke 1999;30:2644.

51. Jung DK, Devuyst G, Maeder P, et al. Atrial fibrillation with small subcortical infarcts. J Neurol Neurosurg Psychiatry 2001;70:344–349.

52. Hachinski VC, Potter P, Merskey H. Leukoaraiosis. Arch Neurol 1987;44:21–23.

53. Breteler MMB, van Swieten JC, Bots ML, et al. Cerebral white matter lesions, vascular risk factors, and cognitive function in a population-based study: the Rotterdam Study. Neurology 1994;44:1246–1252.

54. Lindgren A, Roijer A, Rudling O, et al. Cerebral lesions on magnetic resonance imaging, heart disease, and vascular risk factors in subjects without stroke. Stroke 1994;25:929–934.

55. Manolio TA, Kronmal RA, Burke GL, et al. Magnetic resonance abnormalities and cardiovascular disease in older adults: the Cardiovascular Health Study. Stroke 1994;25:318–327.

56. Pantoni L, Garcia JH. The significance of cerebral white matter abnormalities 100 years after Binswanger's report. Stroke 1995;26:1293–1301.

57. Ylikoski A, Erkinjuntti T, Raininko R, et al. White matter hyperintensities on MRI in the neurologically nondiseased elderly: analysis of cohorts of consecutive subjects aged 55 to 85 years living at home. Stroke 1995;26:1171–1177.

58. Longstreth WT, Manolio TA, Arnold A, et al. Clinical correlates of white matter findings on cranial magnetic resonance imaging of 3301 elderly people: the Cardiovascular Health Study. Stroke 1996;27:1274–1282.

59. Roman GC. From UBOs to Biswanger's disease: impact of magnetic resonance imaging on vascular dementia research. Stroke 1996;27:1269–1273.

60. Watanabe N, Imai Y, Nagai K, et al. Nocturnal blood pressure and silent cerebrovascular lesions in elderly Japanese. Stroke 1996;27:1319–1327.

61. Inzitari D. Age-related white matter changes and cognitive impairment. Ann Neurol 2000;47:141–143.

62. McQuinn BA, O'Leary DH. White matter lucencies on computed tomography, subacute arteriosclerotic encephalopathy (Binswanger's disease), and pressure. Stroke 1987;18:900–905.

63. Bakker SLM, de Leeuw F-E, de Groot JC, et al. Cerebral vasomotor reactivity and cerebral white matter lesions in the elderly. Neurology 1999;52:578–583.

64. Babikian VL, Ropper AH. Binswanger's disease: a review. Stroke 1987;18:2–12.

65. Caplan LR. Binswanger's disease—revisited. Neurology 1995;45:626–633.

66. Bogousslavsky J, Van Melle G, Regli F. The Lausanne Stroke Registry: analysis of 1000 consecutive patients with first stroke. Stroke 1988;19:1083–1092.

67. Bogousslavsky J, Van Melle G, Regli F. Middle cerebral artery pial territory infarcts: a study of the Lausanne Stroke Registry. Ann Neurol 1989;25:555–560.

68. Caplan L. Posterior circulation ischemia: then, now and tomorrow: the Thomas Willis Lecture-2000. Stroke 2000;31:2011–2023.

69. Heinsius T, Bougousslavsky J, Van Melle G. Large infarcts in the middle cerebral artery territory: etiology and outcome patterns. Neurology 1998; 50:1940–1943.

70. Caplan LR, Amarenco P, Rosengart A, et al. Embolism from vertebral artery origin occlusive disease. Neurology 1992;42:1505–1512.

71. Lee L, Kidwell C, Alger J, et al. Impact on stroke subtype diagnosis of early diffusion-weighted magnetic resonance imaging and magnetic resonance angiography. Stroke 2000;31:1081–1089.

72. Ricci S, Celani MG, La Rosa F, et al. Silent brain infarction in patients with first-ever stroke: a community-based study in Umbria, Italy. Stroke 1993;24:647–651.

73. Roh J-K, Kang D-W, Lee S-H, et al. Significance of acute multiple brain infarction on diffusion-weighted imaging. Stroke 2000;31:688–694.

74. Jorgensen L, Torvik A. Ischaemic cerebrovascular diseases in autopsy series, part 2: prevalence, location, pathogenesis and clinical course of cerebral infarcts. J Neurol Sci 1969;9:285–320.

75. Belden JR, Caplan LR, Pessin MS, et al. Mechanisms and clinical features of posterior borderzone infarcts. Neurology 1999;53:1312.

76. Min WK, Park KK, Kim YS, et al. Topographic diversity with common occurrence of concomitant small cortical and subcortical infarcts. Stroke 2000;31:2055–2061.

77. Chaves CJ, Silver B, Schlaug G, et al. Diffusion- and perfusion-weighted MRI patterns in borderzone infarcts. Stroke 2000;31:1090–1096.

78. Heros RC. Surgical treatment of cerebellar infarction. Stroke 1992;23:937–938.

79. Schwab S, Rieke K, Aschoff A, et al. Hemicraniotomy in space-occupying hemispheric infarction: useful early intervention or desperate activism? Cerebrovasc Dis 1996;6:325–329.

80. Roden-Jullig A. Progressing stroke: epidemiology. Cerebrovasc Dis 1997;7[Suppl 5]:2–5.

81. Yamamoto H, Bogousslavsky J, van Melle G. Different predictors of neurological worsening in different causes of stroke. Arch Neurol 1998;55:481–486.

82. Forteza AM, Babikian VL, Hyde C, et al. Effect of time and cerebrovascular symptoms on the prevalence of microembolic signals in patients with cervical carotid stenosis. Stroke 1996;27:687–690.

83. Adams HP, Bendixen BH, Leira E, et al. Antithrombotic treatment of ischemic stroke among patients with occlusion or severe stenosis of the internal carotid artery. Neurology 1999;53:122–125.

84. Dahl T, Sandset PM, Abildgaard U. Heparin treatment in 52 patients with progressive ischemic stroke. Cerebrovasc Dis 1994;4:101–105.

85. Pessin MS, Estol CJ, Lafranchise F, et al. Safety of anticoagulation after hemorrhagic infarction. Neurology 1993;43:1298–1303.

86. Chamorro A, Vila N, Saiz A, et al. Early anticoagulation after large cerebral embolic infarction. A safety study. Neurology 1995;45:861–865.

87. Rordorf G, Koroshetz WJ, Ezzeddine MA, et al. A pilot study of drug-induced hypertension for treatment of acute stroke. Neurology 2001;56:1210–1213.

88. Baron JC. Mapping the ischemic penumbra with PET: implications for acute stroke. Cerebrovas Dis 1999;9:193–201.

89. Oliveira-Filho J, Massaro AR, Yamamoto F, et al. Stroke as the first manifestation of calcific aortic stenosis. Cerebrovasc Dis 2000;10:413–416.

90. Forteza AM, Koch S, Romano JG, et al. Transcranial Doppler detection of fat emboli. Stroke 1999;30:2687–2691.

91. Schwermann M, Seiler C, Lipp E, et al. Relation between directly detected patent foramen ovale and ischemic brain lesions in sport divers. Ann Intern Med 2001;134:21–24.

92. Hinkle DA, Raizen DM, McGarvey ML, et al. Cerebral air embolism complicating cardiac ablation procedures. Neurology 2001;56:792–794.

93. Wijman CAC, Kase CS, Jacobs AK, et al. Cerebral air embolism as a cause of stroke during cardiac catheterization. Neurology 1998;51:318–319.

94. CAST (Chinese Acute Stroke Trial) Collaborative Group. Randomized placebo-controlled trial of early aspirin use in 20,000 patients with acute ischaemic stroke. Lancet 1997;349:1641–1649.

95. International Stroke Trial (IST) Collaborative Group. A randomised trial of aspirin, subcutaneous heparin, both, or neither among 19,435 patients with acute ischaemic stroke. Lancet 1997;349:1569–1581.

96. French Study of Aortic Plaques Stroke Group. Atherosclerotic disease of the aortic arch as a risk factor for recurrent ischemic stroke. N Engl J Med 1996;334: 1216–1221.

97. Barnett HJM, Gunton RW, Eliasziw M, et al. Causes and severity of ischemic stroke in patients with internal carotid artery stenosis. JAMA 2000;283:1429–1436.

98. North American Symptomatic Carotid Endarterectomy Trial Collaborators. Beneficial effect of carotid endarterectomy in symptomatic patients with high-grade stenosis. N Engl J Med 1991;325:445–453.

99. Wennberg DE, Lucas FL, Birkmeyer JD, et al. Variation in carotid endarterectomy mortality in the Medicare population: trial hospitals, volume, and patient characteristics. JAMA 1998;279:1278–1281.

100. Kasper GC, Wladis AR, Lohr JM, et al. Carotid thromboendarterectomy for recent total occlusion of the internal carotid artery. J Vasc Surg 2001;33:242–250.

101. Johnston DC, Goldstein LB. Clinical carotid endarterectomy decision making. Neurology 2001;56: 1009–1015.

102. CAVATAS Investigators. Endovascular versus surgical treatment in patients with carotid stenosis in the carotid and vertebral artery transluminal angioplasty study (CAVATAS): a randomized trial. Lancet 2001;357:1729–1737.

103. Caplan L, Stein R, Patel D, et al. Intraluminal clot of the carotid artery detected radiographically. Neurology 1984;34:1175–1181.

104. Schievink WI. Spontaneous dissection of the carotid and vertebral arteries. N Engl J Med 2001;344: 898–906.

105. Malek AM, Higashida RT, Phatouros CC. Endovascular management of extracranial carotid artery dissection achieved using stent angioplasty. AJNR Am J Neuroradiol 2000;21:1280–1292.

106. Executive Committee for the Asymptomatic Carotid Atherosclerosis Study. Endarterectomy for asymptomatic carotid artery stenosis. JAMA 1995;273: 1421–1428.

107. Ringelstein EB, Sievers C, Ecker S, et al. Noninvasive assessment of CO2 induced cerebral vasomotor response in normal individuals and patients with internal carotid artery occlusions. Stroke 1988;19:963–969.

108. Markus HS, Harrison MJG. Estimation of cerebrovascular reactivity using transcranial Doppler, including the use of breath-holding as the vasodilatory stimulus. Stroke 1992;23:668–673.

109. Ringelstein EB, Van Eyck S, Mertens I. Evaluation of cerebral vasomotor reactivity by various vasodilating stimuli: comparison of CO_2 to acetazolamide. J Cereb Blood Flow Metab 1992;12:162–168.

110. Chimowitz MI, Furlan AJ, Jones SC, et al. Transcranial Doppler assessment of cerebral perfusion reserve in patients with carotid occlusive disease and no evidence of cerebral infarction. Neurology 1993;43: 353–357.

111. Widder B, Kleiser B, Krapf H. Course of cerebrovascular reactivity in patients with carotid artery occlusions. Stroke 1994;25:1963–1967.

112. Silvestrini M, Troisi E, Matteis M, et al. Transcranial Doppler assessment of cerebrovascular reactivity in symptomatic and asymptomatic severe carotid stenosis. Stroke 1996;27:1970–1973.

113. Vernieri F, Pasqualetti P, Passarelli F, et al. Outcome of carotid artery occlusion is predicted by cerebrovascular reactivity. Stroke 1999;30:593–598.

114. Visser GH, van der Grond J, van Huffelen AC, et al. Decreased transcranial Doppler carbon dioxide reactivity is associated with disordered cerebral metabolism in patients with internal carotid artery stenosis. J Vasc Surg 1999;30:252–260.

115. Van der Grond J, Eikelboom BC, Mali WP. Flow-related anaerobic metabolic changes in patients

with severe stenosis of the internal carotid artery. Stroke 1996;27:2026–2032.

116. Markus H, Cullinane M. Severely impaired cerebrovascular reactivity predicts stroke and TIA risk in patients with carotid artery stenosis and occlusion. Brain 2001;124:457–467.

117. Silverstrini M, Vernieri F, Pasqualetti P, et al. Impaired cerebral vasoreactivity and risk of stroke in patients with asymptomatic carotid artery stenosis. JAMA 2000;283:2122–2127.

118. Kleiser B, Widder B. Course of carotid artery occlusions with impaired cerebrovasular reactivity. Stroke 1992;23:171–174.

119. Vernieri F, Pasqualetti P, Matteis M, et al. Effect of collateral blood flow and cerebral vasomotor reactivity on the outcome of carotid artery occlusion. Stroke 2001;32:1552–1558.

120. Dean CC, Johnston MD, Goldstein LB. Clinical carotid endarterectomy decision making: noninvasive vascular imaging versus angiography. Neurology 2001;56:1009–1015.

121. Segura T, Serena J, Castellanos M, et al. Embolism in acute middle cerebral artery stenosis. Neurology 2001;56:497–501.

122. Chimowitz MI, Kokkinos J, Strong J, et al. The warfarin-aspirin symptomatic intracranial disease study. Neurology 1995;45:1488–1493.

123. Thijs VN, Albers GW. Symptomatic intracranial atherosclerosis: outcome of patients who fail antithrombotic therapy. Neurology 2000;55:490–497.

124. Gomez CR, Misr VK, Liu MW, et al. Elective stenting of symptomatic basilar artery stenosis. Stroke 2000;31:95–99.

125. Piotin M, Blanc R, Kothimbakam R, et al. Primary basilar artery stenting: immediate and long-term results in one patient. AJR Am J Roentgenol 2000;175:1367–1369.

126. Wolf PA, Abbott RD, Kannel WB. Atrial fibrillation: a major contributor to stroke in the elderly. Arch Intern Med 1987;147:1561–1564.

127. Petersen P, Godtfredsen J, Boysen G, et al. Placebo-controlled, randomized trial of warfarin and aspirin for prevention of thromboembolic complications in chronic atrial fibrillation. Lancet 1989;1:175–179.

128. Sherman D. Stroke prevention trials in atrial fibrillation. Cerebrovasc Dis 1992;2:14–17.

129. The SPAF III Writing Committee for the Stroke Prevention in Atrial Fibrillation Investigators. Patients with nonvalvular atrial fibrillation at low risk of stroke during treatment with aspirin. JAMA 1998;279:1273–1277.

130. Di Pasquale G, Urbinati S, Pinelli G. New echocardiographic markers of embolic risk in atrial fibrillation. Cerebrovasc Dis 1995;5:315–322.

131. EAFT Study Group. Silent brain infarction in nonrheumatic atrial fibrillation. Neurology 1996;46:159–165.

132. Pullicino PM, Halperin JL, Thompson JLP. Stroke in patients with heart failure and reduced left ventricular ejection fraction. Neurology 2000;54:288–294.

133. Loh E, Sutton MSJ, Wun CC, et al. Ventricular dysfunction and the risk of stroke after myocardial infarction. N Engl J Med 1997;336:251–257.

134. Ferrari E, Vidal R, Chevallier T, et al. Atherosclerosis of the thoracic aorta and aortic debris as a marker of poor prognosis: benefit of oral anticoagulants. J Am Coll Cardiol 1999;33:1317–1322.

135. Saver JL, Johnston KC, Homer D, et al. Infarct volume as a surrogate or auxiliary outcome measure in ischemic stroke clinical trials. Stroke 1999;30:293–298.

136. Baird AE, Benfield A, Schlaug G, et al. Enlargement of human cerebral ischemic lesion volumes measured by diffusion-weighted magnetic resonance imaging. Ann Neurol 1997;41:581–589.

137. Barber PA, Davis SM, Darby DG, et al. Absent middle cerebral artery flow predicts the presence and evolution of the ischemic penumbra. Neurology 1999;52:1125–1132.

138. Darby DG, Barber PA, Gerraty RP, et al. Pathophysiological topography of acute ischemia by combined diffusion-weighted and perfusion MRI. Stroke 1999;30:2043–2052.

139. Karonen JO, Vanninen RL, Liu Y, et al. Combined diffusion and perfusion MRI with correlation to single-photon emission CT in acute ischemic stroke: ischemic penumbra predicts infarct growth. Stroke 1999;30:1583–1590.

140. Neumann-Haefelin T, Wittsack H-J, Wenserski F, et al. Diffusion- and perfusion-weighted MRI: the DWI/PWI mismatch region in acute stroke. Stroke 1999;30:1591–1597.

141. Thijs VN, Lansberg MG, Beaulieu C, et al. Is early ischemic lesion volume on diffusion-weighted imaging an independent predictor of stroke outcome? A multivariable analysis. Stroke 2000;31:2597–2602.

142. Pereira AC, Saunders DE, Doyle VL, et al. Measurement of initial N-acetyl aspartate concentration by magnetic resonance spectroscopy and initial infarct volume by MRI predicts outcome in patients with middle cerebral artery territory infarction. Stroke 1999;30:1577–1582.

143. Parsons MW, Li T, Barber PA, et al. Combined 1H MR spectroscopy and diffusion-weighted MRI improves the prediction of stroke outcome. Neurology 2000;55:498–505.

144. Wild JM, Wardlaw JM, Marshall I, et al. N-Acetylaspartate distribution in proton spectroscopic images of ischemic stroke: relationship to infarct appearance on T2-weighted magnetic resonance imaging. Stroke 2001;32:3008–3014.

145. Powers WJ. Testing a test: a report card for DWI in acute stroke. Neurology 2000;54:1549–1551.

146. Keir SL, Wardlaw JM. Systematic review of diffusion and perfusion imaging in acute ischemic stroke. Stroke 2000;31:2723–2731.

147. Camerlingo M, Casto L, Censori B, et al. Prognostic use of ultrasonography in acute non-hemorrhagic carotid stroke. Ital J Neurol Sci 1996;17:215–218.

148. Halsey JH. Prognosis of acute hemiplegia estimated by transcranial Doppler ultrasonography. Stroke 1988;19:648–649.

149. Alexandrov AV, Bladin CF, Norris JW. Intracranial blood flow velocities in acute ischemic stroke. Stroke 1994;25:1378–1383.

150. Baracchini C, Manara R, Ermani M, et al. The quest for early predictors of stroke evolution: can TCD be a guiding light? Stroke 2000;31:2942–2947.

151. Kushner MJ, Zanette EM, Bastianello S, et al. Transcranial Doppler in acute hemispheric brain infarction. Neurology 1991;41:109–113.

152. Toni D, Fiorelli M, Zanette EM, et al. Early spontaneous improvement and deterioration of ischemic stroke patients. Stroke 1998;29:1144–1148.

153. Wong KS, Li H, Chan YL, et al. Use of transcranial Doppler ultrasound to predict outcome in patients with intracranial large-artery occlusive disease. Stroke 2000;31:2641–2647.

154. Seidel G, Kaps M, Gerriets T. Potential and limitations of transcranial color-coded sonography in stroke patients. Stroke 1995;26:2061–2066.

155. Maurer M, Shambal S, Berg D, et al. Differentiation between intracerebral hemorrhage and ischemic stroke by transcranial color-coded duplex-sonography. Stroke 1998;29:2563–2567.

156. Gerriets T, Stolz E, Modrau B, et al. Sonographic monitoring of midline shift in hemispheric infarctions. Neurology 1999;52:45–49.

157. Gerriets T, Stolz E, Konig S, et al. Sonographic monitoring of midline shift in space-occupying stroke: an early outcome predictor. Stroke 2001;32:442–447.

158. Becker G, Bogdahn U, Strassberg H-M, et al. Identification of ventricular enlargement and estimation of intracranial pressure by transcranial color-coded real-time sonography. J Neuroimaging 1994;4:17–22.

159. Seidel G, Gerriets T, Kaps M, Missler U. Dislocation of the third ventricle due to space-occupying stroke evaluated by transcranial duplex sonography. J Neuroimaging 1996;6:227–230.

160. Stolz E, Gerriets T, Fiss I, et al. Comparison of transcranial color-coded duplex sonography and cranial CT measurements for determining third ventricle midline shift in space-occupying stroke. AJNR Am J Neuroradiol 1999;20:1567–1571.

161. Limburg M, van Royen EA, Hijdra A, et al. Single-photon emission computed tomography and early death in acute ischemic stroke. Stroke 1990;21:1150–1155.

162. Giubilei F, Lenzi GL, Di Piero V, et al. Predictive of brain perfusion single-photon emission computed tomography in acute ischemic stroke. Stroke 1990;21:895–900.

163. Laloux P, Richelle F, Jamart J, et al. Comparative correlations of HMPAO-SPECT indices, neurological score, and stroke subtypes with clinical outcome in acute carotid infarcts. Stroke 1995;26:816–821.

164. Baird AE, Austin MC, McKay WJ, et al. Changes in cerebral tissue perfusion during the first 48 hours of ischemic stroke: relation to clinical outcome. J Neurol Neurosurg Psychiatry 1996;61:26–29.

165. Bowler JV, Wade JPH, Jones BE, et al. Single-photon emission computed tomography using hexamethylpropyleneamine oxime in the prognosis of acute cerebral infarction. Stroke 1996;27:82–86.

166. Mountz JM, Modell JG, Foster NL, et al. Prognostication of recovery following stroke using the comparison of CT and technetium-99m-HMPAO SPECT. J Nucl Med 1990;31:61–66.

167. Davis SM, Chua MG, Lichtenstein M, et al. Cerebral hypoperfusion in stroke prognosis and brain recovery. Stroke 1993;24:1691–1696.

168. Alexandrov AV, Ehrlich LE, Bladin CF, et al. Cerebral perfusion index: a new marker for clinical outcome in acute stroke. J Neuroimaging 1993;3:209–215.

169. Alexandrov AV, Bladin CF, Ehrlich LE, et al. Noninvasive assessment of intracranial perfusion in acute cerebral perfusion. J Neuroimaging 1995;5:76–82.

170. Alexandrov AV, Black SE, Ehrlich LE, et al. Simple visual analysis of brain perfusion on HMPAO-SPECT predicts early outcome in acute stroke. Stroke 1996;27:1537–1542.

CHAPTER

12

Cerebral Venous Thrombosis

Vineeta Singh and Daryl R. Gress

Cerebral venous thrombosis (CVT) is an infrequent but alarming disease characterized clinically by headache, papilledema, seizures, focal deficits, progressive coma, or death. It is recognized pathologically by hemorrhagic infarction.

Before the introduction of cerebral angiography, CVT was diagnosed at autopsy and therefore thought to be most often lethal. Most patients in the present era do not fall into the original description of CVT as a mysterious and lethal disorder. Contemporary brain imaging techniques allow the diagnosis of benign forms of CVT with minimal symptoms and spontaneous recovery. Another reason for this change is that septic thrombosis has, since the use of antibiotics, become far less frequent and severe. Despite the advances in imaging technology and therapeutic options, the wide variety of causes and its unpredictable course leave CVT a challenge for the clinician.

VENOUS ANATOMY

The cerebral venous system is composed of dural sinuses and superficial cortical and deep veins. The cerebral veins carry venous blood from the brain and empty into dural sinuses and are mostly drained by the internal jugular veins.

Dural Sinuses

Superior Sagittal Sinus

The superior sagittal sinus (SSS; Figure 12-1) is a midline structure that lies in the attached border of the falx cerebri. It is lined by endothelium and contains no valves. It starts at the foramen cecum and extends posteriorly to its confluence with the straight and lateral sinuses (LSs) to form the torcular herophili. The SSS's rostral part is narrow or sometimes atretic and is replaced by intradural venous channels receiving prominent tributaries from the cerebral cortex. As a result, the anterior part of the sinus is poorly visualized on angiography, and this anomaly should not be mistaken for pathologic occlusion.[1]

The SSS receives superficial cortical veins and drains the major part of the cerebral cortex. It also receives diploic veins that are connected to the scalp veins via emissary veins, which explains SSS thrombosis in some cases of scalp infection or laceration.

Lateral Sinuses

The LSs consist of two portions: the transverse portion that lies in the border of the tentorium, and the sigmoid portion that runs in the posterolateral wall of the petrous temporal bone and is susceptible to secondary thrombosis in patients with otitis media or mastoiditis. The sigmoid sinuses continue inferiorly into the jugular bulb at the skull base.

Asymmetry of the LS is common (50–80% of the cases), with the right LS usually the dominant drainage pattern. An isolated lack of filling of the left transverse sinus more commonly reflects hypoplasia rather than pathologic occlusion.

Cavernous Sinuses

Cavernous sinuses are complex, multiseptated extradural venous spaces located on each side of the sella tur-

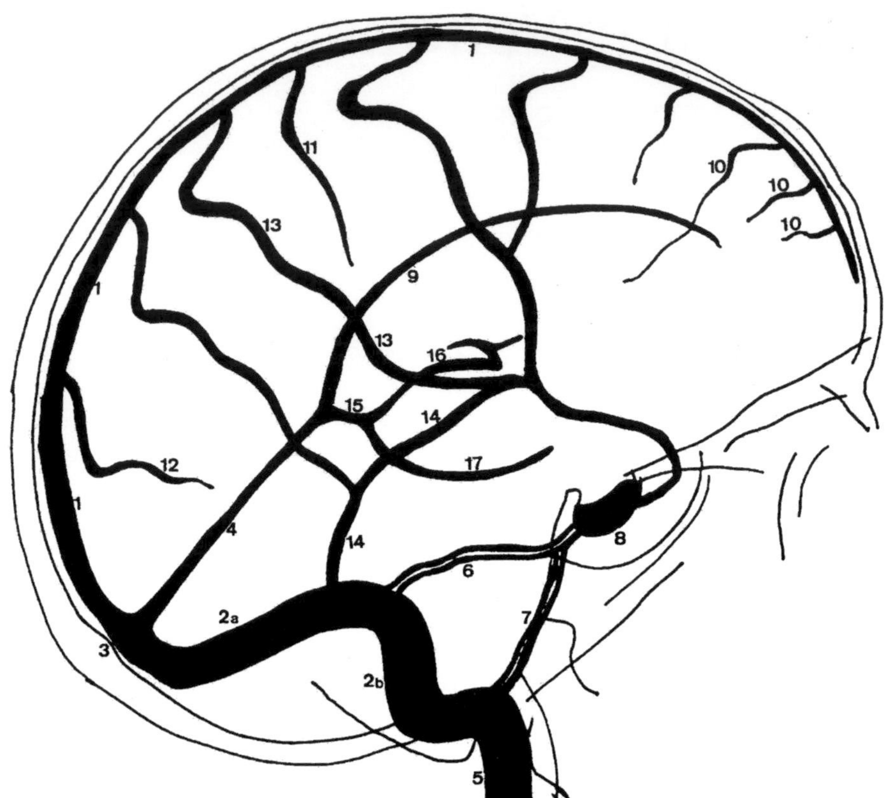

FIGURE 12-1. **1.** Superior sagittal sinus. **2a.** Transverse portion of lateral sinuses. **2b.** Sigmoid portion of lateral sinuses. **3.** Torcular herophili. **4.** Straight sinus. **5.** Internal jugular vein. **6.** Superior petrosal sinus. **7.** Inferior petrosal sinus. **8.** Cavernous sinus. **9.** Inferior sagittal sinus. **10–12.** Superficial cortical veins. **13.** Vein of Trolard. **14.** Vein of Labbé. **15.** Great vein of Galen. **16.** Internal cerebral vein. **17.** Basal vein.

cica. The oculomotor and trochlear-cranial nerves, along with the first two divisions of the trigeminal nerve, traverse along the lateral wall of the cavernous sinuses, whereas the abducens nerve, along with the cavernous portion of the internal carotid artery, lies within the sinus itself.

The cavernous sinuses receive the superior and inferior ophthalmic veins and communicate with each other via intercavernous sinuses. They also drain the anterior part of the base of the brain by the sphenoparietal sinus and middle cerebral veins. They empty into both the superior and inferior petrosal sinuses and finally into the internal jugular veins. Because of their drainage pattern, the cavernous sinuses often become thrombosed. This is usually due to infection of the face or sphenoid sinusitis.[2]

Cerebral Veins

The cerebral veins can be divided into superficial cerebral or cortical veins, deep cerebral veins, and the veins of the posterior fossa.

Superficial Cerebral Veins

Superficial cerebral veins are usually small and highly variable. The frontal, parietal, and occipital superficial cerebral veins drain the cortex superiorly into the SSS, whereas others, mainly the middle cerebral veins, drain inferiorly into the cavernous sinuses. The vein of Trolard is a large, anastomotic vein that courses cephalad from the sylvian fissure to the vertex, connecting the superficial middle cerebral vein to the SSS. Another named cerebral vein that links the superficial middle cerebral vein to the transverse portion of the LS is known as the *vein of Labbé*. These cortical veins possess special features that are important for understanding some of the clinical features of CVT.[3] They are thin-walled and lack muscle fibers and valves, thereby allowing dilatation and reversal of blood flow when the draining sinus is occluded. The veins are interconnected by numerous anastomoses, allowing the development of a collateral circulation recognized angiographically as corkscrew vessels.

Deep Cerebral Veins

The deep cerebral veins include the medullary veins, the subependymal veins, the basal veins, and the vein of Galen. The subcortical and deep white matter are drained by the medullary veins that course centrally toward the subependymal veins surrounding the ventricles. The thalamostriate and septal veins are two named subependymal veins that join near the foramen of Monro to form the internal cerebral vein (ICV). The ICVs receive prominent venous channels from the medial temporal lobes and caudate. The basal veins of Rosenthal arise in the sylvian fissure, receiving drainage from the anterior and deep middle cerebral veins and from small veins draining the insula and cerebral peduncles. The basal veins of Rosenthal course posterosuperiorly in the ambient cistern and, with the ICVs, form the great vein of Galen. The vein of Galen and inferior sagittal sinus unite to form the straight sinus. In contrast to the superficial veins, the deep system is constant and well visualized at angiography, so that a thrombosis of this vessel is easily recognized.

Veins of the Posterior Fossa

The pontomesencephalic vein is a plexus of numerous small tributaries that lie along the surface of the pons and midbrain. The precentral cerebellar vein lies in front of the cerebellar vermis, in proximity to the roof of the fourth ventricle. Superior and inferior vermian veins drain the cerebellar vermis; hemispheric veins drain the hemispheres.

PATHOPHYSIOLOGY

CVT is a multistep process that likely begins when thrombus incompletely occludes a dural sinus, usually the SSS. The thrombosis then progresses, obstructing first the sinus and then extending to involve the bridging veins anterior to the obstruction. Progression of the thrombus from the sinus into bridging and cortical veins plays a key role in the development of cerebral edema, petechial perivascular hemorrhages, and cortical venous infarctions.[4]

The pathophysiology of arterial thrombosis is much better known than for venous thrombosis. For this reason, pathophysiologic features of venous thrombosis are described by comparing it with arterial thrombosis.

Time Course

An arterial stroke is heralded by an arterial occlusion that usually induces sudden decrease in cerebral blood flow and sudden onset of symptoms that frequently are maximal at onset. CVT, on the other hand, has a gradual onset, and the time course of the symptoms depends on a dynamic equilibrium between prothrombotic and thrombolytic processes, and compensation of occlusions by collaterals. Symptoms usually appear when the compensation is no longer sufficient.

Intracranial Pressure

In arterial stroke, the sudden decrease in cerebral blood flow results in a decrease in blood volume. This is followed by cytotoxic edema related to cellular damage and subsequent increases in intracranial pressure (ICP). In CVT, blockade of outflow induces ischemia and increases in blood volume early in the time course of the disease. Therefore, elevated ICP indicates severe tissue injury in arterial stroke, whereas it may indicate reversible increase in blood volume in CVT. The occurrence of intraparenchymal hemorrhage may also lead to elevated ICP in CVT. Involvement of the SSS may impair the cerebrospinal fluid resorption through pacchionian granulations and therefore account for elevated ICP in some cases. However, the exact mechanism by which SSS thrombosis leads to an increase in ICP still is debatable.[5,6]

Intracranial Hemorrhage

Intracranial hemorrhage occurs in arterial stroke and CVT[7] with similar frequency, although the mechanism differs significantly in the two. In arterial stroke, the process starts with reperfusion of the injured area of the brain with subsequent leakage of blood into the tissue. In CVT, the primary reason for subsequent hemorrhage is increased blood volume due to impaired venous drainage and intact arterial inflow. Logically, therapies aiming at removal of thrombus will increase the risk of hemorrhage in arterial stroke and decrease the risk of hemorrhage in CVT.

EPIDEMIOLOGY

The incidence and prevalence of CVT are not known with certainty, although there are data available from case series and autopsy studies. In most autopsy series, the incidence was found to be extremely low. Kalbag and Woolf[3] indicated that CVT was the principal cause of death in only 21.7 persons per year in England and Wales between 1952 and 1961. By contrast, Towbin[8] found CVT in 9% of 182 consecutive autopsies. The publication of a large clinical series[1,9,10] suggests that the true incidence is much higher than thought from autopsy series—possibly 10 times higher, because the present mortality rate is estimated to be less than 10%. All age groups, from the neonate to the very old, may be affected by CVT, with a slight preponderance in young females because of specific causes, such as oral contraceptives, pregnancy, and puerperium.

ETIOLOGY

Numerous conditions can cause or predispose to CVT (Table 12-1). They include all surgical, gyneco-obstetric, and medical causes of deep vein thrombosis, as well as local causes that are either infectious or noninfectious, such as head trauma, brain tumors, and brain surgery. The incidence of infectious causes of CVT has dramatically diminished in developed countries since the introduction of antibiotics.[2,11] In young women, CVT occurs more frequently during puerperium than pregnancy[10,12] and remains very common in developing countries. Studies have provided strong evidence that the intake of oral

TABLE 12-1. Etiologies of Cerebral Venous Thrombosis

General
Postsurgical (with or without deep venous thrombosis)
Gynecologic/obstetric (pregnancy, puerperium, oral contraceptives)
Medical
Coagulation disorders (factor V Leiden mutation; protein C, protein S, and antithrombin III deficiencies; prothrombin gene mutation; circulating anticoagulants; disseminated intravascular coagulation; heparin-induced thrombocytopenia)
Malignancies (visceral carcinomas, lymphomas, leukemia)
Congestive heart failure, congenital heart diseases
Others: systemic lupus erythematosus, sarcoidosis, nephrotic syndrome, inflammatory bowel disease, Behçet's syndrome, severe dehydration of any cause
Local
Head injury
Neurosurgical operations
Brain tumors
Dural arteriovenous fistula
Infectious
Intracranial infections, regional infections (sinusitis, stomatitis, otitis, skin)
Idiopathic

contraceptives is an independent risk factor for CVT, especially in users of third-generation products.[13–15]

Among the various noninfective causes of CVT, inherited thrombophilia—particularly increased resistance to activated protein C with factor V Leiden mutation, which has been found in 10–20% of cases with CVT—is the most frequent.[16–18] Antiphospholipid antibody syndrome has been associated with thrombotic complications, and the best-studied clinical manifestation is venous thrombosis.[19,20] Behçet's syndrome is the single most common etiology in adults from Middle Eastern countries.[21]

Despite the continuous description of new causes for CVT, to date, the fraction of cases with unknown causes is still more than 20%.[14,17,22–26] This stresses the need, when no cause is found, for a prolonged follow-up with repeated investigations.

CLINICAL FEATURES

CVT presents with a remarkably wide spectrum of symptoms and signs. The most frequent signs are headache and papilledema. Headache is the earliest symptom in the majority of cases.[22] It has no specific features and can mimic a vast majority of intracranial disorders. It is usually associated with other neurologic signs, such as papilledema, focal deficits, or seizures. The frequency of papilledema is highly variable, ranging from 7%[27] to 80%.[21] Transient visual obscurations are present in cases with severe papilledema indicating threatened vision. Focal deficits are the presenting symptoms in approximately 15% of cases[24] and are present at some point in the course of disease in approximately 50% of cases. The focal deficits depend on the site and extent of thrombosis; the most frequent are motor and sensory deficits predominantly in the legs. Less frequent deficits include aphasia, cranial neuropathies, and, rarely, visual field deficits. Seizures are the presenting symptom in approximately 15% of cases and present sometime during the course of the disease in approximately 50% of cases. Focal and generalized seizures are equally common. Alteration of consciousness is present in approximately 50% of the patients, usually a late sign and indicative of increased ICP or involvement of deep venous drainage. The mode of onset of symptoms is also highly variable. Acute onset is more common in CVT of infectious or obstetric etiology, whereas a more gradual onset is more frequent in inflammatory or idiopathic cases.

Based on clinical presentation, CVT can be divided into five different clinical subgroups: those with isolated intracranial hypertension, those with focal cerebral signs, those with cavernous sinus syndrome, those with subacute encephalopathy, and those with unusual presentations (Table 12-2).

TOPOGRAPHY

Thrombosis most frequently involves (in order of decreasing frequency) the SSS, LS, and cavernous sinus. In most cases, thrombosis affects several sinuses or sinuses and cerebral veins and, rarely, a sinus or cerebral vein in isolation. The thrombus formation in the SSS often presents with extension into the cerebral veins, transverse sinus, and sigmoid sinuses. ICV thrombosis is an infrequent but clinically devastating event. The clot in the ICV may extend to involve the vein of Galen or straight sinus. Thrombosis of the ICV typically causes bilateral venous infarcts in the deep gray matter nuclei and upper midbrain.[28]

Unlike arterial occlusion, CVTs lack well-defined clinical syndromes. The likely explanation for this difference is frequent association of sinus and cerebral vein thrombosis and extreme variation in the venous anatomy, along with the possibility of flow reversal and development of collateral circulation in the cortical veins.

Superior Sagittal Sinus Thrombosis

When thrombosis is limited to the SSS, patients usually present with isolated intracranial hypertension. Generalized seizures and psychiatric disturbances may occur in isolated SSS thrombosis. Extension to cortical veins is

TABLE 12-2. Various Clinical Presentations of Cerebral Venous Thrombosis

Patterns of presentation of cerebral venous thrombosis	*Symptoms and signs*	*Differential diagnosis*
Isolated intracranial hypertension	Headache, papilledema, sixth nerve palsy	Pseudotumor cerebri
Focal cerebral signs	Sudden hemiplegia, aphasia	Arterial stroke, tumor
Cavernous sinus thrombosis	Chemosis, proptosis, and painful ophthalmoplegia	Carotid cavernous fistula, Graves' disease, lymphoma
Subacute encephalopathy	Altered mentation or features of raised intracranial pressure	Encephalitis, cerebral vasculitis, disseminated intravascular coagulation
Unusual presentations	Headache with aura-like phenomena	Migraine
	Thunderclap headache with stiff neck	Aneurysmal subarachnoid hemorrhage
	Grand mal seizure after delivery	Eclampsia
	Depression, irritability after delivery	Postpartum psychosis

frequent and is heralded by acute or progressive onset of focal motor or sensory deficits, usually more marked in the leg.

Lateral Sinus Thrombosis

Isolated LS thrombosis is usually asymptomatic. In some cases, it may manifest as raised ICP if the dominant sinus is involved, hence the term *otitic hydrocephalus*, given by Symonds[29] to describe the effects of LS thrombosis related to an ear infection. Extension of thrombosis to the superior or inferior petrosal sinuses usually presents with the fifth and sixth cranial neuropathies, respectively.

Cortical Vein Thrombosis

Superior cerebral veins are most commonly involved. The clinical presentation is variable in most cases. In some cases, no parenchymal involvement occurs due to rapid development of collateral circulation. In other cases, an area of focal edema that can still be asymptomatic is found. At a later stage, venous ischemia develops, but the neuronal injury is mostly reversible, as evident by the frequency of totally regressive focal deficits. Even when an infarct confirmed by neuroimaging occurs, clinical recovery remains favorable in most cases. Isolated cortical vein thrombosis is exceedingly rare, with an overall frequency of 2%.[22,30] It presents with focal deficits, focal seizures mimicking stroke, or a space-occupying lesion. In the majority of cases, thrombosis extends to the SSS, resulting in increased ICP; rarely, it extends to the cortical veins on the contralateral side, leading to the classic description of a bilateral parasagittal infarct.

Deep Vein Thrombosis

The classic description of a deep CVT is that of an acute coma with decerebration leading to death in a few days or resolving, but with major deficits such as akinetic mutism, dementia, bilateral athetoid movements, vertical gaze palsy, and dystonia.[31,32] Later reports offered a more benign course of the disease, presenting mainly with confusion.[10,33,34]

RADIOGRAPHIC DIAGNOSIS

Clinical suspicion of CVT warrants further investigations for confirmation or exclusion of the diagnosis. The diagnosis must rely on the demonstration of dural or sinus occlusion due to thrombosis. Another important assessment is involvement of the brain tissue and complications of the thrombosis. The main methods that have been proposed for the confirmation of diagnosis are cranial computed tomography (CT), cerebral angiography, magnetic resonance imaging (MRI), and magnetic resonance venography (MRV). Cranial CT with and without contrast is usually the first neuroimaging examination in the evaluation of patients with headache, focal deficits, or seizures, particularly on an emergency basis. It is extremely useful to rule out the many conditions that CVT can mimic, such as arterial strokes, subarachnoid hemorrhage, tumors, abscesses, sinusitis, and mastoiditis.

CT scanning can reliably show consequences of CVT, such as venous infarcts, intracranial hemorrhage, and brain swelling. It can also provide important hints about the CVT. For instance, the dense sinus sign is characterized by the hyperdense appearance of the thrombosed sinus (Figure 12-2). A thrombosed cortical vein shown in Figure 12-3 is referred to as a *cord sign*. The delta sign, or empty delta sign, denotes a lack of contrast enhancement within the occipital part of the SSS that is surrounded by contrast enhancement of the wall of the sinus due to the presence of collateral tributaries.

In 10–20% of cases, the CT scan is normal in patients with proven CVT,[22,35] more so in those pre-

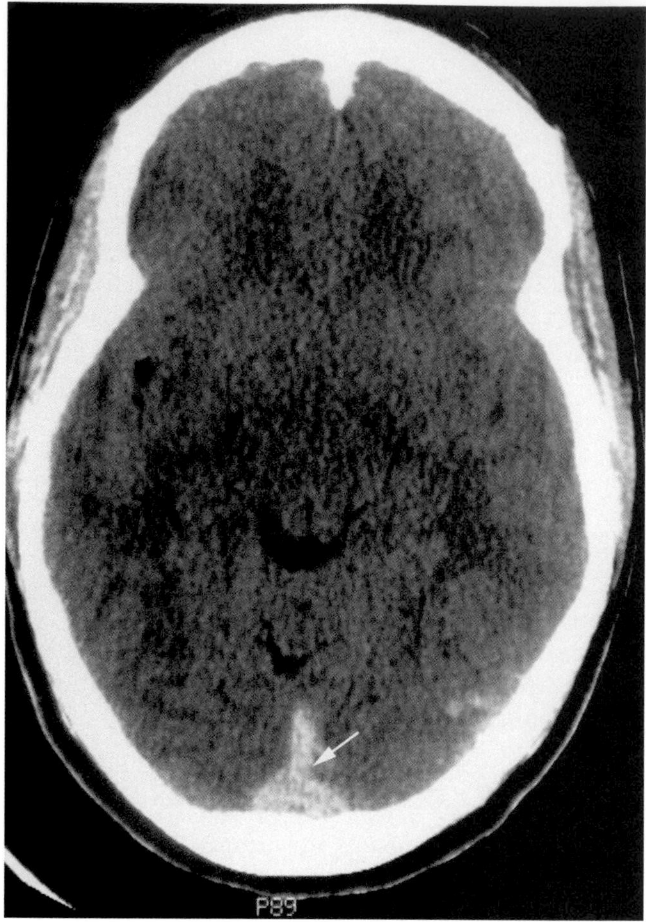

FIGURE 12-2. Unenhanced computed tomographic scan showing a dense triangle (*arrow*) in a patient with recent superior sagittal sinus thrombosis.

senting with isolated intracranial hypertension than in those with focal signs. MRI combined with MRV is a reliable sole examination for this condition.[36,37] It can show the consequences of thrombosis, such as brain swelling, mass effect, cortical sulcal effacement, and hemorrhagic components, as well as the anatomy of the disturbed venous circulation (Figure 12-4). In cases of acute CVT, various stages of parenchymal changes of venous infarction have been shown to correlate with the clinical presentation and outcome. The described stages of CVT result from the varying degree of venous congestion and elevated dural sinus pressure.[27] It has been suggested that diffusion and perfusion-weighted imaging can noninvasively provide valuable information to help triage patients with dural sinus thrombosis between conservative and aggressive management.[38]

MRV has the advantage of being easily repeatable and noninvasive but has a limited role in diagnosing partial thrombosis, cortical vein, and cavernous sinus thrombosis.

Angiography remains the method of reference for evaluation of new methods of neuroimaging. The partial or complete lack of filling of veins or sinuses is the best angiographic sign of CVT (Figure 12-5). The indirect signs of CVT include delayed emptying, collateral venous pathways, venous dilation, and tortuous cortical collateral veins (corkscrew veins) (Figure 12-6).

In summary, it is important in the diagnosis of CVT to clearly demonstrate the thrombotic process in the venous system and to delineate the damage to the brain tissue (Figure 12-7). The proposed methods to most efficiently obtain this information are a combination of cranial CT and angiography and a combination of MRI and MRA (Figures 12-8 and 12-9). The goal should be one of rapid diagnosis. Therefore, by no means is it justified to wait for one of the aforementioned studies when the other may be more rapidly available.

OTHER INVESTIGATIONS

Cerebrospinal fluid (CSF) examination is a useful diagnostic tool, because it is rarely (10% of the time) entirely normal in composition or pressure. It remains important in the appropriate clinical context to rule out meningitis or subarachnoid hemorrhage before the diagnosis of CVT has been established. Its other importance is in patients who are thought to have benign intracranial hypertension, in which the presence of any abnormal findings in the CSF may point toward CVT as the underlying cause of raised pressure.

Coagulation studies should be performed, particularly in young patients with CVT of unknown etiology. Blood should be sent for protein C, protein S, and antithrombin III levels before initiating warfarin therapy. Other tests to detect inherited disorders of coagulation, such as factor V Leiden mutation, prothrombin gene mutation, methylenetetrahydrofolate reductase mutation for homocystinemia, and antiphospholipid antibody, are not affected by warfarin therapy. Studies to exclude possible underlying infectious, inflammatory, or malignant causes should also be sought.

TREATMENT

Treatment for CVT can be summarized in a three-pronged approach: (1) revascularization or removal of the thrombus, (2) etiologic and symptomatic treatment, and (3) prophylaxis after the acute phase.

Revascularization

First advocated in the middle of the twentieth century, heparin has been more and more widely used, because evidence has accumulated that it is both effective and safe to achieve revascularization. However, due to the

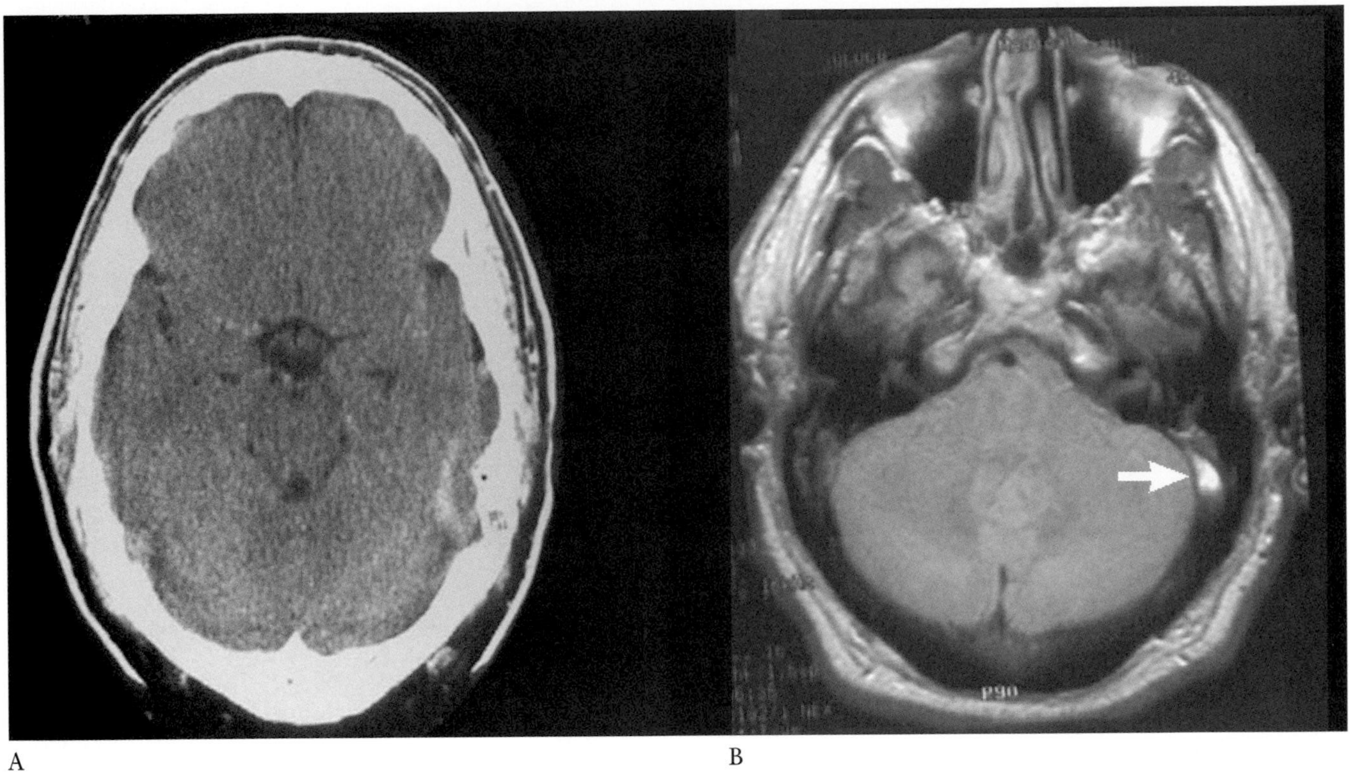

A B

FIGURE 12-3. Unenhanced computed tomographic scan (**A**) and axial magnetic resonance image with gadolinium (**B**) with thrombosed cortical vein (vein of Labbé) (*arrow*).

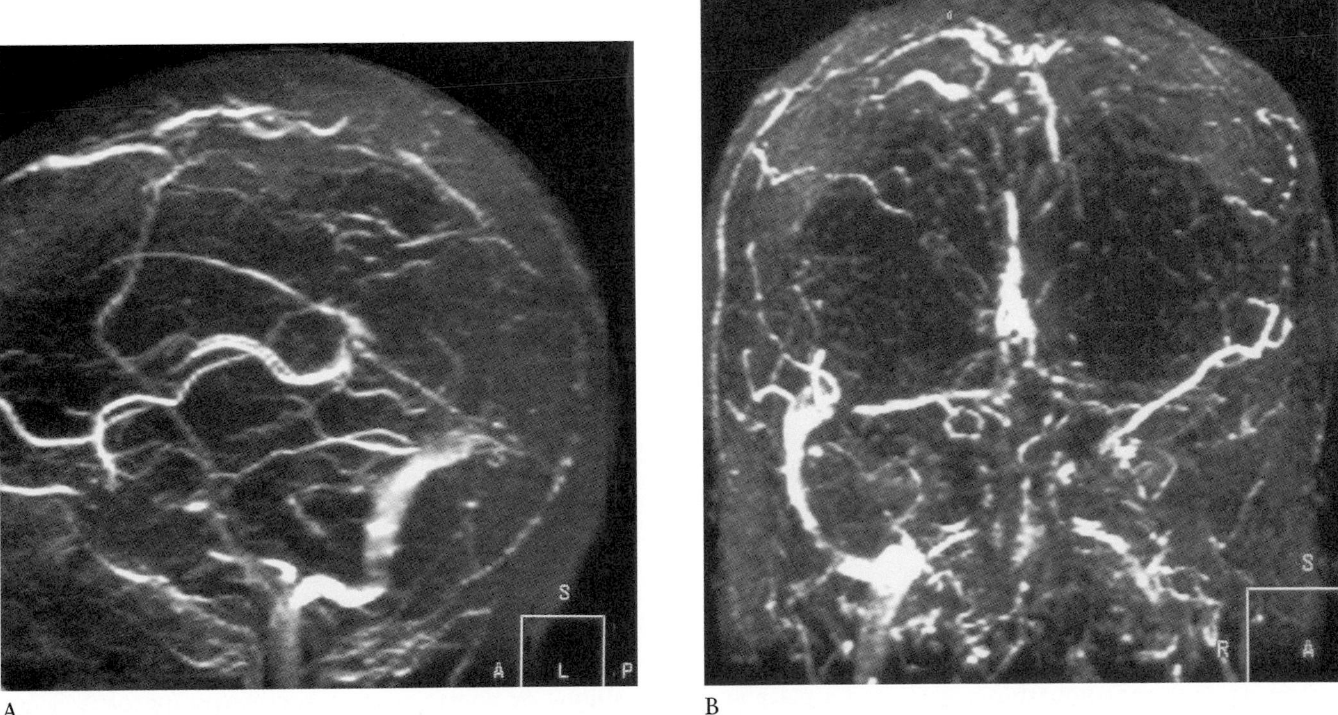

A B

FIGURE 12-4. Sagittal (**A**) and anterior-posterior (**B**) magnetic resonance venography images showing abnormal signal in the superior sagittal sinus, straight sinus, bilateral transverse, and left sigmoid sinus suggestive of extensive venous thrombosis.

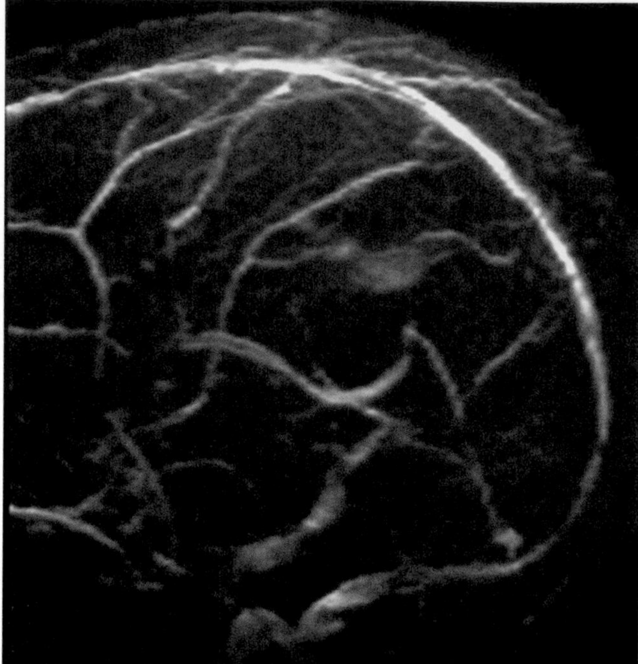

A

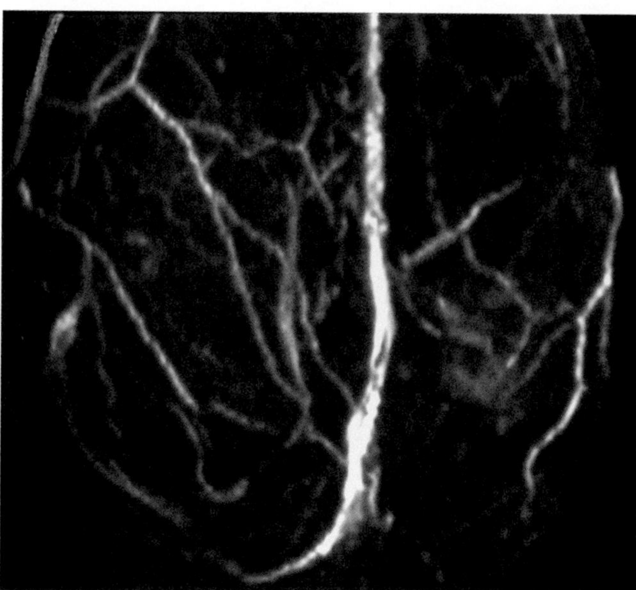

B

FIGURE 12-5. Magnetic resonance venography showing normal flow-related enhancement in the major dural sinuses. There is a dominant right transverse sinus with a diminutive left transverse sinus, a normal variant. **A.** Lateral view. **B.** Axial view.

relative rarity of CVT, there is scarcity of controlled therapeutic trials. The only randomized, double-blind prospective study comparing heparin and a placebo on patients with CVT was performed by Einhaupl et al. in 1991 (Table 12-3).[39] This study was interrupted prematurely after the enrollment of 20 patients because of a

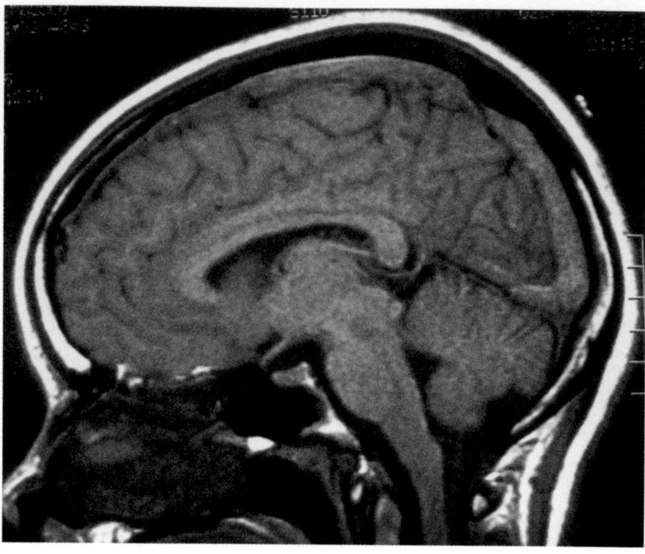

FIGURE 12-6. T1-weighted magnetic resonance image showing sagittal sinus thrombus extending into straight sinus.

significantly better recovery and fewer deaths in the heparin group. These results have been challenged owing to the small number of patients, delay in the start of treatment, and outcome of the grading system.[40] Nevertheless, the results are impressively in favor of heparin.

In 1999, a double-blind, placebo-controlled, randomized trial[41] using low-molecular-weight heparin (nadroparin) on patients showed, once again, that heparin is safe and that its benefit, although not statistically significant, is clinically relevant (Table 12-4)—especially when considered in combination with the results of Einhaupl et al.[39]

There have been several case reports and four larger series of local thrombolysis during venous angiography.[42–45] The need for a multidisciplinary team with expertise limits these treatments to specialized centers. The effect of heparin may be too slow to help the subgroup of patients with rapidly progressing thrombosis that involves large parts of the cerebral venous system and rapidly leads to diffuse brain swelling and hemorrhages. It is in this group of patients that the need for more aggressive local thrombolysis might be considered.[43,46–49] A future randomized trial of heparin alone versus local thrombolysis plus heparin remains extremely controversial. Surgical removal of thrombus alone or in combination with local thrombolytic treatment has not gained wide acceptance.

In summary, intravenous heparin treatment is recommended for patients with CVT. In patients who deteriorate despite heparin treatment or who present with stupor or coma, a more aggressive approach is warranted. Local thrombolytic treatment during venous angiography seems to be the most promising alternative treatment in selected cases.

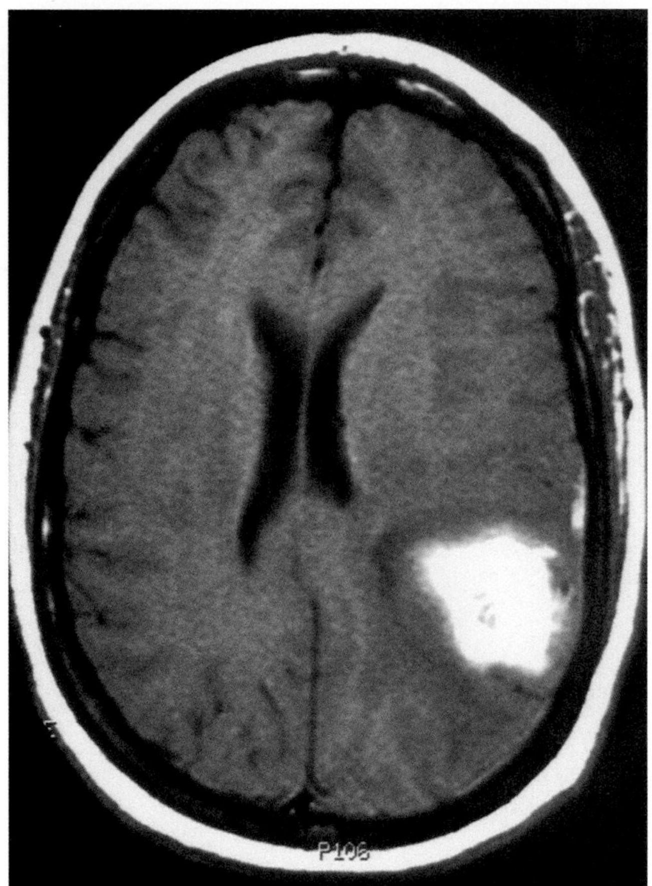

A

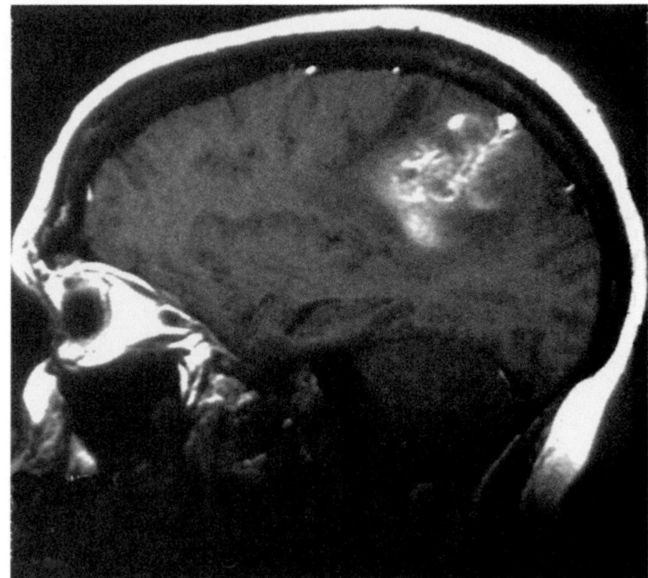

B

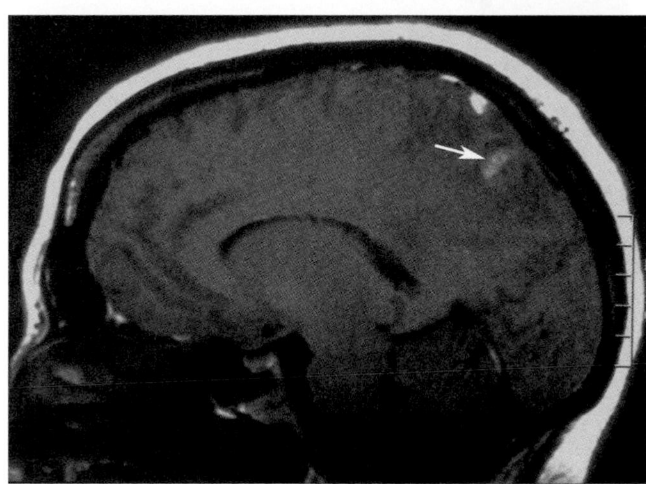

C

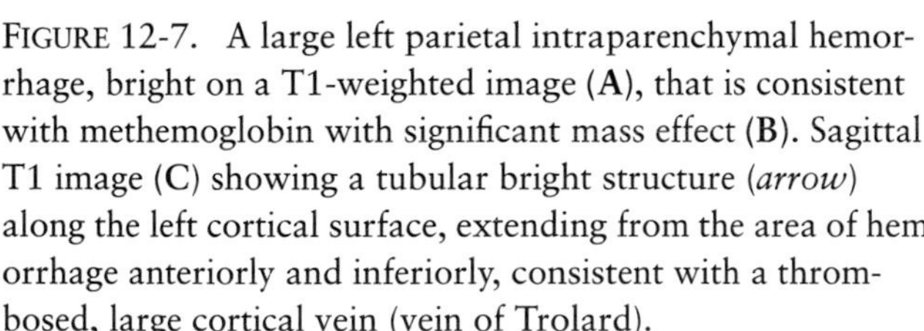

FIGURE 12-7. A large left parietal intraparenchymal hemorrhage, bright on a T1-weighted image (**A**), that is consistent with methemoglobin with significant mass effect (**B**). Sagittal T1 image (**C**) showing a tubular bright structure (*arrow*) along the left cortical surface, extending from the area of hemorrhage anteriorly and inferiorly, consistent with a thrombosed, large cortical vein (vein of Trolard).

Symptomatic Treatment

Elevated Intracranial Pressure

No additional treatment is required for the minor brain swelling that is seen in almost all patients with CVT. In cases of impending herniation, aggressive therapy in the form of intravenous mannitol infusion or pentobarbital-induced coma and invasive ICP monitoring may be necessary. Corticosteroids are not routinely recommended. In patients presenting with isolated intracranial hypertension (pseudotumor cerebri) and threatened loss of vision, one or two spinal taps with removal of large volumes of CSF should be performed before initiating anticoagulation therapy.

Anticonvulsant Therapy

Whether antiepileptic treatment should be given to all patients or only to those who present with seizures is controversial.[50,51]

Other Symptomatic Treatments

Patients with CVT frequently experience headaches. Drugs with antiplatelet activity, such as aspirin, should be avoided, especially in patients receiving intravenous heparin, to reduce the risk of intracranial bleeding. Other symptomatic treatments, such as antibiotics, antiemetics, and analgesia, may be needed, depending on the circumstances.

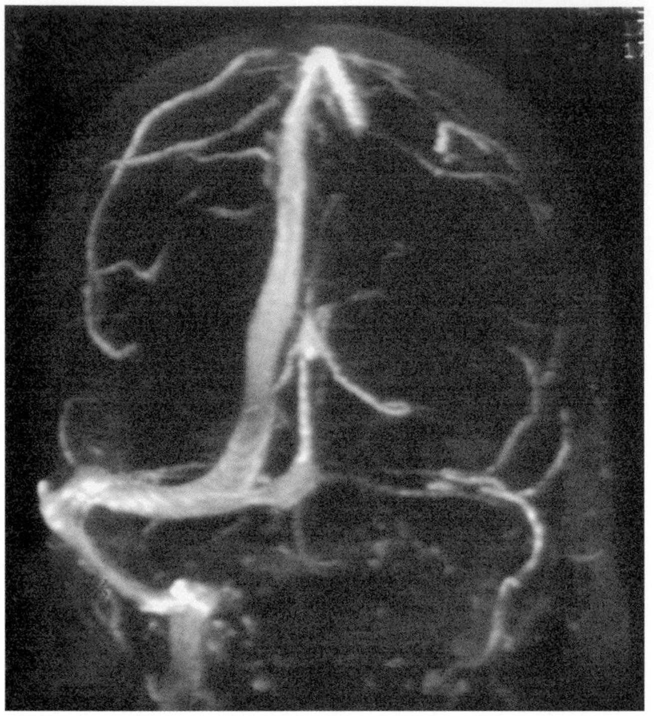

A

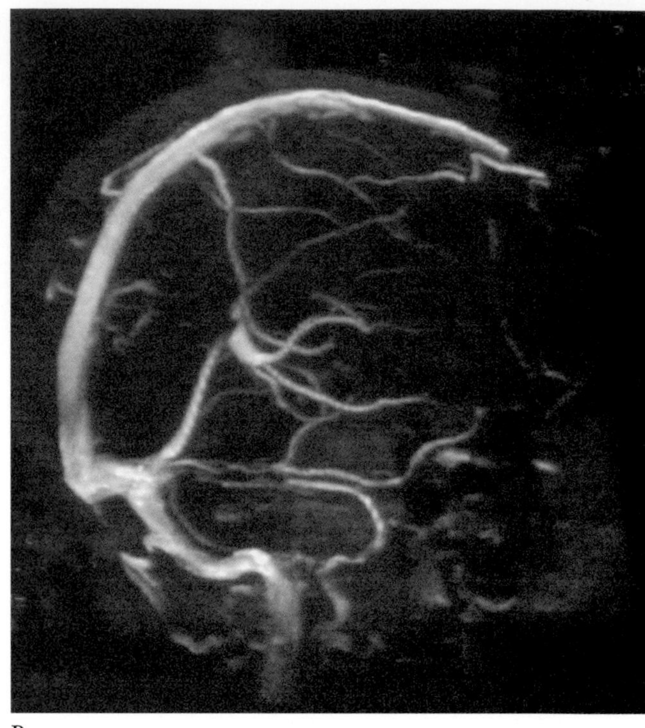

B

FIGURE 12-8. Magnetic resonance venography showing left transverse sinus thrombosis. **A.** Anterior-posterior view. **B.** Sagittal view.

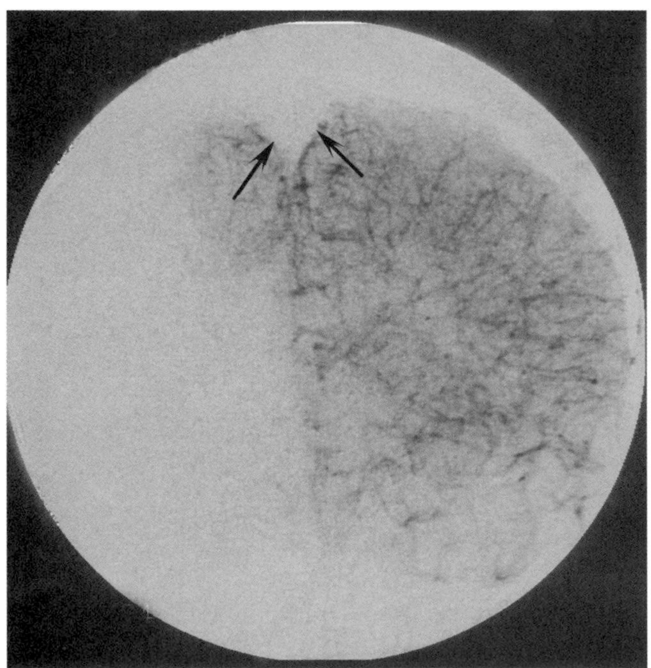

FIGURE 12-9. Venous phase of a cerebral angiography (carotid injection) showing a filling defect (*arrows*) in the superior sagittal sinus.

Prophylaxis after the Acute Phase

The recommended minimum duration of oral anticoagulation is 3–6 months after successful treatment of CVT. In patients who do not have an underlying hypercoagulable disorder, anticoagulation is eventually stopped.

TABLE 12-3. Role of Heparin in the Treatment of Cerebral Venous Thrombosis (CVT)

Outcome	*No deficit*	*Deficit*	*Dead*
20 patients with aseptic CVT: heparin vs. placebo (randomized)			
Heparin*	8	2	0
Placebo*	1	6	3
40 patients with CVT and intracerebral hemorrhage: heparin vs. placebo (nonrandomized)			
Heparin (n = 27)	14 (52%)	9	4 (15%)
Placebo (n = 13)	3 (23%)	1	9 (69%)

*Outcome in 8 months.

Source: Reprinted with permission from KM Einhaupl, A Villringer, W Meister, et al. Heparin treatment in sinus venous thrombosis. Lancet 1991;338(8767):597–600.

TABLE 12-4. Death and Other Poor Outcomes after 3 and 12 Weeks

Outcome	*Nadroparin (n = 30)*	*Placebo (n = 29)*	*Risk difference (95% confidence interval)*
After 3 wks			
Death	2	4	—
BI score <15	4	3	—
Death or BI score <15	6 (20%)	7 (24%)	4% (–25 to 17)
After 12 wks			
Death	2	4	—
Dependence (OHS 3–5)	2	2	—
Death or dependence (OHS 3–5)	4 (13%)	6 (21%)	7% (–26 to 12)

BI = Barthel Index; OHS = Oxford Handicap Score.
Source: Reprinted with permission from SF de Bruijn, J Stam. Randomized, placebo-controlled trial of anticoagulant treatment with low-molecular-weight heparin for cerebral sinus thrombosis. Stroke 1999;30(3):484–488.

OUTCOME

One of the more perplexing aspects of symptomatic CVT is the diversity in outcomes, ranging from complete recovery to death. Thought to be uniformly fatal at the beginning of the twentieth century, mortality still ranged between 30% and 50% in early angiographic series. More recently, the mortality in cases of CVT has decreased to less than 10%.[21,22,24,52] Clearly, increased diagnostic capabilities increase the number of less severe cases reported in clinical series. Coma and intracerebral hemorrhage are independent predictors for poor outcome of CVT.[53] One study assessed the long-term outcome of 77 patients with CVT, of whom 86% had no neurologic sequelae. Twelve percent had a second CVT, and 14% later developed extracranial thrombosis. The outcome of CVT is therefore generally favorable, but these patients are at risk for further thrombosis. Hence, extensive investigation for coagulation disorders should be performed to identify those at highest risk for future thrombotic events.

SUMMARY

CVT is far more common than previously assumed and is extremely variable in its clinical presentation, mode of onset, and outcome. A high index of clinical suspicion is required to diagnose this challenging condition so that appropriate therapy can be instituted in a timely fashion. Heparin is the medical treatment of choice. Early institution of heparin should be combined with etiologic (antibiotics in septic CVT) and symptomatic (reduction of raised ICP, analgesic, and anticonvulsant) treatment as necessary.

REFERENCES

1. Krayenbuhl HA. Cerebral venous and sinus thrombosis. Clin Neurosurg 1966;14:1–24.

2. DiNubile MJ. Septic thrombosis of the cavernous sinuses. Arch Neurol 1988;45(5):567–572.

3. Kalbag RM. Dural sinus thrombosis. J Neurol Neurosurg Psychiatry 1967;30(6):586.

4. Fries G, Wallenfang T, Hennen J, et al. Occlusion of the pig superior sagittal sinus, bridging and cortical veins: multistep evolution of sinus-vein thrombosis. J Neurosurg 1992;77(1):127–133.

5. Greitz D, Hannerz J. A proposed model of cerebrospinal fluid circulation: observations with radionuclide cisternography. AJNR Am J Neuroradiol 1996;17(3):431–438.

6. Kristensen B, Malm J, Markgren P, Ekstedt J. CSF hydrodynamics in superior sagittal sinus thrombosis. J Neurol Neurosurg Psychiatry 1992;55(4):287–293.

7. Villringer A, Mehraein S, Einhaupl KM. Pathophysiological aspects of cerebral sinus venous thrombosis (SVT). J Neuroradiol 1994;21(2):72–80.

8. Towbin A. The syndrome of latent cerebral venous thrombosis: its frequency and relation to age and congestive heart failure. Stroke 1973;4(3):419–430.

9. Thron A, Wessel K, Linden D, et al. Superior sagittal sinus thrombosis: neuroradiological evaluation and clinical findings. J Neurol 1986;233(5):283–288.

10. Bousser MG, Chiras J, Bories J, Castaigne P. Cerebral venous thrombosis—a review of 38 cases. Stroke 1985;16(2):199–213.

11. Southwick FS, Richardson EP, Swartz MN. Septic thrombosis of the dural venous sinuses. Medicine (Baltimore) 1986;65(2):82–106.

12. Bansal BC, Gupta RR, Prakash C. Stroke during pregnancy and puerperium in young females below the age of 40 years as a result of cerebral venous/venous sinus thrombosis. Jpn Heart J 1980;21(2):171–183.

13. de Bruijn SF, Stam J, Vandenbroucke JP. Increased risk of cerebral venous sinus thrombosis with third-generation oral contraceptives. Cerebral Venous Sinus Thrombosis Study Group. Lancet 1998;351 (9113):1404.

14. de Bruijn SF, Stam J, Koopman MM, Vandenbroucke JP. Case-control study of risk of cerebral sinus thrombosis in oral contraceptive users and in [correc-

tion of who are] carriers of hereditary prothrombotic conditions. The Cerebral Venous Sinus Thrombosis Study Group. BMJ 1998;316(7131):589–592.

15. Martinelli I, Taioli E, Palli D, Mannucci PM. Risk of cerebral vein thrombosis and oral contraceptives. Lancet 1998;352(9124):326.

16. Bertina RM, Koeleman BP, Koster T, et al. Mutation in blood coagulation factor V associated with resistance to activated protein C. Nature 1994;369(6475):64–67.

17. Martinelli I, Landi G, Merati G, et al. Factor V gene mutation is a risk factor for cerebral venous thrombosis. Thromb Haemost 1996;75(3):393–394.

18. Zuber M, Toulon P, Marnet L, Mas JL. Factor V Leiden mutation in cerebral venous thrombosis. Stroke 1996;27(10):1721–1723.

19. Bacharach JM, Stanson AW, Lie JT, Nichols DA. Imaging spectrum of thrombo-occlusive vascular disease associated with antiphospholipid antibodies. Radiographics 1993;13(2):417–423.

20. Brey RL, Escalante A. Neurological manifestations of antiphospholipid antibody syndrome. Lupus 1998;7(Suppl 2):S67–S74.

21. Daif A, Awada A, al-Rajeh S, et al. Cerebral venous thrombosis in adults. A study of 40 cases from Saudi Arabia. Stroke 1995;26(7):1193–1195.

22. Ameri A, Bousser MG. Cerebral venous thrombosis. Neurol Clin 1992;10(1):87–111.

23. Heistinger M, Rumpl E, Illiasch H, et al. Cerebral sinus thrombosis in a patient with hereditary protein S deficiency: case report and review of the literature. Ann Hematol 1992;64(2):105–109.

24. Cantu C, Barinagarrementeria F. Cerebral venous thrombosis associated with pregnancy and puerperium. Review of 67 cases. Stroke 1993;24(12):1880–1884.

25. Brey RL, Coull BM. Cerebral venous thrombosis. Role of activated protein C resistance and factor V gene mutation [editorial comment]. Stroke 1996;27(10):1719–1720.

26. Deschiens MA, Conard J, Horellou MH, et al. Coagulation studies, factor V Leiden, and anticardiolipin antibodies in 40 cases of cerebral venous thrombosis. Stroke 1996;27(10):1724–1730.

27. Tsai FY, Wang AM, Matovich VB, et al. MR staging of acute dural sinus thrombosis: correlation with venous pressure measurements and implications for treatment and prognosis. AJNR Am J Neuroradiol 1995;16(5):1021–1029.

28. Rahman NU, al-Tahan AR. Computed tomographic evidence of an extensive thrombosis and infarction of the deep venous system. Stroke 1993;24(5):744–746.

29. Symonds C. Hydrocephalic and focal cerebral symptoms in relation to thrombophlebitis of the dural sinuses and cerebral veins. Brain 1937;50:531.

30. Einhaupl KM, Masuhr F. [Cerebral sinus and venous thrombosis]. Ther Umsch 1996;53(7):552–558.

31. Bots GT. Thrombosis of the galenic system veins in the adult. Acta Neuropathol 1971;17(3):227–233.

32. Johnsen S, Greenwood R, Fishman MA. Internal cerebral vein thrombosis. Arch Neurol 1973;28(3):205–207.

33. Eick JJ, Miller KD, Bell KA, Tutton RH. Computed tomography of deep cerebral venous thrombosis in children. Radiology 1981;140(2):399–402.

34. Hanigan WC, Rossi LJ, McLean JM, Wright RM. MRI of cerebral vein thrombosis in infancy: a case report. Neurology 1986;36(10):1354–1356.

35. Buonanno FS, Moody DM, Ball MR, Laster DW. Computed cranial tomographic findings in cerebral sinovenous occlusion. J Comput Assist Tomogr 1978;2(3):281–290.

36. Vogl TJ, Bergmann CU, Villringer A, et al. [Venous MR angiography for the primary diagnosis and follow-up of sinus venous thrombosis. The correlation with the clinical picture and DSA]. Rofo Fortschr Geb Rontgenstr Neuen Bildgeb Verfahr 1993;159(1):78–85.

37. Wang AM. MRA of venous sinus thrombosis. Clin Neurosci 1997;4(3):158–164.

38. Manzione J, Newman GC, Shapiro A, Santo-Ocampo R. Diffusion- and perfusion-weighted MR imaging of dural sinus thrombosis. AJNR Am J Neuroradiol 2000;21(1):68–73.

39. Einhaupl KM, Villringer A, Meister W, et al. Heparin treatment in sinus venous thrombosis. Lancet 1991;338(8767):597–600.

40. Stam J, Lensing AW, Vermeulen M, Tijssen JG. Heparin treatment for cerebral venous and sinus thrombosis. Lancet 1991;338(8775):1154.

41. de Bruijn SF, Stam J. Randomized, placebo-controlled trial of anticoagulant treatment with low-molecular-weight heparin for cerebral sinus thrombosis. Stroke 1999;30(3):484–488.

42. Horowitz M, Purdy P, Unwin H, et al. Treatment of dural sinus thrombosis using selective catheterization and urokinase. Ann Neurol 1995;38(1):58–67.

43. Smith TP, Higashida RT, Barnwell SL, et al. Treatment of dural sinus thrombosis by urokinase infusion. AJNR Am J Neuroradiol 1994;15(5):801–807.

44. Kim SY, Suh JH. Direct endovascular thrombolytic therapy for dural sinus thrombosis: infusion of alteplase. AJNR Am J Neuroradiol 1997;18(4):639–645.

45. Frey JL, Muro GJ, McDougall CG, et al. Cerebral venous thrombosis: combined intrathrombus rtPA and intravenous heparin. Stroke 1999;30(3):489–494.

46. Tsai FY, Higashida RT, Matovich V, Alfieri K. Acute thrombosis of the intracranial dural sinus: direct

thrombolytic treatment. AJNR Am J Neuroradiol 1992;13(4):1137–1141.

47. Barnwell SL, Higashida RT, Halbach VV, et al. Direct endovascular thrombolytic therapy for dural sinus thrombosis. Neurosurgery 1991;28(1):135–142.

48. Higashida RT, Helmer E, Halbach VV, Hieshima GB. Direct thrombolytic therapy for superior sagittal sinus thrombosis. AJNR Am J Neuroradiol 1989;10(5 Suppl):S4–S6.

49. Scott JA, Pascuzzi RM, Hall PV, Becker GJ. Treatment of dural sinus thrombosis with local urokinase infusion. Case report. J Neurosurg 1988;68(2): 284–287.

50. Bousser MG. Cerebral Venous Thrombosis. In HJM Barnett (ed), Stroke: Pathophysiology, Diagnosis and Management (2nd ed). New York: Churchill Livingstone, 1992;517–537.

51. Villringer A, Einhaupl KM. Dural sinus and cerebral venous thrombosis. New Horiz 1997;5(4): 332–341.

52. Brucker AB, Vollert-Rogenhofer H, Wagner M, et al. Heparin treatment in acute cerebral sinus venous thrombosis: a retrospective clinical and MR analysis of 42 cases. Cerebrovasc Dis 1998;8(6):331–337.

53. de Bruijn SF, de Haan RJ, Stam J. Clinical features and prognostic factors of cerebral venous sinus thrombosis in a prospective series of 59 patients. For The Cerebral Venous Sinus Thrombosis Study Group. J Neurol Neurosurg Psychiatry 2001;70(1):105–108.

SECTION

IV

Hemorrhagic Cerebrovascular Disease

CHAPTER 13

Intraparenchymal Hemorrhage

Robert W. Tarr

Intraparenchymal hemorrhage (IPH) is a cataclysmic and often life-threatening neurologic event. It accounts for approximately 10% of all cases of stroke.[1] The mortality of IPH has decreased in recent years due to improved management of associated hypertension and medical therapy. However, mortality from IPH remains disproportionately high compared to ischemic stroke, with case fatality rates approaching 40–60%.[2–4]

The clinical presentation of IPH is the sudden onset of an acute, new neurologic deficit. The type and extent of the deficit depend on the location of the hemorrhage. The onset of the deficit is often accompanied by a headache. As opposed to the usual symptoms from an acute ischemic stroke, IPH is often accompanied by a diminished level of consciousness at the onset due to an abrupt increase in intracranial pressure. Seizure at the time of the initial ictus is rare, unless the hemorrhage is lobar.

The gold standard for imaging in the diagnosis of an acute IPH remains the noncontrast computed tomography (CT) examination. The extreme sensitivity of CT to acute blood allows rapid identification of the hemorrhage as well as accurate anatomic localization. Magnetic resonance imaging (MRI) is more accurate than CT in diagnosing the hemorrhagic nature of lesions presenting in a subacute form. Additionally, MRI may provide valuable information regarding the etiology of the hemorrhage, if this is unclear based on the initial CT examination.

The most common etiologies of IPH include hemorrhage associated with chronic hypertension, cerebral congophilic angiopathy (CCA), hemorrhage into an area of ischemic infarction, neoplastic hemorrhage, coagulopathies, hemorrhage associated with drug abuse, and infectious related hemorrhage. Two other common etiologies of IPH, vascular malformations and veno-occlusive disease, are covered in separate chapters.

PATHOPHYSIOLOGY OF INTRAPARENCHYMAL HEMORRHAGE

IPH can be divided pathologically into six stages:

I. Hyperacute—first 6 hours
II. Acute—7 hours to 3 days
III. Subacute—4 days to 10 days
IV. Early chronic—11 days to 6 weeks
V. Late chronic—7 weeks to 6 months
VI. Ancient—greater than 6 months[5–7]

In the hyperacute stage (I), within seconds after extravasation of blood, a platelet plug forms at the bleeding site, and a fibrin strand thrombus begins to form. Erythrocyte aggregation then occurs, and the cells begin to lose their natural biconcave shape and become spherical. This cellular deformation begins in the central portion of the clot due to rapid depletion of the glucose energy substrate. In addition, in the central portion of the clot, the red blood cells become progressively dehydrated and oxyhemoglobin begins to transform into deoxyhemoglobin.

In the acute stage (II), edema begins to develop in the brain, adjacent to the hematoma due to a breakdown in the blood-brain barrier. The edema typically peaks at approximately 72 hours after the initial hemorrhage. Infiltration of new capillaries and macrophages into the hematoma bed is then initiated. The spherical change in the shape of the red blood cells becomes irreversible. There is progressive dehydration of red blood cells and deoxygenation of hemoglobin that occurs in a centripetal manner within the clot. Natural fibrinolysis may change the shape of the clot during this stage.

In the subacute stage (III), neocapillary growth and microglial infiltration peak. In addition, reactive astrocytosis is evident in the surrounding parenchyma. During this stage, red blood cell lysis begins in the center of the clot. Oxidative conversion of intracellular deoxyhemoglobin to intracellular methemoglobin begins at the clot periphery.

In the early chronic stage (IV), edema in the adjacent brain parenchyma subsides and is replaced by gliosis. There is progressive phagocytosis of red blood cells by microglia. Reactive astrocytosis peaks in the adjacent brain tissue. Vascular proliferation also peaks at the peripheral margin of the hematoma. Hemosiderin-laden macrophages accumulate at the periphery of the hematoma. There is an oxidative reduction of deoxyhemoglobin from lysed red blood cells in the central portion of the clot to extracellular methemoglobin.

In the late chronic stage (V), a dense collagenous capsule forms around the hematoma cavity. Hemosiderin-laden macrophages and less well-organized collagen are found within the hematoma. The hematoma cavity contains predominantly free extracellular methemoglobin.

In the ancient stage (VI), the reactive scar surrounding the hematoma contracts. Hemosiderin-laden astrocytes are present at the periphery of the scar, and residual hemosiderin-laden macrophages are trapped within the central portion.

COMPUTED TOMOGRAPHY APPEARANCE OF INTRAPARENCHYMAL HEMORRHAGE

The CT appearance of IPH mimics the pathologic changes. In the acute stage (II), a nonenhanced CT scan demonstrates a well-marginated, hyperdense mass due to the high protein content of the intact red blood cells. The degree of hyperdensity may be affected by the patient's hematocrit at the time of the initial hemorrhage. Surrounding the hyperdense clot, there may be a small rim of hypodensity in the adjacent brain parenchyma due to the development of perivascular inflammation and vasogenic edema. In the subacute stage (III), as the red blood cells lyse and progressively lose hemoglobin, the hematoma approaches isodensity to the normal brain parenchyma. If contrast is administered in the subacute stage, a complete or almost complete thin rim of enhancement may be seen around the rim of the hematoma cavity. In the early chronic stage (IV), filling of the acellular hematoma cavity with a vascularized matrix may cause the hematoma to again be slightly hyperdense compared to brain parenchyma. During this stage, the developing neovascularity contributes to the ring enhancement pattern on a contrast-enhanced CT brain scan. Eventually, in the late chronic stage (V), the ring pattern of enhancement is replaced by a more nodular pattern due to advancement of the developing neovascularity toward the center of the hematoma cavity. Eventually, in the ancient stage (VI), the hematoma cavity has contracted, and a variably sized area of encephalomalacia is left behind. At this point, there should be no more enhancement after contrast administration.

On contrast-enhanced CT examinations in the subacute to chronic stages, the enhancement pattern of non-neoplastic hemorrhage may mimic the pattern seen with hemorrhagic neoplasms. This is especially true of the nodular pattern, which may be seen in the chronic stage. Typically, there is less mass effect with a non-neoplastic hemorrhage than with a tumoral hemorrhage in the subacute to chronic stage. In addition, the total volume of enhancement decreases over time with non-neoplastic hemorrhages, as opposed to the volume of enhancement seen with neoplastic hemorrhages, which may increase over time (Figure 13-1).[7,8]

MAGNETIC RESONANCE APPEARANCE OF INTRAPARENCHYMAL HEMORRHAGE

The magnetic resonance (MR) appearance of IPH is complex and somewhat variable among individual patients. The basis for the MR appearance of IPH is multifactorial, depending on imaging variables such as field strength and pulse sequences used. In addition, biophysical variables affected by the age and state of the hematoma—such as clot structure (including both intra- and extracellular proton density and protein concentration) as well as the concentration and distribution of various oxidative states of hemoglobin—drastically affect the MRI characteristics of IPH. General guidelines for the MR appearance of IPH are stated here, based on the temporal and pathophysiologic properties described previously. However, it must be kept in mind that the general appearance in individual patients may differ somewhat from these guidelines due to the complex interaction between multiple variables.

In general, the temporal signal intensity changes seen at high field strengths (1.0–1.5 T) are somewhat more gradual and detailed than those seen at intermediate (0.3–0.6 T) and low field (0.12–0.17 T) strengths but are otherwise similar. The guidelines that are outlined below are based on the appearance of IPH at high field strengths with spin echo sequences.

In the first several hours after onset of an IPH, the freshly extravasated erythrocytes contain fully oxygenated hemoglobin. In this hyperacute stage (I), the oxygenated red blood cells have diamagnetic properties.

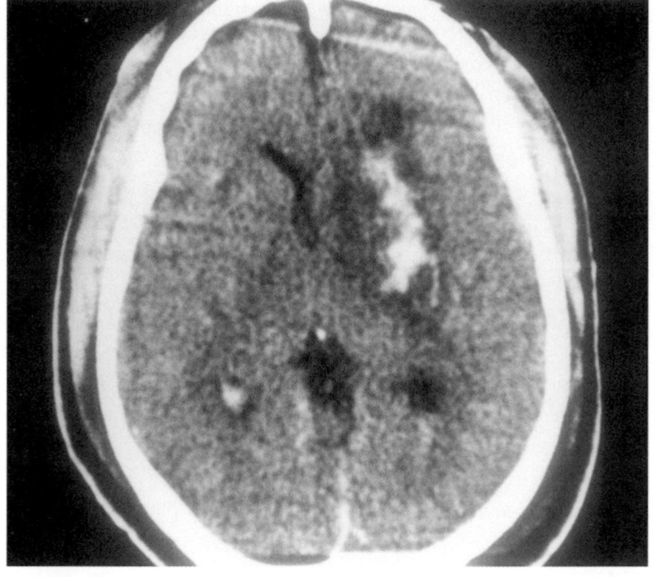

A

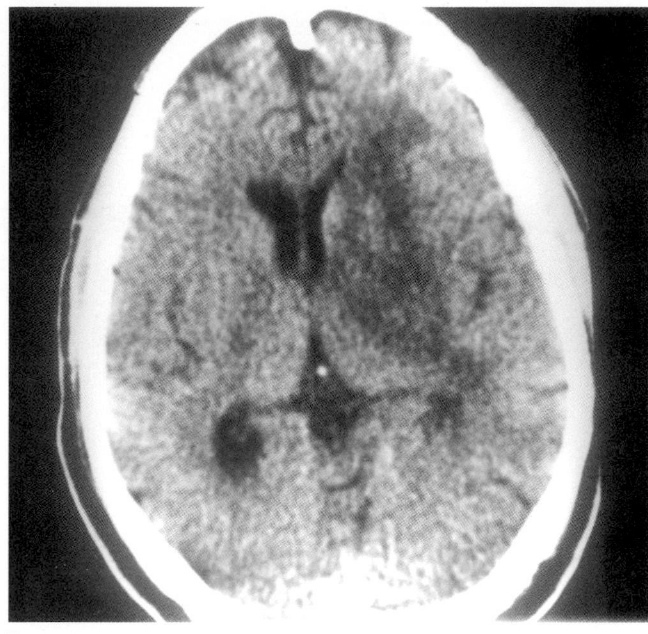

B

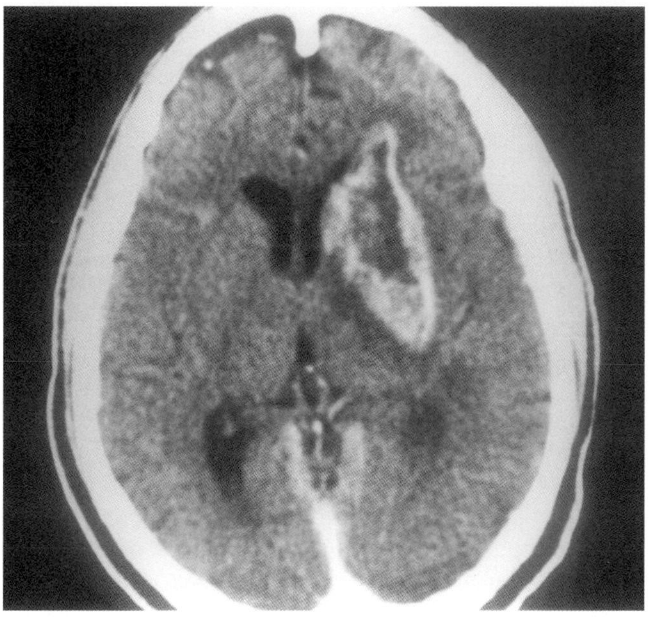

C

FIGURE 13-1. **A.** Noncontrast computed tomography head scan 48 hours after a left lenticular nucleus intraparenchymal hemorrhage. The central area of the hematoma is hyperdense. Peripheral vasogenic edema causes mass effect on the lateral ventricle. **B.** Early chronic stage (2 weeks). Noncontrast computed tomography head scan demonstrates focal areas of isodensity in the center of the hematoma cavity at this stage due to developing vascularized matrix. **C.** Early chronic stage (2 weeks). Postcontrast computed tomography head scan. There is an irregular rim of enhancement at the periphery of the hematoma cavity. Additionally, there is slight nodular enhancement of the central vascularized matrix.

Therefore, they have no significant direct effect on MR signal intensity. Similarly, other components of the hyperacute IPH, including serum proteins and platelets, probably contribute little to the MRI characteristics.[9,10] Thus, a hyperacute hematoma may appear nearly identical to many other brain lesions on MR. Predominantly, it will be slightly hypointense to gray matter on short TR/TE sequences and hyperintense to gray matter on long TR/TE sequences due to the high spin density characteristics of freshly extravasated red blood cells. At times, a markedly hypointense rim can be seen at the periphery of the hematoma, which demarcates the hematoma from the adjacent parenchymal edema. This finding can help distinguish hyperacute IPH from other cerebral pathologies. The hypointense rim is secondary to the rapid diffusion of oxygen at the clot tissue interface and the production of deoxyhemoglobin, which diminishes signal intensity on long TR/TE sequences due to its magnetic susceptibility properties (Figure 13-2).[11]

In the acute stage (II) (7 hours to 3 days), there is progressive deoxygenation of hemoglobin within intact erythrocytes. The deoxygenation occurs due to hypoperfusion of the surrounding tissue, diminished local pH, and elevated local CO_2 concentrations—all of which

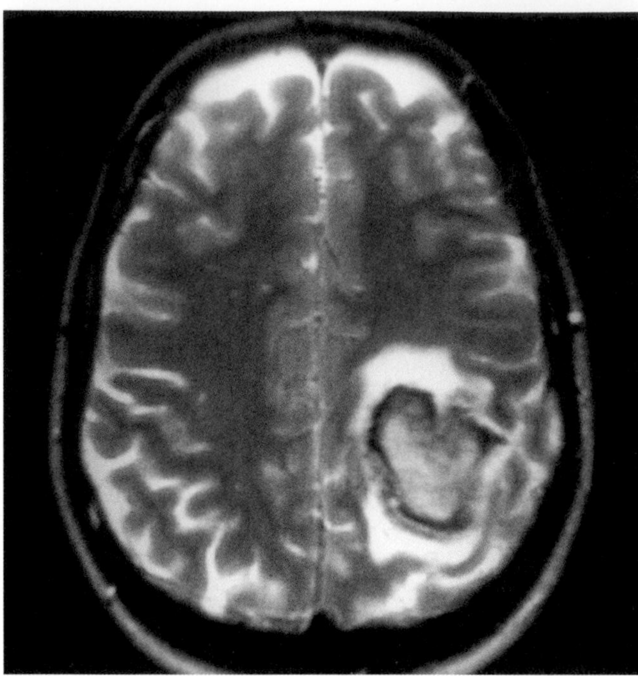

FIGURE 13-2. Hyperacute (6 hours) left parietal intraparenchymal hemorrhage. Note the hypointense rim at the periphery of the hematoma due to early production of deoxyhemoglobin.

promote oxygen dissociation from hemoglobin. Whereas the deoxyhemoglobin is contained within the erythrocytes, the intracellular magnetic susceptibility is different than the surrounding matrix. This field of inhomogeneities causes T2*-shortening but does not affect T1-relaxation properties. Therefore, in the acute stage, the IPH appears as a markedly hypointense mass with surrounding hyperintense vasogenic edema on long TR/TE sequences. The hematoma remains slightly hypointense to gray matter on short TR/TE sequences.

In the subacute stage (III) (4–10 days), hemoglobin becomes oxidized to methemoglobin. Additionally, erythrocyte lysis begins in this stage due to enzymes released by inflammatory cell infiltrates. The conversion of hemoglobin to methemoglobin begins at the periphery of the clot and progresses radially inward over time.[12] Due to its paramagnetic effect, methemoglobin causes increased signal intensity on short TR/TE sequences. Therefore, early in the subacute stage there is a hyperintense periphery surrounding a slightly hypointense center on short TR/TE sequences. In the early subacute stage, the hematoma remains hypointense on long TR/TE sequences due to the paramagnetic effects of methemoglobin at the periphery of the hematoma and the field inhomogeneity effects of intracellular deoxyhemoglobin in the center of the clot (Figure 13-3).

Erythrocyte lysis in the subacute stage begins in the central portion of the hematoma and progresses in a centrifugal manner towards the periphery. As a consequence of red blood cell lysis, extracellular methemoglobin accumulates within the clot. On long TR/TE sequences, the hematoma becomes hyperintense due to the loss of the field inhomogeneity-inducing properties of intracellular deoxyhemoglobin and the marked T1-shortening properties of extracellular methemoglobin.[13–15] Because of its T1-shortening properties, extracellular methemoglobin causes the hematoma to remain hyperintense on short TR/TE sequences.

In the chronic (IV) to ancient stages (VI) (2 weeks to more than 6 months), hemosiderin accumulates at the periphery of the hematoma cavity (Figure 13-4). Hemosiderin causes marked T2*-shortening and, therefore, causes marked hypointensity on long TR/TE sequences. Over time, the methemoglobin in the cavity is slowly broken down into smaller degradation products, and its T1-shortening properties are eventually lost.[16] The hematoma cavity therefore becomes progressively hypointense on short TR/TE sequences. Rarely, methemoglobin can persist for years, yielding residual high signal on short TR/TE sequences. However, its presence after several years should lead one to suspect rebleeding or an underlying vascular malformation such as a cavernous angioma as the etiology of the initial hemorrhage.[17] In the ancient stage (VI), a residual cleft of marked hypointensity on long TR/TE images and slight hypointensity on short TR/TE images due to hemosiderin staining may be all that is seen as evidence of a previous hemorrhage.

HYPERTENSIVE HEMORRHAGE

Chronic and poorly controlled or unrecognized hypertension is the most common presumed etiology of nontraumatic ICH. The location of hypertensive hemorrhages is usually where the brain parenchyma is supplied by small perforating arteries. In 1868, Charcot and Bouchard recognized during autopsies the presence of microaneurysms on perforating arteries in close proximity to deep cerebral hemorrhages.[18] It is currently widely accepted that rupture of a perforating artery microaneurysm is the inciting incident in hypertensive hemorrhages. The microaneurysms probably form secondary to angionecrosis as the result of fibrinoid degeneration of the vessel wall due to the effects of chronic hypertension.[19–21] Large hypertensive hemorrhages may occur either due to rupture of multiple perforating vessels simultaneously, or alternatively, the initial hemorrhage may cause vasospasm and increased permeability of adjacent vessels.[19,22] Spontaneous intracerebral hemorrhage due to chronic hypertension is usually a monophasic event with a brief period of active bleeding.[23,24] However, hematoma expansion with clinical deterioration can be seen within the first 24 hours of the initial ictus. In a series of 419 patients, Fuji et al. found a 14.3% incidence of clot

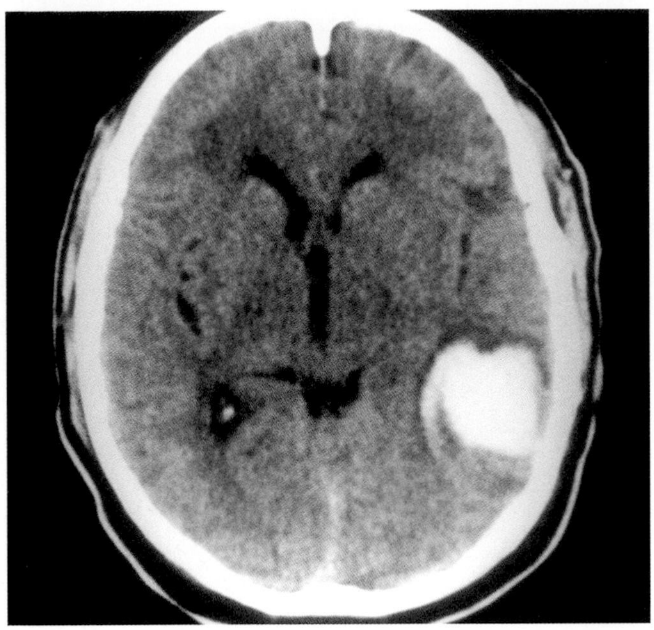

A

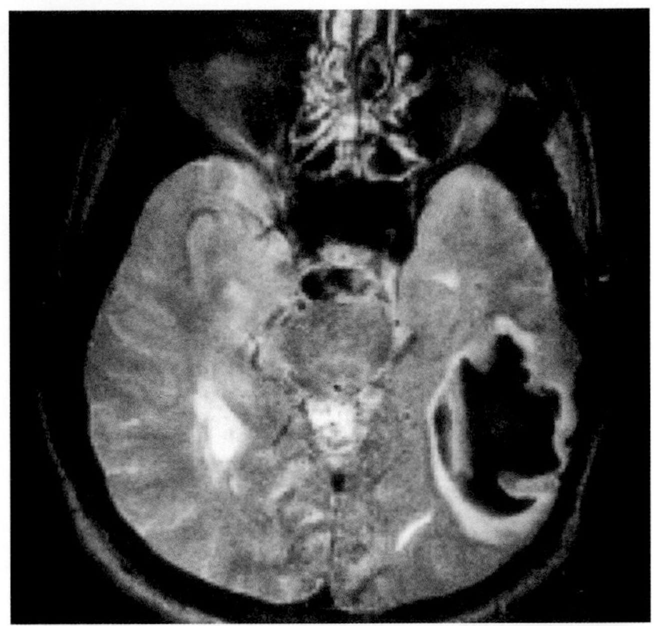

B

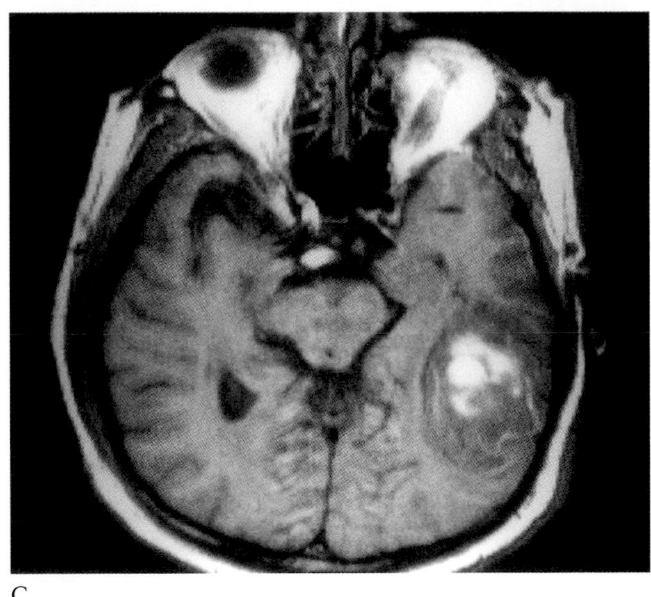

C

FIGURE 13-3. Intraparenchymal hemorrhage, subacute stage of 4–10 days. **A.** Noncontrast computed tomography. **B.** Long TR/long TE magnetic resonance image. The center of the hematoma shows decreased signal intensity due to the paramagnetic effects of methemoglobin at the periphery of the hematoma and field inhomogeneity effects of intracellular deoxyhemoglobin in the center. **C.** Short TR/short TE magnetic resonance demonstrates increased signal intensity in the center of the hematoma due to T1 shortening of methemoglobin.

expansion.[25] Clot expansion was seen more frequently when the initial hematoma was irregularly shaped. In addition, enlargement was significantly increased in patients with evidence of liver dysfunction.

The distribution of hypertensive IPH reflects the territorial supply of the causative perforating arteries. Fifty-five percent occur within the lentiform nuclei, 15% are subcortical, 10% are thalamic, 10% occur within the pons, and 10% occur within the deep cerebellar white matter.[26] The overall mortality from a hypertensive IPH is approximately 20–30%, regardless of whether surgical intervention or medical management is used. However, surgical therapy does appear to improve mortality rates for patients who initially present in a poor clinical grade.[21] Large hematoma size, pontine location, intraventricular extension, and older age at presentation tend to correlate with poorer prognosis (Figure 13-5).[27]

CEREBRAL CONGOPHILIC ANGIOPATHY

In the elderly population, deposition of amyloid protein within the cerebral arteriolar walls can occur. This amyloid deposition can lead to injury, separation, or frank necrosis of smooth muscle cells within the arterial wall,

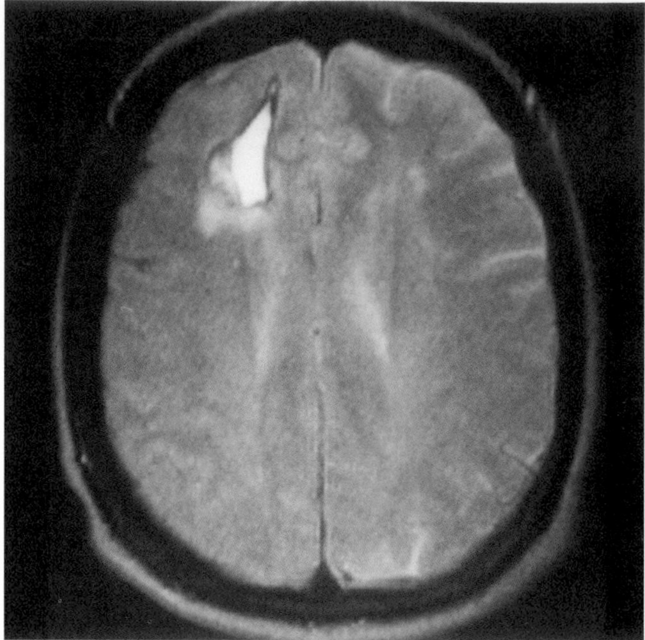

A

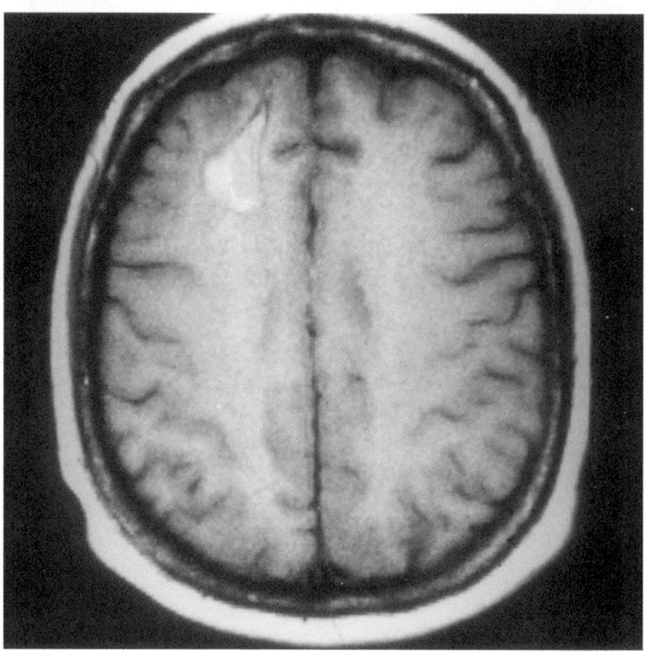

B

FIGURE 13-4. Right frontal intraparenchymal hemorrhage, chronic to ancient stage (2 months). **A.** Long TR/long TE magnetic resonance image. Note the hypointense rim due to hemosiderin deposition. **B.** Short TR/short TE magnetic resonance image. Residual central hypointensity is due to retained extracellular methemoglobin.

which causes the affected arteries to become weak and prone to rupture.[28] This pathologic process related to aging is termed *cerebral congophilic angiopathy.* CCA is an important cause of nontraumatic IPH in the elderly.

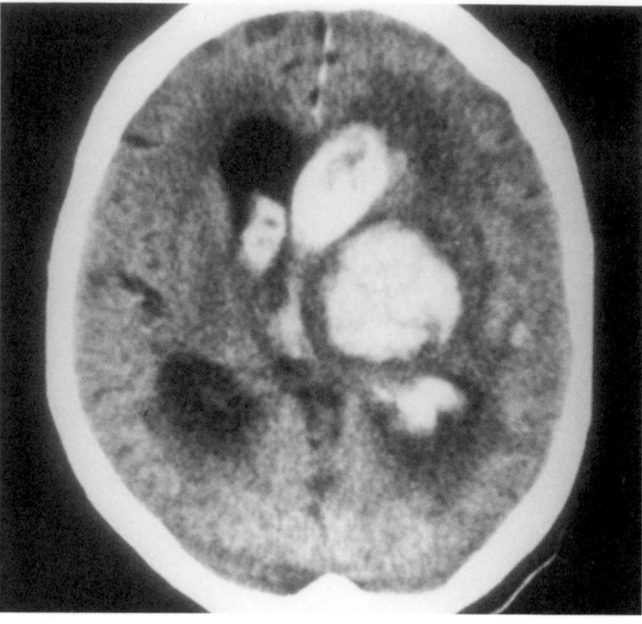

FIGURE 13-5. Left thalamic hypertensive intraparenchymal hemorrhage with intraventricular extension and hydrocephalus on noncontrast computed tomography head scan.

CCA has been implicated as the probable causative factor in 15% of patients older than age 60 years with IPH and in almost 20% of patients older than age 70 years with IPH.[29] The microangiopathy seen in hemorrhages associated with CCA is also a significant component of the neuropathologic changes that are associated with senile dementia of the Alzheimer type. In fact, approximately 70% of patients with presumed CCA-related IPH have clinical dementia.[30] The mean age of CCA-related hemorrhages is approximately 72 years. The male to female distribution of the hemorrhages is approximately equal.

Patients with CCA are at increased risk for developing IPH when being treated with anticoagulant or thrombolytic drugs.[31,32] Although initial reports with small numbers of patients suggested that attempts at surgical clot decompression in patients with CCA were often associated with disastrous hemorrhagic complications, more recent reports suggest that clot decompression can be performed when necessary with relative safety.[33,34] Classically, the hemorrhages seen with CCA are lobar in location. The frequency and distribution of the hemorrhages are as follows: frontal lobe in 35.1%; temporal lobe in 14.0%; parietal lobe in 26.3%; occipital lobe in 18.7%; deep gray matter in 4.1%; and cerebellum in 1.8%.[30] The hemorrhages associated with CCA are usually large in size and often demonstrate irregular borders. At times, multiple hemorrhages can be seen during the initial presentation (Figure 13-6). Alternatively, areas of encephalomalacia or leukomalacia may be seen as evidence of previous hemorrhagic epi-

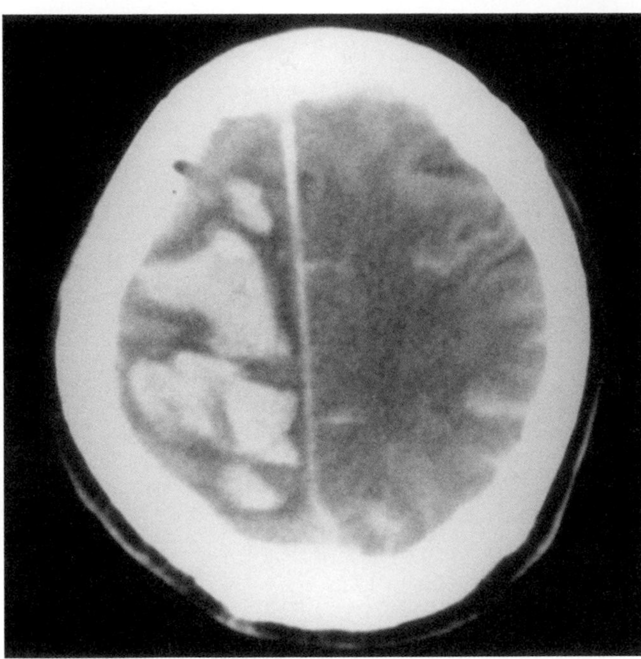

FIGURE 13-6. Noncontrast computed tomography in a patient with intraparenchymal hemorrhage due to cerebral congophilic angiopathy. Note the multiple irregular hemorrhages in the right hemisphere.

sodes.[35] Rarely, CCA can present as a mass lesion without evidence of an acute hemorrhage.[36,37]

HEMORRHAGE INTO INFARCTION

There is a neuropathologic spectrum of hemorrhagic infarction that ranges from microscopic petechial hemorrhage to frank intraparenchymal hematoma. At autopsy, approximately 51–71% of infarctions are found to have some hemorrhagic component.[38] The majority of these autopsy findings are small petechial hemorrhages that are probably secondary to a breakdown of the endothelial tight junctions and diapedesis of red blood cells.

Frank IPH with associated mass effect into an infarct bed is a less common but clinically more significant event, which portends a worse prognosis for the patient.[39] IPH into an infarction is thought to occur when an area of ischemia-damaged endothelium is suddenly reperfused. The etiology of the infarct that transforms into a hemorrhage is usually a cerebral embolus. Thus, either there is autolysis of the embolus after sufficient ischemic damage has occurred, or leptomeningeal collaterals reperfuse the infarct bed with sufficient perfusion pressure to cause IPH into the infarcted region. The transformation of a bland infarct into an IPH infarct can occur from hours to weeks after the initial ictus. Typically, IPH that occurs secondary to clot autolysis occurs within 48 hours of the initial ictus, whereas IPH caused by luxury perfusion usually occurs more than 1 week after the initial ictus.[40]

IPH into an infarct is found more often in association with large infarcts that have mass effect. Patients whose infarcts become hemorrhagic have statistically more severe neurologic deficits, greater disturbances of consciousness, and a poorer prognosis than those patients with nonhemorrhagic infarcts.[39] Though the types of infarctions that are prone to develop IPH are associated with a worse prognosis, the actual event of hemorrhage into an infarct is associated with clinical worsening in only approximately 10% of patients. If clinical deterioration occurs as the result of hemorrhage into an infarct, it is more likely that the hemorrhage occurs early after the initial ictus.[39]

IPH into an infarct may mimic other etiologies of IPH on CT and MRI. The presence of an edema pattern in a typical vascular territory distribution or a gyriform-like component associated with the IPH is a clue of an IPH into an infarct (Figure 13-7). In addition, the timing of MR signal intensity changes in hemorrhagic cortical infarction differs somewhat from that of other causes of IPH. This is most likely due to differences in local oxygen concentration and the presence of free radicals in the infarcted tissue (Figure 13-8).[41]

One of the main medical therapies for an acute ischemic stroke is anticoagulation. The rationale of instituting anticoagulation therapy is the prevention of clinical worsening due to recurrent embolic phenomena. Although anticoagulation therapy probably does not increase the frequency of hemorrhage into infarction, it may worsen the outcome if hemorrhage does occur. Whereas most nonan-

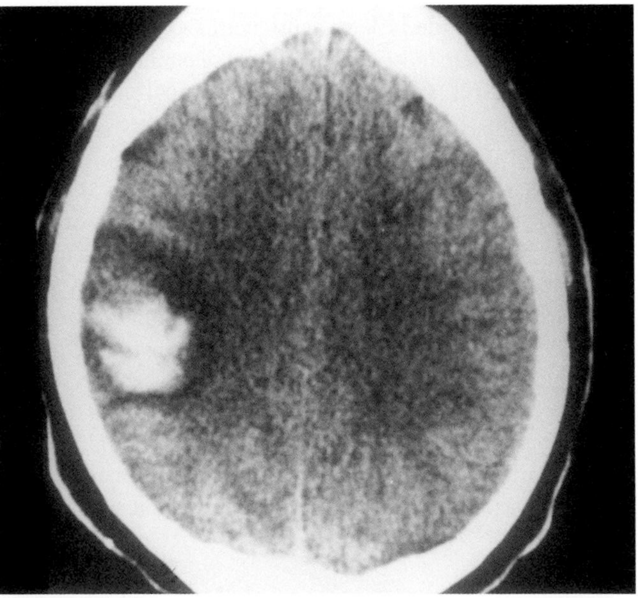

FIGURE 13-7. Intraparenchymal hemorrhage into an infarct. Noncontrast computed tomography head scan demonstrates gyriform hemorrhage within a wedge-shaped lucent infarct bed.

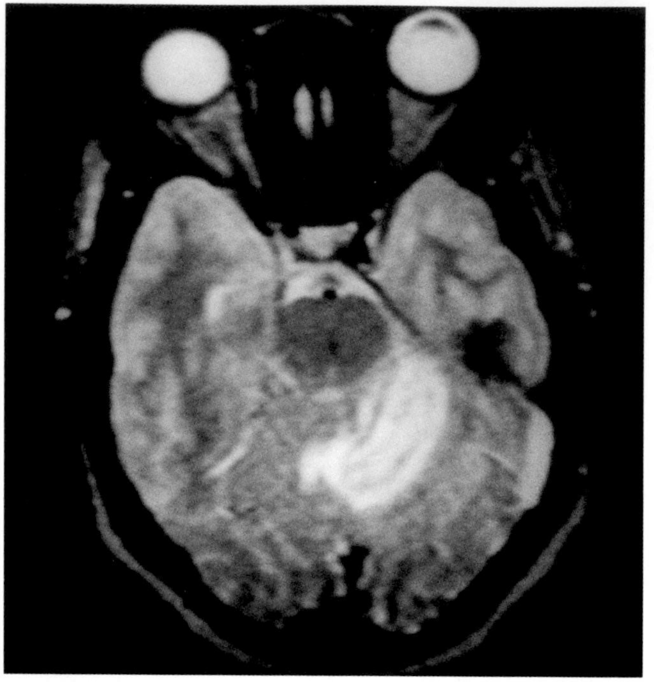

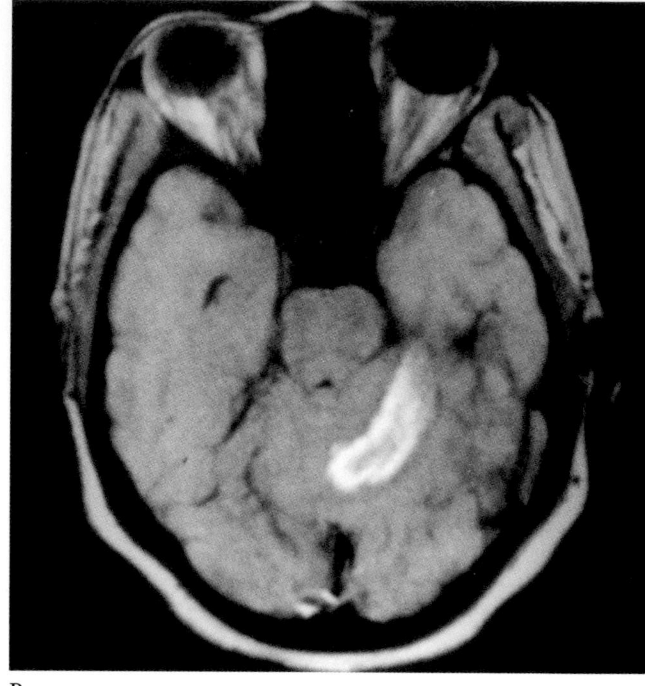

FIGURE 13-8. Subacute hemorrhage left cerebellar infarct. **A.** Magnetic resonance imaging done with long TR/long TE. **B.** Short TR/short TE. Note the gyriform nature of the hemorrhage. Also, the signal intensity pattern exhibits extracellular methemoglobin peripherally and centrally, in addition to a central band of residual deoxyhemoglobin.

ticoagulated patients who experience hemorrhage into an infarct do not demonstrate clinical deterioration, anticoagulation may accentuate the extent of hemorrhage and increase the likelihood of clinical decline.[42,43] Therefore, delaying anticoagulation for several days, avoiding excessive anticoagulation, and controlling hypertension have been recommended for patients with large infarcts.[44]

Although intravenous tissue plasminogen activator (t-PA) has been shown to improve clinical outcome when given within three hours after the onset of stroke, and there is cumulative evidence of improved clinical outcome with intra-arterial thrombolysis up to 6 hours after stroke onset, both of these regimens increase the frequency of hemorrhage into infarction compared to the natural history of an ischemic stroke. In the National Institute of Neurological Disorders and Stroke (NINDS) recombinant t-PA trial, the incidence of symptomatic hemorrhage in the population treated with intravenous t-PA was 6.1% compared to 0.6% in the placebo-controlled group. However, despite this increased risk of hemorrhage in the treated group, these patients demonstrated significantly improved clinical outcome compared to the placebo group at 90 days after therapy.[45,46]

TUMORAL HEMORRHAGE

IPH related to an underlying neoplasm is a relatively less common but not rare occurrence. Four main factors are involved in the pathophysiology of neoplastic hemorrhage: (1) structural abnormalities in tumor vessels, (2) tumor invasion of blood vessel walls, (3) tumor or brain necrosis, and (4) associated coagulation defects.[47] Kondziolka et al. reported an incidence of intratumoral hemorrhage of 14.6%.[48] The majority of these hemorrhages was microscopic (9.2%), whereas 5.4% were macroscopic. Intratumoral hemorrhage is more common in metastatic tumors than primary tumors. Hemorrhage occurs in approximately 10% of metastatic tumors to the brain. Approximately 5% of primary tumors exhibit intratumoral hemorrhage.[47] In approximately 24% of cases, intratumoral hemorrhage is the initial clinical manifestation of a brain neoplasm.[49] In regard to metastatic tumors, melanoma carries the highest risk of intratumoral hemorrhage. Up to 40% of metastatic melanoma lesions exhibit bleeding (Figure 13-9).[48,50,51] Vascular metastatic neoplasms such as renal cell carcinoma, thyroid carcinoma, and choriocarcinoma are also prone to hemorrhage. Additionally, intratumoral hemorrhage can be seen with metastatic bronchogenic carcinoma. Of the primary cerebral neoplasms, glioblastoma is the most common type to bleed. Oligodendrogliomas have the second highest frequency of intratumoral hemorrhage, followed by astrocytomas. Uncommonly, intratumoral hemorrhage may be seen with ependymomas and medulloblastomas.

On CT brain scans, there are several characteristics of tumoral hemorrhage, which distinguish it from

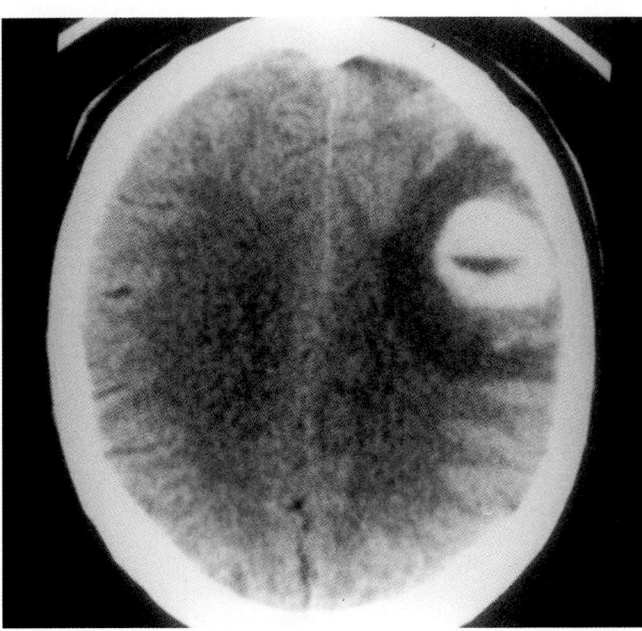

FIGURE 13-9. Hemorrhage into a metastatic melanoma tumor on noncontrast head computed tomography scan. Note the fluid/hemorrhage level within the tumor.

other etiologies of IPH. Multiple hemorrhagic lesions at the gray-white junction are suggestive of metastatic disease. In addition, hemorrhage in an unusual location, accompanied by abundant mass effect, and exhibiting irregular enhancement pattern are features that suggest tumoral hemorrhage.[52] At times, the hemorrhage may encompass the entire neoplasm, making it difficult to distinguish from other causes of IPH. In these instances, follow-up imaging may provide the proper diagnosis. Inhomogeneous perihematoma enhancement, which is present greater than 8–12 weeks after the initial ictus, helps to distinguish tumoral hemorrhage from hypertensive hemorrhage due to hemorrhagic infarction.

MR is often helpful to determine that neoplasm is the underlying cause of an IPH. Usually the hematoma does not encompass the entire neoplasm and there is marked signal heterogeneity in the hemorrhagic mass (Figure 13-10). The nonhemorrhagic portion of the tumor may appear nearly isointense to gray matter. After contrast administration, there is usually enhancement of the solid nonhemorrhagic portions of the tumor. In addition, compared to non-neoplastic hemorrhage, intratumoral hemorrhage may have a diminished, irregular, or absent peripheral hemosiderin rim; pronounced and persistent edema; as well as delayed hematoma evolution.[53,54]

Patients with systemic neoplasms are also prone to develop hemorrhage into infarction. There may be direct tumoral invasion of the dural sinuses or cerebral vessels. Coagulation disorders such as hyperviscosity syndromes and nonbacterial endocarditis can also predispose to hemorrhage into infarction. In addition, treatment regimens such as L-asparaginase therapy for leukemia can cause sinus thrombosis and IPH.[55]

COAGULOPATHY-INDUCED INTRAPARENCHYMAL HEMORRHAGE

Hemostasis is the result of a complex balance between coagulation, fibrinolysis, platelets, and vascular endothelium. This system is composed of a number of inter-related enzymatic regulatory steps. Functional abnormalities may be caused by inherent genetically determined disorders or acquired through infectious or drug-related exposure. Coagulopathies related to these functional abnormalities predispose to IPH occurring either spontaneously or in relation to minor trauma.

Two of the more common noniatrogenic bleeding disorders include idiopathic thrombocytopenic purpura (ITP) and hemophilia. ITP is an autoimmune disorder in which antiplatelet antibodies cause platelet destruction. The disorder may be self-limited or chronic and is often preceded by a viral illness.[56] The incidence of intracranial hemorrhage in chronic ITP is reported at 1%.[57] Platelet counts below 20,000/mm^3 increase the risk of spontaneous IPH.[58]

Hemophilia is a sex-linked blood dyscrasia resulting in deficiencies in either clotting factor VIII or factor IX. Intracranial hemorrhage is the leading cause of death in hemophiliacs, occurring in 2.2–10.9% of patients and having a mortality rate of 20–64%.[59,60] Although the most common location of intracranial hemorrhage in hemophiliacs is a subdural hematoma, IPH is not uncommon. Intracranial hemorrhage is usually accompanied by a history of at least minor head trauma (Figures 13-11 and 13-12). Clinically, there may be a delay between the onset of hemorrhage and the development of symptoms presumably due to the slow progressive nature of the bleeding.[59,60]

The most common exogenous iatrogenic coagulopathies associated with IPH are anticoagulation and thrombolytic therapy. In general, the risk of intracranial hemorrhage is greater for patients treated with warfarin than those treated with heparin. The incidence of intracranial hemorrhage in patients on long-term warfarin therapy is between 0.4% and 1.6%, which represents an eight- to tenfold increase in risk compared to an untreated population.[61,62] The risk of hemorrhage during anticoagulation therapy is greater when the prothrombin time is greater than 1.5 times control and is higher with increasing patient age and associated hypertension.[63,64]

DRUG-ASSOCIATED INTRAPARENCHYMAL HEMORRHAGE

Sympathomimetic drug abuse is the fourth most common etiology for nontraumatic intracranial hemorrhage

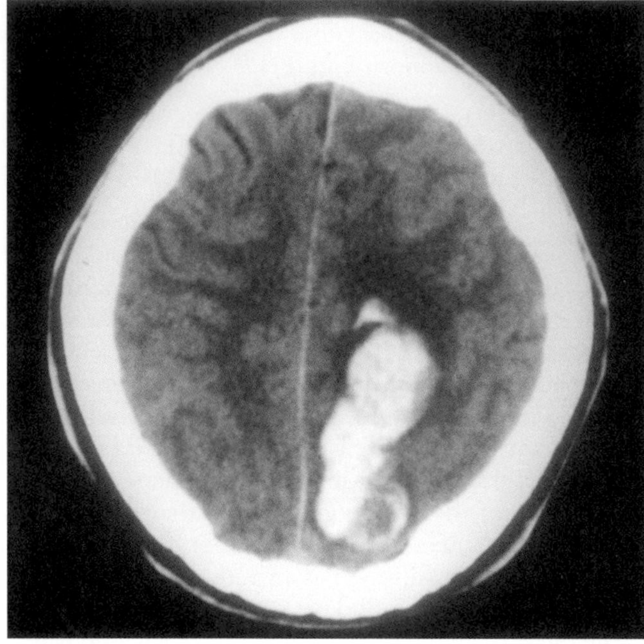

A

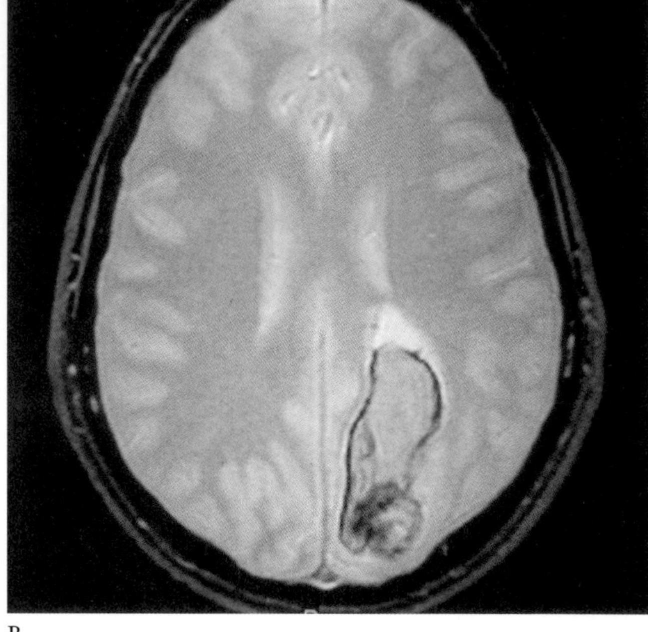

B

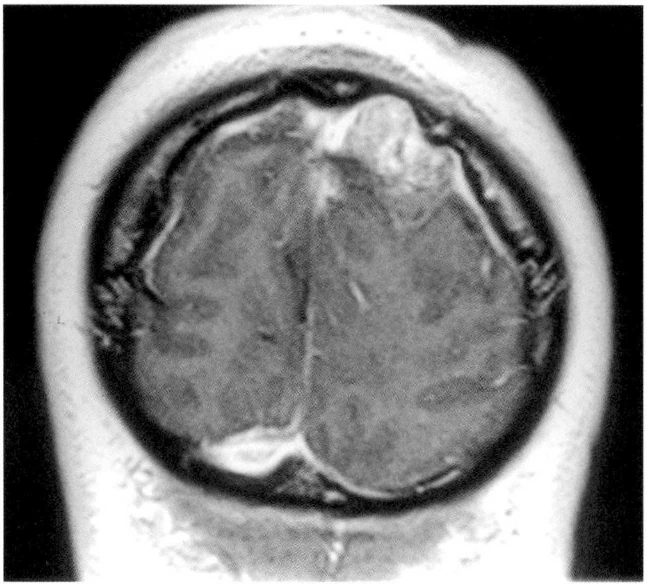

C

FIGURE 13-10. Primary leptomeningeal melanotic neoplasm with intraparenchymal hemorrhage. **A.** Noncontrast computed tomography head scan demonstrates a left parietal intraparenchymal hemorrhage and an associated hemorrhagic tumor nodule adjacent to the posterior aspect of the hematoma cavity. **B.** Long TR/long TE magnetic resonance scan demonstrates heterogeneous signal intensity of the posterior located tumor nodule. **C.** Postcontrast short TR/short TE coronal magnetic resonance imaging scan demonstrates enhancement of the tumor nodule.

in young adults between the ages of 15 and 45.[65] The most common drugs associated with IPH include cocaine, amphetamine, phenylpropanolamine, phencyclidine, ephedrine, and pseudoephedrine.[66–68] These drugs predispose to hemorrhage either due to their direct effects on cerebral blood vessels or through the induction of systemic hypertension.

Cocaine-induced hemorrhages are usually secondary to the elevation of systemic blood pressure caused by the drug. There may be an underlying vascular lesion such as an aneurysm or vascular malformation, which hemorrhages as the result of a drastic rise in systemic blood pressure.[69] The location of cocaine associated IPH, which occurs without evidence of an underlying lesion, is often similar to the location of IPH seen in association with chronic hypertension. That is, the basal ganglia, internal capsule, and deep cerebellum are often involved.[69] There is no evidence that cocaine results in a vasculitis. However, cocaine can cause multifocal narrowing and focal occlusions of intracerebral vessels secondary to the vasospasm. The vasospasm may be secondary to the uptake block of serotonin that cocaine causes.[69–71]

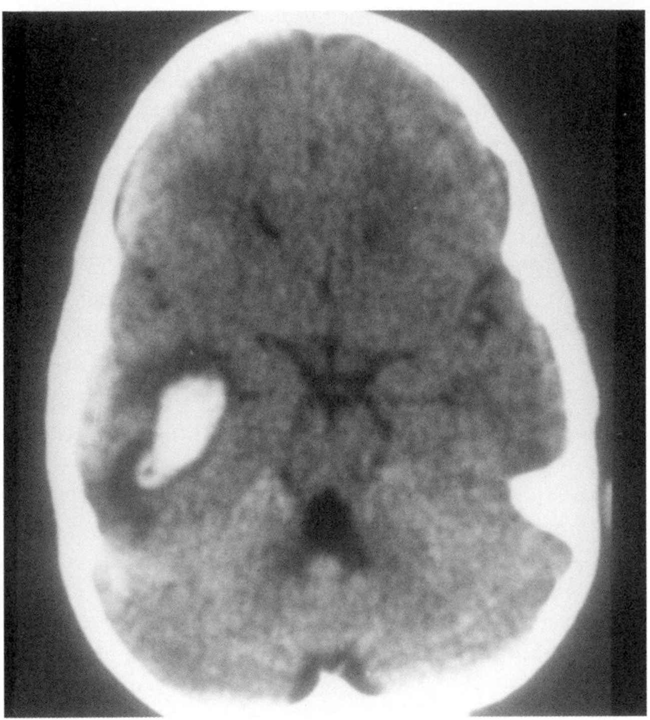

FIGURE 13-11. Hemophiliac patient with a history of minor head trauma. Noncontrast computed tomography head scan demonstrates a right temporal lobe intraparenchymal hemorrhage.

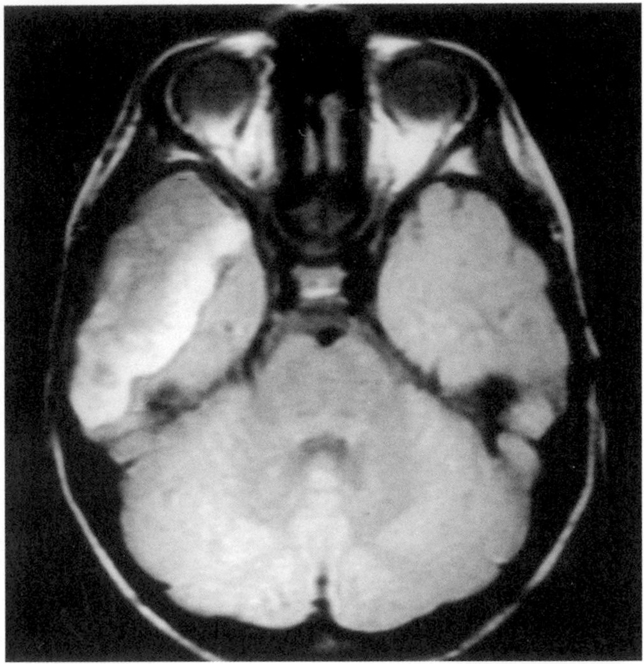

FIGURE 13-12. Patient with von Willebrand's disease and a history of minor head trauma. The magnetic resonance imaging scan demonstrates a hemorrhage within the right temporal lobe lesion.

Like cocaine, amphetamine abuse may result in IPH due to the temporary hypertensive effects of the drug. However, unlike cocaine, amphetamines are known to cause endothelial damage and cerebral vasculitis. The pathology of the early vascular changes within the vessel wall include a fibrinoid angiitis, necrosis of the media and intima, and a leukocytic infiltrate with marked intimal proliferation. These changes are often irreversible and may result in the delayed onset of IPH, even after abstinence from the drug.[72,73]

IPH is less common after the ingestion of phenylpropanolamine or phencyclidine. When seen in association with these drugs, the mechanism is most likely due to the pressor effects of the drugs.[74,75]

INTRAPARENCHYMAL HEMORRHAGE IN INFECTIOUS DISEASE

Infective endocarditis is the most common cause of IPH related to infectious diseases. Neurologic complaints are the presenting symptoms in approximately 29–38% of patients with infective endocarditis. Of those patients who develop neurologic symptoms, 50–58% die.[76,77] Neurologic manifestations in patients with endocarditis may be nonspecific and include stroke-like symptoms, toxic encephalopathy, meningitis, brain abscess, visual loss, seizures, headaches, back pain, or a mononeuropathy.[78] Siekert found that multiple crescendo transient ischemic attacks were the presenting neurologic symptoms in 75% of patients in their series. Thirty percent of these patients developed subsequent cerebral hemorrhages and died. Clues to the septic nature of these embolic events include the presence of fever, malaise, and an elevated erythrocyte sedimentation rate.[79]

Subarachnoid hemorrhage or IPH (or both) occurs in 5–10% of patients with infective endocarditis who have neurologic manifestations.[77] There are three potential mechanisms of IPH in patients with endocarditis. Hemorrhage can occur due to septic erosion of arterial walls secondary to focal arteritis. This phenomenon occurs frequently with *Staphylococcus aureus* endocarditis and can occur without aneurysm formation.[80] A second important mechanism of bleeding is hemorrhage into a bland infarct. Infarction may be due either to focal arteritis or secondary to septic emboli arising from the infected heart valve. Third, IPH may result from aneurysm rupture.

The incidence of mycotic aneurysms in patients with infective endocarditis who develop neurologic symptoms is approximately 5–12%.[77,79] However, a significant number of patients with bacterial endocarditis without neurologic signs or symptoms present with a life-threatening hemorrhage from an infectious aneurysm. Ten of 12 patients (83%) reported by Barrow and

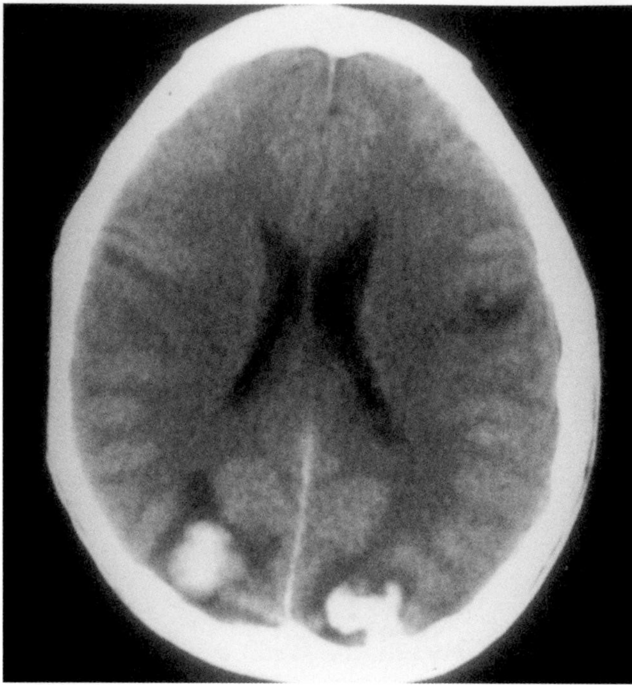

A

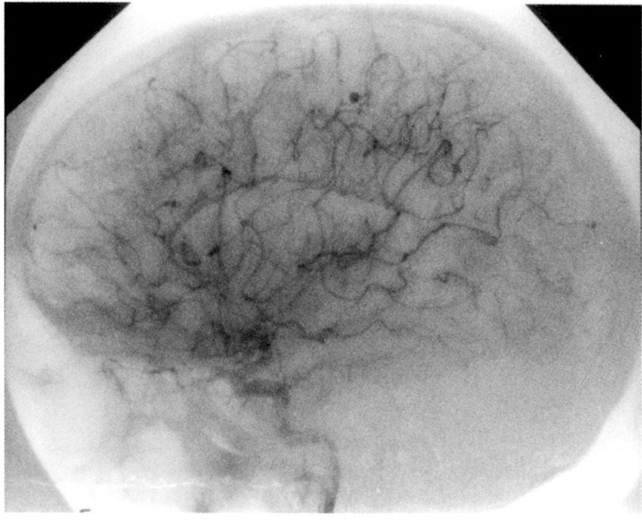

B

FIGURE 13-13. Fifteen-year-old boy with staphylococcal bacterial endocarditis. **A.** Noncontrast computed tomography head scan demonstrates biparietal intraparenchymal hemorrhages as well as an ischemic focus in the left posterior lobe. **B.** Lateral left internal carotid angiogram demonstrates multiple peripheral mycotic aneurysms.

Prats bled as the initial neurologic manifestation (Figure 13-13).[81]

The majority of mycotic aneurysms associated with infectious endocarditis is caused by *Streptococcus* or *Staphylococcus*. Ojemann, in a review of 81 cases, found the following incidence of causative organisms: *Streptococcus* (44%), *Staphylococcus* (18%), multiple organisms (4.8%), and negative cultures (10%).[82] Mycotic aneurysms due to anaerobic bacterial and fungal infections are increasing in prevalence, possibly due to more widespread use of antibiotics, corticosteroids, and other immunosuppressant agents.[83]

As opposed to berry aneurysms, which tend to be predominantly located near the circle of Willis, mycotic aneurysms tend to arise distally in secondary or tertiary branches of the intracranial vasculature. Due to their peripheral location, mycotic aneurysm rupture is more likely to have an associated IPH component than berry aneurysm rupture. Not uncommonly, mycotic aneurysms associated with infective endocarditis are multiple. Bohnfalk et al. reported a 17.6% incidence of multiple mycotic aneurysms in patients with endocarditis.[84]

There are two main theories regarding the mechanism of formation of mycotic aneurysms. Nakata et al. believed that stasis and sepsis in the vasa vasorum cause local inflammation and weakening of the arterial wall.[85] Molinari et al., however, argued that the vasa vasorum are rarely present in the distal cerebral arterial branches where mycotic aneurysms are usually found. Using experimentally produced aneurysms with infected emboli, they found that bacteria penetrate the vessel wall and produce an inflammatory focus in the Virchow-Robin space. This inflammatory reaction subsequently invades the adventitia and spreads to involve the media of the vessel wall.[86]

IPH associated with bacterial intracerebral abscess is rare. However, more recently, IPH has been associated with infections in the immunocompromised host. The most common organisms involved in this immunocompromised setting are *Aspergillus* and *Toxoplasma*. Enzmann found that two of eight immunocompromised patients with cerebral aspergillosis had small hemorrhages in the center of their lesions.[87] The mechanism of IPH is most likely due to direct vessel wall invasion by the organism with resultant thrombosis, hemorrhage, and cerebral infarction. Although rare, hemorrhage has also been documented in toxoplasmosis lesions in the setting of acquired immunodeficiency syndrome.[88] The mechanism of hemorrhage is most likely a combination of vascular proliferation and vascular necrosis associated with these lesions.

SUMMARY

IPH is an acute, life-threatening phenomenon that may occur secondary to a multitude of etiologies. Rapid diagnosis with appropriate imaging is imperative for proper patient management. Along with pertinent clinical information, the pattern of IPH on CT or MRI may provide important clues regarding the underlying causative factor for the hemorrhage.

REFERENCES

1. Mohr JP, Caplan LR, Melski JW, et al. The Harvard Cooperative Stroke Registry: a prospective registry. Neurology 1978;28:754–761.

2. Bamford J, Sandercock P, Dennis M, et al. A prospective study of acute cerebrovascular disease in the community: the Oxfordshire Stroke Project: 1981–1986. 2. Incidence, case fatality rates and overall outcome at one year of cerebral infarction, primary intracerebral and subarachnoid haemorrhage. J Neurol Neurosurg Psychiatry 1990;53:16–22.

3. Garraway WM, Whisnant JP, Durry I. The changing pattern of survival following stroke. Stroke 1983;14:699–703.

4. Kojima S, Omura T, Wakamatsu W, et al. Prognosis and disability of stroke patients after 5 years in Akita, Japan. Stroke 1990;21:72–77.

5. Kirkpatrick JB, Hayman A. Pathophysiology of Intracranial Hemorrhage. In LA Hayman, KH Taber (eds), Neuro Imaging Clinics of North America: Nontraumatic Intracranial Hemorrhage. Philadelphia: Saunders, 1992;11–23.

6. Davis KR. Computed tomography of cerebral infarction: hemorrhagic contrast enhancement and time of appearance. Comput Tomogr 1977;71–76.

7. Lee Y, Moser R, Bruner JM, Van Tassel P. Organized intracerebral hematoma with acute hemorrhage: CT patterns and pathologic correlations. AJR Am J Roentgenol 1986;147:111–118.

8. Enzmann DR. Natural history of experimental intracerebral hemorrhage: sonography, computed tomography, and neuropathology. AJNR Am J Neuroradiol 1981;2:517–526.

9. Clark RA, Watanabe AT, Bradley WG, Roberts JD. Acute hematomas: effects of deoxygenation, hematocrit, and fibrin-clot formation and retraction on T2 shortening. Radiology 1990;175:201–206.

10. Bunn HF, Forget BG. Hemoglobin Structure. In HF Bunn (ed), Hemoglobin: Molecular, Genetic and Clinical Aspects. Philadelphia: WB Saunders; 1986;13–35.

11. Fullerton GD, Potter JL, Dornbluth NC. NMR relaxation of protons in tissues and other macromolecular water solutions. Magn Reson Imaging 1982;1:209–228.

12. Gomori JM, Grossman RI, Goldberg HI, et al. Intracranial hematomas: imaging by high-field MR. Radiology 1985;157:1019–1026.

13. Hackney D, Atlas SW, Grossman RI, et al. Subacute intracranial hemorrhage: contribution of spin density to appearance on spin echo MR images. Radiology 1987;165:199–202.

14. Gomori JM, Grossman RI, Yu-Ip C, et al. NMR relaxation times of blood: dependence on field strength, oxidation state and cell integrity. J Comput Assist Tomogr 1987;11:684–690.

15. Bradley WGJ, Schmidt PG. Effect of methemoglobin formation on the MR appearance of subarachnoid hemorrhage. Radiology 1985;156:99–103.

16. Blumberg WE. Spectroscopic Properties of Hemoglobins: The Study of Hemoglobin by Electron Paramagnetic Resonance Spectroscopy. In C Ho (ed), Methods in Enzymology. New York: Academic Press, 1981:312–329.

17. Gomori JM, Grossman RI, Goldberg HI, et al. Occult cerebral vascular malformations: high field MR imaging. Radiology 1986;158:707–717.

18. Charcot JM, Bouchard CH. Nouvelles recherches sur la pathogenie de hemorrhagie cerebrale. Harch Physical Norm Pathol 1868;1:110.

19. Matsuoka S. Morphological pathology of apoplexia cerebri based on vascular changes. Trans Soc Path Japan 1950;39:1–10.

20. Ooneda G , Kishi M, Oka K, et al. The nature and morphogenesis of the so-called angionecrosis of cerebral vessels as the direct cause of apoplectic cerebral hemorrhage. Gunma J Med Soc 1959;8:1–13.

21. Yoshica Y, Ooneda G, Sekiguchi I, et al. Pathology of hypertensive intracerebral hemorrhage. Saishinigaku 1970;16:320–321.

22. Mizukami M. Surgical Treatment of Hypertensive Intracerebral Hemorrhage. In JM Fein, ES Flamm (eds), Cerebrovascular Surgery, Volume IV. New York: Springer, 1985;1259–1282.

23. Herbstein DJ, Schaumberg HH. Hypertensive intracerebral hematoma. An investigation of the initial hemorrhage and rebleeding using chromium Cr 51-labeled erythrocytes. Arch Neurol 1974;30:412–414.

24. Mohr JP, Caplan LR, Melski JW, et al. The Harvard Cooperative Stroke Registry: a prospective registry. Neurology 1978;28:754–762.

25. Fuji Y, Tanaka R, Takeuchi S, et al. Hematoma enlargement in spontaneous intracerebral hemorrhage. J Neurosurg 1994;80:51–54.

26. Fisher CM. Pathology and Pathogenesis of Intracerebral Hemorrhage. In WS Fields (ed), Pathogenesis and Treatment of Cerebrovascular Disease. Springfield, IL: Charles C Thomas, 1961;295–310.

27. Cahill DW, Ducker TB. Spontaneous intracerebral hemorrhage. Clin Neurosurg 1982;29:722–729.

28. Vinters HV. Amyloid and the Central Nervous System: The Neurobiology, Genetics and Immunocytochemistry of a Process Important in Neurodegenerative Diseases and Stroke. In PA Cancilla, FS Vogel, N Kaufman (eds), Neuropathology. Baltimore: Williams & Wilkins, 1990;55.

29. Nadeau SE. Stroke. Med Clin North Am 1989;73:1351–1369.

30. Vinters HV. Cerebral amyloid angiopathy: a critical review. Stroke 1987;18:311–324.

31. Franke CL, de Jonge J, van Swieten JC, et al. Intracerebral hematomas during anticoagulant treatment. Stroke 1990;21:726–730.

32. Pendlebury WW, Iole ED, Tracy RP, et al. Intracerebral hemorrhage related to cerebral amyloid angiopathy and t-PA treatment. Ann Neurol 1991; 29:210–213.

33. Torak RM. Congophilic angiopathy complicated by surgery and massive hemorrhage. Am J Pathol 1975;81:349–365.

34. Matkovic Z, Davis S, Gonzales M, et al. Surgical risk of hemorrhage in cerebral amyloid angiopathy. Stroke 1991;22:456–461.

35. Brown RT, Coates RK, Gilbert JJ. Radiographic-pathologic correlation in cerebral amyloid angiopathy. A review of 12 patients. J Can Assoc Radiol 1985;36:308–311.

36. Briceno CE, Resch L, Bernstain M. Cerebral amyloid angiopathy presenting as a mass lesion. Stroke 1987;18:234–239.

37. Hendricks HT, Franke CL, Theunissen PHM. Cerebral amyloid angiopathy: diagnosis by MRI and brain biopsy. Neurology 1990;40:1308–1310.

38. Lodder J, Krijne-Kubat B, Broekman J. Cerebral hemorrhagic infarction at autopsy: cardiac embolic cause and the relationship to the cause of death. Stroke 1986;17:626–632.

39. Hornig CR, Dorndorf W, Agnoli AL. Hemorrhagic cerebral infarction: a prospective study. Stroke 1986;17:179–185.

40. Hart RG, Easton JD. Hemorrhagic infarcts. Stroke 1986;17:586–593.

41. Grain MR. Cerebral ischemia: evaluation with contrast enhanced MR imaging. AJNR Am J Neuroradiol 1991;12:631–639.

42. Hakim AM, Furlan AJ, Hart RG, et al. Immediate anticoagulation of embolic stroke: a randomized trial. Stroke 1983;14:668–676.

43. Ott BR, Zamani A, Kleefield J. The clinical spectrum of hemorrhagic infarction. Stroke 1986; 17:630–637.

44. Hart RG, Lockwood KI, Hakim AM, et al. Immediate anticoagulation of embolic stroke: brain hemorrhage and management options. Stroke 1984; 15:779–789.

45. The National Institute of Neurological Disorders and Stroke rt-PA Stroke Study Group. Tissue plasminogen activator for acute ischemic stroke. N Engl J Med 1995;333:1581–1587.

46. Furlan A, Higashida RT, Wechsler L, et al. Intra-arterial prourokinase for acute ischemic stroke: the PROACT II Study: a randomized controlled trial. JAMA 1999;282:2003–2011.

47. Nutt SH, Patchell RA. Intracranial hemorrhage associated with primary and secondary tumors. Neurosurg Clin North Am 1992;3:591–599.

48. Kondziolka D, Bernstein M, Resch L, et al. Significance of hemorrhage into brain tumors: clinicopathological study. J Neurosurg 1987;67:852–857.

49. Wakai S, Yamakawa K, Manaka S, et al. Spontaneous intracranial hemorrhage caused by brain tumor: its incidence and clinical significance. Neurosurgery 1982;10:437–444.

50. Mandybur TI. Intracranial hemorrhage in metastatic tumors. Neurology 1977;27:650–655.

51. Scott M. Spontaneous intracerebral hematoma caused by cerebral neoplasms. J Neurosurg 1975;42: 338–342.

52. Zimmerman RA, Bilanicik LT. Computed tomography of intratumoral hemorrhage. Radiology 1980;135:355–359.

53. Atlas SW, Grossman RI, Gomori JM, et al. Hemorrhagic intracranial malignant neoplasms: spin echo MR imaging. Radiology 1987;164:71–77.

54. Sze F, Krol G, Olsen WL, et al. Hemorrhagic neoplasms: MR mimics of occult vascular malformations. AJNR Am J Neuroradiol 1987;8:795–802.

55. Gras F, Rogers LA, Posner JB. Cerebrovascular complications in patients with cancer. Medicine 1985;1:16–35.

56. Karpatkin S. Autoimmune thrombocytopenic purpura. Blood 1980;56:329–343.

57. Brenner B, Guiburd JN, Tatarsky I, et al. Spontaneous intracranial hemorrhage in immune thrombocytopenic purpura. Neurosurgery 1988;22: 761–764.

58. Ratner L. Human immunodeficiency virus-associated autoimmune thrombocytopenic purpura: a review. Am J Med 1989;86:194–202.

59. Andes WA, Wulff K, Smith B. Head trauma in hemophilia: a prospective study. Arch Intern Med 1984;144:1981–1983.

60. Eyster ME, Gill FM, Blatt PM, et al. Central nervous system bleeding in hemophiliacs. Blood 1978;51:1179–1188.

61. Foffar JC. A 7-year analysis of haemorrhage in patients on long-term anticoagulant treatment. Br Heart J 1979;42:128–132.

62. Franke CL, de Jonge J, van Sweiten JC, et al. Intracerebral hematomas during anticoagulant treatment. Stroke 1990;21:726–730.

63. Kase CS, Robinson K, Stein RW, et al. Anticoagulant related intracerebral hemorrhage. Neurology 1985;35:943–945.

64. Kase CS. Intracerebral hemorrhage: non-hypertensive causes. Stroke 1986;17:590–594.

65. Toffol GJ, Biller J, Adams HP. Nontraumatic intracerebral hemorrhage in young adults. Arch Neurol 1987;44:483–485.

66. Garcia-Albea E. Subarachnoid haemorrhage and nasal vasoconstrictor abuse. J Neurol Neurosurg Psychiatry 1983;46:875–876.

67. Stoessl AJ, Young GB, Feasby TE. Intracerebral haemorrhage and angiographic beading following ingestion of catecholaminergics. Stroke 1985;16:734–736.

68. Loizou LA, Hamilton JG, Tsementzis SA. Intracranial haemorrhage in association with pseudoephedrine overdose. J Neurol Neurosurg Psychiatry 1982;45:471–472.

69. Jacobs IF, Roszler MH, Kelly JK, et al. Cocaine abuse: neurovascular complications. Radiology 1989;170:223–227.

70. Mangiardi JR, Daras M, Geller ME, et al. Cocaine related intracranial hemorrhage. Report of nine cases and review. Acta Neurol Scand 1988; 77:177–180.

71. Green RM, Kelly KM, Gabrielson T, et al. Multiple intracerebral hemorrhages after smoking "crack" cocaine. Stroke 1990;21:957–962.

72. Citron BP, Halpern M, McCarron M, et al. Necrotizing angiitis associated with drug abuse. N Engl J Med 1970;283:1003–1011.

73. Harrington H, Heller HA, Dawson D, et al. Intracerebral hemorrhage and oral amphetamine. Arch Neurol 1983;40:503–507.

74. Kase CS, Foster TE, Reed JE, et al. Intracerebral hemorrhage and phenylpropanolamine use. Neurology 1987;37:399–404.

75. Bessen HA. Intracranial hemorrhage associated with phencyclidine abuse. JAMA 1982;248:585–586.

76. Garvey GJ, Neu HC. Infective endocarditis—an evolving disease: a review of endocarditis at the Columbia-Presbyterian Medical Center, 1968–1973. Medicine 1978;57:105–127.

77. Pruitt AA, Rubin RH, Karchmer AW, et al. Neurologic complications of bacterial endocarditis. Medicine 1978;57:329–343.

78. Jones HR, Siekert RG. Neurologic manifestations of bacterial endocarditis. Brain 1989;112:1295–1315.

79. Siekert RG, Jones HR. Transient cerebral ischemic attacks associated with subacute bacterial endocarditis. Stroke 1970;1:178–183.

80. Hart RG, Kagan-Hallet K, Joern SE. Mechanisms of intracranial hemorrhage in infective endocarditis. Stroke 1987;18:1048–1056.

81. Barrow DL, Prats AR. Infectious intracranial aneurysms: comparison of groups with and without endocarditis. Neurosurgery 1990;27:562–572.

82. Ojemann RG. Infectious Intracranial Aneurysms. In JM Fein, ES Flamm (eds), Cerebrovascular Surgery. New York: Springer, 1984;3:1047–1060.

83. Ahuja GK, Jain N, Vijayaraghavan M, et al. Cerebral mycotic aneurysms of fungal origin. J Neurosurg 1978;49:107–110.

84. Bohnfalk GL, Story JL, Wissinger JP, et al. Bacterial intracranial aneurysm. J Neurosurg 1978;48: 369–382.

85. Nakata Y, Shionoya S, Kamiya K. Pathogenesis of mycotic aneurysm. Angiology 1968;19:593–601.

86. Molinari GF, Smith L, Goldstein MN, et al. Pathogenesis of cerebral mycotic aneurysms. Neurology 1973;23:325–332.

87. Enzmann DR, Britt RH, Pacone R. Staging of human brain abscess by computed tomography. Radiology 1983;146:703–708.

88. Chaudhair AB, Singh A, Jundal S, et al. Haemorrhage in cerebral toxoplasmosis: a report on a patient with the acquired immunodeficiency syndrome. South Afr Med J 1989;76:272–274.

CHAPTER

14

Subarachnoid Hemorrhage

Nafi Aygun and John Perl II

Spontaneous subarachnoid hemorrhage (SAH) is a common and often devastating occurrence affecting approximately 30,000 Americans annually.[1] Population-based incidence rates vary from 6 to 16 per 100,000 persons.[2,3] The adverse consequences of SAH are protean. Overall, there is 25–30% mortality with substantial morbidity in 50% of the survivors.[4] Approximately one-half of the patients with "favorable" outcomes experience substantial neuropsychological or cognitive deficits.[5]

Due to its high incidence, trauma is the most common cause of SAH. Nontraumatic SAH accounts for 5–10% of all strokes, with aneurysm rupture being the most common cause, comprising approximately 70–80% of the cases.[6] The differential diagnosis of nonaneurysmal SAH is broad, including perimesencephalic nonaneurysmal SAH (PNSAH), arteriovenous malformations (AVMs), tumors, pituitary apoplexy, vasculopathies (including amyloid angiopathy), vasculitis associated with collagen vascular diseases, arterial dissections, hematologic conditions (including leukemia and coagulopathies), central nervous system vasculitis, and drugs (including cocaine, ephedrine, and amphetamine). PNSAH constitutes approximately 70% of the nonaneurysmal SAH cases.[7] The classic clinical presentation of spontaneous SAH is an acute onset of severe headache with nuchal rigidity. A small group of patients may have focal neurologic findings that may help localizing the aneurysm. Approximately 45% of the patients experience a brief episode of loss of consciousness.[8] Of the patients who present to an emergency department describing "the worst headache" of their lives, only 12% have SAH.[9] This increases to 25% when "the worst headache" of a patient's life is accompanied by a neurologic abnormality.

About one-third of SAH patients describe "warning signs,"[1] and one-half of these seek medical attention less than 2 weeks before a major SAH. The sentinel signs and symptoms, including sudden headache, vomiting, and dizziness, may be attributable to minor SAH, hemorrhage into the aneurysm wall, rapid expansion of the aneurysm sac, or ischemia. Early diagnosis can drastically decrease mortality and morbidity in these patients.[8]

IMAGING OF SUBARACHNOID HEMORRHAGE

Computed Tomography

Because of its high sensitivity and widespread availability, the initial imaging evaluation of patients presenting with signs and symptoms of acute SAH is computed tomography (CT). The sensitivity, however, is technique dependent. The optimal study protocol consists of 5-mm-thick images from the foramen magnum to the base of the sella turcica, followed by 3-mm-thick images extending 2–3 cm cephalad from the base of the sella turcica through the region of the circle of Willis, followed by 10-mm-thick images to the vertex.[10] A thin layer of SAH may be overlooked if only routine 8- or 10-mm-thick slices are used. Unenhanced CT is approximately 92–98% sensitive in detecting SAH within the first 24 hours of ictus.[11,12] SAH appears as increased attenuation coefficient ("bright") in the cerebrospinal fluid (CSF) spaces. This increased attenuation is related to the protein (globin) component of the hemoglobin molecule. Therefore, the appearance of SAH on CT depends on the hemoglobin concentration, the hematocrit value, the volume of blood, and the timing of the CT scan in relation to hemorrhage.[10] The CT attenuation value of whole blood with a hematocrit of 45% is 56 Hounsfield units (HU), and that of cerebral cortex is 37–41 HU. Blood with a hemoglobin value of less than 10 g/dl may be isodense with the cerebral cortex on CT.[13] The sensitivity for detection of SAH decreases with time and falls below 50% 1 week after the initial event. If the initial CT is unrevealing for SAH, a lumbar puncture with spectrophotometric analysis of the CSF is still needed.[11,12] No correlation has been found between the number of red blood cells in the CSF collected by lumbar puncture and the amount and extent of SAH detected by CT.[14]

Parenchymal hemorrhage, intraventricular hemorrhage, and subdural hematoma are found in 19.0%, 20.0%, and 1.8% of all cases of SAH secondary to aneurysm rupture, respectively.[12] Rarely, an isolated subdural hematoma may be the only finding of a ruptured aneurysm (Figure 14-1).

The location of the SAH detected on CT is often predictive of the location of the ruptured aneurysm. However, due to overlap of different hemorrhage patterns, the distribution of subarachnoid blood is not pathognomonic for a specific site of a ruptured aneurysm.[15–17] Some patterns of SAH may imply nonaneurysmal etiology.[18] A report by Davis et al.[19] did not show any correlation between the ruptured aneurysm site and CT findings in a prospective study of 168 patients. van der Jagt et al.[20] found that a parenchymal hematoma (when present) was an excellent predictor of the location of ruptured aneurysm (Figure 14-2). They predicted the anterior cerebral artery as the site of aneurysm rupture on the basis of SAH in the interhemispheric fissure distribution on CT with a very high positive predictive value, but, for other sites, the results were poor, with high interobserver variability.[20] Nevertheless, patterns described in Table 14-1 may focus attention on specific sites (see Figure 14-2; Figures 14-3 and 14-4). Occasionally, larger aneurysms and surrounding hematoma can be directly visualized on noncontrast CT studies (Figure 14-5).

In addition to diagnosing SAH and predicting the location of a ruptured aneurysm, CT can provide important information on potential complications of SAH and patient outcome. In the International Cooperative Study on the Timing of Aneurysm Study (ICSTAS),[12] multivariate analysis showed that the amount of SAH on CT was a significant predictive factor, in addition to clinical grade, for death and disability. In a smaller prospective study, the amount of SAH on CT was found to be a powerful independent predictor for the occurrence of vasospasm and subsequent cerebral ischemia, although its predictive value was not equally strong for patient outcome.[21] Fisher et al.[22] evaluated 47 SAH patients for development and severity of vasospasm relative to the distribution of SAH on CT. Patients with focal or diffuse layers of SAH less than 1 mm thick or with intraparenchymal or intraventricular bleed did not develop macroscopic cerebral ischemia, although a few patients showed evidence of angiographic vasospasm. On the other hand, a majority of patients with localized clot or vertical layers of SAH greater than 1 mm thick developed vasospasm and ischemia.

Approximately 20% of the SAH patients develop acute ventricular dilatation due to impaired CSF flow through the basal subarachnoid cisterns, the outlets of the fourth ventricle, or subarachnoid cisterns around the tentorial incisura.[8] Chronic hydrocephalus develops in 10% of the aneurysmal SAH survivors, requiring permanent diversion of CSF with a ventricular shunt. CT is very accurate in the assessment of these patients.

Magnetic Resonance Imaging

Initially, in addition to higher cost and limited availability, the "insensitivity" of conventional magnetic resonance imaging (MRI) to the detection of acute SAH restricted its use in the evaluation of SAH patients. With improved hardware capabilities and new pulse sequence designs, such as fast fluid-attenuated inversion recovery (FLAIR) and susceptibility-weighted gradient echo (GRE), MRI is now an acceptable modality in selected clinical scenarios. Perl et al.[23] reported 85% combined accuracy for detection of acute SAH with a combination of conventional spin echo T1-weighted, spin density (SD)–weighted, T2*-weighted GRE and FLAIR sequences in their model of iatrogenically created SAH in dogs. In an in vitro study, Noguchi et al.[24] demonstrated that FLAIR imaging is more sensitive than CT in the detection of small amounts of simulated SAH. In a series of 20 patients, FLAIR imaging was found to be 100% sensitive for acute SAH.[25] In a smaller patient group, Singer et al.[26] reported similar results (Figure 14-6). It must be pointed out, however, that the specificity of FLAIR imaging for SAH is quite low. This is improved by the addition of GRE and SD sequences.[23,27] Although the first imaging study in the clinical setting of suspected SAH is frequently CT, the appearance of SAH on MRI should be known because SAH patients may be triaged to the ischemic stroke clinical pathway, where MRI may be the first study performed. Prospective studies involving larger patient groups are needed to establish the role of MRI in the setting of acute SAH.

MRI is superior to CT in the detection of subacute and chronic SAH.[28,29] MRI can demonstrate SAH up to 45 days after the ictus as areas of increased signal on T1-, T2-, and SD-weighted images and fast FLAIR images (Figure 14-7). The FLAIR sequence is more sensitive to subacute SAH than the other pulse sequences; however, no statistically significant difference was found among

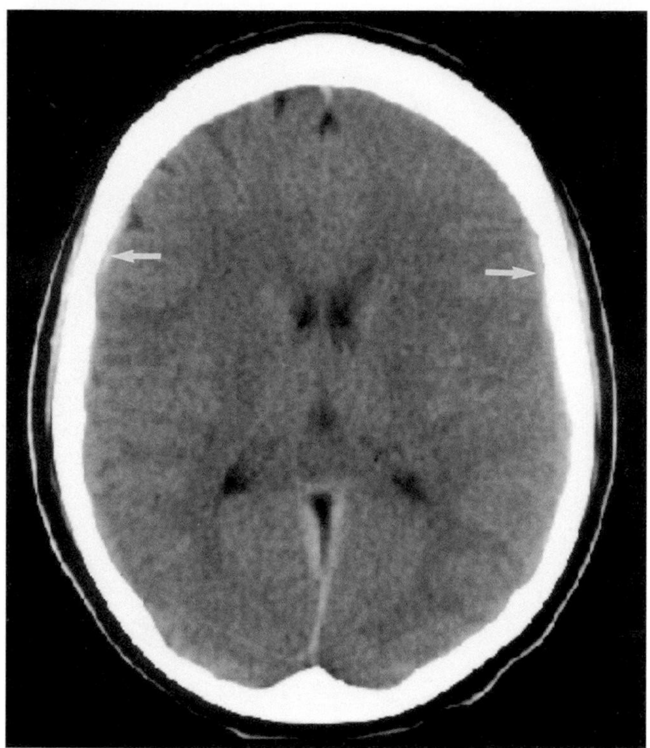

A

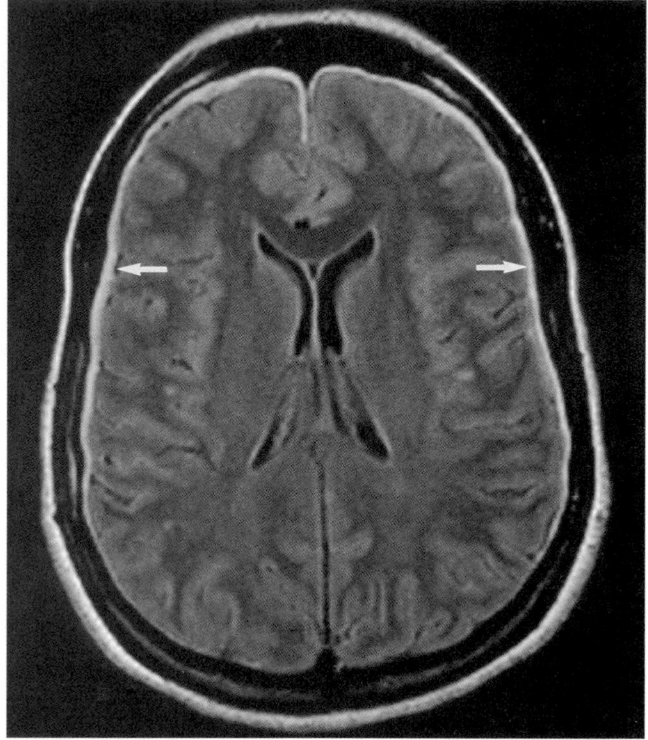

B

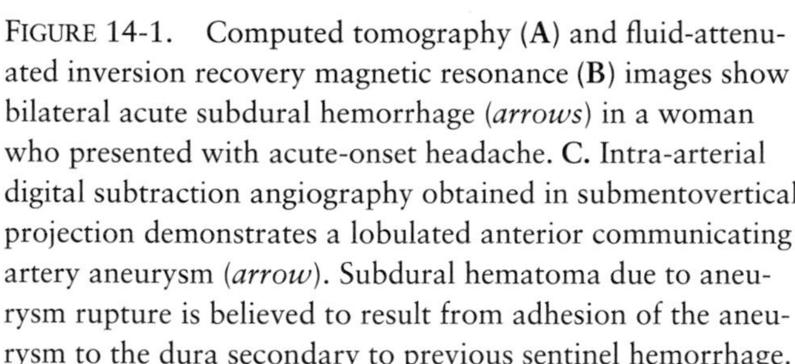

FIGURE 14-1. Computed tomography (**A**) and fluid-attenuated inversion recovery magnetic resonance (**B**) images show bilateral acute subdural hemorrhage (*arrows*) in a woman who presented with acute-onset headache. **C.** Intra-arterial digital subtraction angiography obtained in submentovertical projection demonstrates a lobulated anterior communicating artery aneurysm (*arrow*). Subdural hematoma due to aneurysm rupture is believed to result from adhesion of the aneurysm to the dura secondary to previous sentinel hemorrhage.

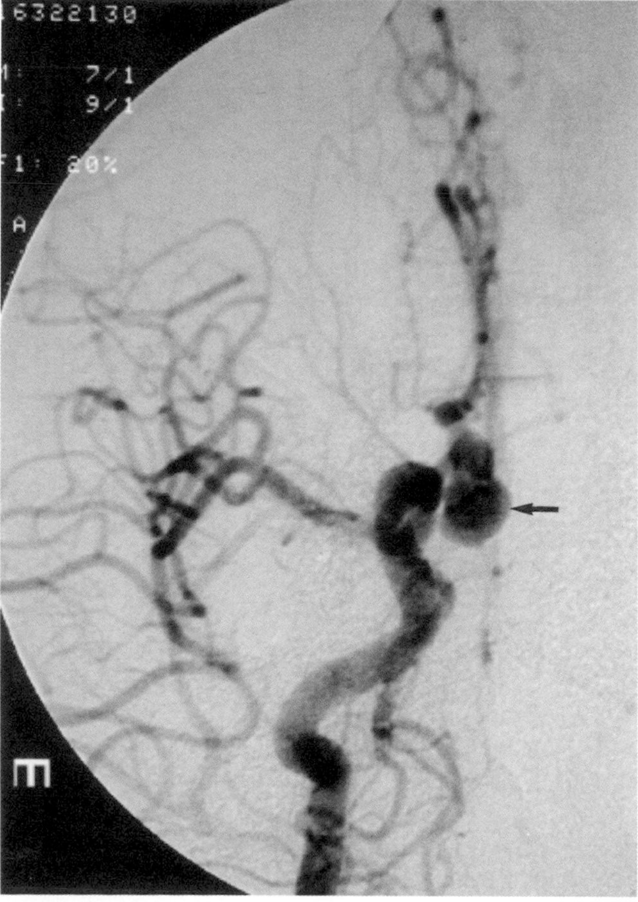

C

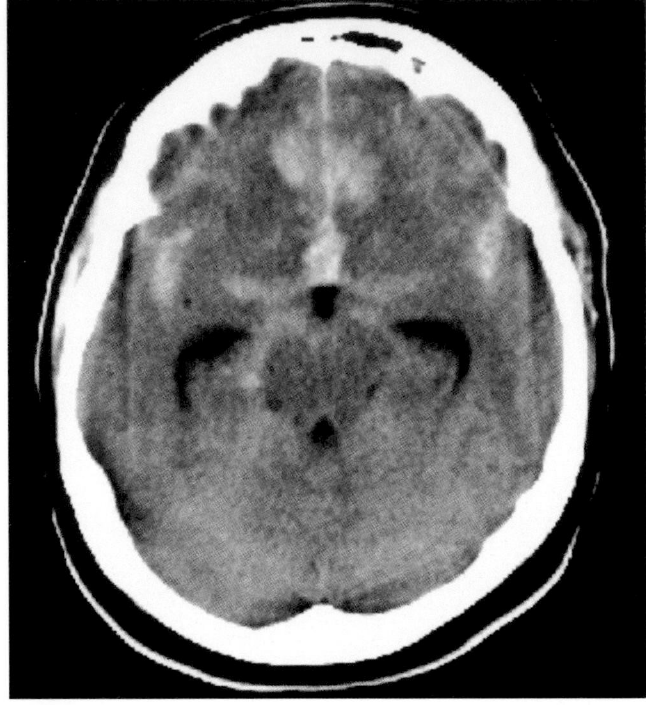
A

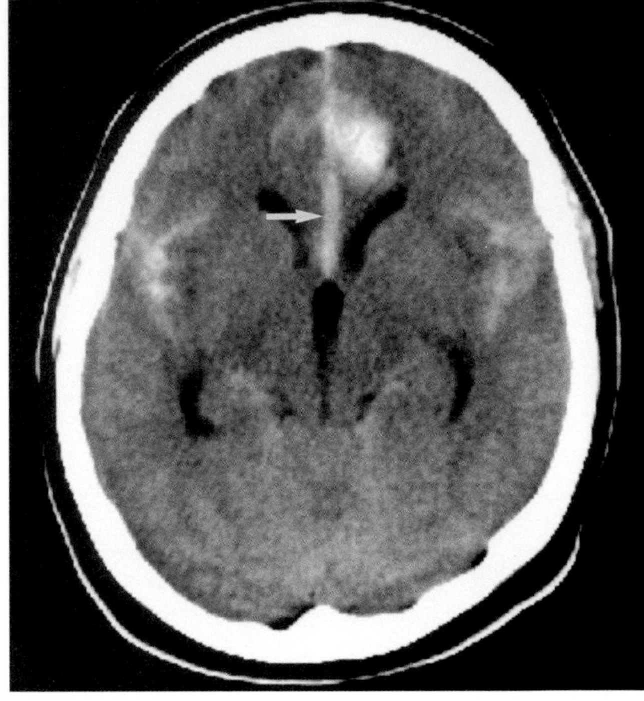
B

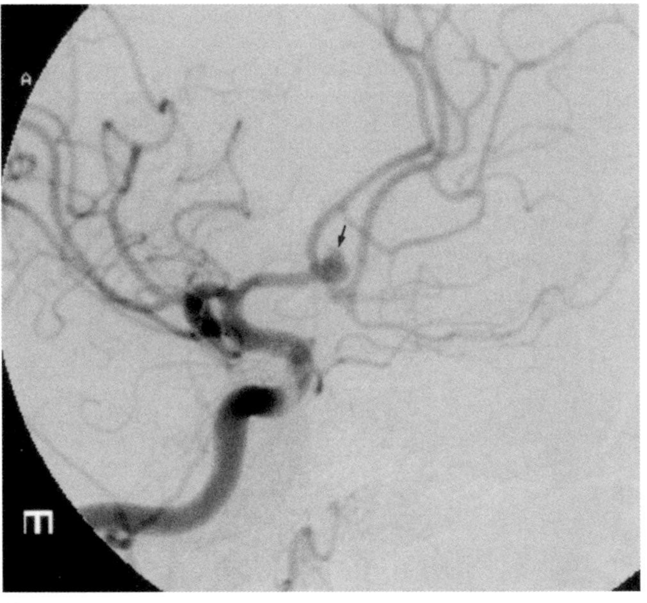

C

FIGURE 14-2. Acute subarachnoid hemorrhage due to a ruptured anterior communicating artery aneurysm. **A,B.** Anterior interhemispheric fissure (*arrow*) and gyrus rectus hematoma. Note the mild ventricular dilatation. **C.** Anterior communicating artery aneurysm with a "nipple" sign (*arrow*) indicating acute rupture. The left A1 segment is hypoplastic (not shown).

the various MRI pulse sequences for the detection of chronic SAH.[28] Caution must be exercised, however, because the specificity of MRI for SAH is reduced, because any subarachnoid space disease with increased CSF protein concentration may mimic the appearance of SAH. In addition to pathologic processes, other causes of increased signal intensity may be due to artifact from field inhomogeneity or from anesthetics such as propofol. Increased signal in CSF spaces on FLAIR images performed after gadolinium administration should not be mistaken for SAH.[30]

ANEURYSMAL SUBARACHNOID HEMORRHAGE

The true incidence of SAH is difficult to determine because of differences in study design, population characteristics, definition of aneurysm, and autopsy tech-

TABLE 14-1. Location of Aneurysm and Its Relationship to the Distribution of Subarachnoid Hemorrhage

Aneurysm site	*Distribution of subarachnoid hemorrhage*
Anterior communicating artery complex	Anterior-inferior interhemispheric fissure, septum ± suprasellar cistern or third ventricle, gyrus rectus hematoma
Middle cerebral artery	Sylvian fissure ± temporal lobe hematoma
Internal carotid/posterior communicating artery	Lateral, anterior suprasellar and ambient cisterns ± proximal sylvian fissure, basal ganglia hematoma
Tip of the basilar artery	Prepontine, interpeduncular, perimesencephalic, and chiasmatic cisterns
Posterior-inferior cerebellar artery	Fourth ventricle ± aqueduct and third ventricle
Perimesencephalic nonaneurysmal	Perimesencephalic cistern ± interpeduncular, prepontine cisterns and middle cerebral artery fissure

niques.[2,3,5,31–34] It varies between 6 and 16 per 100,000 person/year. A recent meta-analysis of the prospective population-based studies of SAH reported a worldwide incidence of 10.5 per 100,000 person/year that has remained stable over many decades.[35] Approximately 70–80% of these cases are related to aneurysm rupture.[36] The prevalence of aneurysms is much higher than the incidence of SAH; however, autopsy studies and angiographic studies done for reasons other than aneurysm and SAH suggest that approximately 1–5% of adults harbor an intracranial aneurysm.[4,36–45] Of these cases, 90% are in the anterior circulation, and 80–85% are solitary.

The incidence of aneurysmal SAH increases with age and is higher in women.[46] Smoking is widely recognized as a risk factor for SAH,[47] and hypertension may also be a risk factor.[48,49] First- and second-degree relatives of patients with ruptured aneurysms are at a four- to sixfold increased risk for SAH.[50,51] Excessive ethanol use is an independent risk factor for aneurysm rupture.[51] Other risk factors include race, previous SAH, physical exertion, and illicit drug use.[52–54] Hereditary disorders of connective tissue are linked to higher rates of aneurysm formation and rupture.[55,56] Autosomal-dominant polycystic kidney disease, sickle cell anemia, neurofibromatosis I, and α_1-antitrypsin deficiency are associated with SAH.[56] Systemic inflammatory vasculopathies such as systemic lupus erythematosus, giant cell arteritis, Takayasu's disease, fibromuscular dysplasia, and polyarteritis nodosa may lead to aneurysm formation and rupture.[57–60]

Classification of aneurysms is often based on either the histologic and morphologic architecture or the etiology of the aneurysm. The morphologic appearance is commonly classified as saccular (berry) or fusiform. The etiologies of aneurysms include congenital (berry), atherosclerotic, inflammatory, mycotic, dissecting, traumatic, and neoplastic. The majority of intracranial aneurysms are saccular aneurysms and are believed to have both a congenital and developmental etiology arising from a combination of intrinsic arterial wall weakness and hemodynamic stress.[61]

Anatomic Locations of Saccular Aneurysms

Intracranial aneurysms are located intradurally or extradurally. Extradural aneurysms involve the internal carotid arteries (ICAs) below the ophthalmic segment and virtually never cause SAH as the first clinical manifestation. They frequently attain relatively larger sizes, and mass effect may cause cranial neuropathy. Intradural aneurysms usually involve the distal ICAs, arteries of the circle of Willis, the middle cerebral artery (MCA) bifurcations, and the vertebrobasilar trunk. Intradural aneurysms often present with SAH and are generally amenable to surgical clipping, endovascular treatment, or both.[62] Determining whether an aneurysm located adjacent to or just below the ophthalmic artery is extradural or intradural is often difficult because direct visualization of the dural ring is not possible with any imaging modality. The origin of the ophthalmic artery is intradural in more than 90% of patients and provides a reasonably reliable anatomic landmark to differentiate the intra- from extradural location.

ICA aneurysms arising opposite of the ophthalmic artery origin are named *paraclinoid aneurysms*.[63] Some authors define the intradural portion of the ICA from the dural ring to the origin of the posterior communicating artery (PCOM) as the ophthalmic segment.

Approximately 1–5% of all intradural aneurysms arise from this segment of the ICA that is divided into five subsites. *Transitional aneurysms* arise from outside the dural ring but insinuate partially or entirely through the ring into the subarachnoid space.[64] The intradural component of these aneurysms can produce SAH. *Carotid cave aneurysms* arise at the level of the dural ring[65] in the potential space created by the redundant dura between the medial wall of the ICA and bony wall of the carotid sulcus. Occasionally, cave aneurysms breach the dura and bulge into the cavernous sinus to

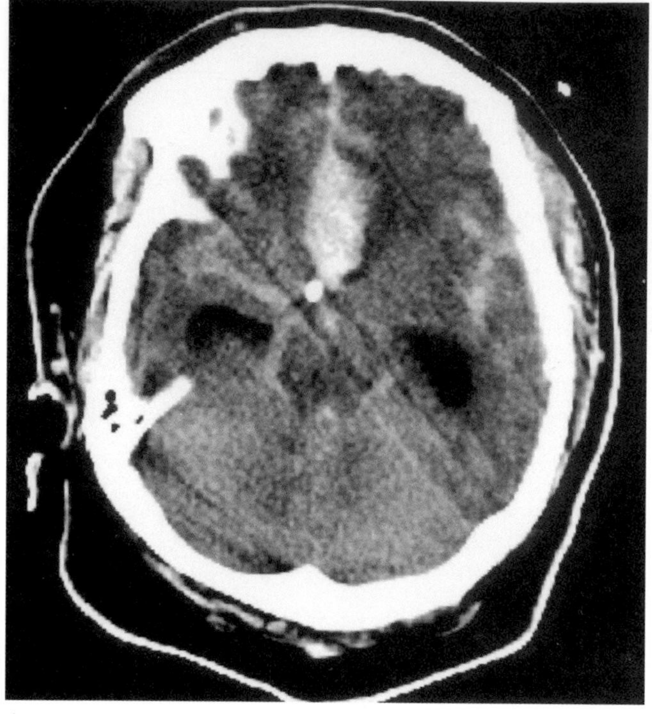

A

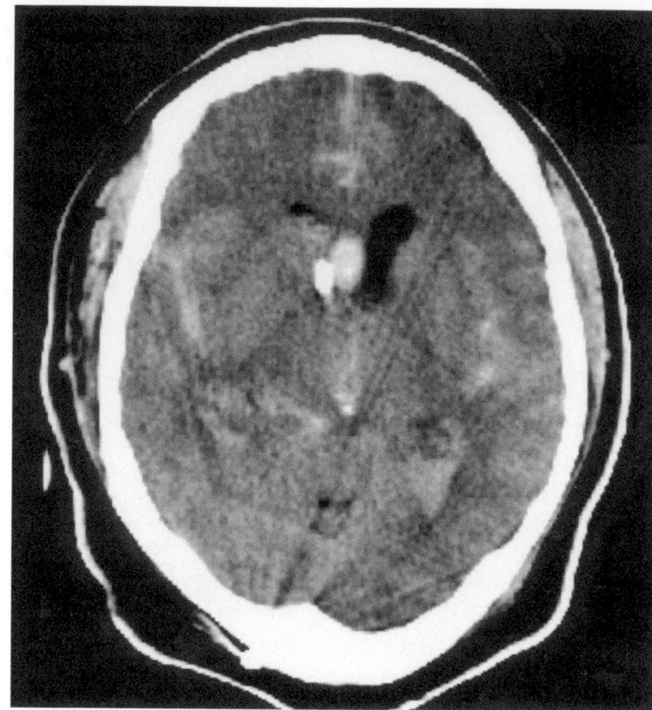

B

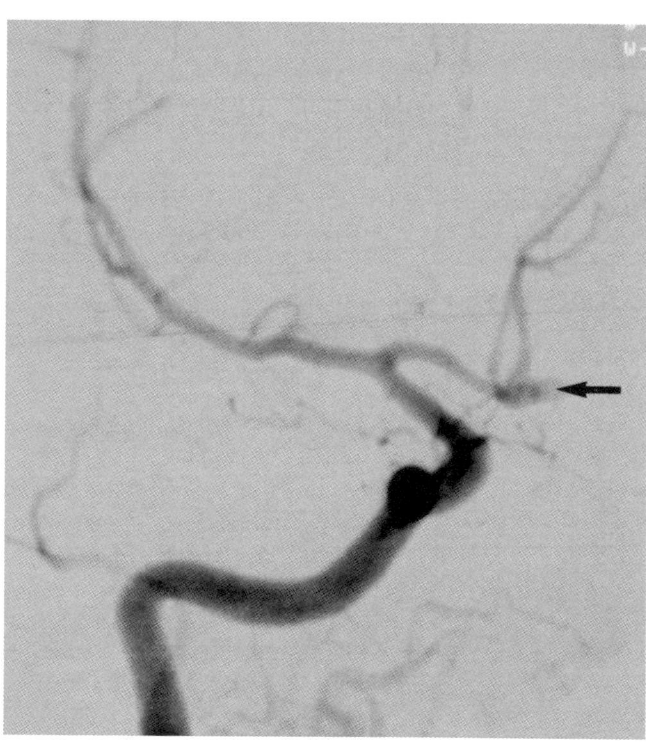

C

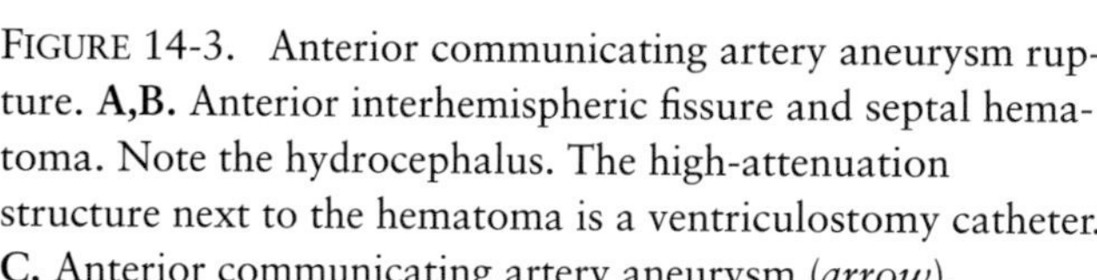

FIGURE 14-3. Anterior communicating artery aneurysm rupture. **A,B.** Anterior interhemispheric fissure and septal hematoma. Note the hydrocephalus. The high-attenuation structure next to the hematoma is a ventriculostomy catheter. C. Anterior communicating artery aneurysm (*arrow*).

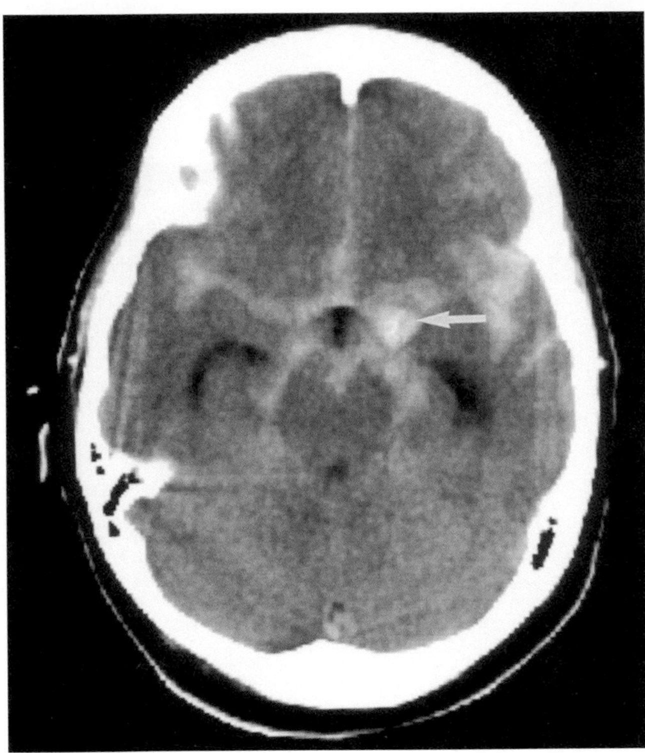

FIGURE 14-4. Acutely ruptured left posterior communicating artery aneurysm with diffuse subarachnoid hemorrhage and a suprasellar cistern hematoma (*arrow*) at the aneurysm site.

add further confusion about their origin. *Carotid-ophthalmic aneurysms* arise from the vicinity of the ophthalmic artery origin and usually project cranially, potentially producing visual symptoms by optic nerve compression.[66,67] These aneurysms are more common in women. *Posterior carotid wall* (*ventral paraclinoid*) *aneurysms* usually extend into the cavernous sinus. *Superior hypophyseal aneurysms* arise between the ophthalmic and PCOM origin and project medially and inferomedially to give the erroneous angiographic impression that they extend into the cavernous sinus.

Up to 20% of the intracranial aneurysms arise from the communicating segment of the ICA just distal to the origin of the PCOM and project posteriorly, slightly inferiorly, and laterally. Ninety percent of these aneurysms present with SAH.[68] Third nerve palsy, invariably involving the pupil, is the presenting symptom in the remainder of the cases. Aneurysms of the PCOM should be differentiated from an infundibulum that represents dilatation of the vessel origin. The infundibulum is funnel shaped, is never larger than 3 mm, and has a vessel arising from its apex (Figure 14-8). Although the prevailing opinion is that the infundibulum is benign, adherence to strict criteria is important, because some authors have reported cases of SAH secondary to "infundibulum" rupture.[69,70] Progression of infundibulum to aneurysm has also been reported.[70]

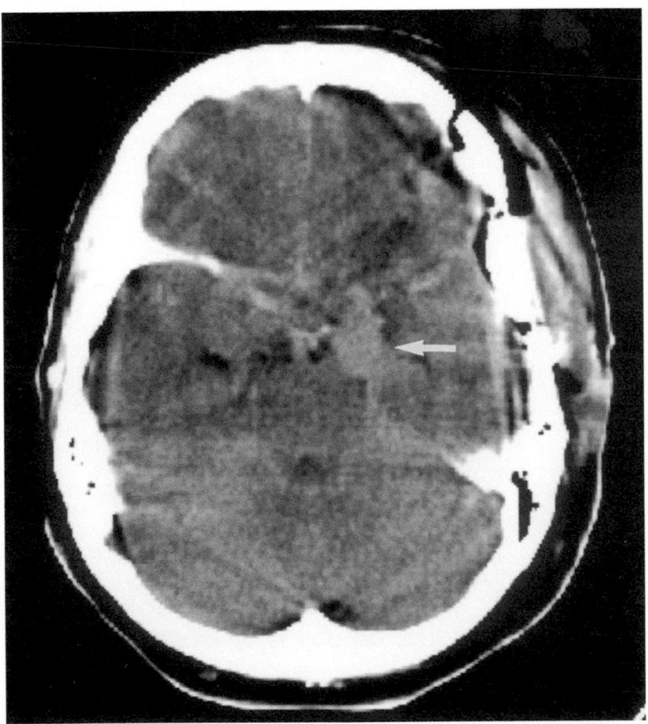

A

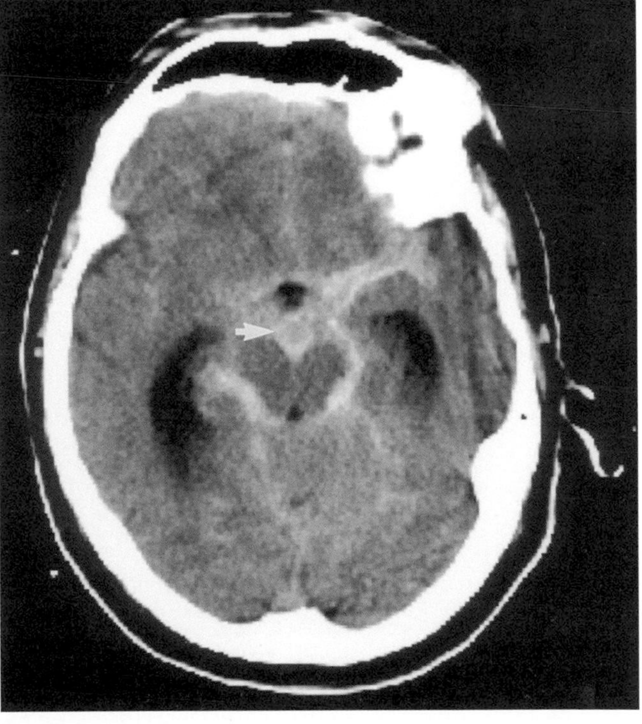

B

FIGURE 14-5. Subarachnoid hemorrhage in a patient with posterior communicating artery (*arrow*) (**A**) and basilar artery (*short arrow*) (**B**) aneurysms. The patient first underwent an unsuccessful surgical clipping procedure. The aneurysms were successfully treated with endovascular coiling.

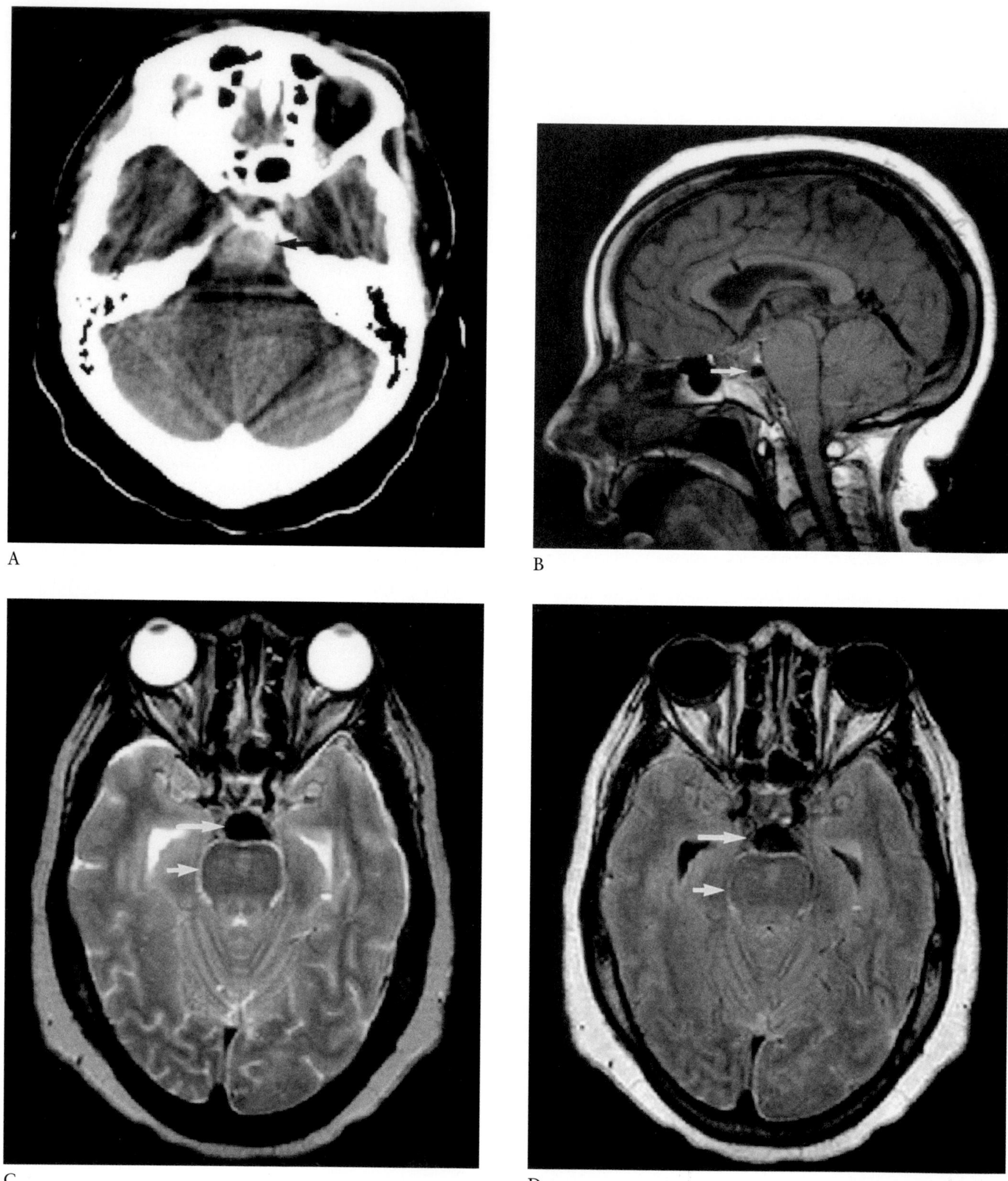

FIGURE 14-6. Mid-basilar artery aneurysm rupture. **A.** Acute hemorrhage in the prepontine cistern (*arrow*). T1-weighted (**B**), T2-weighted (**C**), and fluid-attenuated inversion recovery (**D**) images show the aneurysm as a flow void (*arrows*). Notice that the subarachnoid hemorrhage is better seen on the fluid-attenuated inversion recovery image (*short arrows*). (*continued*)

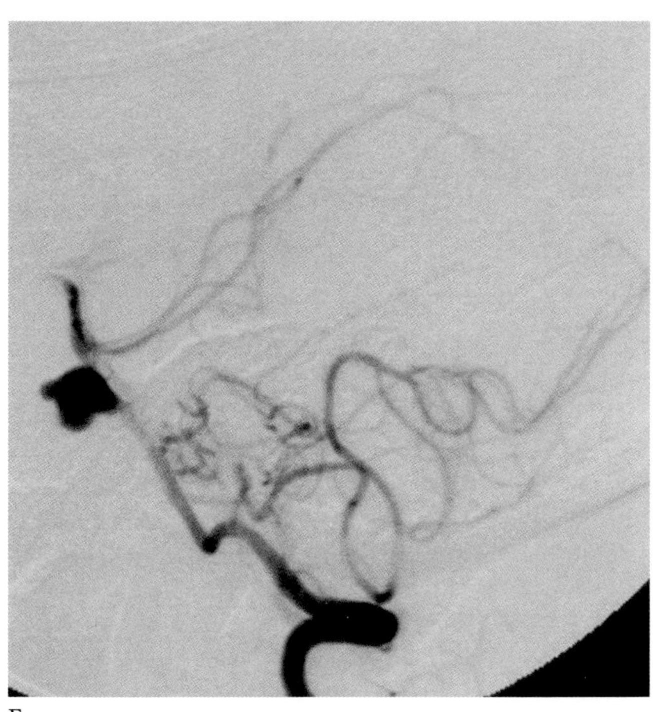
E

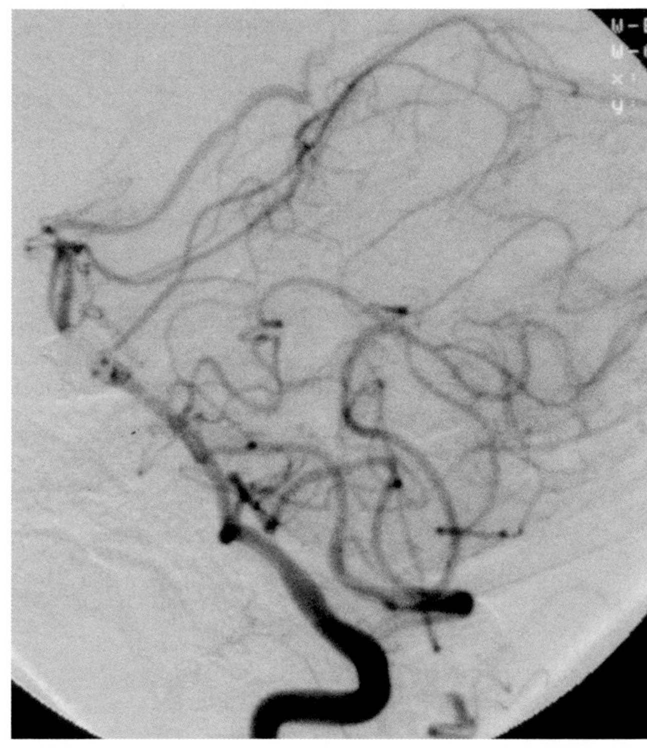
F

FIGURE 14-6. *Continued.* **E.** Lobulated nature of the aneurysm is best appreciated on intra-arterial digital subtraction angiography. **F.** Almost complete exclusion of the aneurysm after Guglielmi detachable coiling.

Anterior choroidal artery aneurysms morphologically resemble PCOM aneurysms (Figure 14-9) and almost always present with SAH. Because they originate just beyond the anterior choroidal artery origin and project posteriorly above the tentorium and oculomotor nerve, associated third nerve palsy is uncommon.[68]

Carotid bifurcations, also called *carotid terminus aneurysms*, represent approximately 5% of all the intracranial aneurysms (Figure 14-10). Ninety-four percent of these aneurysms present with SAH.[67,68] Intraparenchymal hematoma is not uncommon and closely mimics hypertensive basal ganglia bleeds. The majority of childhood aneurysms occur at this location.

The anterior communicating artery (ACOM) complex is the most common site for aneurysm formation. Approximately 35–40% of all intradural aneurysms arise from the ACOM and its branches.[12] Usually, there is an associated anatomic variation, such as hypoplastic contralateral A1 (85%), fenestration, azygos artery, or duplication. SAH is the clinical presentation in 97% of the patients.[68] A minority of the ACOM aneurysms arise distally from the bifurcation points of the callosomarginal and pericallosal arteries.

Most saccular aneurysms of the MCA occur at the bifurcation and constitute 20–22% of all intradural aneurysms (Figure 14-11).[12] Ninety percent of the aneurysms at this location present with SAH.[52] Associated parenchymal hematoma is relatively common (30–50% of the patients).

The majority of the aneurysms arising from the posterior circulation (approximately 8% of all intradural aneurysms) involve the tip of the basilar artery (Figure 14-12).[12] These are associated with higher morbidity and mortality.

Other Aneurysms

Aneurysms involving more peripheral cerebral vessels are less common and usually are due to inflammatory, infectious, traumatic, or tumoral etiology.[44,71–73]

Mycotic aneurysms result from the invasion of the arterial wall by micro-organisms causing subsequent inflammation and destruction. The most common offending agent is *Streptococcus viridans*. Invasion occurs in the context of infective endocarditis. Meningitis and cavernous sinus thrombophlebitis can cause mycotic aneurysms, which are invariably associated with regional cerebritis. The mode of presentation is SAH in 90% of the cases, with 20% of the patients harboring multiple aneurysms. Treatment consists of intravenous antibiotics and often surgical resection. Serial angiograms are often performed to measure the response to antibiotics.[74]

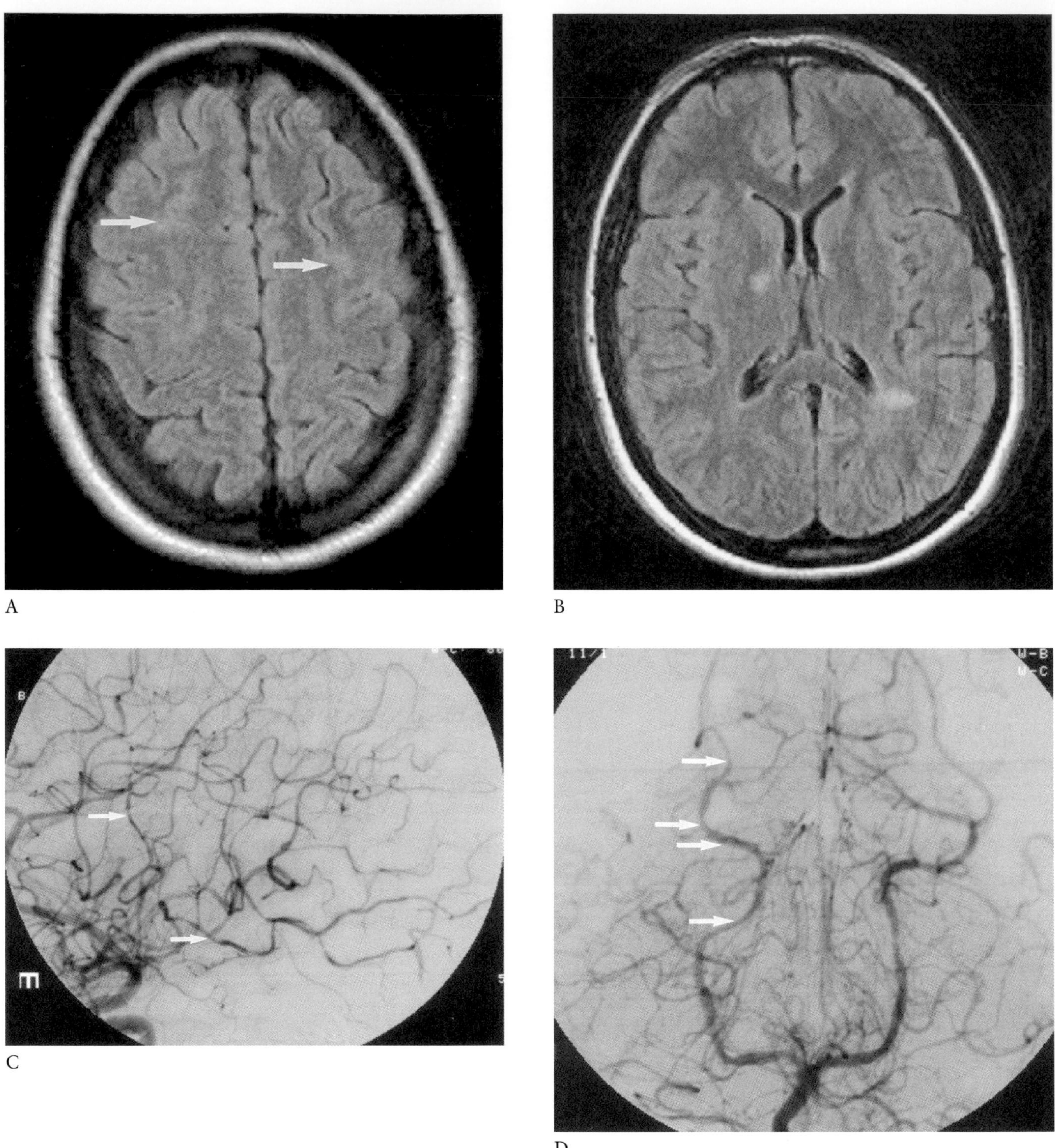

FIGURE 14-7. Primary central nervous system vasculitis. A young female patient presented with worsening headaches over 1 week. **A.** Subtle increased signal on fluid-attenuated inversion recovery image in the dorsal aspects of the superior frontal sulci (*arrows*). Lumbar puncture confirmed subarachnoid hemorrhage. Computed tomography was negative. **B.** Scattered white matter lesions. **C,D.** Multiple alternating stenoses (*arrows*) in the anterior and posterior circulations.

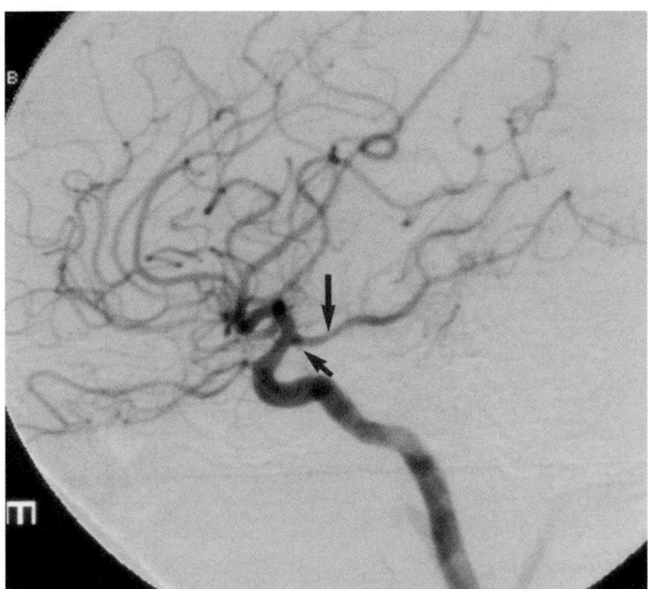

FIGURE 14-8. Small posterior communicating artery aneurysm (*short arrow*). Notice that the posterior communicating artery (*arrow*) does not arise from the apex of the outpouching, excluding the possibility of an infundibulum.

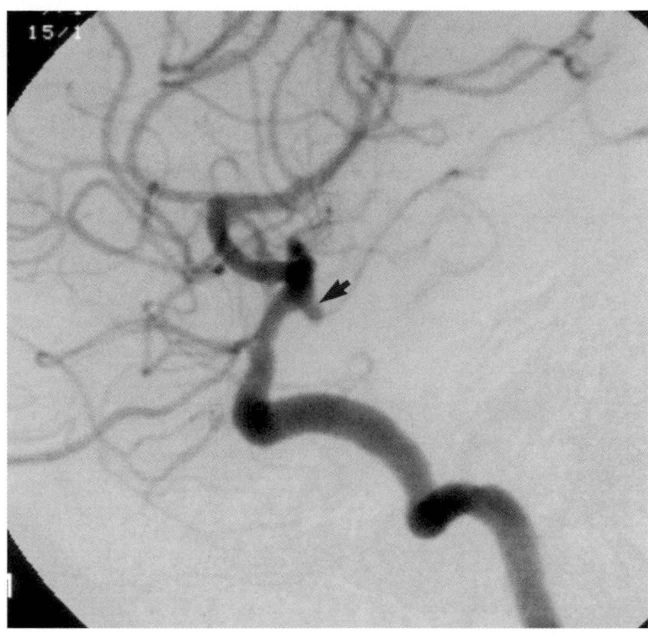

FIGURE 14-9. Anterior choroidal artery aneurysm (*arrow*).

Atrial myxoma and choriocarcinoma emboli may also cause intracranial aneurysm.[75,76] Neoplastic aneurysms most commonly involve the MCA territory due to the relatively higher proportion of blood flow.

Traumatic aneurysms are associated with skull base fractures or penetrating injuries that typically involve the MCA along the sphenoid ridge, pericallosal artery along the falx, or posterior circulation vessels along the tentorium.[77,78]

Fusiform aneurysms usually develop on the setting of atherosclerosis and hypertension. They involve a large segment of the artery and frequently contain thrombi, producing ischemic symptoms due to emboli or small perforator vessel occlusion (Figure 14-13). Symptoms secondary to mass effect are also common. SAH occurs but rarely is the initial symptom. The vertebrobasilar vessels are the most frequent site for fusiform aneurysm formation. These patients usually have ectatic tortuous intracranial vessels.[79,80]

Serpentine aneurysms are rare and are usually seen in younger patients. The MCA is the most common site, with angiography demonstrating a large, irregular vessel with different entrance and exit points on the parent artery. The flow is usually very slow in the aneurysm. Evaluation of collateral circulation is important, because treatment usually involves a reconstructive bypass procedure.[81]

Dissecting aneurysms are being recognized with an increasing frequency. They are formed by the penetration of blood between the layers of the arterial wall. Although they are more common in the anterior circulation, SAH-producing dissecting aneurysms generally arise from the vertebrobasilar arteries.[82,83] The angiographic findings of dissection and dissecting aneurysm include irregular narrowing proximal or distal to the aneurysm ("pearl and string" appearance), retention of contrast in the aneurysm due to slow flow, double lumen, and a rapidly changing appearance on serial studies.[84] Dissecting aneurysms may spontaneously heal; however, because of

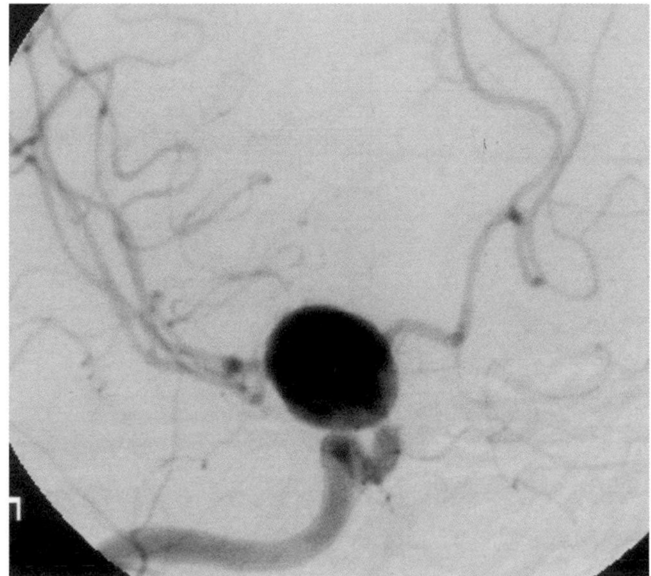

FIGURE 14-10. Large carotid bifurcation aneurysm.

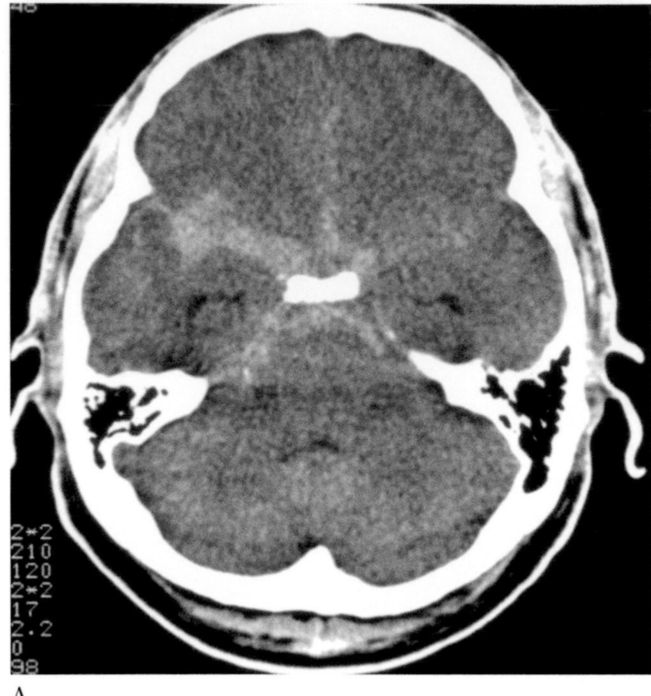

A

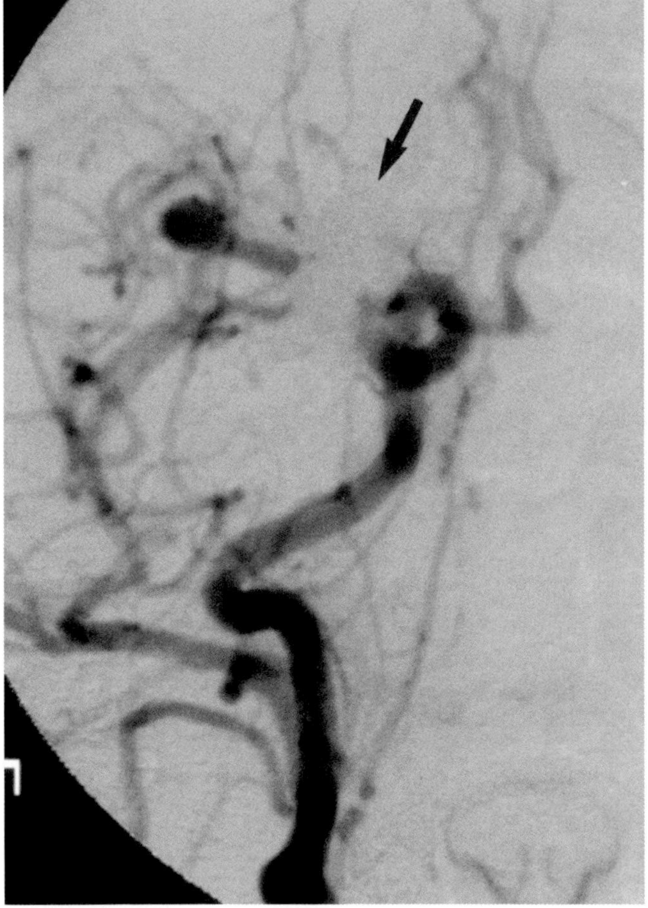
C

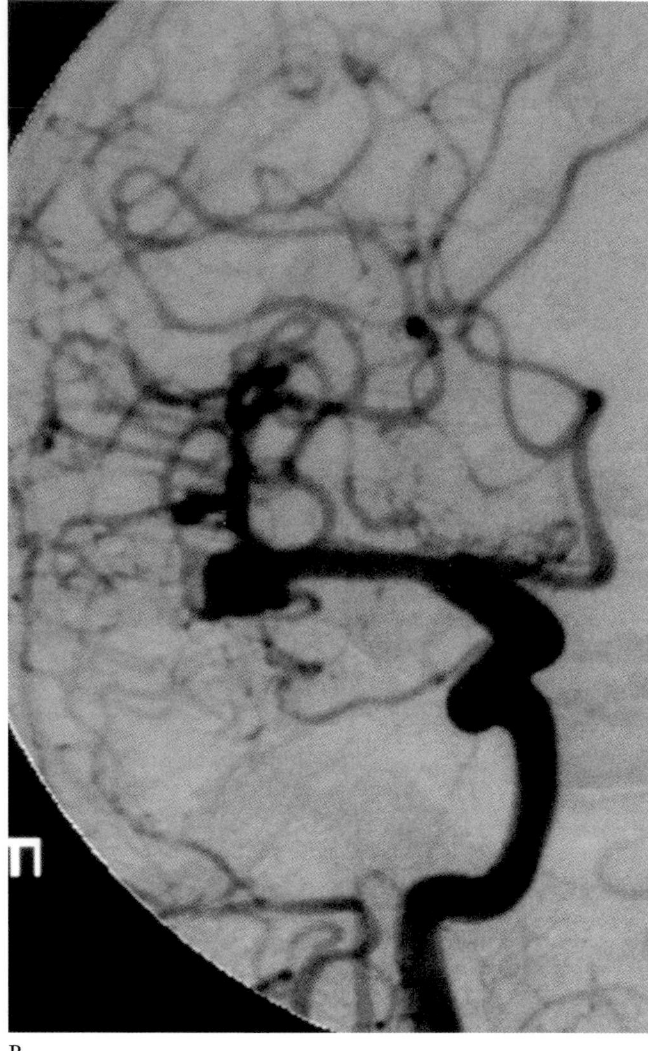
B

FIGURE 14-11. Right middle cerebral artery aneurysm rupture. **A.** The greatest volume of subarachnoid hemorrhage is in the right sylvian fissure, suggesting the site of hemorrhage. **B,C.** The middle cerebral artery bifurcation aneurysm. A submentovertical view (**C**) demonstrates the aneurysm neck best. Note the subtraction artifact from the dental fillings (*arrow*).

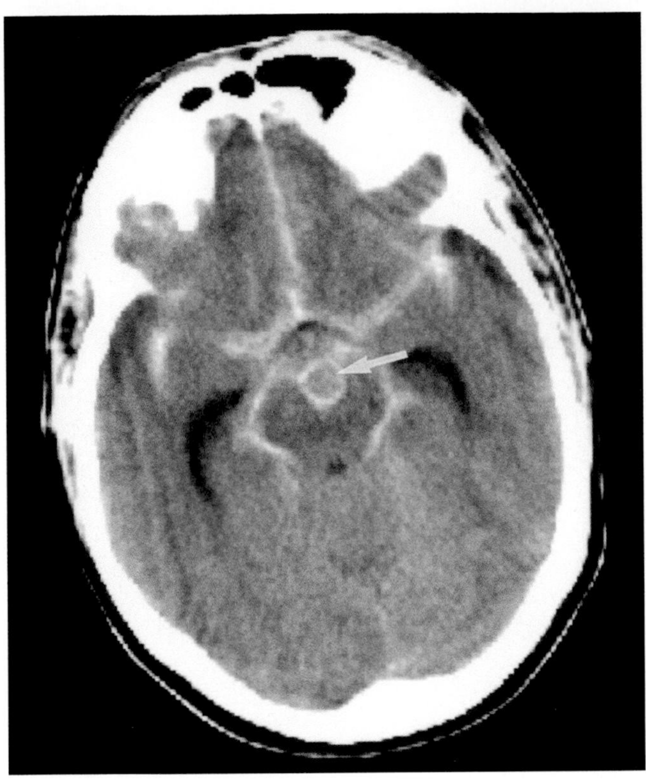

A

FIGURE 14-12. Basilar tip aneurysm rupture. **A.** Subarachnoid hemorrhage delineates the aneurysm (*arrow*) in the interpeduncular cistern. **B.** Complete exclusion of the aneurysm from the arterial circulation with densely packed aneurysm coils (*arrow*).

B

rebleed risk in cases of SAH, early treatment, usually by parent vessel occlusion, is advocated.[85]

Approximately 2.5–7.0% of all intracranial aneurysms are classified as giant aneurysms (greater than 25 mm in size).[86] In contrast to small aneurysms, patients with giant aneurysms present most frequently with symptoms related to mass effect.[87,88] Giant aneurysms are often partially thrombosed, occluding a fraction of the aneurysm lumen, explaining the discrepancy between size on angiography and cross-sectional imaging (Figure 14-14). The morphology can be saccular or fusiform, which alters the decision for therapy with a reconstructive procedure or Hunterian (proximal) occlusion of the supplying artery.[88] The circle of Willis and pial collateral flow need to be evaluated before parent artery occlusion, as does the patient's clinical tolerance to test-occlusion of the vessel.

Imaging of Aneurysms

Imaging evaluation of the aneurysms should include more than a simple demonstration of a presence of an aneurysm. The size, shape, and orientation of the aneurysm; size and extent of the aneurysm neck relative to the parent vessel; aneurysm dome size and configuration; anatomic variations of the parent vessel; collateral blood supply; and presence or absence of thrombus, vasospasm, and associated vascular malformations should all be demonstrated to facilitate surgical or endovascular treatment.

ANGIOGRAPHY

Intra-arterial digital subtraction angiography (IADSA) is the diagnostic gold standard for the evaluation of intracranial aneurysms. Angiography provides the most accurate assessment of the aneurysm's location, size, geometry, relationship to the adjacent vessels, and potential multiplicity.

Although film screen angiography traditionally has been thought to provide superior spatial but worse contrast resolution when compared to IADSA, modern digital subtraction angiography (DSA) units with smaller focal spot size and 1,024 × 1,024 digital matrix provide a resolution comparable or superior to conventional film screen angiography.

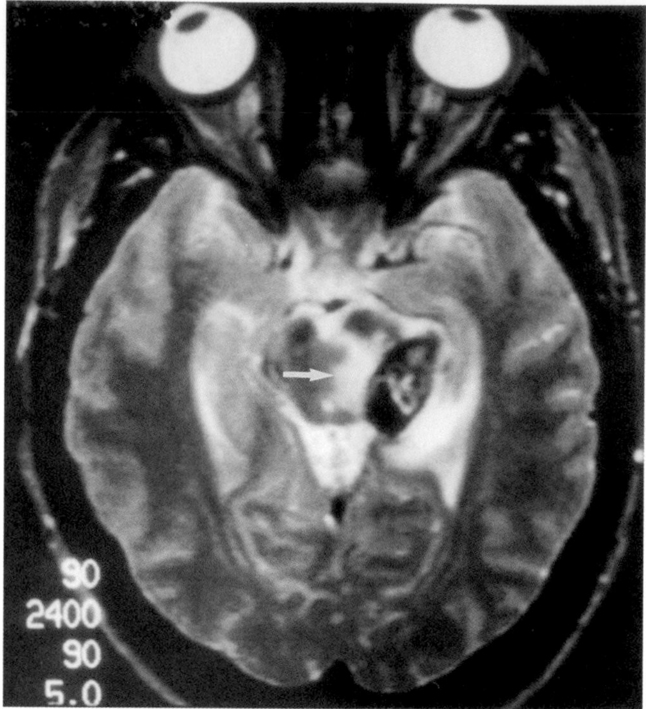

A

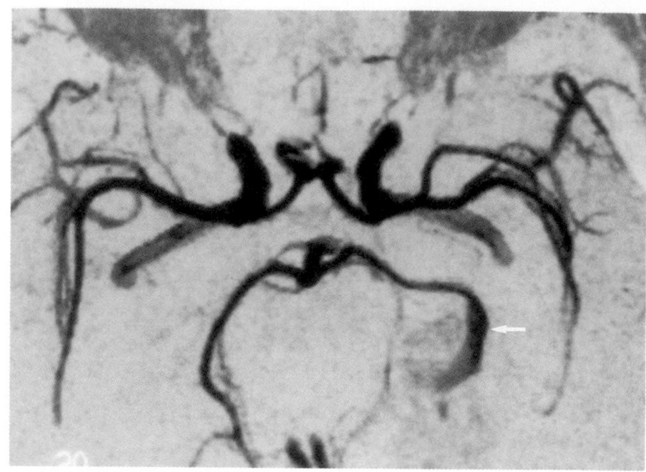

B

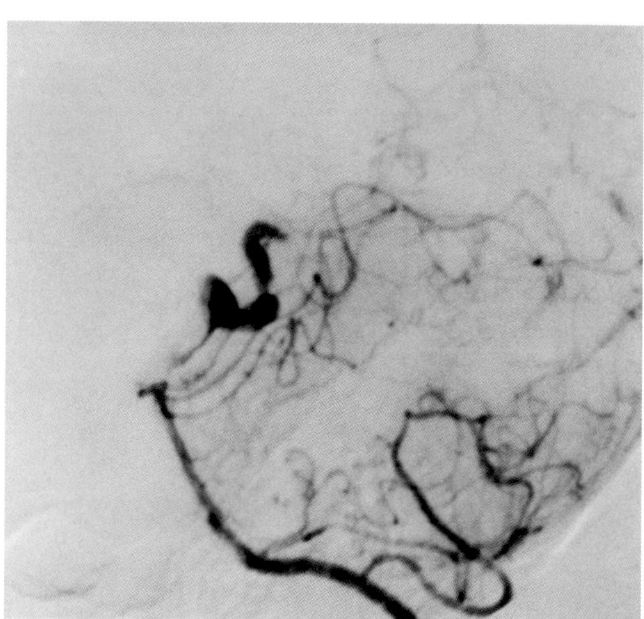

C

FIGURE 14-13. Unruptured, partially thrombosed, fusiform aneurysm of the left posterior cerebral artery. **A.** T2-weighted magnetic resonance image shows increased signal (*arrow*) in the mesencephalon due to mass effect. **B.** Incomplete demonstration of the aneurysm (*arrow*) on magnetic resonance angiography due to slow flow and saturation. **C.** Intra-arterial digital subtraction angiography demonstrating the lumen of the aneurysm.

IADSA has several advantages for aneurysm analysis as compared to film screen angiography. Fast frame rate allows the assessment of flow dynamics within the aneurysm. By using fast frame rates (four to six frames per second), a jet of contrast medium entering the aneurysm usually can be seen. Visualization of this jet is often useful in determining the morphology of the neck of an aneurysm. Rapid image acquisition allows multiple projections to be obtained in a short time, permitting accurate determination of aneurysm orientation. In addition, postprocessing capabilities of IADSA, such as use of a delayed mask technique, can give more specific information regarding the location and direction of an aneurysm neck as well as the size of the neck relative to the aneurysm.[89] High-resolution road mapping is very helpful for safe catheterization of vessels. Recently, rotational angiography has been implemented with DSA, providing superior assessment of aneurysm morphology with three-dimensional reconstruction capabilities.[90] The full impact of this technology on aneurysm therapy is not yet appreciated.

A pancerebral angiogram, including bilateral carotid and vertebral artery injections, should be performed whenever possible. If this is unrevealing, investigation of external carotid and extracranial vertebral arteries should follow to exclude dural fistulas and spinal AVMs or dissections. In the setting of acute SAH, it is recommended that the investigation of the vascular territory most likely to harbor the offending abnormality be performed first. Subtotal angiography may be appropriate in cases of unstable patients who require immediate intervention. The possibility of an erroneous

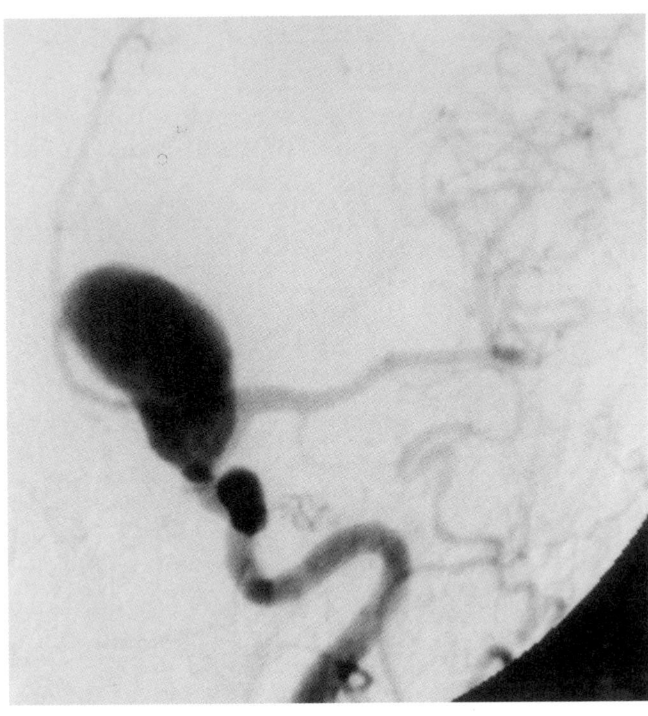

A

B

FIGURE 14-14. **A.** Partially thrombosed giant aneurysm of the ophthalmic segment of the internal carotid artery. **B.** Notice the concentric layers of thrombus within the aneurysm and much larger size on the magnetic resonance image.

exploration is low in the presence of a CT suggestive of the rupture site and a corresponding documented aneurysm on single vessel angiography.[91] Incomplete studies are not advocated given the high frequency of multiplicity and its impact on therapeutic planning and postoperative management of the vasospasm.

Typically, certain radiographic projections are helpful in evaluating aneurysms in specific locations. Table 14-2 provides positioning guidelines for the most common intracranial aneurysms.[92] Improvised projections are often needed because of the anatomic variations of the skull and vessels, differences in head positioning on the table, and exact projection of the aneurysm.

Current recommendations for managing aneurysmal rupture include early clipping or endovascular treatment of most aneurysms and aggressive treatment of vasospasm.[12,93] The angiogram should be performed promptly, and the rate of rerupture during angiography is not higher than the spontaneous rerupture rate.[94,95] However, the outcome of reruptured cases during angiography is worse.[94,95]

False-Negative Angiogram

The exact sensitivity of IADSA for aneurysm detection is difficult to determine, because most patients with negative angiograms do not undergo surgical exploration and are assumed to have nonaneurysmal hemorrhage. The sensitivity of IADSA is estimated to exceed 90%. Recent angiographic techniques have probably increased sensitivity.[96] False-negative rates on initial pancerebral angiography vary from 2% to 23%, with more recent series estimating initial false-negative rates ranging from 11.7% to 16.0%.[97–100] The proposed etiologies of false-negative angiograms include vasospasm, peculiar flow patterns, thrombosis of the aneurysm or parent vessel, microaneurysms, technically inadequate studies, and inaccurate interpretation.[98,101–104] A second or third angiogram may visualize an aneurysm that was angiographically occult despite a technically satisfactory study.[13]

Because of the grim consequences of aneurysmal SAH, an exhaustive search should be undertaken to ensure that SAH is nonaneurysmal when the first angiogram is negative.[105] A general guideline is to obtain a second angiogram within the first 2 weeks after a negative angiogram in the setting of SAH. If the first angiogram is technically inadequate, it should be repeated immediately. MRI of the brain obtained after a negative angiogram may provide further insight as to the source of SAH. A third angiogram may be indicated if the critical evaluation of the initial CT reveals a highly suspicious pattern for aneurysmal SAH or if there is evidence of vasospasm. Other sources for SAH may arise from the spine, which also should be considered in a negative workup of the intracranial contents. If the initial CT shows a pattern consistent with PNSAH and a technically adequate

TABLE 14-2. Angiographic Projections for Cerebral Aneurysms

Aneurysm location	*AP tube projection*	*Lateral tube projection*	*Comments*
ICA cavernous, ICA-dural ring	AP, Caldwell, submental-vertex, paraorbital: 55 degrees CL AO	Cranial/caudal angulation obliques ± 25 degrees	Elongating different segments of the ICA siphon
Ophthalmic segment, superior hypophyseal ICA	AP, Caldwell, submental-vertex, transorbital: 15–30 degrees CL AO; oblique: 10–15 degrees IL or CL AO	Cranial/caudal angulation obliques ± 25 degrees	—
Posterior communicating artery	AP, paraorbital: 55 degrees CL AO; oblique: 25–35 degrees IL AO (Caldwell's or Waters' angulation)	Cranial/caudal angulation	Depends on ICA course
ICA bifurcation	AP, submental-vertex, transorbital: 15–30 degrees CL AO	Cranial/caudal angulation with oblique ± 25–40 degrees	—
Middle cerebral artery bifurcation	AP, Waters', submental-vertex, transorbital: 10–15 degrees CL AO; oblique: 10–20 degrees IL AO	Various obliques	IL AO elongates the M1 segment, CL AO foreshortens the M1 segment
Anterior communicating artery	AP, Caldwell's, Waters', transorbital: 10–30 degrees CL AO; oblique: 40–60 degrees IL AO	Obliques 40–60 degrees	CL AO elongates the A1 segment
Distal ACA	AP, Caldwell's, Towne's for pericallosal, oblique: 25–45 degrees CL AO	Obliques ± 10–20 degrees	Obliques in lateral to separate right and left distal ACA
Posterior inferior cerebellar artery, distal vertebral artery	Waters', submental-vertex, Towne's oblique: 25–35 degrees CL AO	Obliques 25–45 degrees	—
Vertebro-basilar or vertebro-vertebral junction	Caldwell's, Waters', submental-vertex, oblique: 25–45 degrees IL or CL AO	Obliques 25–60 degrees	—
Basilar artery, anterior inferior cerebellar artery basilar	Waters', submental-vertex, oblique: 10–25 degrees IL or CL AO	Caudal angulation elongates artery while foreshortening PCAs	—
Upper basilar, basilar apex	Towne's, AP, Caldwell's, Waters', oblique: 10–25 degrees IL or CL AO	Cranial/caudal angulation, obliques ± 10–30 degrees	Caudal angulation to visualize the PCA origin; obliques in lateral to separate right and left PCAs
PCA	Towne's, AP oblique: 10–25 degrees IL or CL AO	Cranial/caudal angulation obliques ± 10–30 degrees	Obliques in lateral to separate right and left PCAs

ACA = anterior cerebral artery; AO = anterior oblique; AP = anterior-posterior; CL = contralateral; ICA = internal carotid artery; IL = ipsilateral; PCA = posterior cerebral artery.

Source: Reprinted with permission from A Setton, AJ Davis, A Bose, et al. Angiography of cerebral aneurysms. Neuroimaging Clin North Am 1996;6(3):705–738.

angiogram is normal with absence of vasospasm, a repeat study yield is low.[7,97,105]

Multiple Aneurysms

In the scenario of SAH with multiple aneurysms, certain angiographic features may help determine the ruptured aneurysm. These findings include focal mass effect on the adjacent vessels, focal vasospasm, or a small outpouching from the aneurysm dome that may represent a defect in the aneurysm wall.[106] A multilobulated aneurysm is a less reliable sign that may incriminate the specific aneurysm. Moreover, an additional clue to determining the ruptured aneurysm is the aneurysm size. In a study by Wood[107] of 105 cases with multiple aneurysms, the largest of the aneurysms had ruptured in 87% of the patients.[108] If there are several aneurysms identified on the same parent vessel, the more proximal aneurysm, unless thrombosed, ruptures most frequently.[86]

Risks of Cerebral Angiography

One meta-analysis that evaluated the risks of cerebral angiography in patients with SAH, aneurysms, and AVMs demonstrated that persistent neurologic deficits occurred in approximately 0.07% of the patients undergoing IADSA.[109] This figure is lower than previously quoted and lower than the risk for patients with ischemic symptoms (transient ischemic attack or stroke). The reduced complication rate in comparison with earlier studies may be related to the decreased examination time with DSA, as well as to the use of new iso-osmolar contrast media.

Intraoperative and Postoperative Angiography

The frequency of incomplete aneurysm clipping ranges from 4% to 15%.[110,111] Unexpected occlusion of a major artery after aneurysm clipping occurs in up to 12% of patients.[112] Previously, residual necks or outpouchings at the site of the clip have been thought to be inconsequential. However, it is now known that recurrent aneurysms and subsequent SAH from these rests do occur.[99,113] Feuerberg et al.[114] found that the incidence of rebleeding from an aneurysm rest was 0.38–0.79% per year during the 4- to 13-year observation period. Currently, postclipping angiography is the only way to ensure that the entire aneurysm is obliterated.[17] The common practice of opening the aneurysm after clipping does not exclude a residual neck.[17] Postoperative or intraoperative angiography should be performed in all patients in whom placement of the aneurysm clip across the neck cannot be visualized completely at surgery.

An intraoperative IADSA achieves many of the same goals as a postoperative angiogram and allows adjustment of the aneurysm clip in the event of suboptimally treated aneurysm. It allows recognition and correction of many technical defects, potentially reducing the operative complications and eliminating the need for a reoperation.[111,115,116] Intraoperative angiography also allows for evaluation of adjacent or parent vessels to ensure that they are not being compromised or occluded by the clip.

Perhaps the most important aspect of an intraoperative angiogram is presurgical planning of the intraoperative study. Specifically, patient preparation and positioning are of paramount importance to ensure a safe and expeditious examination. The operating suite must be organized so that manipulation of the angiography unit will not contaminate the surgical field or limit the motion of the angiographic unit. Use of a radiolucent headholder and table is also helpful.

In a patient with a small residual aneurysm, an immediate reoperation is not indicated, and a follow-up angiogram in 3–5 years is probably in order.[17]

MAGNETIC RESONANCE ANGIOGRAPHY

Signal changes produced by flow of blood through a magnetic field gradient can be exploited to produce blood vessel images. This is primarily accomplished by two techniques: The time-of-flight (TOF) technique relies on the high signal from unsaturated flowing blood on the background of low signal from saturated stationary tissues; the phase contrast (PC) technique exploits the phase shift accrued by moving spins in a magnetic field. In spite of several advantages of PC technique over TOF, it is not used routinely because of its inherently low spatial resolution. Both PC and TOF data sets can be postprocessed to produce "angiographic-type" images. Because a complete discussion on the physical principles of these techniques is beyond the scope of this chapter, the reader is referred to other sources.[117,118]

The spatial resolution of current three-dimensional TOF magnetic resonance angiography (MRA) is approximately 0.8 × 0.8 × 0.8 mm less than catheter angiography but is high enough to detect aneurysms as small as 2–3 mm. Although there is no size threshold below which an aneurysm will not rupture, most aneurysms of clinical concern are large enough to be detected by current MRA techniques.

Lateral saccular aneurysms project nearly perpendicularly from the side of the parent artery. The characteristic flow pattern in these aneurysms is a discrete inflow zone along the distal edge of the aneurysm ostium. The blood flows in a circular fashion about the dome of the aneurysm and exits adjacent to the proximal edge of the aneurysm ostium. Centrally, recirculation of the blood results in a vortex flow pattern.[87,119] Both PC and TOF MRAs demonstrate the vortex flow as a region of central lower signal intensity.[87] The decreased signal intensity is primarily due to saturation effect rather than intravoxel dephasing. The slow central flow can be visualized best with a PC technique with a low-velocity encoding.[119] The accumulation of platelets and leukocytes along the intimal surface due to the flow stasis in the aneurysm reduces the oxygen diffusion and delivery of metabolites to the aneurysm wall.[120] These factors have been proposed to lead to thrombus formation, thickening of the aneurysm wall, and aneurysm growth.[121] Thus, the following are the two main flow features of lateral aneurysms that have an impact on the MRA appearance: (1) The flow velocity is greatest within the inflow stream along the periphery of the aneurysm wall, and the maximum flow velocity and shear stress are at the neck, not at the dome, of the aneurysm. (2) Thrombus formation within the aneurysm is a dynamic process that tends to occur in concentric layers and is flow related.

Therefore, aneurysms may appear substantially different on sequential MRI/MRA examinations in the absence of intervening therapy.

The flow characteristics of bifurcation aneurysms have also been well documented in experimental models.[87] Inflow into the aneurysm occurs at the margin of the ostium nearest to the long axis of the parent artery. Rapid helical flow is present most commonly in these aneurysms, with rotation of flow within and in the direction of the vascular outflow branch. All these flow patterns maintain a nearly laminar and relatively coherent flow profile. Because outflow is predominantly into one distal vessel, it can be difficult to visualize small branch vessels adjacent to the aneurysm. The high-flow conditions within these aneurysms are sensitive to detection by 3D TOF MRA techniques. Whereas loss of signal may occur from intravoxel dephasing, the relatively high inflow into these aneurysms adequately defines the contour.

The flow into terminal aneurysms is determined by a portion of the aneurysm ostium closest to a straight line drawn through the center of the parent artery. Similar to bifurcation aneurysms, flow within terminal aneurysms is rapid and rotary in nature, with no evidence of slow central vortex patterns.[122] Outflow is along the opposite edge of the aneurysm ostium and typically passes almost exclusively into the vessel nearest the outflow stream.

It is important to note that turbulent or chaotic flow is not commonly present in most aneurysms. In all cases, flow within the aneurysm—although not always laminar—is seldom chaotic. Perktold et al.,[123] using mathematic models and computer simulations to predict flow in an axisymmetric aneurysm model, noted complex and consistent intra-aneurysmal flow fields, with varying shear stresses in different portions of the aneurysm. Strother et al.[87] also showed that the geometric relationship between an aneurysm and its parent artery is the principal factor that determines the intra-aneurysmal flow pattern. Flow is highly predictable and varies according to the geometric relationship of the aneurysm to the parent artery. Flow transitions that represent intermediate stages between laminar flow and turbulence were observed in all three aneurysm geometries. In light of the complex flow conditions, occasional difficulties may be encountered in adequately visualizing the aneurysms using MRA techniques.

The predominant feature of fusiform and giant aneurysms is slow flow along the wall, often resulting in laminated mural thrombus. Because of saturation effects, the slow flow commonly makes these aneurysms difficult to identify by 3D TOF MRA, and in fact, the artery may appear normal in caliber on PC MRA if the mural thrombus has sufficiently reduced the aneurysm lumen. Therefore, the aneurysm size and associated thrombus can be evaluated best on spin echo MRI (see Figure 14-13).

Acute Subarachnoid Hemorrhage and Magnetic Resonance Angiography

IADSA, as the exclusive vascular modality of evaluation of patients with acute SAH, is being challenged. In a case report of a patient with SAH, MRA demonstrated an ACOM aneurysm that was undetected by catheter angiography.[124] The results of a study comparing MRA to IADSA in the setting of SAH are also encouraging.[125] Fourteen patients with acute SAH were evaluated with both modalities. In three of the 14 patients, no abnormalities were detected on either diagnostic test, and two patients had two aneurysms each. MRA detected all the aneurysms with the exception of one, a 2-mm MCA aneurysm. IADSA also failed to detect a 5-mm MCA aneurysm. More recently, Anzalone et al.[126] and Sankhla et al.[127] evaluated MRA in the setting of acute SAH in a larger series, and both reported high sensitivity and specificity. Twenty of 51 patients in Sankhla's[127] series were operated on based on MRA alone. Several other studies reported high accuracy rates for MRA. However, it should be emphasized that, before replacing IADSA with another imaging test, one must take into account the extremely high (60–70%) fatality rate in untreated ruptured aneurysms. Currently, MRA is far from replacing IADSA in the setting of acute SAH because of its low sensitivity for small aneurysms and vessels.

Detection

Many studies have shown consistent detection of unruptured aneurysms using MRA with high sensitivity, specificity, and accuracy.[128] Some of these studies are flawed by small patient numbers and other methodologic inaccuracies. On the other hand, a substantial number of these studies used MRA techniques that are not state-of-the-art. It can be safely presumed that with modern, high-field magnetic resonance equipment, state-of-the-art pulse sequence designs, and postprocessing algorithms, the accuracy of MRA for the detection of aneurysms of the circle of Willis larger than 5 mm approaches that of IADSA. MRA is not as robust for the detection of aneurysms smaller than 3 mm.

Screening

For routine screening to be recommended, screening tests should have a high sensitivity and specificity, the prevalence and natural history of the disease must be known, and the risks of the test and treatment need to be low. These conditions are not always satisfied in asymptomatic patients at high risk for saccular aneurysms.

Although aneurysmal SAH is a condition of high morbidity and mortality, there is no consensus today regarding the natural history and risk of rupture of intact intracranial aneurysms.[129–134] Calculating the risk of rupture is confounded by the poor discrimination between symptomatic and asymptomatic aneurysms in most studies.[123,129,133–136] Symptomatic unruptured aneurysms are associated with a significantly higher risk of hemorrhage, and these aneurysms rupture at a rate of at least 4% per year.[129,132,133,136] The rate of rupture of a previously unruptured aneurysm has been the subject of many investigations and speculations. The findings of two recently published and credible studies are in concordance with the previous estimates that the long-term risk of rupture for an incidentally discovered aneurysm is 1–2% per year.[137–140] The size of the aneurysm and the age of the patient at the time of diagnosis are the predictors of rupture. A more recent, larger, multicenter study (International Study of Unruptured Intracranial Aneurysms)[141] assessed the natural history and treatment-related morbidity and mortality of unruptured aneurysms in a total of 2,621 patients. The cumulative rupture rate of aneurysms smaller than 10 mm was less than 0.05% per year in patients with no history of another previously ruptured aneurysm (group 1). The rate was 0.5% for patients who had a history of previous aneurysm rupture and subsequent repair in another location (group 2). The rupture rate was less than 1% per year for aneurysms that were larger than 10 mm in both groups. A rupture rate of 6% the first year was reported for giant aneurysms (25 mm or larger). In this study, the surgical mortality and morbidity rates were remarkably higher than previously reported. These results have been criticized, however, because of significant patient selection bias, relatively short follow-up (the study is ongoing), and inclusion of cavernous and some paraclinoid aneurysms, which are known to have a lower rupture rate, resulting in underestimation of the rupture rate of free intradural aneurysms.[142]

In addition to the risk of rupture, the prevalence of aneurysms is an important predictor of the benefit and cost effectiveness of screening, yet studies of the prevalence of aneurysms in asymptomatic subjects have been limited by small numbers of patients.[143]

Two early studies assessed the prevalence of aneurysms in asymptomatic subjects with a history of autosomal-dominant polycystic kidney disease. Schievink et al.[144] used MRA to identify six patients with aneurysms among 27 patients with a family history of aneurysm or SAH; the 95% confidence interval for the prevalence of aneurysms based on this study was 0.08–0.42. Ruggieri et al.[145] also used MRA to identify five patients with saccular intracranial aneurysms among 27 patients with a family history or suspected family history of aneurysm; the 95% confidence interval for the prevalence of aneurysms based on this study was 0.09–0.42 (adjusted for the estimated false-negative rate of MRA).

In a study of patients without polycystic kidney disease, Aoki et al.[146] used a combination of catheter angiography and MRA to screen 400 Japanese patients with a family or clinical history of cerebrovascular disease; 26 patients (6.5%) had aneurysms. Volunteers with a family history of SAH within the second degree of consanguinity showed a higher incidence of aneurysms (17.9%). A more recent study from Finland evaluated 400 asymptomatic individuals with a family history of aneurysm; 37 MRAs demonstrated aneurysms, and 32 of these subjects underwent IADSA that revealed no aneurysm in four subjects.[147] The false-negative rate is unknown, because IADSA was not performed on subjects with normal MRA. The smallest aneurysm detected was 2.5 mm.

Several, but not all, detailed decision analyses advocated MRA screening.[148–153] Using MRA, Raaymakers et al.[154] screened 626 individuals who had a first-degree relative with a history of spontaneous SAH and found 25 aneurysms in 25 individuals. Eighteen underwent surgery, and the outcome was assessed 6 months postoperatively. In their analysis, the estimated increase in life expectancy did not offset the risk of postoperative sequelae.[153] The conflicting results may be due to overestimation of the accuracy of MRA and underestimation of the surgical risk by earlier studies, as suggested by more recent and vigorous trials.[128,141] Although it is known that small aneurysms and aneurysms in certain locations, namely the ACOM complex, are associated with a lower surgical complication rate as well as lower rupture risk, there is no study designed to investigate the impact of a screening program on these subsets. In addition, there is currently no evidence-based opinion as to frequency and duration of MRA screening to exclude de novo aneurysm formation and enlargement of previously detected or undetected small aneurysms.

With the controversial data available, it is difficult to establish recommendations regarding screening. A large randomized trial of medical therapy (i.e., cessation of smoking, control of hypertension) versus intervention (clipping/coiling) may provide further insight into this complex matter.

COMPUTED TOMOGRAPHIC ANGIOGRAPHY

Recently, CT angiography (CTA) has emerged as a very powerful tool for aneurysm imaging. It can be obtained immediately after unenhanced CT and requires a relatively rapid intravenous infusion of iodinated contrast material. Helical image acquisition starts 25–60 seconds after the start of contrast material infusion from the level of the foramen magnum in a plane parallel to the orbitomeatal line and extends cranially with a table speed of 1.0–1.5 mm per second and a pitch of 1. The total acquisition time is approximately 1 minute. Images can be displayed as simple multiplanar reconstructions, more sophisticated postprocessing algorithms such as MIP, or a surface-shaded display that can be used to produce angiography-like images (the latter is time consuming, however, and generally requires an offline work station). Most authors agree that evaluation of MIP images in conjunction with source images increases the accuracy.[155] Unwanted bone detail may be removed from the image with additional postprocessing, but bones often serve as anatomic landmarks (Figure 14-15).

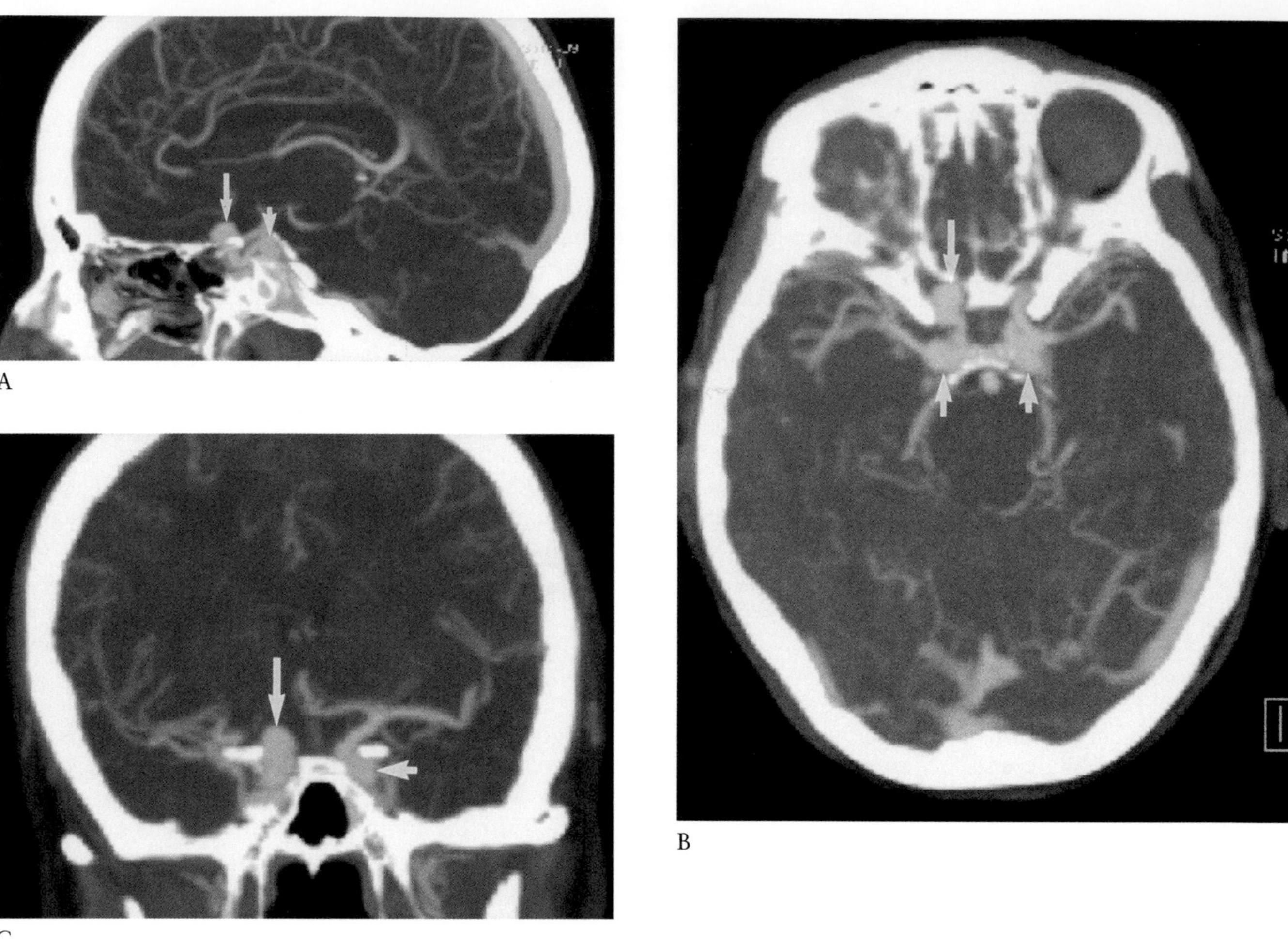

FIGURE 14-15. **A–C.** Demonstration of a right paraophthalmic (intradural [*arrows*]) and bilateral proximal cavernous internal carotid artery (extradural [*short arrows*]) aneurysms with computed tomographic angiography. Ability to display the relation of bony landmarks to the aneurysm can be helpful in treatment planning.

The advantages of CTA include the short acquisition time, the ease of obtaining it immediately after unenhanced CT, and compatibility with life-support devices. It is also less affected by flow than MRA. Several studies demonstrated accuracy rates comparable to MRA in the detection of aneurysms.[155–166] However, as with MRA, CTA is not suitable for aneurysms smaller than 3 mm. Aneurysms close to the bony structures may not be evaluated optimally. In early studies, aneurysms outside the imaging volume were the biggest source of false-negative results; however, this is not a substantial problem with currently available, multidetector helical scanners. Perhaps the most important current clinical use of CTA is in the characterization of the aneurysm and neck morphology in anatomically difficult locations. CTA, because of its ability to reconstruct and view the image from different angles, is a very helpful tool in planning treatment of complex aneurysms and in visualization of the neck and dome.[160,161,165] Presence of thrombus and aneurysm wall calcification is also evaluated better with CTA than IADSA. Precise size and volume measurements is extremely helpful before coiling procedures.

NONANEURYSMAL SUBARACHNOID HEMORRHAGE

Approximately 20% of the initial angiograms in acute SAH patients fail to identify a cause for SAH.[7] Repeated angiographic studies provide identification of a causative lesion in a small number of these patients. Inadequate angiographic technique, vasospasm, occult aneurysms, and vascular malformations may account for an additional small group of unidentified causes. A substantial number of these remain idiopathic and may be due to coagulopathy, drug use/abuse, trauma, dissection, sickle cell disease or, most commonly, PNSAH. PNSAH refers to a benign form of SAH, in which the center of the extravasated blood is in the cisterns in front of the brain stem, and the IADSA is negative. The source of hemorrhage is proposed to be nonarterial, such as capillary leak or venous rupture.[167] PNSAH may stem from anterior longitudinal pontine, interpeduncular or posterior communicating veins, lenticulostriate or thalamoperforate arteries, or cryptic AVMs of the brain stem.

In their prospective study, van Gijn et al.[167] demonstrated the differences in the outcome of aneurysmal and PNSAH, with no death or rebleed seen in the latter group. Several other studies revealed similar results with no mortality or significant morbidity.[7] A recent study, however, reported considerable psychosocial sequelae in a majority of these patients, although no neurologic deficit was seen in accordance with previous studies.[168] One patient in this series had a recurrent PNSAH 31 months later.

Rinkel et al.[169] analyzed the pattern of distribution of SAH in 52 patients with nonaneurysmal hemorrhage. All of these patients had blood in the prepontine and interpeduncular cisterns with or without extension to the ambient or quadrigeminal cisterns and the basal portion of the sylvian fissure. There was no complete filling of the anterior interhemispheric fissure and no extension to the lateral sylvian fissure except for a minute amount of blood. There was no frank intraventricular hemorrhage. The predictive value of these criteria for a negative angiogram was 0.95 (Figure 14-16). Interobserver agreement was high, but both observers mistook a basilar artery aneurysm rupture for PNSAH. Therefore, an IADSA should be performed to exclude an aneurysm. Most authors believe that a technically adequate and negative angiogram with typical CT findings should complete the workup of these patients, and that no further investigation is needed.[7,105,167,169] Aneurysmal SAH may mimic the pattern of PNSAH on delayed CT scans due to washout, redistribution, and absorption of blood. CT scans obtained 48 hours after the ictus should be interpreted very cautiously.

Surgical intervention requiring hydrocephalus, although less common, does occur after PNSAH. Clinical vasospasm is very rare.

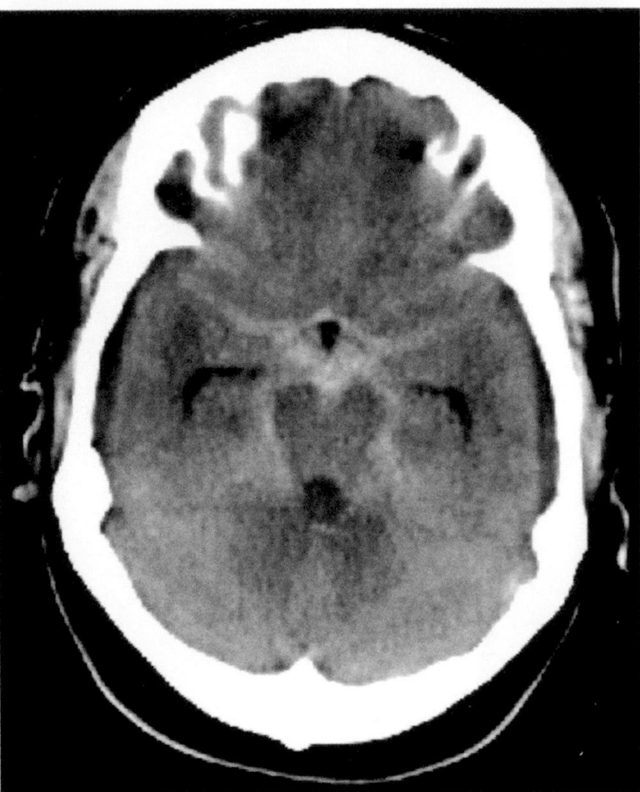

FIGURE 14-16. Nonaneurysmal perimesencephalic subarachnoid hemorrhage. The blood is centered in the interpeduncular cistern, with marginal extension into the proximal sylvian fissures and perimesencephalic cisterns.

VASOSPASM

Defined as the delayed narrowing of large capacitance intracranial arteries, *vasospasm* is the greatest source of mortality and morbidity in the SAH patients who survive the ictus. Approximately 32% of the hospitalized SAH patients develop delayed ischemic neurologic deficits (DIND) that may progress to infarction or resolve.[12] Decreased cerebral blood flow through the narrowed vessel at the circle of Willis as the presumed mechanism for neurologic deterioration in SAH patients has been challenged. However, the CT, positron emission tomography, and autopsy evidence of ischemia in the distribution of involved vessels support this notion.[170,171] The exact pathophysiology of vasospasm has not been resolved, and multiple factors, such as release of numerous vasoactive agents, changes in endothelial morphology and permeability, structural alterations in the muscular cells of the vessel wall, and inflammatory response, may play roles.[172] Several clinical trials are under way to determine the clinical efficacy of different pharmacologic agents that interact with the proposed molecular mechanisms.

The amount of SAH and the duration of exposure of cisternal vessels to SAH are accurate predictors of the development of vasospasm. Therefore, initial CT scans are very critical in determining the risk of vasospasm and outcome.[11,22,173] One study, however, reported a large interobserver variability in grading the amount and distribution of SAH.[174] This may limit the value of CT.

Promptly recognized, vasospasm can be treated very effectively. Oral nimodipine is proven to be effective in reducing the poor outcome due to vasospasm, although the vessel caliber on angiography is not affected by this therapy.[93] Traditionally, the "triple H" (*h*ypertension, *h*emodilution, *h*ypervolemia) therapy has

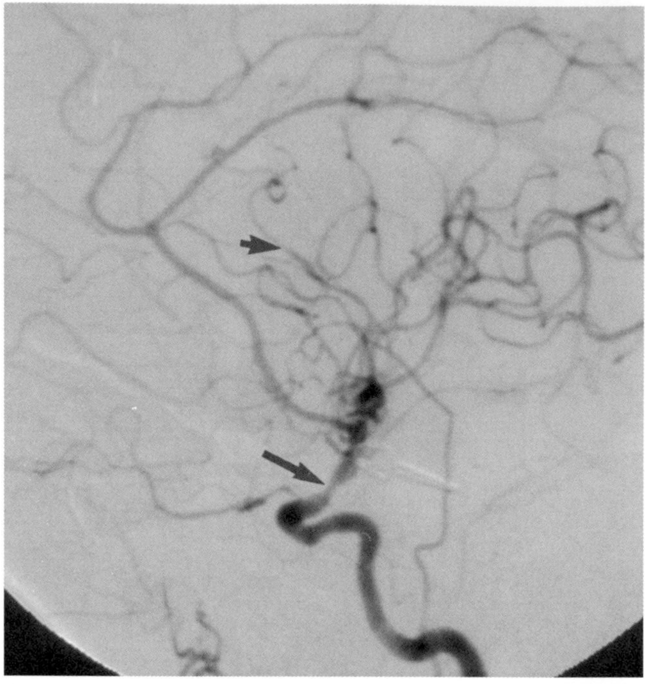

A

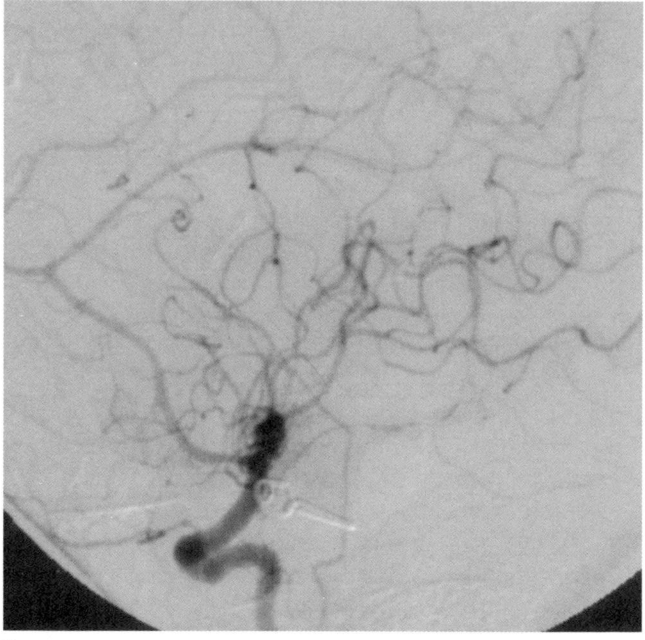

B

FIGURE 14-17. Neurologic deterioration 10 days after subarachnoid hemorrhage due to a ruptured posterior communicating artery aneurysm that was clipped. **A.** Vasospasm in the contralateral supraclinoid internal carotid artery (*arrow*) and distal middle cerebral artery (*short arrow*). **B.** Intra-arterial digital subtraction angiography after balloon angioplasty.

been used in prevention of complications of vasospasm.[175,176] Although the efficacy of "triple H" therapy has not been tested in large randomized trials, it is recommended by the Stroke Council of the American Heart Association.[93] Mechanical disruption and thrombolysis of cisternal clot and antioxidant and anti-inflammatory agents are other potentially useful tools. Transluminal angioplasty is recommended in patients for whom conventional therapy has failed and provides profound improvement in 60–80% of patients with no significant recurrent vasospasm (Figure 14-17). Similar results have been reported with intra-arterial papaverine injection; however, the recurrence rate is much higher with the latter.[177–179] Half of SAH patients show evidence of vasospasm on IADSA. Typically, angiographic vasospasm appears 3–5 days after the ictus, peaks at 5–14 days, and resolves gradually at 2–4 weeks.[12] DIND associated with vasospasm presents shortly after the onset of angiographic vasospasm. Not all patients with angiographic evidence of vasospasm develop cerebral ischemia, and observed neurologic deterioration may be due to hydrocephalus, seizures, rebleeding, electrolyte alterations, drug reactions, or cardiorespiratory failure. In fact, approximately one-half of the patients with angiographic vasospasm do not demonstrate any change in neurologic status.

The diagnostic standard for vasospasm is IADSA, but, currently, it is used uncommonly because of its invasiveness and the difficulty in obtaining repeated studies in critically ill patients.

Transcranial Doppler (TCD) ultrasound is used extensively to diagnose and monitor vasospasm in the setting of SAH. Ability to obtain repeated studies at the bedside with no known side effects, high sensitivity, and low cost of TCD are the main advantages. Systolic, diastolic, and mean arterial flow velocities (FVs) are recorded by using a 2-MHz transducer and transtemporal, transorbital, and suboccipital acoustic windows. In approximately 5% of the patients, the temporal bones are too thick to allow sound transmission. Occasionally, the suboccipital window may be limited for the evaluation of the basilar artery in its entirety, but an experienced operator can obtain a high-quality study in the majority of SAH patients. Any decrease in the vessel caliber results in increased FV, which precedes the neurologic deterioration in the SAH setting and correlates well with the changes seen in IADSA. Normative values are established for anterior circulation vessels, and any value above 80 cm per second is abnormal for MCA.[180] It is, however, very unusual for FV in the range of 120–140 cm per second to result in ischemia. Nonetheless, FV above 120 cm per second should alert the clinician to the possibility of impending ischemia.[180] An FV above 200 cm per second correlates closely with severe angiographic vasospasm. To differentiate hyperemia from truly increased FV, the MCA/ICA index can be calculated with a small addition to examination time; ratios greater than 3 indicate vasospasm.[181] The normative values in the vertebrobasilar system are less well defined; an early and sharp increase in FV should be treated with a high index of suspicion. Soustiel et al.[182] observed more ischemic symptoms above a threshold of 85 cm per second.

It must be emphasized that TCD measures FV (not the blood volume) in the arteries, and FV measurement does not provide any direct evidence for decreased tissue perfusion. Moreover, development of ischemia is affected by other factors, such as metabolic demand and collateral supply. Therefore, before making the presumptive diagnosis of ischemia due to vasospasm on the basis of increased FV, other causes of neurologic deterioration should be excluded. Other imaging techniques that measure the tissue perfusion and metabolism, such as single-photon emission CT, xenon-enhanced CT, positron emission tomography, and MRI perfusion imaging, can be used in difficult cases.

A baseline TCD examination before the vasospasm develops is very valuable to recognize the early changes and to differentiate other potential causes of increased FV, such as atherosclerotic stenosis.

Wardlaw et al.[183] assessed the impact of serial TCD monitoring on the diagnosis, management, and outcome of DIND complicating SAH in 186 patients. They found that TCD made a positive contribution to the diagnosis in 72% of the patients and changed the management in 43% of the cases.[183]

MRA does not seem to be a practical alternative in imaging of vasospasm after SAH because of the logistical difficulties and artifacts arising from the aneurysm clips.[184] CTA is used with success in imaging vasospasm. A very high correlation was reported with IADSA in detection of no spasm and severe spasm in proximal arterial locations; however, the accuracy dropped for mild and moderate vasospasm.[185,186]

REFERENCES

1. Detailed Diagnoses and Procedures, National Hospital Discharge Survey, 1990. Hyattsville, MD: US Department of Health and Human Services; 1992. DHHS publication PHS 92-1774, Series 13.
2. Broderick JP, Brott T, Tomsick T, et al. Intracerebral hemorrhage more than twice as common as subarachnoid hemorrhage. J Neurosurg 1993;78(2):188–191.
3. Davis PH, Hachinski V. Epidemiology of Cerebrovascular Disease. In DW Anderson (ed), Neuroepidemiology: A Tribute to Bruce Schoenberg. Boca Raton, FL: CRC Press, 1991.
4. Ingall TJ, Wiebers DO. Natural History of Subarachnoid Hemorrhage. In JP Whisnant (ed), Stroke: Populations, Cohorts, and Clinical Trials. Boston: Butterworth–Heinemann, 1993.
5. Nakayama T, Date C, Yokoyama T, et al. A 15.5-year follow-up study of stroke in a Japanese provincial city. The Shibata Study. Stroke 1997;28(1);45–52.
6. Walton JN. Subarachnoid Hemorrhage. London: Churchill Livingstone, 1956.
7. Schwartz TH, Solomon RA. Perimesencephalic nonaneurysmal subarachnoid hemorrhage: review of the literature. Neurosurgery 1996;39(3):433–440.
8. Macdonald RL, Weir B. Pathophysiology and Clinical Evaluation of Subarachnoid Hemorrhage. In JR Youmans (ed), Neurological Surgery (4th ed). Philadelphia: Saunders, 1997.
9. Linn FH, Wijdicks EF, van der Graaf Y, et al. Prospective study of sentinel headache in aneurysmal subarachnoid hemorrhage. Lancet 1994;344(8922):590–593.
10. Latchaw RE, Silva P, Falcone SF. The role of CT following aneurysmal rupture. Neuroimaging Clin North Am 1997;7(4):693–708.
11. van der Wee N, Rinkel GJ, Hasan D, van Gijn J. Detection of subarachnoid haemorrhage on early CT: is lumbar puncture still needed after a negative scan? J Neurol Neurosurg Psychiatry 1995;58(3):357–359.
12. Kassell NF, Torner JC, Haley EC Jr, et al. The international cooperative study on the timing of aneurysm surgery. Part 1: overall management results. J Neurosurg 1990;73(1):18–36.
13. Smith WP Jr, Batnitzky S, Rengachary SS. Acute isodense subdural hematomas: a problem in anemic patients. AJR Am J Roentgenol 1981;136(3):543–546.
14. Davis JM, Ploetz J, Davis KR, et al. Cranial computed tomography in subarachnoid hemorrhage: relationship between blood detected by CT and lumbar puncture. J Comput Assist Tomogr 1980;4(6):794–796.
15. Ishii R, Koike T, Ohsugi S, et al. Ruptured cerebral aneurysms not diagnosed by the initial cerebral angiography. Clinical and radiological study. Neurol Med Chir 1983;23(6):471–477.
16. Drake CG, Friedman AH, Peerless SJ. Failed aneurysm surgery. Reoperation in 115 cases. J Neurosurg 1984;61(5):848–856.
17. Lin T, Fox AJ, Drake CG. Regrowth of aneurysm sacs from residual neck following aneurysm clipping. J Neurosurg 1989;70(4):556–560.
18. Graeb DA, Robertson WD, Lapointe JS, et al. Computed tomographic diagnosis of intraventricular hemorrhage. Etiology and prognosis. Radiology 1982;143(1):91–96.
19. Davis KR, Kistler JP, Heros RC, Davis JM. A neuroradiologic approach to the patient with a diagnosis of subarachnoid hemorrhage. Radiol Clin North Am 1982;20(1):87–94.
20. van der Jagt M, Hasan D, Bijvoet HW, et al. Validity of prediction of the site of ruptured intracranial aneurysms with CT. Neurology 1999;52(1):34–39.
21. Brouwers PJ, Dippel DW, Vermeulen M, et al. Amount of blood on computed tomography as an independent predictor after aneurysm rupture. Stroke 1993;24(6):809–814.
22. Fisher CM, Kistler JP, Davis JM. Relation of

cerebral vasospasm to subarachnoid hemorrhage visualized by computerized tomographic scanning. Neurosurgery 1980;6(1):1–9.

23. Perl J 2nd, Tkach JA, Porras-Jimenez M, et al. Hemorrhage detected using MR imaging in the setting of acute stroke: an in vivo model. AJNR Am J Neuroradiol 1999;20(10):1863–1870.

24. Noguchi K, Seto H, Kamisaki Y, et al. Comparison of fluid-attenuated inversion-recovery MR imaging with CT in a simulated model of acute subarachnoid hemorrhage. AJNR Am J Neuroradiol 2000; 21(5):923–927.

25. Noguchi K, Ogawa T, Inugami A, et al. Acute subarachnoid hemorrhage: MR imaging with fluid-attenuated inversion recovery pulse sequences. Radiology 1995;196(3):773–777.

26. Singer MB, Atlas SW, Drayer BP. Subarachnoid space disease: diagnosis with fluid-attenuated inversion-recovery MR imaging and comparison with gadolinium-enhanced spin-echo MR imaging—blinded reader study. Radiology 1998;208(2):417–422.

27. Gustafsson O, Rossitti S, Ericsson A, Raininko R. MR imaging of experimentally induced intracranial hemorrhage in rabbits during the first 6 hours. Acta Radiol 1999;40(4):360–368.

28. Noguchi K, Ogawa T, Seto H, et al. Subacute and chronic subarachnoid hemorrhage: diagnosis with fluid-attenuated inversion-recovery MR imaging. Radiology 1997;203(1):257–262.

29. Ogawa T, Inugami A, Fujita H, et al. MR diagnosis of subacute and chronic subarachnoid hemorrhage: comparison with CT. AJR Am J Roentgenol 1995;165(5):1257–1262.

30. Lev MH, Schaefer PW. Subarachnoid gadolinium enhancement mimicking subarachnoid hemorrhage on FLAIR MR images. Fluid-attenuated inversion recovery. AJR Am J Roentgenol 1999;173(5):1414–1415.

31. Inagawa T, Tokuda Y, Ohbayashi N, et al. Study of aneurysmal subarachnoid hemorrhage in Izumo City, Japan. Stroke 1995;26(5):761–766.

32. Jerntorp P, Berglund G. Stroke registry in Malmö, Sweden. Stroke 1992;23(3):357–361.

33. Knekt P, Reunanen A, Aho K, et al. Risk factors for subarachnoid hemorrhage in a longitudinal population study. J Clin Epidemiol 1991;44(9):933–939.

34. Reunanen A, Aho K, Aromaa A, Knekt P. Incidence of stroke in a Finnish prospective population study. Stroke 1986;17(4):675–681.

35. Linn FH, Rinkel GJ, Algra A, van Gijn J. Incidence of subarachnoid hemorrhage: role of region, year, and rate of computed tomography: a meta-analysis. Stroke 1996;27(4):625–929.

36. Pakarinen S. Incidence, etiology, and prognosis of primary subarachnoid haemorrhage: a study based on 589 cases diagnosed in a defined urban population during a defined period. Acta Neurol Scand 1967;43[suppl 29]:1–28.

37. Inagawa T, Hirano A. Autopsy study of unruptured incidental intracranial aneurysms. Surg Neurol 1990;34(6):361–365.

38. Stehbens WE. Aneurysms and anatomic variations of cerebral arteries. Arch Pathol 1963;75:45–64.

39. Wiebers DO, Torner JC, Meissner I. Impact of unruptured intracranial aneurysms on public health in the United States. Stroke 1992;23(10):1416–1419.

40. Atkinson JL, Sundt TM, Houser OW, Whisnant JP. Angiographic frequency of anterior circulation intracranial aneurysms. J Neurosurg 1989;70(4):551–555.

41. Nakagawa T, Hashi K. The incidence and treatment of asymptomatic, unruptured cerebral aneurysms. J Neurosurg 1994;80(2):217–223.

42. Jellinger K. Pathology and Aerology of Intracranial Aneurysms. In HW Pia, L Langmaid, J Zierski (eds), Advances in Diagnosis and Therapy. New York: Springer, 1979;5–19.

43. Bannerman RM, Ingall GB, Graf CJ. The familial occurrence of intracranial aneurysms. Neurology 1979;29(3):283–292.

44. Housepian EM, Pool JL. A systematic analysis of intracranial aneurysms from the autopsy file of Presbyterian Hospital. J Neuropathol Exp Neurol 1958;17:409–423.

45. McCormick WF. Problems and Pathogenesis of Intracranial Arterial Aneurysms. In JF Toole, J Moosey, R Janeway (eds), Cerebrovascular Disorders (2nd ed). New York: Grune & Stratton, 1971;219–231.

46. Ingall TJ, Whisnant JP, Wiebers DO, O'Fallon WM. Has there been a decline in subarachnoid hemorrhage mortality? Stroke 1989;20(6):718–724.

47. Shinton R, Beevers G. Meta-analysis of relation between cigarette smoking and stroke. BMJ 1989;298(6676):789–794.

48. Wiebers DO, Whisnant JP, O'Fallon WM. The natural history of unruptured intracranial aneurysms. N Engl J Med 1981;304(12):696–698.

49. Winn HR, Almaani WS, Berga SL, et al. The long-term outcome in patients with multiple aneurysms. Incidence of late hemorrhage and implications for treatment of incidental aneurysms. J Neurosurg 1983;59(4): 642–651.

50. Schievink WI, Schaid DJ, Michels VV, Piepgras DG. Familial aneurysmal subarachnoid hemorrhage: a community-based study. J Neurosurg 1995;83(3):426–429.

51. Longstreth WT Jr, Nelson LM, Koepsell TD, van Belle G. Cigarette smoking, alcohol use, and subarachnoid hemorrhage. Stroke 1992;23(9):1242–1249.

52. Miller CA, Hill SA, Hunt WE. "De novo" aneurysms. A clinical review. Surg Neurol 1985;24(2): 173–180.

53. Schievink WI, Karemaker JM, Hageman LM, van der Werf DJ. Circumstances surrounding aneurysmal subarachnoid hemorrhage. Surg Neurol 1989; 32(4):266–272.

54. Lichtenfeld PJ, Rubin DB, Feldman RS. Subarachnoid hemorrhage precipitated by cocaine snorting. Arch Neurol 1984;41(2):223–224.

55. Beighton P. Ehler-Danlos Syndrome. In P Beighton (ed), McKusick's Heritable Disorders of Connective Tissue. St. Louis: Mosby, 1993;189–251.

56. Schievink WI, Michels VV, Piepgras DG. Neurovascular manifestations of heritable connective tissue disorders. A review. Stroke 1994;25(4):889–903.

57. Harvey AM, Schulman LE, Tumulty PA, et al. Systemic lupus erythematosus: review of the literature and clinical analysis of 138 cases. Medicine 1954;33: 291–437.

58. Griffin J, Price DL, Davis L, McKhann GM. Granulomatous angiitis of the central nervous system with aneurysms on multiple cerebral arteries. Trans Am Neurol Assoc 1973;98:145–148.

59. Parker HL, Kernohan JW. The central nervous system in periarteritis nodosa. Proc Staff Meet Mayo Clin 1949;24:43–48.

60. Masuzawa T, Kurokawa T, Oguro K, et al. Pulseless disease associated with multiple intracranial aneurysms. Neuroradiology 1986;28(1):17–22.

61. Campbell GJ, Roach MR. Fenestrations in the internal elastic lamina at bifurcations of human cerebral arteries. Stroke 1981;12(4):489–496.

62. Iwanaga H, Wakai S, Ochiai C, et al. Ruptured cerebral aneurysms missed by initial angiographic study. Neurosurgery 1990;27(1):45–51.

63. Fox JL. Microsurgical treatment of ventral (paraclinoid) internal carotid artery aneurysms. Neurosurgery 1988;22[1 Part 1]:32–39.

64. al-Rodhan NR, Piepgras DG, Sundt TM Jr. Transitional cavernous aneurysms of the internal carotid artery. Neurosurgery 1993;33(6):993–996.

65. Yasargil MG, Fox JL. The microsurgical approach to intracranial aneurysms. Surg Neurol 1975;3(1):7–14.

66. Day AL. Aneurysms of the ophthalmic segment. A clinical and anatomical analysis. J Neurosurg 1990;72(5):677–691.

67. Yasargil MG. Microneurosurgery. New York: Thieme, 1987.

68. Fox AL. Intracranial Aneurysms. Berlin: Springer, 1983;419–431, 1453–1455.

69. Koike G, Seguchi K, Kyoshima K, Kobayashi S. Subarachnoid hemorrhage due to rupture of infundibular dilation of a circumflex branch of the posterior cerebral artery: case report. Neurosurgery 1994;34(6):1075–1077.

70. Marshman LA, Ward PJ, Walter PH, Dossetor RS. The progression of an infundibulum to aneurysm formation and rupture: case report and literature review. Neurosurgery 1998;43(6):1445–1448.

71. Buckingham MJ, Crone KR, Ball WS, et al. Traumatic intracranial aneurysms in childhood: two cases and a review of the literature. Neurosurgery 1988;22(2):398–408.

72. Messina AV, Chernik NL. Computed tomography: the "resolving" intracerebral hemorrhage. Radiology 1976;118(3):609–613.

73. Ross JS, Masaryk TJ, Modic MT, et al. Intracranial aneurysms: evaluation by MR angiography. AJNR Am J Neuroradiol 1990;11(3):449–455.

74. Brust JC, Dickinson PH, Hughes JE, Holtzman RN. The diagnosis and treatment of cerebral mycotic aneurysms. Ann Neurol 1990;27(3):238–246.

75. Roeltgen DP, Weimer GR, Patterson LF. Delayed neurologic complications of left atrial myxoma. Neurology 1981;31(1):8–13.

76. Murata J, Sawamura Y, Takahashi A, et al. Intracerebral hemorrhage caused by a neoplastic aneurysm from small-cell lung carcinoma: case report. Neurosurgery 1993;32(1):124–126.

77. Parkinson D, West M. Traumatic intracranial aneurysms. J Neurosurg 1980;52(1):11–20.

78. Herman JM, Rekate HL, Spetzler RF. Pediatric intracranial aneurysms: simple and complex cases. Pediatr Neurosurg 1991;17(2):66–72.

79. Echiverri HC, Rubino FA, Gupta SR, Gujrati M. Fusiform aneurysm of the vertebrobasilar arterial system. Stroke 1989;20(12):1741–1747.

80. Nishizaki T, Tamaki N, Takeda N, et al. Dolichoectatic basilar artery: a review of 23 cases. Stroke 1986;17(6):1277–1281.

81. Segal HD, McLaurin RL. Giant serpentine aneurysm. Report of two cases. J Neurosurg 1977; 46(1):115–120.

82. Berger MS, Wilson CB. Intracranial dissecting aneurysms of the posterior circulation. Report of six cases and review of the literature. J Neurosurg 1984;61(5):882–894.

83. Friedman AH, Drake CG. Subarachnoid hemorrhage from intracranial dissecting aneurysm. J Neurosurg 1984;60(2):325–334.

84. Shimoji T, Bando K, Nakajima K, Ito K. Dissecting aneurysm of the vertebral artery. Report of seven cases and angiographic findings. J Neurosurg 1984;61(6):1038–1046.

85. Mizutani T, Aruga T, Kirino T, et al. Recurrent subarachnoid hemorrhage from untreated ruptured vertebrobasilar dissecting aneurysms. Neurosurgery 1995;36(5):905–911.

86. Crompton MR. Mechanism of growth and rupture in cerebral berry aneurysms. BMJ 1966;5496: 1138–1142.

87. Strother CM, Eldevik P, Kikuchi Y, et al. Thrombus formation and structure and the evolution of

mass effect in intracranial aneurysms treated by balloon embolization: emphasis on MR findings. AJNR Am J Neuroradiol 1989;10(4):787–796.

88. Sundt TM Jr, Piepgras DG. Surgical approach to giant intracranial aneurysms. Operative experience with 80 cases. J Neurosurg 1979;51(6):731–742.

89. Lanzieri CR, Tarr RF, Selman WR, et al. Use of the delayed mask for improved demonstration of aneurysms on intraarterial DSA. AJNR Am J Neuroradiol 1992;13(6):1589–1593.

90. Tanoue S, Kiyosue H, Kenai H, et al. Three-dimensional reconstructed images after rotational angiography in the evaluation of intracranial aneurysms: surgical correlation. Neurosurgery 2000;47(4):866–871.

91. Mizoi K, Suzuki J, Yoshimoto T. Surgical treatment of multiple aneurysms. Review of experience with 372 cases. Acta Neurochir (Wien) 1989;96(1–2):8–14.

92. Setton A, Davis AJ, Bose A, et al. Angiography of cerebral aneurysms. Neuroimaging Clin North Am 1996;6(3):705–738.

93. Mayberg MR, Batjer HH, Dacey R, et al. Guidelines for the management of aneurysmal subarachnoid hemorrhage. A statement for healthcare professionals from a special writing group of the Stroke Council, American Heart Association. Stroke 1994; 25(11):2315–2328.

94. Saitoh H, Hayakawa K, Nishimura K, et al. Rerupture of cerebral aneurysms during angiography. AJNR Am J Neuroradiol 1995;16(3):539–542.

95. Yasui T, Kishi H, Komiyama M, et al. Very poor prognosis in cases with extravasation of the contrast medium during angiography. Surg Neurol 1996; 45(6):560–564.

96. Locksley HB. Natural history of subarachnoid hemorrhage, intracranial aneurysms and arteriovenous malformations. Based on 6368 cases in the cooperative study. J Neurosurg 1966;25(2):219–239.

97. Duong H, Melancon D, Tampieri D, Ethier R. The negative angiogram in subarachnoid hemorrhage. Neuroradiology 1996;38(1):15–19.

98. Forster DM, Steiner L, Hakanson S, Bergvall U. The value of repeat pan-angiography in cases of unexplained subarachnoid hemorrhage. J Neurosurg 1978;48(5):712–716.

99. Hove B, Andersen BB, Christiansen TM. Intracranial oncotic aneurysms from choriocarcinoma. Case report and review of the literature. Neuroradiology 1990;32(6):526–528.

100. Juul R, Fredriksen TA, Ringkjob R. Prognosis in subarachnoid hemorrhage of unknown etiology. J Neurosurg 1986;64(3):359–362.

101. Bohmfalk GL, Story JL. Intermittent appearance of a ruptured cerebral aneurysm on sequential angiograms. Case report. J Neurosurg 1980;52(2):263–265.

102. Di Lorenzo N, Guidetti G. Anterior communicating aneurysm missed at angiography: report of two cases treated surgically. Neurosurgery 1988;23(4):494–499.

103. Gilbert JW, Lee C, Young B. Repeat cerebral pan-angiography in subarachnoid hemorrhage of unknown etiology. Surg Neurol 1990;33(1):19–21.

104. Shellock FG, Curtis JS. MR imaging and biomedical implants, materials, and devices: an updated review. Radiology 1991;180(2):541–550.

105. Tatter SB, Crowell RM, Ogilvy CS. Aneurysmal and microaneurysmal "angiogram-negative" subarachnoid hemorrhage. Neurosurgery 1995;37(1):48–55.

106. Allock JM. Aneurysms. In TH Newton, DG Potts (eds), Radiology of the Skull and Brain. St. Louis: Mosby, 1974;2445–2559.

107. Wood EH. Angiographic identification of the ruptured lesion in patients with multiple cerebral aneurysms. J Neurosurg 1964;21:182–198.

108. Wilson FM, Jaspan T, Holland IM. Multiple cerebral aneurysms—a reappraisal. Neuroradiology 1989;31(3):232–236.

109. Cloft HJ, Joseph GJ, Dion JE. Risk of cerebral angiography in patients with subarachnoid hemorrhage, cerebral aneurysm, and arteriovenous malformation: a meta-analysis. Stroke 1999;30(2):317–320.

110. Barrow DL, Boyer KL, Joseph GJ. Intraoperative angiography in the management of neurovascular disorders. Neurosurgery 1992;30(2):153–159.

111. Heiserman JE, Bird CR. Cerebral aneurysms. Neuroimaging Clin North Am 1994;4(4):799–822.

112. Macdonald RL, Wallace MC, Kestle JR. Role of angiography following aneurysm surgery. J Neurosurg 1993;79(6):826–832.

113. Davis JM, Davis KR, Crowell RM. Subarachnoid hemorrhage secondary to ruptured intracranial aneurysm: prognostic significance of cranial CT. AJR Am J Roentgenol 1980;134(4):711–715.

114. Feuerberg I, Lindquist C, Lindqvist M, Steiner L. Natural history of postoperative aneurysm rests. J Neurosurg 1987;66(1):30–34.

115. Hackney DB, Lesnick JE, Zimmerman RA, et al. MR identification of bleeding site in subarachnoid hemorrhage with multiple intracranial aneurysms. J Comput Assist Tomogr 1986;10(5):878–880.

116. Martin NA, Bentson J, Vinuela F, et al. Intraoperative digital subtraction angiography and the surgical treatment of intracranial aneurysms and vascular malformations. J Neurosurg 1990;73(4):526–533.

117. Edelman RR. Basic principles of magnetic resonance angiography. Cardiovasc Intervent Radiol 1992;15(1):3–13.

118. Seibert JE, Pernicone JR, Potchen EJ. Physical principles and application of magnetic resonance angiography. Semin Ultrasound CT MR 1992;13(4):227–245.

119. Jellinger K. Vascular malformations of the central nervous system: a morphological overview. Neurosurg Rev 1986;9(3):177–216.

120. Strother CM, Graves VB, Rappe A. Aneurysm hemodynamics: an experimental study. AJNR Am J Neuroradiol 1992;13(4):1089–1095.

121. Garretson H. Intracranial Arteriovenous Malformations. In R Wilkins, S Rengachary (eds), Neurosurgery. New York: McGraw-Hill, 1985;1448–1457.

122. Brown RD Jr, Wiebers DO, Forbes GS. Unruptured intracranial aneurysms and arteriovenous malformations: frequency of intracranial hemorrhage and relationship of lesions. J Neurosurg 1990;73(6):859–863.

123. Perktold K. On the paths of fluid particles in an axisymmetrical aneurysm. J Biomech 1987;20(3):311–317.

124. Rosenorn J, Eskesen V, Schmidt K. Unruptured intracranial aneurysms: an assessment of the annual risk of rupture based on epidemiological and clinical data. Br J Neurosurg 1988;2(3):369–377.

125. Wiebers DO, Whisnant JP, Sundt TM Jr, O'Fallon WM. The significance of unruptured intracranial saccular aneurysms. J Neurosurg 1987;66(1):23–29.

126. Anzalone N, Triulzi F, Scotti G. Acute subarachnoid hemorrhage: 3D time-of-flight MR angiography versus intra-arterial digital angiography. Neuroradiology 1995;37(4):257–261.

127. Sankhla SK, Gunawardena WJ, Coutinho CM, et al. Magnetic resonance angiography in the management of aneurysmal subarachnoid hemorrhage: a study of 51 cases. Neuroradiology 1996;38(8):724–729.

128. White PM, Lindsay KW, Teasdale E, et al. Should we screen for familial intracranial aneurysm? Stroke 1999;30(10):2241–2242.

129. Turski PA, Korosec FR. Phase Contrast Angiography. In CM Anderson, RR Edelman, PA Turski (eds), Clinical Magnetic Resonance Angiography. New York: Lippincott–Raven, 1993;43–72.

130. Artmann H, Vonofakos D, Muller H, Grau H. Neuroradiologic and neuropathologic findings with growing giant intracranial aneurysm. Review of the literature. Surg Neurol 1984;21(4):391–401.

131. Steiger HJ, Liepsch DW, Poll A, Reulen HJ. Hemodynamic stress in terminal saccular aneurysms: a laser-Doppler study. Heart Vessels 1988;4(3):162–169.

132. McCormick WF, Acosta-Rua GJ. The size of intracranial saccular aneurysms. An autopsy study. J Neurosurg 1970;33(4):422–427.

133. Sevick RJ, Tsuruda JS, Schmalbrock P. Three-dimensional time-of-flight MR angiography in the evaluation of cerebral aneurysms. J Comput Assist Tomogr 1990;14(6):874–881.

134. Huston J 3rd, Rufenacht DA, Ehman RL, Wiebers DO. Intracranial aneurysms and vascular malformations: comparison of time-of-flight and phase-contrast MR angiography. Radiology 1991;181(3):721–730.

135. Runge VM, Kirsch JE, Lee C. Contrast-enhanced MR angiography. J Magn Reson Imaging 1993;3(1):233–239.

136. Demaerel P, Marchal G, Casteels I, et al. Intracavernous aneurysm. Superior demonstration by magnetic resonance angiography. Neuroradiology 1990;32(4):322–324.

137. Jane JA, Kassell NF, Torner JC, Winn HR. The natural history of aneurysms and arteriovenous malformations. J Neurosurg 1985;62(3):321–323.

138. Juvela S, Porras M, Heiskanen O. Natural history of unruptured intracranial aneurysms: a long-term follow-up study. J Neurosurg 1993;79(2):174–182.

139. Yasui N, Suzuki A, Nishimura H, et al. Long-term follow-up study of unruptured intracranial aneurysms. Neurosurgery 1997;40(6):1155–1159.

140. Adams HP Jr, Kassell NF, Torner JC, et al. Early management of aneurysmal subarachnoid hemorrhage. A report of the Cooperative Aneurysm Study. J Neurosurg 1981;54(2):141–145.

141. International Study of Unruptured Intracranial Aneurysms Investigators. Unruptured intracranial aneurysms—risk of rupture and risks of surgical intervention. N Engl J Med 1998;339(24):1725–1733.

142. Berenstein A, Flamn ES, Kupersmith MJ. Unruptured intracranial aneurysms. N Engl J Med 1999;340(18):1439–1440.

143. Wiebers DO, Torres VE. Screening for unruptured intracranial aneurysms in autosomal dominant polycystic kidney disease. N Engl J Med 1992;327(13):953–955.

144. Schievink WI, Limburg M, Dreissen JJ, et al. Screening for unruptured familial intracranial aneurysms: subarachnoid hemorrhage 2 years after angiography negative for aneurysms. Neurosurgery 1991;29(3):434–437.

145. Ruggieri PM, Poulos N, Masaryk TJ, et al. Occult intracranial aneurysms in polycystic kidney disease: screening with MR angiography. Radiology 1994;191(1):33–39.

146. Aoki S, Sasaki Y, Machida T, et al. Cerebral aneurysms: detection and delineation using 3D-CT angiography. AJNR Am J Neuroradiol 1992;13(4):1115–1120.

147. Ronkainen A, Puranen MI, Hernesniemi JA, et al. Intracranial aneurysms: MR angiographic screening in 400 asymptomatic individuals with increased familial risk. Radiology 1995;195(1):35–40.

148. Leblanc R, Worsley KJ, Melanson D, Tampieri D. Angiographic screening and elective surgery of familial cerebral aneurysms: a decision analysis. Neurosurgery 1994;35(1):9–18.

149. King JT Jr, Glick HA, Mason TJ, Flamn ES. Elective surgery for asymptomatic, unruptured intracra-

nial aneurysms: a cost-effectiveness analysis. J Neurosurg 1995;83(3):403–412.

150. Obuchowski NA, Modic MT, Magdinec M. Current implications for the efficacy of noninvasive screening for occult intracranial aneurysms in patients with a family history of aneurysms. J Neurosurg 1995; 83(1):42–49.

151. Kallmes DF, Kallmes MH, Cloft HJ, Dion JE. Guglielmi detachable coil embolization for unruptured aneurysms in nonsurgical candidates: a cost-effectiveness exploration. AJNR Am J Neuroradiol 1998;19(1):167–176.

152. Crawley F, Clifton A, Brown MM. Should we screen for familial intracranial aneurysm? Stroke 1999;30(2):312–316.

153. The Magnetic Resonance Angiography in Relatives of Patients with Subarachnoid Hemorrhage Study Group. Risks and benefits of screening for intracranial aneurysms in first-degree relatives of patients with sporadic subarachnoid hemorrhage. N Engl J Med 1999;341(18):1344–1350.

154. Raaymakers TW. Aneurysms in relatives of patients with subarachnoid hemorrhage: frequency and risk factors. MARS Study Group. Magnetic Resonance Angiography in Relatives of patients with Subarachnoid hemorrhage. Neurology 1999;53(5):982–988.

155. Kuszyk BS, Beauchamp NJ Jr, Fishman EK. Neurovascular applications of CT angiography. Semin Ultrasound CT MR 1998;19(5):394–404.

156. Lenhart M, Bretschneider T, Gmeinwieser J, et al. Cerebral CT angiography in the diagnosis of acute subarachnoid hemorrhage. Acta Radiologica 1997; 38(5):791–796.

157. Zouaoui A, Sahel M, Marro B, et al. Three-dimensional computed tomographic angiography in detection of cerebral aneurysms in acute subarachnoid hemorrhage. Neurosurgery 1997;41(1):125–130.

158. Hope JK, Wilson JL, Thomson FJ. Three-dimensional CT angiography in the detection and characterization of intracranial berry aneurysms. AJNR Am J Neuroradiol 1996;17(3):439–445.

159. Imakita S, Onishi Y, Hashimoto T, et al. Subtraction CT angiography with controlled-orbit helical scanning for detection of intracranial aneurysms. AJNR Am J Neuroradiol 1998;19(2):291–295.

160. Ochi T, Shimizu K, Yasuhara Y, et al. Curved planar reformatted CT angiography: usefulness for the evaluation of aneurysms at the carotid siphon. AJNR Am J Neuroradiol 1999;20(6):1025–1030.

161. Villablanca JP, Martin N, Jahan R, et al. Volume-rendered helical computerized tomography angiography in the detection and characterization of intracranial aneurysms. J Neurosurg 2000;93(2):254–264.

162. Kato Y, Sano H, Katada K, et al. Application of three-dimensional CT angiography (3D-CTA) to cerebral aneurysms. Surg Neurol 1999;52(2):113–121.

163. Young N, Dorsch NW, Kingston RJ. Pitfalls in the use of spiral CT for identification of intracranial aneurysms. Neuroradiology 1999;41(2):93–99.

164. Velthuis BK, Van Leeuwen MS, Witkamp TD, et al. Computerized tomography angiography in patients with subarachnoid hemorrhage: from aneurysm detection to treatment without conventional angiography. J Neurosurg 1999;91(5):761–767.

165. Strayle-Batra M, Skalej M, Wakhloo AK, et al. Three-dimensional spiral CT angiography in the detection of cerebral aneurysm. Acta Radiologica 1998;39(3):233–238.

166. Ng SH, Wong HF, Ko SF, et al. CT angiography of intracranial aneurysms: advantages and pitfalls. Eur J Radiology 1997;25(1):14–19.

167. van Gijn, van Dongen KJ, Vermeulen M, Hijdra A. Perimesencephalic hemorrhage: a nonaneurysmal and benign form of subarachnoid hemorrhage. Neurology 1985;35(4):493–497.

168. Marquardt G, Niebauer T, Schick U, Lorenz R. Long term follow up after perimesencephalic subarachnoid hemorrhage. J Neurol Neurosurg Psychiatry 2000;69(1):127–130.

169. Rinkel GJ, Wijdicks EF, Vermeulen M, et al. Nonaneurysmal perimesencephalic subarachnoid hemorrhage: CT and MR patterns that differ from aneurysmal rupture. AJNR Am J Neuroradiol 1991;12(5):829–834.

170. Powers WJ, Grubb RL Jr, Baker RP, et al. Regional cerebral blood flow and metabolism in reversible ischemia due to vasospasm. Determination by positron emission tomography. J Neurosurg 1985; 62(4):539–546.

171. Crompton MR. The comparative pathology of cerebral aneurysms. Brain 1966;89(4):789–796.

172. Mayberg MR. Cerebral vasospasm. Neurosurg Clin North Am 1998;9(3):615–627.

173. Jarus-Dziedzic K, Zub W, Wronski J, et al. The relationship between cerebral blood flow velocities and the amount of blood clots in computed tomography after subarachnoid haemorrhage. Acta Neurochir (Wien) 2000;142(3):309–318.

174. van der Jagt M, Hasan D, Bijvoet HW, et al. Interobserver variability of cisternal blood on CT after aneurysmal subarachnoid hemorrhage. Neurology 2000;54(11):2156–2158.

175. Dorsch NW. The effect and management of delayed vasospasm after aneurysmal subarachnoid hemorrhage. Neurol Med Chir (Tokyo) 1998;38 [Suppl]:156–160.

176. Pasqualin A. Epidemiology and pathophysiology of cerebral vasospasm following subarachnoid hemorrhage. J Neurosurg Sci 1998;42[1 Suppl 1]:15–21.

177. Firlik AD, Kaufmann AM, Jungreis CA, Yonas H. Effect of transluminal angioplasty on cerebral blood flow in the management of symptomatic vasospasm fol-

lowing aneurysmal subarachnoid hemorrhage. J Neurosurg 1997;86(5):830–839.

178. Elliott JP, Newell DW, Lam DJ, et al. Comparison of balloon angioplasty and papaverine infusion for the treatment of vasospasm following aneurysmal subarachnoid hemorrhage. J Neurosurg 1998;88(2):277–284.

179. Firlik KS, Kaufmann AM, Firlik AD, et al. Intra-arterial papaverine for the treatment of cerebral vasospasm following aneurysmal subarachnoid hemorrhage. Surg Neurol 1999;51(1):66–74.

180. Seiler RW, Grolimund P, Aaslid R, et al. Cerebral vasospasm evaluated by transcranial ultrasound correlated with clinical grade and CT-visualized subarachnoid hemorrhage. J Neurosurg 1986;64(4):594–600.

181. Lindegaard KF, Nornes H, Bakke SJ, et al. Cerebral vasospasm after subarachnoid haemorrhage investigated by means of transcranial Doppler ultrasound. Acta Neurochir Suppl 1988;42:81–84.

182. Soustiel JF, Bruk B, Shik B, et al. Transcranial Doppler in vertebrobasilar vasospasm after subarachnoid hemorrhage. Neurosurgery 1998;43(2):282–291.

183. Wardlaw JM, Offin R, Teasdale GM, Teasdale EM. Is routine transcranial Doppler ultrasound monitoring useful in the management of subarachnoid hemorrhage? J Neurosurg 1998;88(2):272–276.

184. Tamatani S, Sasaki O, Takeuchi S, et al. Detection of delayed cerebral vasospasm, after rupture of intracranial aneurysms, by magnetic resonance angiography. Neurosurgery 1997;40(4):748–753.

185. Anderson GB, Ashforth R, Steinke DE, Findlay JM. CT angiography for the detection of cerebral vasospasm in patients with acute subarachnoid hemorrhage. AJNR Am J Neuroradiol 2000;21(6):1011–1015.

186. Takagi R, Hayashi H, Kobayashi H, et al. Three-dimensional CT angiography of intracranial vasospasm following subarachnoid haemorrhage. Neuroradiology 1998;40(10):631–635.

CHAPTER

15

Epidural and Subdural Hematomas

Robert J. Bert

SUBDURAL HEMATOMAS

Cross-sectional imaging has been the universal method of diagnosing subdural hematomas (SDHs) for 15–20 years. Until the early 1980s,[1–3] cerebral angiography and clinical methods were used to diagnose SDHs. The multiplicity of presenting symptoms, each with low specificity, makes clinical detection less than rewarding. Cerebral angiography has associated risks that are far greater than cross-sectional imaging; it also provides considerably less information.

SDHs have been studied for several centuries.[4] Despite the long history of this investigation, some controversies remain regarding their pathophysiology. The elaborate pathophysiology of these entities and their multiple etiologies and age-related variations produce several pitfalls for interpreting diagnostic imaging studies. If the interpreting physician applies imaging principles correctly, computed tomography (CT) and magnetic resonance imaging (MRI) can contribute significantly to understanding the timing of the occurrence of an SDH and can often elucidate its etiology. Knowledge of the mechanism of occurrence and timing of the inciting event, in turn, allows the diagnostician to make important contributions to patient management.

Pathophysiology of Subdural Hematomas

The radiologic appearance of all SDHs is ultimately derived not only from the general pathophysiology of these entities, but also from particular elements of the pathophysiology of the individual event. If the pathophysiology of SDHs is understood, one can then understand the underpinnings of the radiologic features that are observed.

To understand the pathophysiology of SDHs, it is necessary to review the ultrastructure of the meninges. The outer layer of the meninges, the dura, is made up of multiple layers. The outer fibrous layer is also the periosteum of the inner table of the skull. This, in turn, joins the meningeal dura. These two layers are composed of fibrous material, including fibroblasts and interwoven collagen fibers, and are resistant to disruption.[5–7] The deepest portion of the dura, the dural border layer, is composed of a loose collection of cells with numerous extracellular spaces, few cell junctions, and no tight junctions.[5,7–9] This tissue is in contact with the arachnoid barrier layer of the arachnoid membrane. The barrier layer cells adhere tightly to one another with desmosomes, intermediate junctions, tight junctions, and gap junctions, providing structural stability. These cells are further lined by a strong basement membrane at their deepest border. The dural border cell layer provides a weak link in the meningeal continuum. The introduction of blood produces cleavage of this layer, creating a plane bordered on either side by dural cells.[8,9] Similarly, relatively minor shear forces disrupt this membrane. Different means of disruption may explain the various mechanisms associated with SDH formation.

Clinically[1,10,11] and radiographically,[12–14] SDHs are classified as acute, subacute, and chronic. This classification is based on the clinically perceived need for evacuation[1] or the development of symptoms[2] within 24–72 hours (acute), 1–3 days to 3 weeks (subacute), or more than 3 weeks (chronic) since the occurrence of trauma. Radiographically, the divisions into acute (<1 week), subacute (1–4 weeks), and chronic (>4 weeks) are based on cross-sectional imaging criteria.[12–14] A simplistic view presented in many radiologic texts assumes that acute hematomas evolve into subacute hematomas, and, later, chronic hematomas. Whereas this may be the case in some or even the majority of cases, there is enough variation in the etiologies, pathophysiologies, clinical features, and imaging findings to justify separate treatment of these divisions. They are, therefore, reviewed separately.

Acute Subdural Hematomas

The origins of acute SDHs are varied, resulting from trauma, ruptured aneurysms, cerebrospinal fluid (CSF) hypotension, nosocomial procedures, and "spontaneous" forms associated with coagulopathies.[1–3,15–27] The majority of acute SDHs, however, is caused by trauma. The type of traumatic injury that produces acute SDHs varies with patient age. In some inner-city hospital series, the majority of cases was the result of nonvehicular blunt trauma.[1,3] High-speed motor vehicle accidents (53%) and falls (37%) produced the majority of SDHs in a rural level-1 trauma center.[15] The role of shear forces in producing acute SDHs is controversial, and incorrect definitions of what constitutes a "shear force" are found. Furthermore, data have been interpreted by conjecture rather than by hypothesis testing. Historically, the tearing of bridging veins that join the dural sinuses and the cortical veins (and hang in the subarachnoid space) has been proposed as a major contributor to subdural bleeding based on ultrastructural evaluation and mathematic models. Ultrastructural studies suggest fragility of these vessels. Modeling has suggested a sensitivity of the vessels to injuries with high strain rates.[28–31] This disruption has been described as occurring by shear forces, displacement (tensile forces), and direct traumatic injury. There is evidence challenging the theory that shear forces play an important role in acute SDH formation, suggesting instead that bridging-vein disruption by tensile forces or contusion is the major cause. Using finite element analysis, models predict that the shear forces needed for disrupting these veins are unusually high.[30–32] Additionally, cadaveric measurement of the forces necessary to disrupt these veins failed to confirm model results regarding the sensitivity of these veins to strain rate.[33] Furthermore, the disruption of bridging veins during blunt trauma produces only one small SDH in five cases.[34] Finally, clinical series have shown arterial or cortical vein disruption as the source of hemorrhage in the majority of cases,[1,3] with bridging vein disruption in the minority. It would be conservative to presume that the hemorrhage in SDHs can be derived from arteries, cortical veins, and, in some cases, bridging veins.

The exact role of shear force injury in nonaccidental infant trauma has not been determined. Evidence of bridging vein rupture resulting from shaking is substantial.[35] The role played by shear forces in these injuries, however, has become more controversial. It is likely that impact injury in infants plays a more significant role than previously thought.[36] Modeling suggests that stretching (tensile forces) of bridging veins may be a contributing factor and explain the increased frequency of SDHs in external hydrocephalus.[37] It has also been proposed that tensile forces play a role in the development of vacuum-extraction–related SDHs[27] and in the age-related increased prevalence of SDH formation.[38–40] Other predisposing conditions that can produce tensile forces in the dura and have been associated with SDHs are CSF hypotension/hypovolemia[41,42] and masses that invade the dura, such as meningiomas[43–45] and lymphoma.[46]

In addition to trauma, SDHs can be seen in other conditions. Although rare, acute SDHs have been described in utero. The prognosis for these fetuses is poor, but some do survive.[47,48] The etiology of SDHs in this context has not been established. SDHs resulting from ruptured berry aneurysms may occur with or without associated subarachnoid hemorrhage.[16,25,49,50] Ruptured aneurysms can produce extremely high-velocity jets capable of tearing though cellular layers, including the arachnoid barrier layer. The dense fibrous periosteal and meningeal layers of the dura are more resistant to this jet of blood and presumably direct it to dissect through the loose cellular inner border of the dura.

The idea of subdural infection inciting subdural hemorrhage was proposed by Virchow and was included as a consideration by Cushing.[4] This etiology is extremely rare, even for chronic SDHs. Only a few documented cases of acute SDH formation from hemorrhagic infections are found in the online literature, and, in these cases, the subdural hemorrhage resulted from ruptured mycotic aneurysms.[51–53]

The outcome of acute SDHs can take different courses.[54–57] Some SDHs have been shown to resolve.[55–57] Large, acute SDHs caused by trauma or aneurysm rupture have a poor prognosis unless drained. They are associated with increased intracranial pressure and can enlarge. The causes of morbidity and mortality in this setting include associated parenchymal injuries (Figure 15-1), increased intracranial pressure and herniation (Figure 15-2), and ischemic injury.[1–3,54,58,59] The mechanisms by which SDHs produce ischemia are unclear, although increased metabolic demand, decreased cerebral blood flow unrelated to increased intracranial pressure, and uncoupling of cerebral blood flow and oxidative metabolism have been observed in animal models.[58,59] Finally, some small to moderate acute SDHs evolve into subacute and chronic subdural SDHs. It has been proposed that resolution of acute SDHs may be related to the absence of dural cells on the inner margin of the hematoma, whereas the presence of such a layer

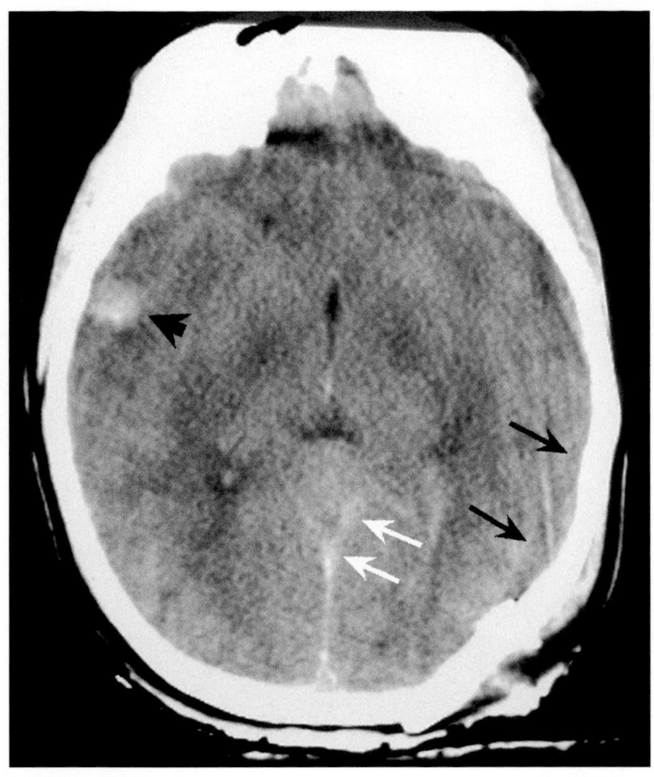

A

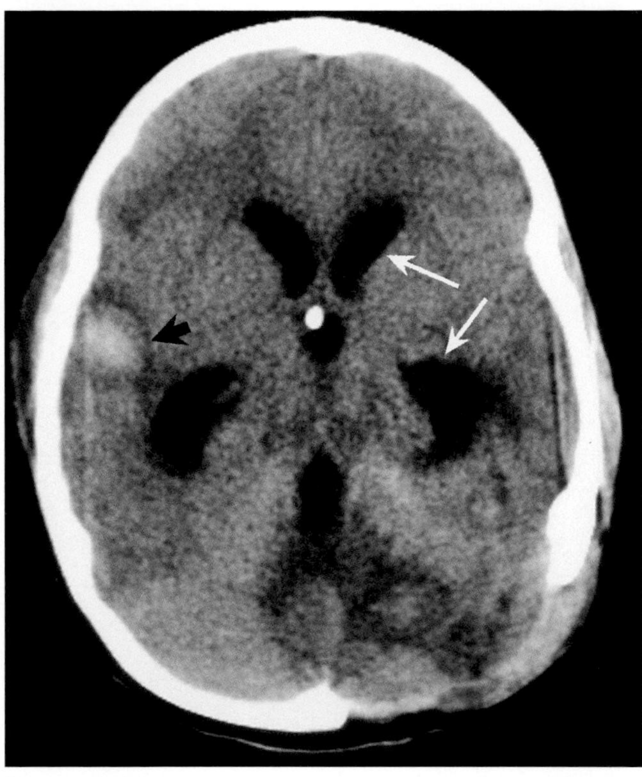

B

FIGURE 15-1. Acute traumatic subdural hematoma with associated contusion. **A.** Contusion (*black arrowheads* in **A,B**), isodense hyperacute subdural hematoma associated with depressed skull fracture (*black arrows*), and subdural and subarachnoid blood layering along the tentorium (*white arrows*). **B.** On the following day, the posterior fossa is decompressed, and the subdural hematoma is evacuated, but hydrocephalus has developed (*white arrows*).

of cells increases the probability of evolution to subacute and chronic stages.[8,60]

Subacute Subdural Hematomas

When related to trauma, subacute SDHs have been clinically defined as hematomas presenting symptomatically or requiring evacuation after 24–72 hours and before 3 weeks.[1,2] Radiologically, the subacute stage has been defined as older than 1 week but younger than 4 weeks of age.[12–14] In these trauma-related cases, hematomas evolve as blood products change over time (Figure 15-3; see Figures 15-10 through 15-12). During this stage, a hematoma undergoes clot lysis and either is resorbed[55–57] or develops a pair of boundary membranes. Outer membrane formation, which has been shown to begin as early as 24 hours after hematoma formation, is completed in approximately 1 week, whereas a thin inner membrane forms by approximately 3 weeks.[60,61]

In a small series of patients with subacute SDHs, imaging findings were correlated with those at surgical exploration.[38,62] The patients in this series demonstrated atypical pathology and imaging findings and had no inner membranes and only one outer membrane. Based on imaging findings in other patients,[63] the authors have postulated that effusion into the hematoma accounts for the increasing mass effect that causes symptoms. A separate small series presented mixed support for this mechanism, with the observation of thin membranes and a CSF-like fluid mixed with clot at surgery.[64] Thus, it is reasonable to conclude that the pathophysiology of subacute SDH formation may be multifactorial. Regardless of their exact mechanisms, subacute SDHs have better outcomes than acute SDHs.[2]

Chronic Subdural Hematomas

Trauma-related chronic SDHs are defined clinically as those presenting symptomatically or requiring surgical evacuation no earlier than 3 weeks after the traumatic event.[1] Radiographically, they are defined as hematomas imaged at least 4 weeks after the initiating traumatic event; the age is sometimes estimated based on MR and CT imaging findings.[12–14] This may represent an oversimplification of the development of these lesions.

The etiology of chronic SDHs is more variable than that of acute SDHs. It is also more controversial. The most widely accepted mechanism is that chronic

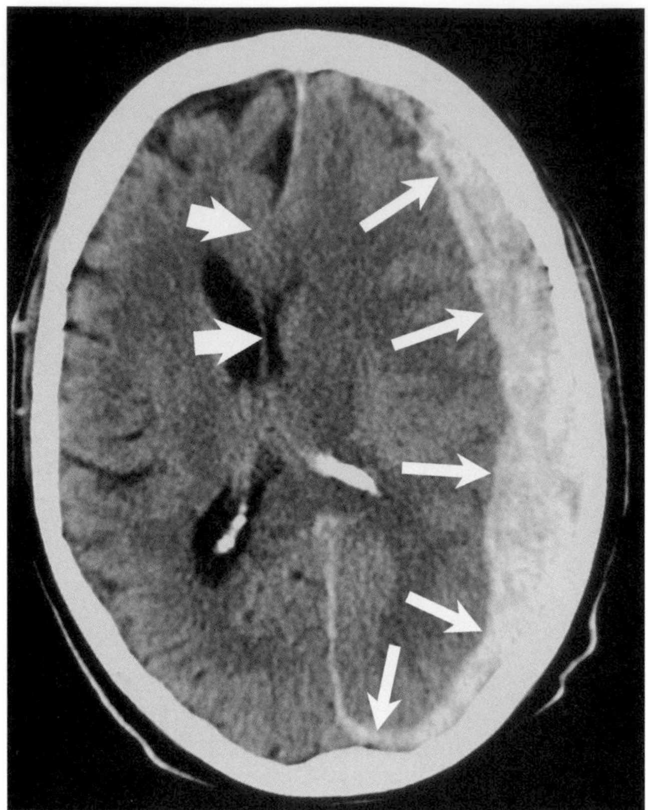

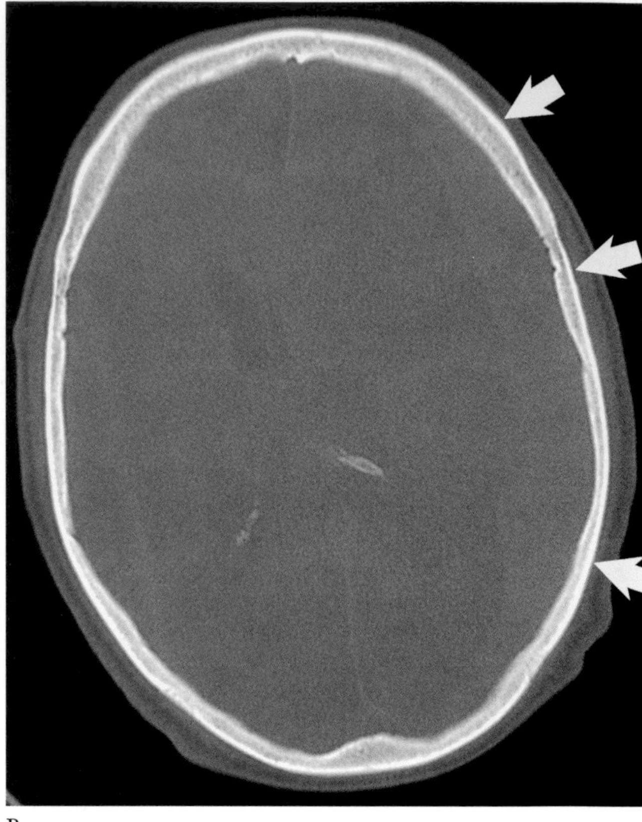

A B

FIGURE 15-2. Acute subdural hematoma with crescentic features and associated midline shift. **A.** Typical crescentic appearance of subdural hematoma (*long arrows*) crossing sutures and layering along the tentorium. Subfalcine herniation (*short arrows*) has occurred. **B.** Calvarium remains intact (*white arrows*).

SDHs evolve from trauma-related acute SDHs after passing through a subacute phase. By definition, these hematomas do not produce symptoms sufficient to require evacuation during the acute and subacute stages. Evidence for the evolution of acute SDHs to chronic SDHs has predominantly been corollary in nature. CT imaging and MRI findings have demonstrated that imaging findings obtained in the acute, subacute, and chronic hematoma periods correlate with the imaging features of evolving hematomas.[13,65–67] Most of these studies, however, were performed retrospectively.

Some serial studies have brought the proposed mechanism into question. Several reports document the development of chronic SDHs from subdural hygromas.[68–72] This progression has been described for hygromas associated with trauma, CSF hypotension,[70,73,74] and ruptured arachnoid cysts.[72] In some animal models, chronic SDH formation occurs only in the presence of CSF in the fluid collection.[75,76] Although these results have been contested,[77] it has been proposed that the majority of chronic SDHs originate not by evolution from acute SDHs but by evolution from subdural hygromas.[70,78] It is conceivable that chronic SDHs associated with CSF hypotension or arachnoid cysts could begin as hygromas. As cited previously, even trauma can produce chronic SDHs from hygromas. Neoplasms that involve the meninges are also associated with chronic SDH formation.[44,46,79,80] Whether these chronic SDHs evolve from acute SDHs or hygromas has not been determined. The age-related variation in occurrence of chronic SDHs is significantly more pronounced than the age-related variation in acute SDHs. This may be related to the widening of the CSF space in infants and adults as well as to other factors associated with aging, such as increased number of falls, the friability of vessels, the increased presence of coagulopathies (especially in alcoholics), and changes in the dura itself.[81]

In the model in which chronic SDHs evolve from acute ones, the hematoma's composition is thought to change in the classic evolutionary pattern described for intra-axial hematomas. After initial vessel rupture, extravasated blood becomes clotted as the stagnant blood is exposed to the extrinsic pathway clotting factors. As the clot ages, clot lysis begins and liquefaction occurs. Although it has been proposed that lysing blood develops elevated oncotic pressures, direct measurements have

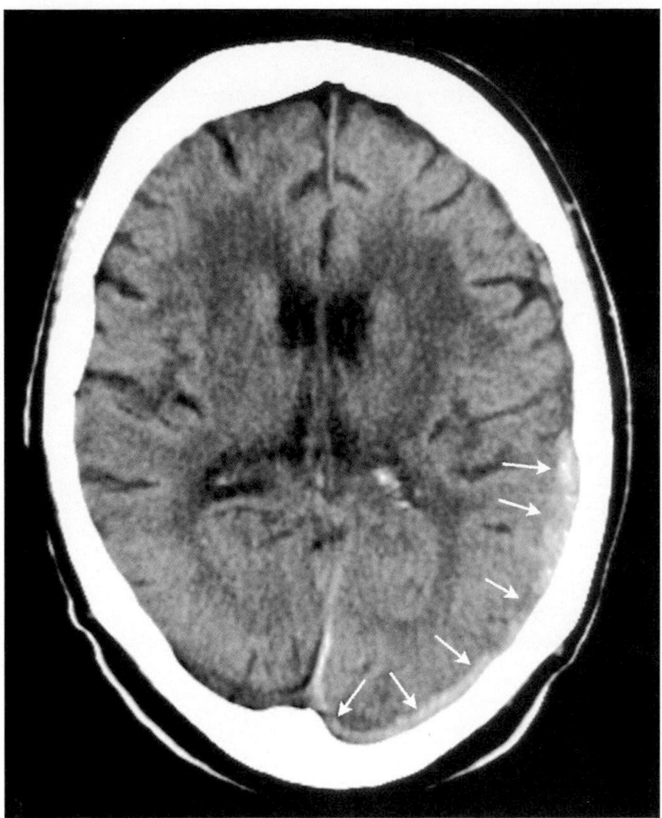

A

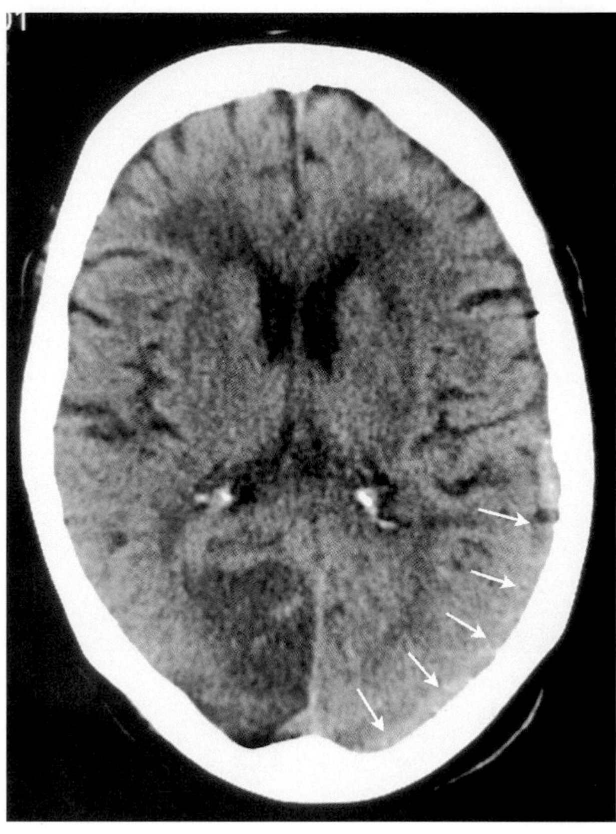

B

FIGURE 15-3. Evolution of hyperdense subdural hematoma to isodense subdural hematoma. **A.** The small acute post-traumatic subdural hematoma imaged the first day is mildly hyperdense (*arrows*). **B.** Subdural hematoma becoming more isodense 3 days later (*arrows*). It was imaged because of evolving right posterior cerebral artery distribution infarct (hypodense region in the right occipital lobe).

shown that these pressures remain normal.[82,83] Instead, enlargement of chronic SDHs has been attributed to the development of inner and outer membranes,[5,6,60,84–86] whereby fragile veins in the outer membrane cause recurrent[6,84,86] and possibly ongoing[85,87] hemorrhage. Fibrinolytic factors play an important role in perpetuating the liquefied state of chronic SDHs.[88–90] Clot lysis factors released from eosinophiles in the inner membrane cause liquefaction of the existing clot, whereas eosinophiles in the outer membrane regulate blood resorption, thereby controlling or inhibiting clot retraction and resolution.[60] Significant blood turnover in chronic SDHs indicates that they are dynamic entities.[87] This idea is further supported by the observation that simple drainage can be a highly successful means of treating chronic SDHs without the need for membrane stripping.[91,92] In addition to frank hemorrhage, there is likely fluid and small molecule exchange through the membranes, as demonstrated by the accumulation of gadolinium contrast in hematomas (Figures 15-4 and 15-5).

As chronic SDHs enlarge, they can reach a volume large enough to produce neurologic deficits. At this stage, brain compression, displacement, and even herniation occur. In addition to the deficit attributable to mass effect, significant deficits also occur as a result of ischemia. Multiple studies have been performed on blood flow–related changes in this setting.[93–100] The findings are contradictory. In patients with unilateral hematomas and headaches, Okuyama et al.[93] have demonstrated reduced cerebral blood flow in the frontal and occipital lobes as well as the cerebellum on the nonhematoma side. When hemiparesis was present, cerebral blood flow was reduced bilaterally in cortical regions and in the putamen and thalamus on the hematoma side. The degree of blood flow reduction was unrelated to midline shift. Obtunded patients had globally reduced cerebral blood flow. In a different study, Ishikawa et al.[99] have shown reductions in cerebral blood flow and metabolic rate in the caudate nucleus and cingulate gyrus on the side of hemiparesis. In the same population, they failed to show significant reductions in the ipsilateral and contralateral cortical cerebral blood flow. Ishikawa et al. also demonstrated elevations in oxygen extraction fraction in the lentiform nuclei and central white matter

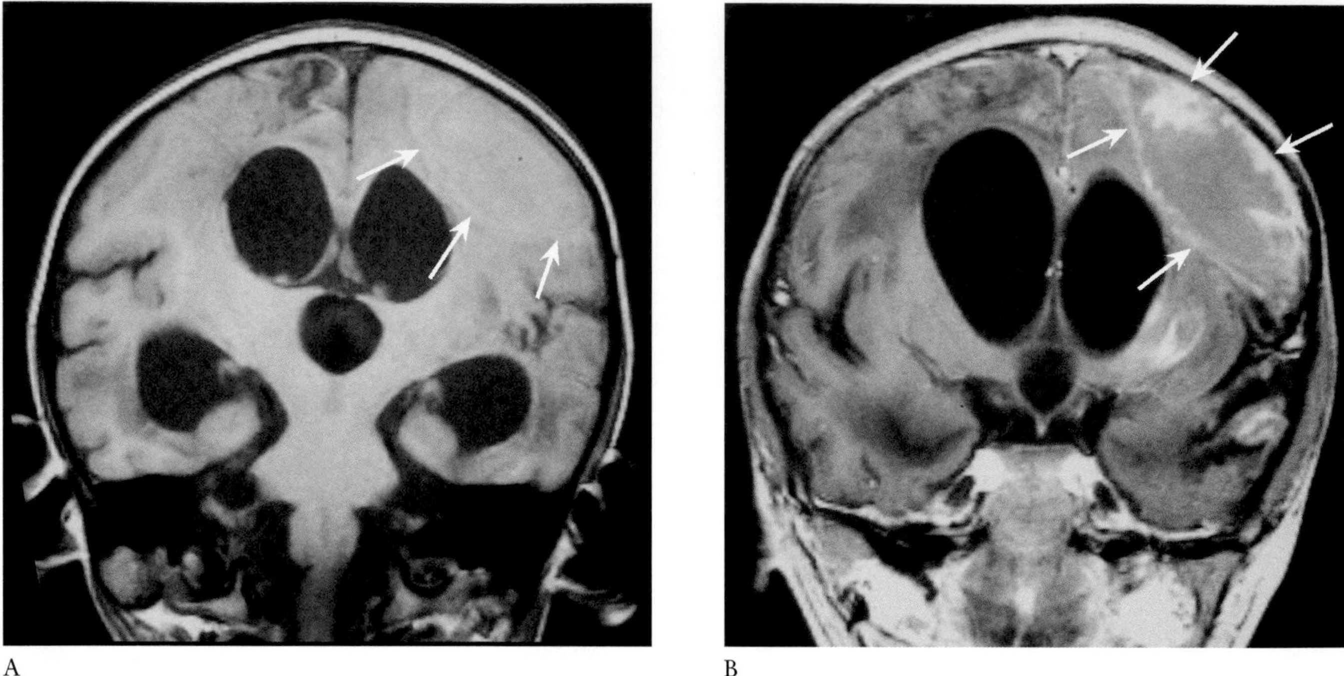

FIGURE 15-4. Contrast enhancement in late subacute hematoma. **A.** Mildly hyperintense hematoma (*arrows*) on a noncontrast, T1-weighted magnetic resonance image. **B.** Peripheral contrast enhancement along inner and outer membranes (*arrows*) on post-contrast, T1-weighted image.

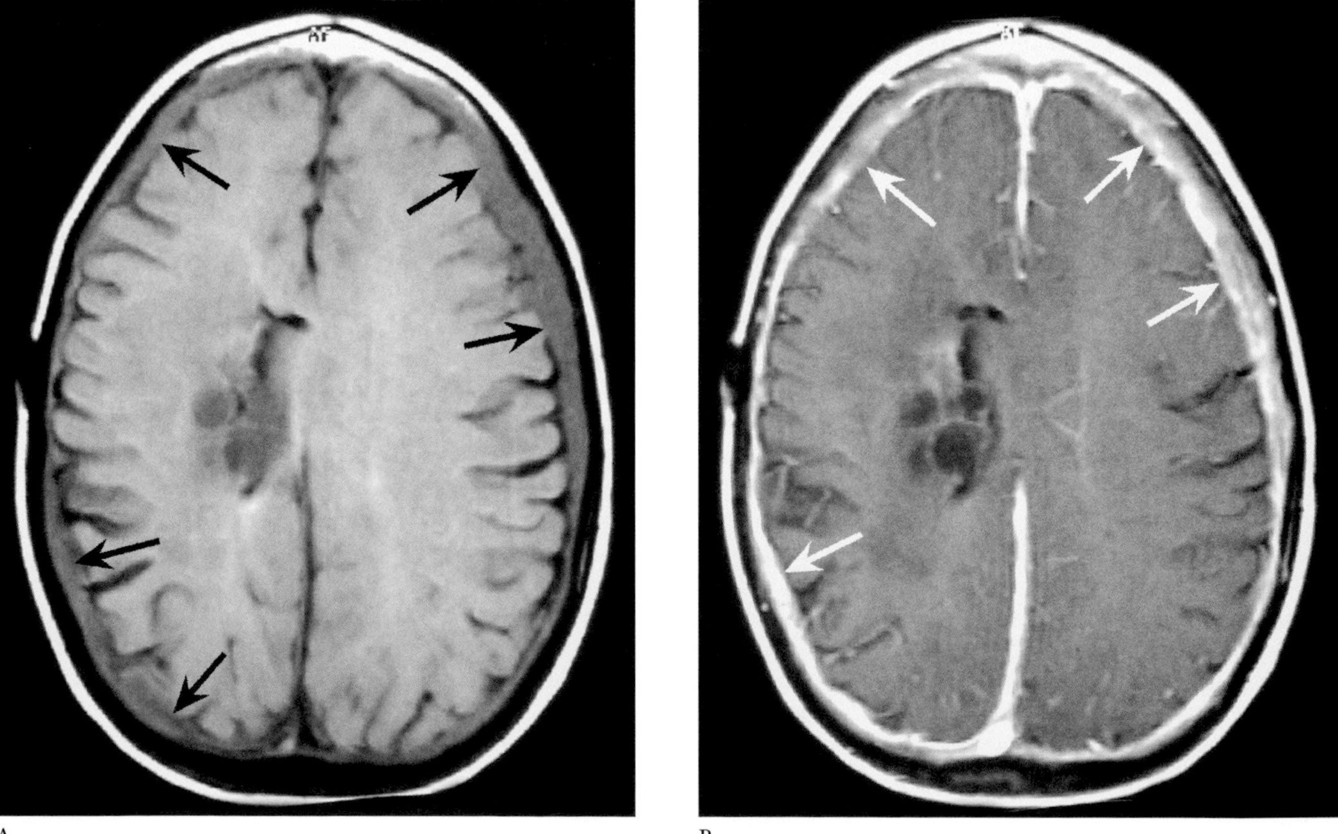

FIGURE 15-5. Contrast enhancement in chronic subdural hematoma. **A.** Nonenhanced T1-weighted magnetic resonance image showing isodense chronic subdural hematomas (*arrows*). **B.** Contrast-enhanced T1-weighted magnetic resonance image showing contrast enhancement along the inner membrane of the subdural hematomas (*arrows*).

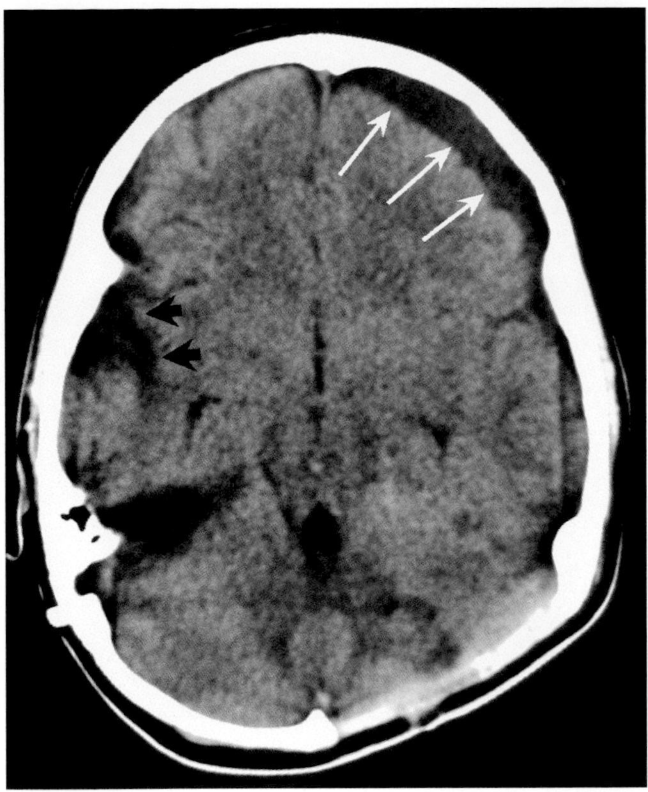
A

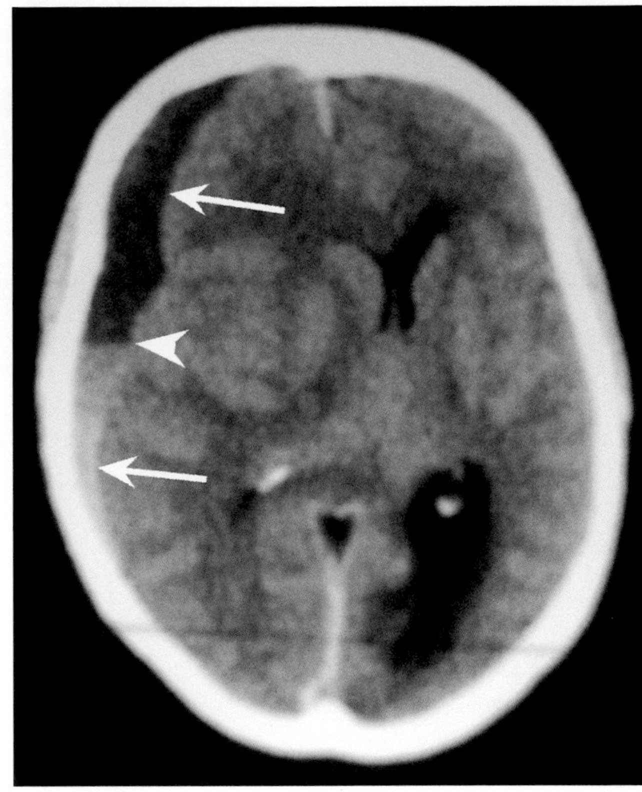
B

FIGURE 15-6. Computed tomographic scan of subdural hygroma versus chronic subdural hematoma. **A.** Same patient as in Figure 15-1, approximately 1 week later with new subdural hygroma (*white arrows*) that developed as a consequence of shunting. The previously seen contusion is resolving (*black arrowheads*). **B.** Different patient presenting with worsening mental status. A chronic subdural hematoma (*arrows*) with a hematocrit level (*arrowhead*) that was found on computed tomography examination.

on both sides of the brain, and in the frontal gray matter underneath the SDH. Other studies suggest that ipsilateral reductions in thalamic blood flow are linearly correlated with thalamic deformation and reduced brain activity as determined by electroencephalography.[97] The electroencephalographic activity is depressed bilaterally. Hemispheric cerebral blood flow correlates with decreased activity on the contralateral but not ipsilateral sides. The depression of brain activity may be related to thalamic deformation rather than reduced hemispheric cerebral blood flow.[97] Cerebral blood flow remains depressed, and vascular CO_2 reactivity remains elevated during the postoperative period despite clinical improvement. Finally, a postoperative hyperperfusion syndrome with increased cerebral blood flow has been described after SDH evacuation.[101]

It is challenging to coordinate the findings of these reports. A conservative assessment suggests that the contribution of cerebral blood flow changes to the pathophysiology of chronic SDH formation is not completely understood. The discrepancies between the various studies could be attributed to a multiplicity of factors, such as differences in the populations studied, in the various parameters measured, and in the sensitivities of the techniques. For instance, the most consistently studied group in these studies included patients with hemiparesis. This finding occurs in a minority of patients at the time of initial presentation.[102]

There are many possible outcomes of chronic SDHs. In addition to becoming symptomatic and requiring evacuation, they can resolve spontaneously,[56,103,104] develop erythropoietic activity,[105,106] or calcify.[39,46,107]

Subdural Hygromas

Subdural hygromas are initially nonhemorrhagic fluid collections thought to arise from either tears in the arachnoid space[13,71] or separation of the dura-arachnoid layers.[69] The inciting event can be trauma,[13,69,70] CSF hypotension[73,74] (Figure 15-6), or rupture of an arachnoid cyst.[72,108]

MRI has played an important role in the pre-operative diagnosis of subdural hygromas, allowing differentiation from SDHs (Figure 15-7).[13,109] Before MRI, it was not always possible to distinguish between these two entities, because SDHs that remain stable over time eventually become hypodense on CT, mimicking subdural

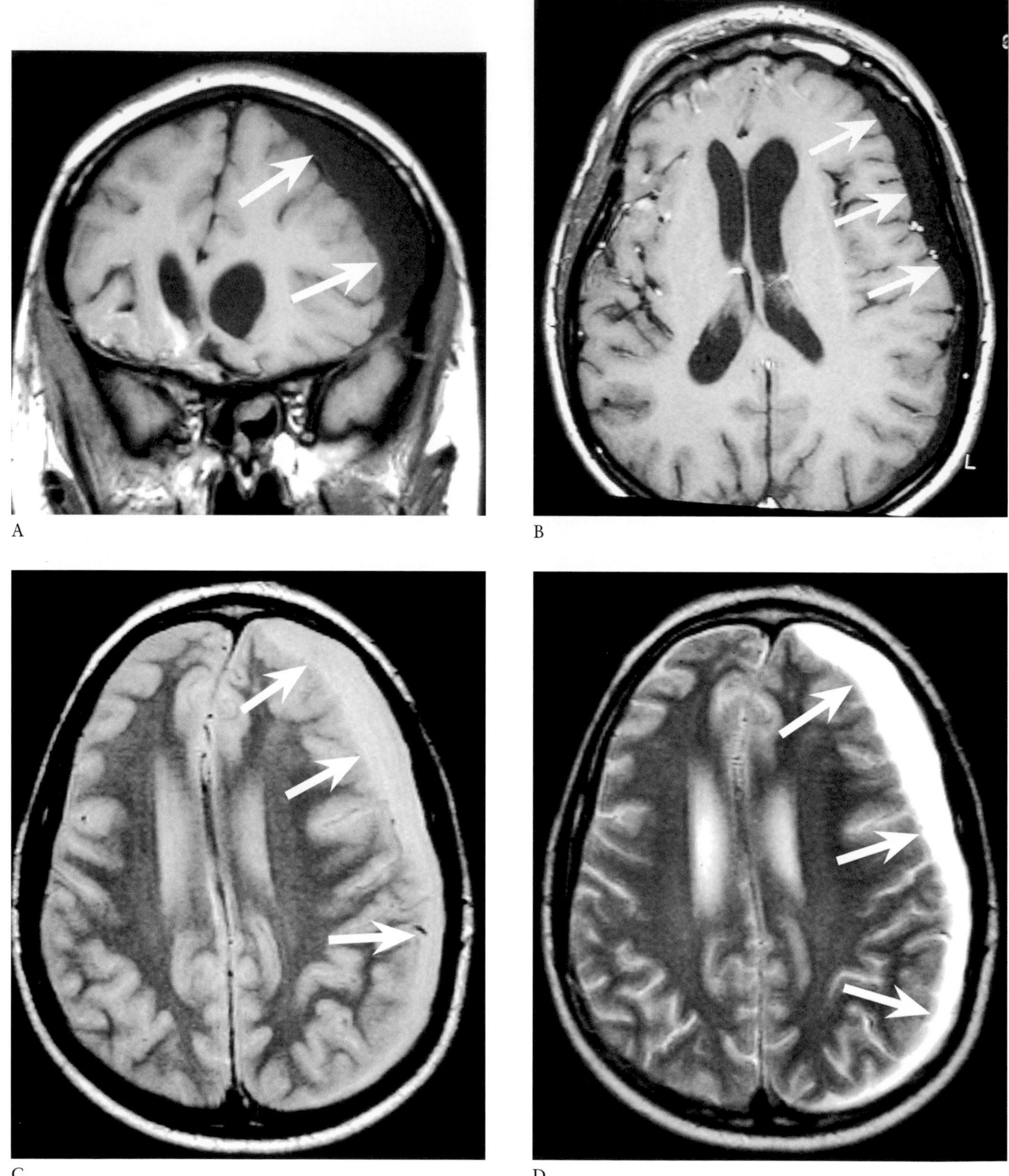

FIGURE 15-7. Magnetic resonance images of subdural hygromas (*arrows*). **A.** Noncontrast T1-weighted image. **B.** Contrast-enhanced T1-weighted image. **C.** Proton density–weighted image. **D.** T2-weighted image.

hygromas. The distinction is important, as the prognosis and management of subdural hygromas varies from those of SDHs. A high percentage of subdural hygromas gradually resolve, and some evolve into chronic SDHs.[68–70,78]

IMAGING SUBDURAL HEMATMOAS

Computed Tomography

The physics of CT imaging is described in other texts. In brief, CT measures the relative electron density of a material. The latter is related to the tissue density and is expressed in Hounsfield units (HU). Zero is arbitrarily set as the density of water. HU can be either positive or negative, so zero is the center point of the range of values obtained. Images are presented with different windows and levels that set the grayscale range and center point of the grayscale images. The narrower the window, the greater the contrast presented between adjacent tissues that differ in HU. The lower the level, the brighter a given HU will appear on the film or screen. Acute blood has typical HU values of 50–100.[110,111] Typical brain soft tissue windows present acute blood as very bright, referred to as *hyperdense*.

Over time, there is a graded decrease in the HU of blood, as it first reaches a density similar to brain and then becomes hypodense.[65,66] When compared to gray matter, hematomas become isodense in approximately 1 week, and 75% become hypodense in approximately 3 weeks. Hence, hyperdense blood overlaps the surgically defined stages of acute (>3 days) and subacute (3 days to approximately 3 weeks) SDH, whereas isodense blood overlaps subacute and chronic (>3 weeks) stages. Very early, before clot retraction occurs, blood may also have an isodense appearance. This has been called the *hyperacute stage* and is thought to represent active bleeding.[112] Although this is usually the case, bleeding occurring in patients with coagulopathy or anemia can present as isodense blood,[112–114] mimicking active bleeding. Based on the tendency for blood to remain hyperdense for approximately a week, radiologists often define this time span as the *acute period*.[110] This can lead to confusion between radiologists and other clinicians.

Acute Subdural Hematomas

On cross-sectional imaging, SDHs are crescentic collections that lie adjacent to the calvarium (see Figure 15-2). Because these collections are bounded by the meningeal and periosteal dura, they typically do not cross the falx cerebri or tentorium. They can, however, occur bilaterally and extend to the falx from both hemispheres. They may also cover the entire convexity of a hemisphere as well as a layer adjacent to the falx cerebri and tentorium. Because these collections occur in the loose inner dural layer that is readily separable from the arachnoid, the collections often remain concave during the acute stage. Occasionally, adhesions between the dura and arachnoid may allow for the collections to become biconvex (Figure 15-8). This appearance is uncommon in acute SDHs. In these cases, it can be difficult to distinguish a subdural from an epidural hematoma. Finally, the convex appearance can occur at some distinct locations, particularly the anterior aspect of the middle cranial fossa adjacent to the anterior pole of the temporal horn.

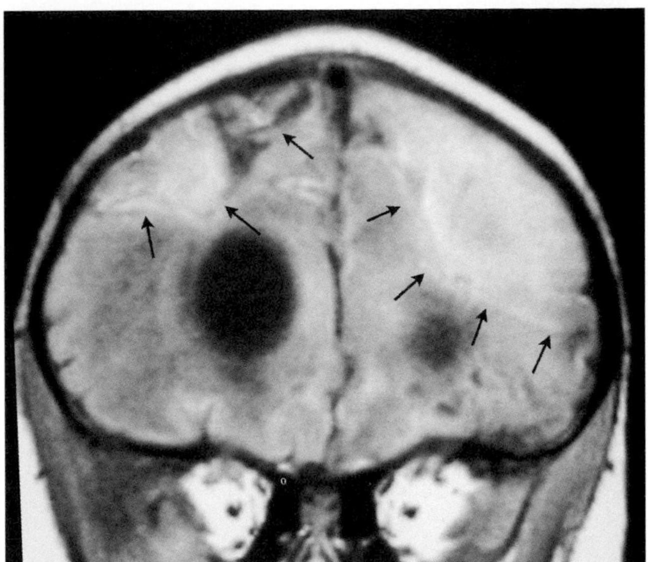

FIGURE 15-8. Biconvex appearance of subdural hematomas. T1-weighted image with near isointense bilateral subdural hematomas (*arrows*).

Subacute Subdural Hematomas

As the clotted hematoma begins to lyse, it decreases in density, becoming isodense (see Figure 15-3) and hypodense relative to gray matter. Isodense clots can be difficult to detect on CT examination. To detect isodense hematomas with CT at this stage, care must be taken to follow the sulci and gyri to the calvarial surface. If they are displaced from the calvarium, an isodense SDH should be suspected. The administration of contrast or coronal CT angiography can aid in detection.[115,116] Although a substantial number of subacute SDHs can be hypodense on CT,[110] a large percentage of chronic hematomas remain isodense because of recurrent bleeding.

Chronic Subdural Hematomas and Subdural Hygromas

During the chronic phase, the subdural collection can be isodense to gray matter or CSF (i.e., hypodense to gray matter). At this phase, it can be difficult to distinguish a chronic SDH from a subdural hygroma (see Figure 15-6)

TABLE 15-1. T1 and T2 Signal Changes Associated with Hemoglobin Deoxygenation and Degradation*

Stage of hemoglobin	*T1 changes from relaxivity*	*T2 changes from relaxivity*	*T2 changes from susceptibility*	*Overall T1 signal*	*Overall T2 signal*
Oxyhemoglobin	—	—	—	—	↑
Deoxyhemoglobin	—	—	↓	—	↓↓
Intracellular methemoglobin	↓	↑	↓↓	↑↑	↓
Extracellular methemoglobin	↓	↑	—	↑↑	↑↑
Hemosiderin	—	—	↓↓	—	↓↓

*Arrows indicate an increase or decrease in signal intensity.

or, when bilateral, a widened subarachnoid space. Chronic SDHs contain membranes and occasionally septations, which are sometimes hyperdense to CSF and enhance. Identifying these structures can allow differentiation. Observing vessels extending from the cortical surface to the dural sinuses has also been described as a means to allow differentiation.[117] However, bridging veins can span the fluid collections, rendering this observation unreliable. Because dural membranes and septations enhance, contrast administration might aid in distinguishing chronic SDHs from subdural hygromas, but the technique has not been systematically studied. MRI has become the method of choice in distinguishing these entities.[13,109,118]

Magnetic Resonance Imaging

The physics of MRI are described in other texts, as are the effects of hemorrhage on the T1 and T2 relaxation coefficients of tissues. In brief, as blood undergoes deoxygenation and eventual degradation, chemical and conformational changes occur, whereby diamagnetic oxyhemoglobin changes to paramagnetic deoxyhemoglobin and then to conformationally altered paramagnetic methemoglobin.[118] As hemoglobin changes from the diamagnetic to the paramagnetic form, it shortens T1 and increases T2* relaxation times of the adjacent protons. T1 is affected more significantly than T2* by this relaxivity effect, although this effect occurs only over extremely short distances. In the deoxyhemoglobin stage, however, the conformation of the molecule prohibits T1 relaxation effects. The compartmentalization of the paramagnetic substance produces a second effect known as *magnetic susceptibility* that shortens only T2*. This effect is less dependent on distance, so that deoxyhemoglobin causes T2* shortening.

As the molecular conformation evolves into the methemoglobin molecule, T1 shortening occurs. The compartmentalization continues to produce T2* shortening, which becomes more pronounced, until cell membranes lyse and compartmentalization-induced susceptibility changes are lost. Finally, as iron is removed from hemoglobin and stored intracellularly as hemosiderin, compartmentalization effects creating T2* shortening recur, but the paramagnetic effects on T1 shortening are again prohibited by the inaccessibility of the paramagnetic iron to protons. The net result of these effects, in a simplified model, is to produce signal changes in overall T1 and T2 signals, as described in Table 15-1.

These signal changes have been used to categorize the MRI characteristics of hematomas as acute, subacute, and chronic (Figures 15-9 through 15-11).[12–14]

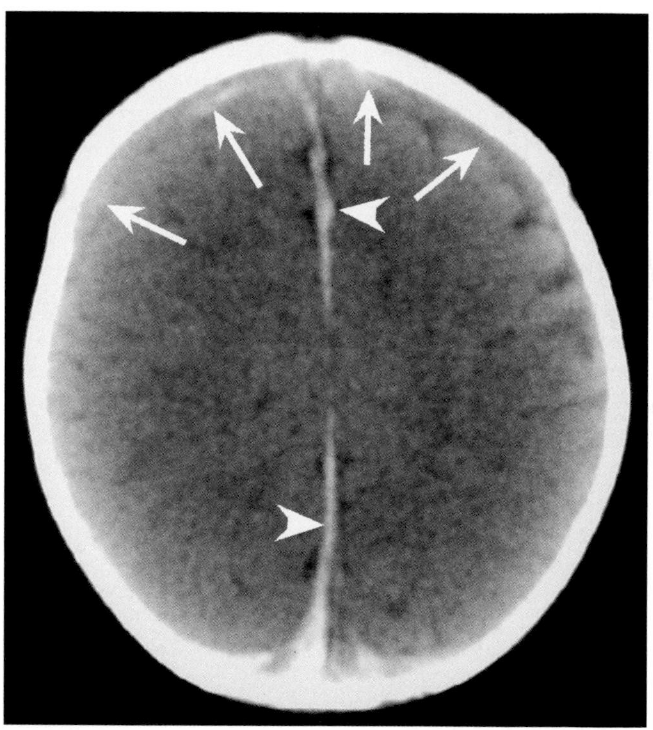

A

FIGURE 15-9. Computed tomographic and magnetic resonance images of acute and subacute subdural hematomas (SDHs) along the convexity (*arrows*) and acute SDHs along the falx cerebri (*arrowheads*) in a case of suspected nonaccidental trauma. **A.** Computed tomography shows scattered areas of isodensity (subacute SDH) and hyperdensity to gray matter (acute SDH). (*continued*)

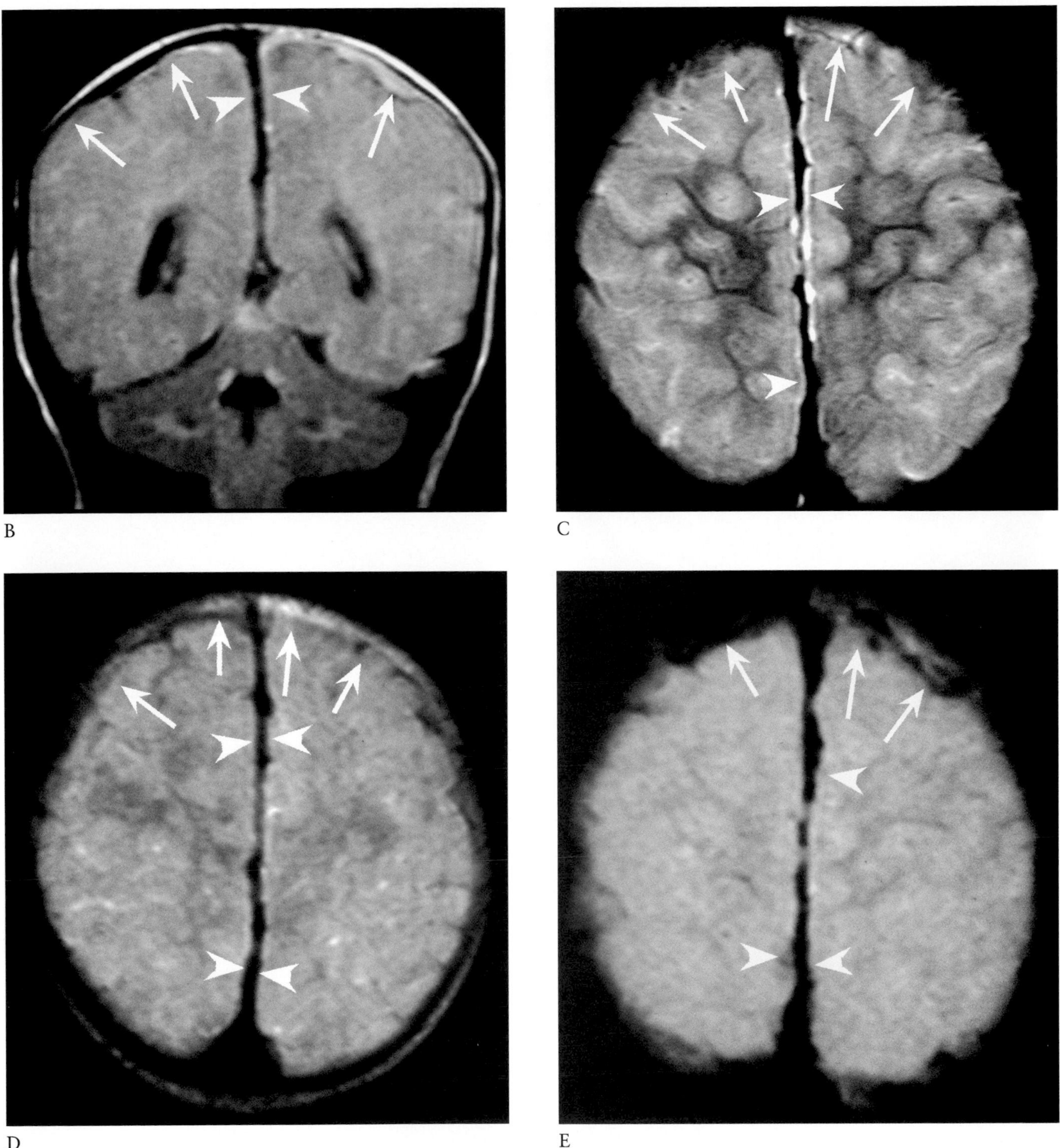

FIGURE 15-9. *Continued*. **B.** T1-weighted image shows areas of hypointensity to isointensity (acute SDH) and hyperintensity (early subacute SDH) to gray matter. **C–E.** T2-weighted turbo spin echo, T2-weighted fluid-attenuated inversion recovery, and T2-weighted gradient-echo images showing regions of hypointensity (acute SDH, deoxyhemoglobin) and isointensity (early subacute SDH, intracellular methemoglobin). Note the hypointense (*black*) region along the falx correlates with the hyperdense (*white*) region on computed tomography.

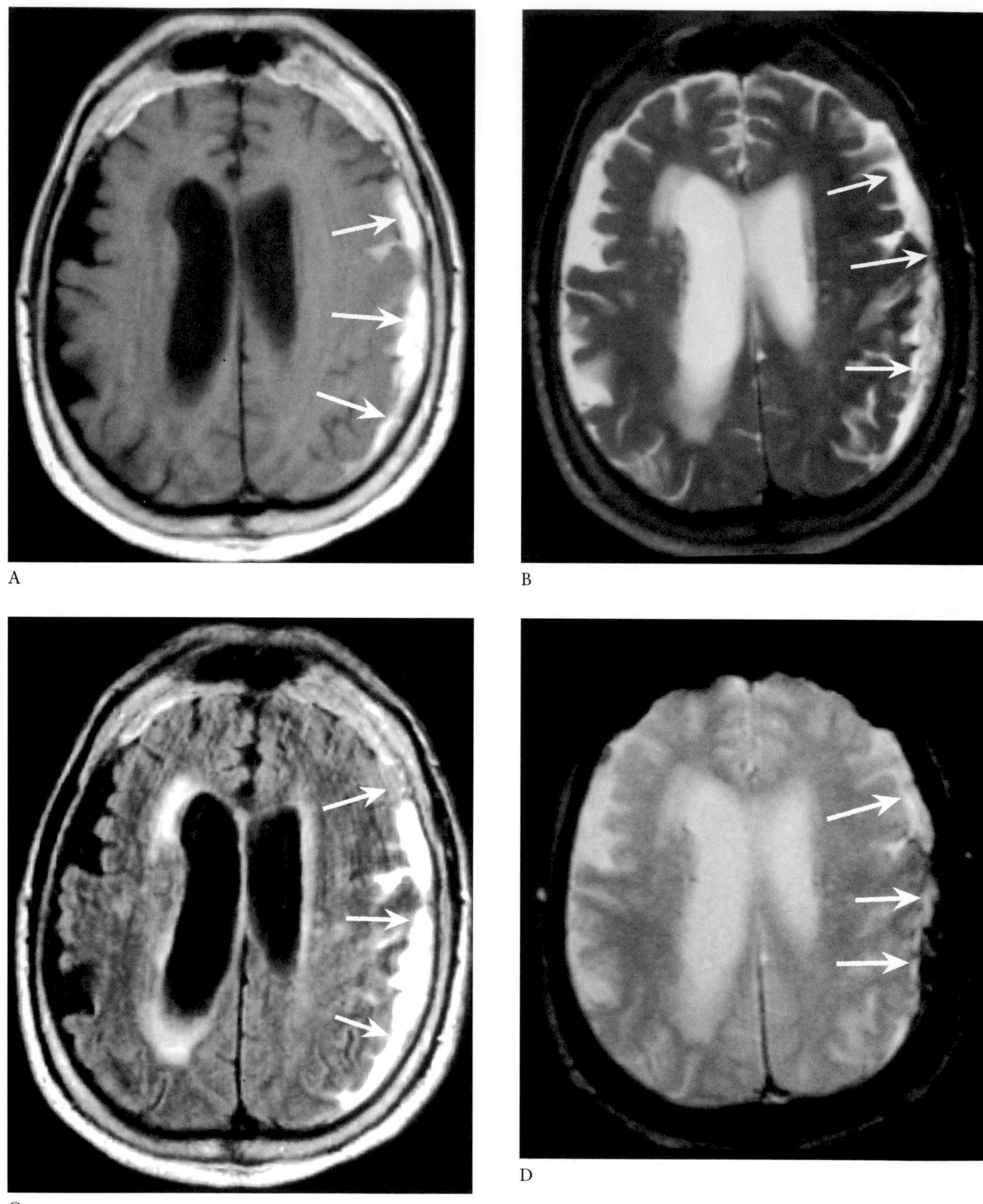

FIGURE 15-10. Magnetic resonance images of an early subacute subdural hematoma (*arrows*), with findings consistent with intracellular methemoglobin. **A.** T1-weighted image. **B.** T2-weighted turbo spin echo image. **C.** T2-weighted fluid-attenuated inversion recovery image. **D.** T2-weighted gradient-echo image. Note that heterogeneity such as this is typical.

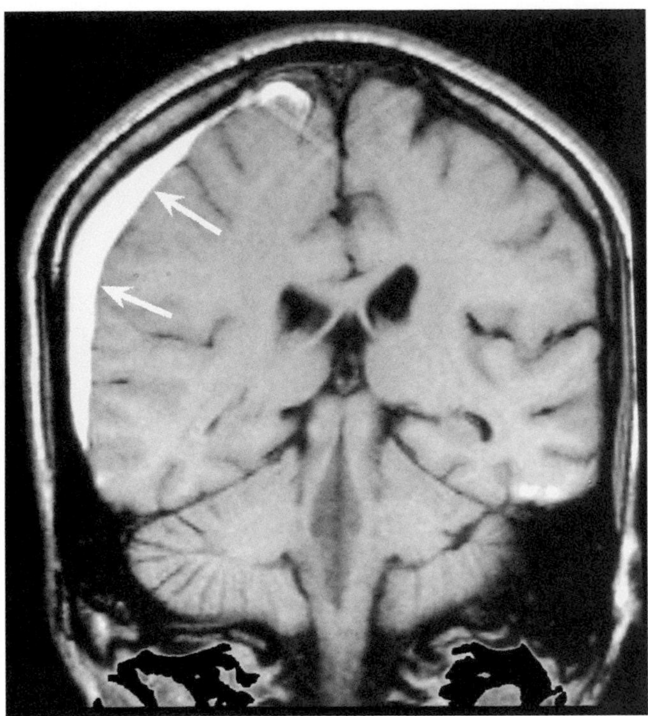

A

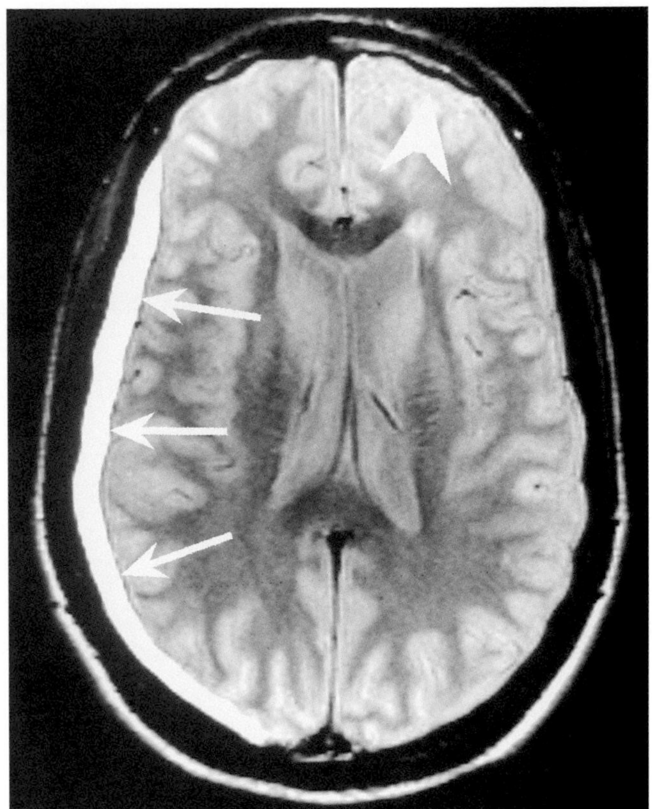

B

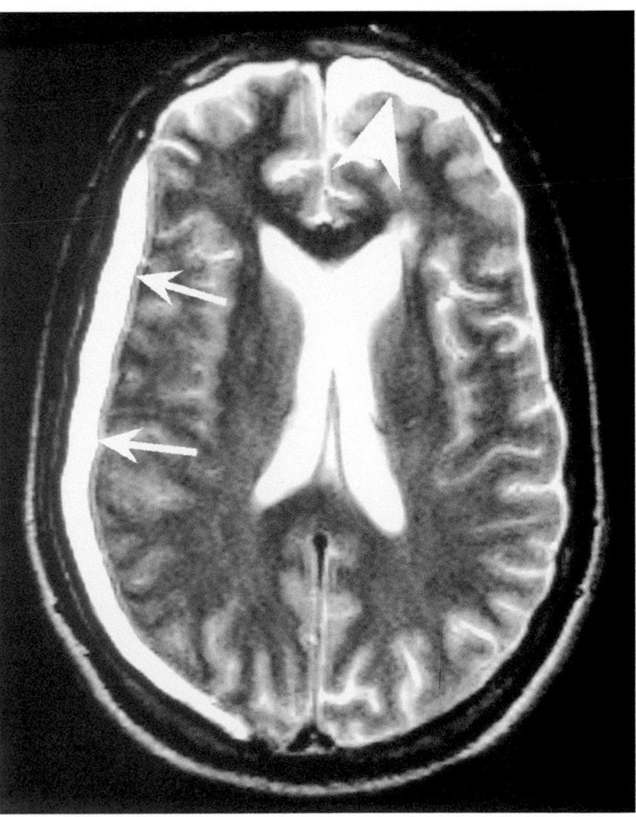

C

FIGURE 15-11. Magnetic resonance imaging of late subacute (**A–C**) versus chronic (**D–F**) subdural hematomas consistent with extracellular methemoglobin. **A–C.** The white arrows depict the right-sided late subacute subdural hematoma. **B,C.** Additionally, white arrowheads depict a small left-sided subdural hygroma. *(continued)*

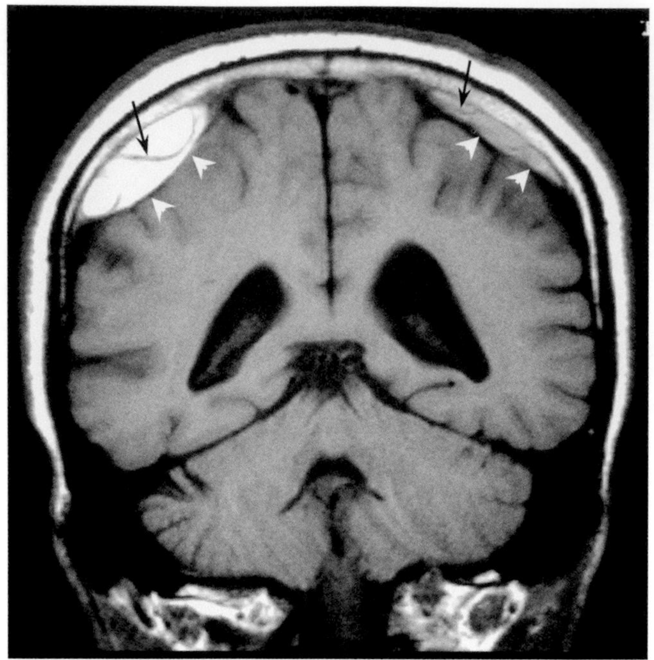

D

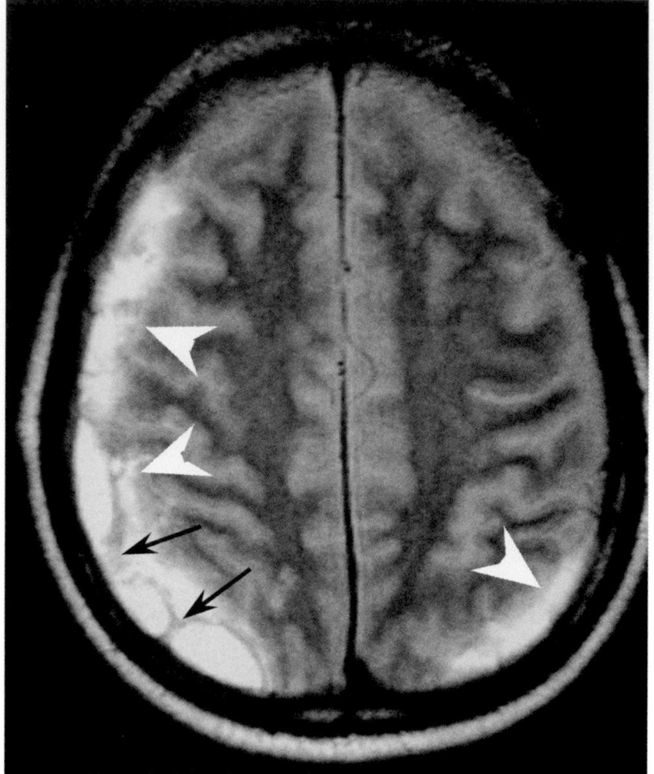

E

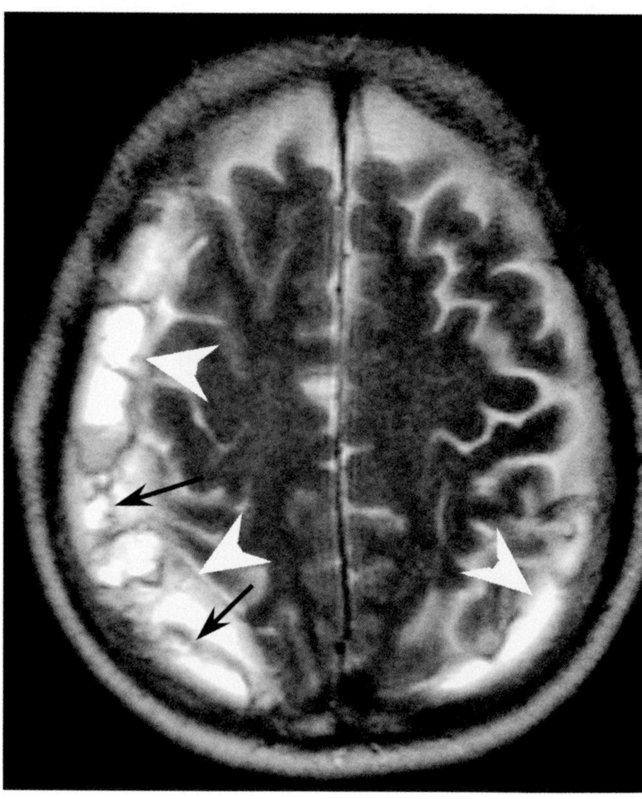

F

FIGURE 15-11. *Continued.* With a different patient (**D–F**), arrowheads depict bilateral chronic subdural hematomas. Black arrows depict septations (membranes). **A,D.** T1-weighted images. **B,E.** Proton density–weighted images. **C,F.** T2-weighted images.

However, there are problems in applying this simple model in a strict manner to SDHs. First, this classification system varies from the surgical classification system described previously, leading to confusion in discussions between radiologists and clinicians. Furthermore, there is variability in the magnetic resonance signal during the subacute stage[14] as a result of the chemical evolution presented in the preceding paragraphs. Additionally, chronic SDHs rarely show hemosiderin deposition compared to subarachnoid and intraparenchymal hematomas (Figure 15-12) and may have either hypointense or hyperintense T1 signals.[109,119] Finally, the simple spin echo sequences used for the development of this classification are seldom used.

Modern MRI is considerably more complex than simple spin echo imaging, because more exotic pulse sequences provide variations regarding the imaging of the intrinsic tissue properties. Inversion recovery is a means to null (drop out) the T1 signal of a specific tissue and is used extensively. For instance, one of the most useful modern pulse sequences is the fluid-attenuated inversion recovery (FLAIR) sequence. In this sequence, the inversion recovery time is chosen such that fluid with T1 relaxation identical to CSF produces no signal. The pulse repetition time and echo times are typically chosen to produce a T2-weighted or a proton density–weighted image. Any tissue that has a T1 relaxation time identical to that of CSF will not produce a significant signal despite a T2 relaxation time that would produce a bright signal. Intrinsic tissue paramagnetic substances, which can change the proton T1 relaxation a small amount from that of CSF, will produce a detectable and possibly bright T2-weighted signal. FLAIR imaging sequences have been shown to produce significantly better detection of SDHs (see Figure 15-12).[120]

Fast spin echo pulse sequences produce images that have many features in common with the older, conventional techniques. Differences do exist, however. The fast spin echo techniques use multiple 180-degree refocusing pulses, which, while improving speed, also reduce susceptibility effects from magnetic field inhomogeneities. This compensates for the signal reduction resulting from susceptibility in acute hematomas and decreases their detectability. Gradient-echo imaging is sometimes used to compensate for this problem. Gradient-echo imaging is used extensively in modern MRI because of its speed in image acquisition. Because it does not compensate for magnetic field inhomogeneities, gradient-echo imaging, especially when T2-weighted, is well known for enhancing T2*-related magnetic susceptibility. This property, which is problematic under some circumstances, becomes an advantage in detecting deoxyhemoglobin and hemosiderin (see Figure 15-9; Figure 15-13).

Finally, echo-planar imaging is a very rapid signal acquisition technique that is used predominantly for producing images that emphasize changes in free water diffusion within tissues. It does, however, have other applications. The appearance of blood on this pulse sequence involves multiple factors. Because echo-planar imaging is primarily used as a variation of the gradient-echo technique, susceptibility artifact contributes to the overall signal characteristics. Finally, blood clotting alters the tissue diffusion coefficients, which contributes to the signal characteristics. The role of diffusion-weighted imaging in SDHs has not yet been fully understood as a result of these compounding factors.

As one can see, contemporary MRI of hemorrhage is quite complex. This complexity can be understood, however, if the factors contributing to the signal are appropriately considered. The different pulse sequences can optimize imaging features. Example applications are given in the following sections.

Hyperacute Subdural Hematomas

A hematoma is classified as *hyperacute* when it is a few hours to 1 day old. Hyperacute blood has a T1 relaxation time similar, but not identical, to that of brain. It has been reported as mildly hypointense to mildly hyperintense.[121–124] Acute hemorrhage has a high fluid content and, therefore, has a high T2 relaxation time similar to CSF when in the oxyhemoglobin state. In hyperacute hematomas, however, there can be a mixture of states even at a few hours of age. The signal can be isointense to CSF, making detection difficult on T2-weighted images. In summary, hyperacute blood has a high T2 signal, even on susceptibility images, and a low T1 signal. Therefore, it can be difficult to differentiate from brain on T1 images and difficult to distinguish from CSF on T2-weighted images. FLAIR images, however, can be quite advantageous in imaging hyperacute SDHs, because the signal is more readily distinguishable from both CSF and gray matter.

Acute Subdural Hematomas

As hemoglobin gives up its oxygen and converts to deoxyhemoglobin, it produces susceptibility effects. It remains isointense to mildly hypointense to gray matter on T1-weighted images but becomes hypointense to gray matter and, more significantly, to CSF on T2-weighted images. The drop in T2 signal is less pronounced. Because of the effects resulting from magnetic susceptibility at this stage, pulse sequences, such as gradient-echo or echo-planar imaging that emphasize this effect, can be very useful at improving detection. Hemorrhage on a T2-weighted gradient-echo sequence

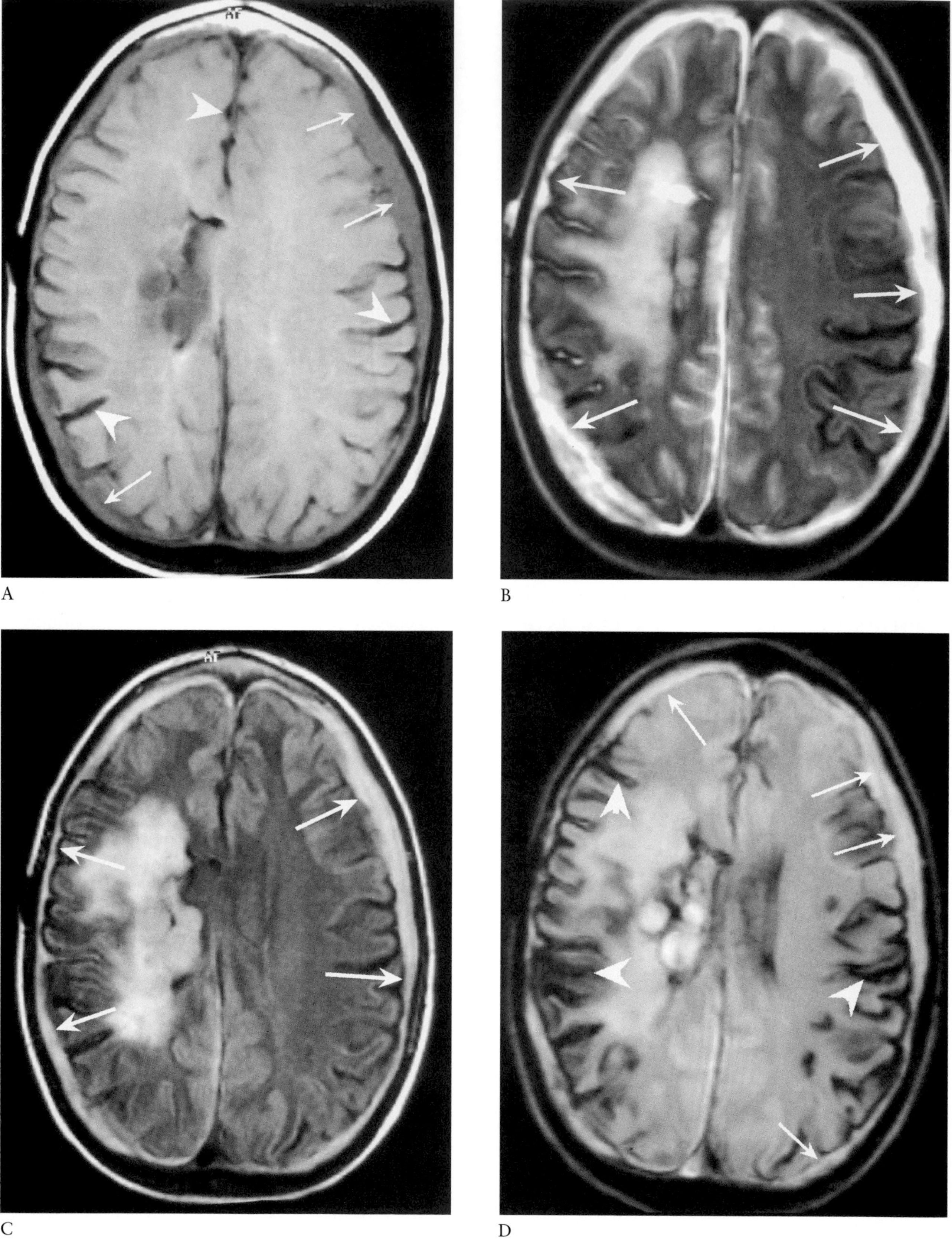

FIGURE 15-12. Chronic subdural and subarachnoid hemorrhages. Note the hypointense hemosiderin deposition predominantly in the subarachnoid space (*arrowheads* in **A,D**), rather than the subdural space (*arrows*), where the subdural fluid roughly follows cerebrospinal fluid signal, except on the T2 fluid-attenuated inversion recovery image. **A.** T1-weighted image. **B.** T2-weighted turbo spin echo image. **C.** T2-weighted fluid-attenuated inversion recovery image. **D.** T2-weighted gradient-echo image.

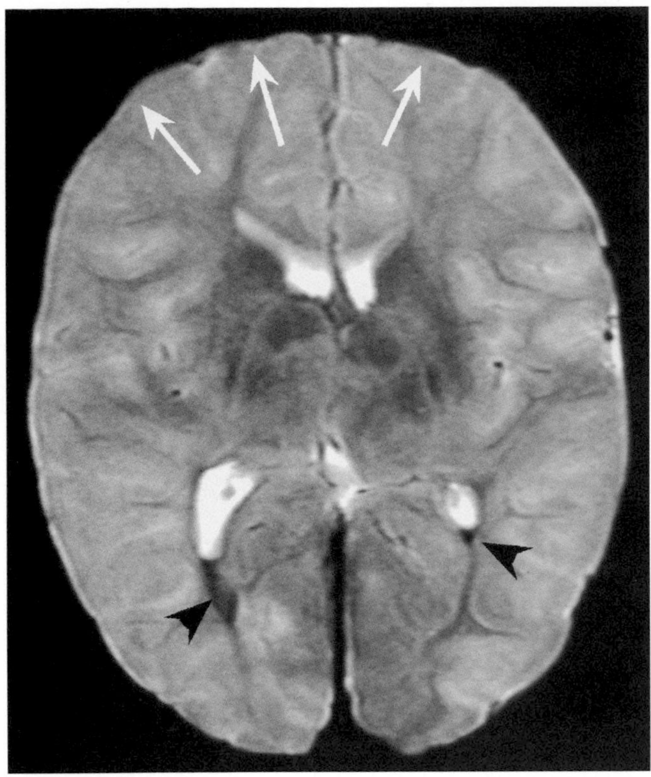

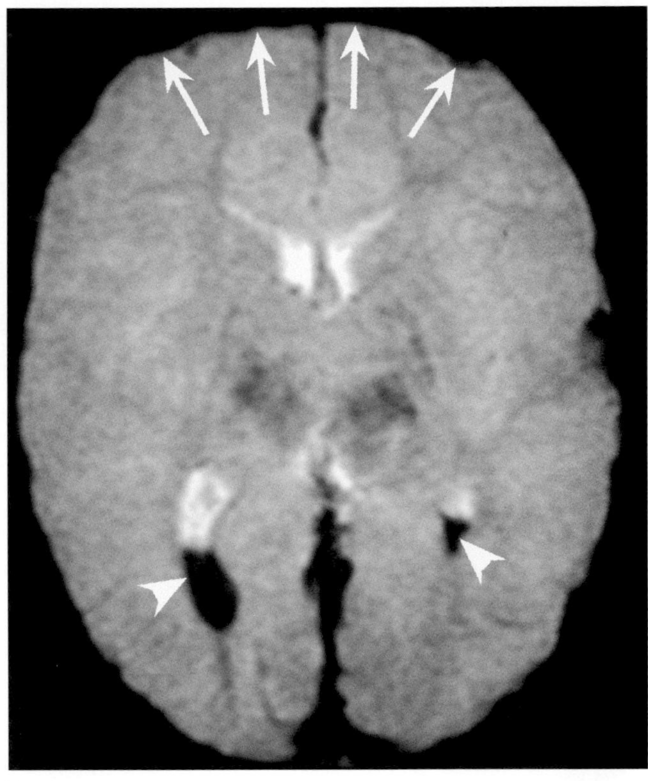

FIGURE 15-13. Comparison of gradient-echo and turbo spin echo sequences in detecting susceptibility changes associated with deoxyhemoglobin and intracellular methemoglobin. **A.** T2-weighted turbo spin echo image. **B.** Gradient-echo T2-weighted image. Note the ease of identification when the hemorrhage lies adjacent to cerebrospinal fluid in the subdural space (*arrows* in **A,B**) or intraventricular space (*arrowheads* in **A,B**).

becomes markedly hypointense to both gray matter and CSF, becoming highly detectable (see Figure 15-12).

Subacute Subdural Hematomas

As hemoglobin continues to age, conformational changes occur that allow relaxivity effects to shorten T1. This results in a very bright signal on T1-weighted images. Early in the subacute phase, hemoglobin remains intracellular. The paramagnetic effects of hemoglobin on T2 relaxation are offset by susceptibility changes from compartmentalization of altered local magnetic fields that change T2*. Other variables, such as clot lysis, might also contribute to T2 changes. The net effect is that T2-weighted images remain slightly hypointense to slightly hyperintense to gray matter, even using susceptibility sequences (see Figure 15-10).

As the red cell membranes begin to deteriorate, methemoglobin extravasates into interstitial fluid. At this point, the relaxivity effects of paramagnetic methemoglobin dominate, affecting T1 and T2 sequences. Disruption of the compartmentalization interrupts the magnetic susceptibility. The hematoma becomes bright on T1- and all T2-weighted images, including FLAIR and susceptibility-weighted images.

Chronic Subdural Hematomas

The MRI appearance of chronic SDHs is variable,[13,109] especially with regard to T1-weighted images. The T1 signal can vary from very bright to isointense to hypointense to gray matter, depending on recurrent bleeding. T2 signal remains elevated on FLAIR and susceptibility images. There is a paucity of hemosiderin (see Figures 15-11 and 15-12). Membrane and septation formation in chronic SDHs can usually be detected on MRI (see Figure 15-11; Figure 15-14).[39] Both membranes and septations can be seen to enhance (see Figures 15-4 and 15-5). Membrane thickness has been linked to the tendency to rebleed and may have prognostic significance.[92]

Subdural Hygromas

MRI may be the best means of distinguishing subdural hygromas from chronic SDHs (see Figures 15-7, 15-11,

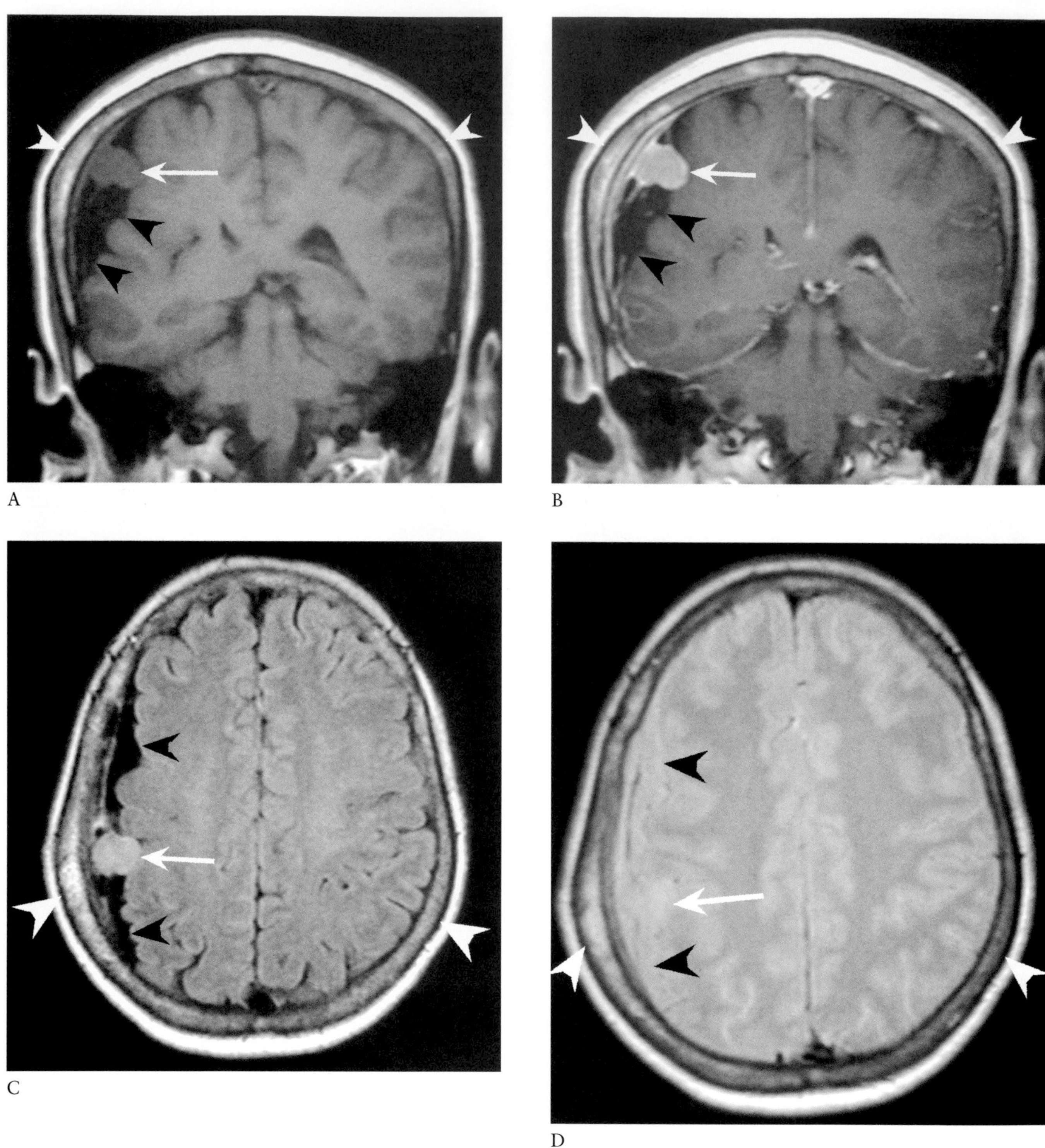

FIGURE 15-14. Chronic subdural hematoma (*black arrowheads*) associated with extra-axial mass (*arrows*). Note the hyperostosis typical for meningioma (*white arrowheads*, compare hyperostotic right side with normal left side of calvarium) and septations (unlabeled). **A.** T1-weighted image. **B.** T1-weighted postcontrast image. **C.** T2 fluid-attenuated inversion recovery image. **D.** Proton density–weighted image. (*continued*)

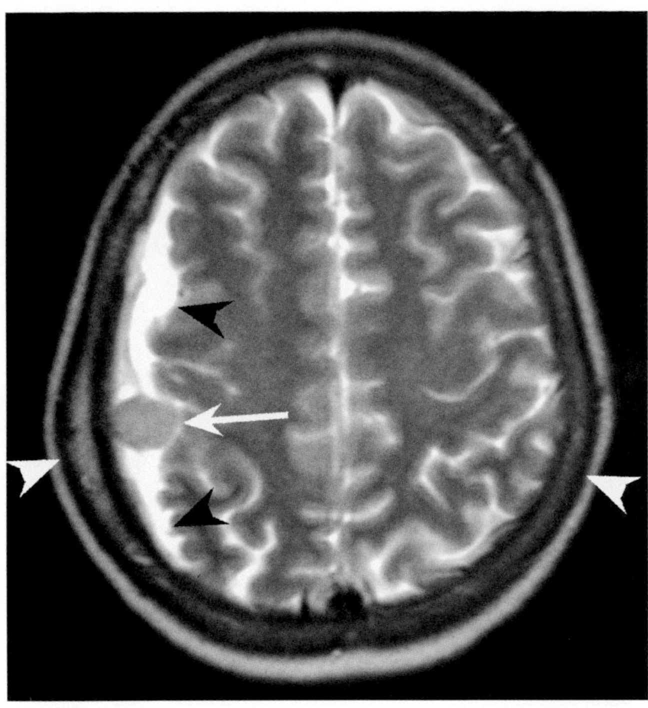
E

FIGURE 15-14. *Continued.* E. T2-weighted image.

and 15-12).[13,109,118] Unless hygromas develop hemorrhage, they tend to show subdural signal isointense to CSF on all pulse sequences, including FLAIR. The FLAIR sequences can be misleading, however, if there is proteinaceous material within the fluid. Although this usually indicates prior hemorrhage, this is not always the case.

Summarizing these effects, a table can be created that shows the stages of hematoma evolution versus T1-weighted and T2-weighted fast spin echo, T2-weighted FLAIR, and gradient-echo T2-weighted signal characteristics (Table 15-2). In combination, these four pulse sequences allow detection of SDHs in virtually all stages. Very early (hyperacute) SDHs are best detected with the FLAIR sequence. Deoxyhemoglobin (acute) is best detected with gradient-echo imaging. Extracellular methemoglobin (early subacute) is best detected with T1-weighted imaging. Intracellular methemoglobin (late subacute) is well detected with T1-weighted and FLAIR images. The chronic subdural collections are variable but probably best detected with the FLAIR or T1 imaging sequence. The persistence of signal that is isointense to CSF on all pulse sequences is consistent with a diagnosis of hygroma.

EPIDURAL HEMATOMAS

Pathophysiology of Epidural Hematomas

Epidural hematomas, by definition, lie superficial to the dura. Because the outer layer of the dura is the periosteum of the inner table of the calvarium, hemorrhage at this location is analogous to subperiosteal hemorrhage elsewhere. The periosteum, being adherent to the bone, does not cross bony sutures. Epidural hematomas, then, are usually contained by the margins of the suture.[125,126] This containment is an important feature helping to differentiate epidural hematomas from SDHs. Furthermore, as blood continues to collect beneath the periosteum, the containment results in a convex deep margin of the hematoma.[125–128] The biconvex appearance is also a feature that differentiates epidural hematomas from SDHs (Figure 15-15).

As with other bones, subperiosteal hemorrhage commonly occurs with fractures. In some series, the occurrence of fracture with epidural hematoma is very high.[125,126,129,130] The most common causes of clinically significant epidural hematomas involve fractures of the temporal bone.[129–131] The squamous portion of the temporal bone is the thinnest portion of the skull, which

TABLE 15-2. Signal Strength Relative to Gray Matter versus Stage of Hematoma Formation for Commonly Used Pulse Sequences

Stage of subdural hematoma	*T1 turbo spin echo*	*T2 turbo spin echo*	*Proton density*	*Fluid-attenuated inversion recovery*	*Gradient-echo*
Hyperacute (oxyhemoglobin)	Isointense	Hyperintense	Hyperintense	Hyperintense*	Hyperintense
Acute (deoxyhemoglobin)	Isointense	Minimally hypointense	Hypointense	Minimally hypo-intense	Very hypointense*
Early subacute (intracellular methemoglobin)	Hyperintense*	Iso- to mildly hypointense	Iso- to mildly hypointense	Iso- to mildly hypointense	Hypointense
Late subacute-chronic (extra-cellular methemoglobin)	Hyperintense*	Hyperintense	Hyperintense*	Hyperintense*	Hyperintense
Hemosiderin (usually absent)	Hypointense	Hypointense	Hypointense	Hypointense	Very hypointense*
Hygroma (fluid)	Hypointense	Hyperintense	Hyperintense	Hypointense	Hyperintense

*The preferred pulse sequence for best overall detection.

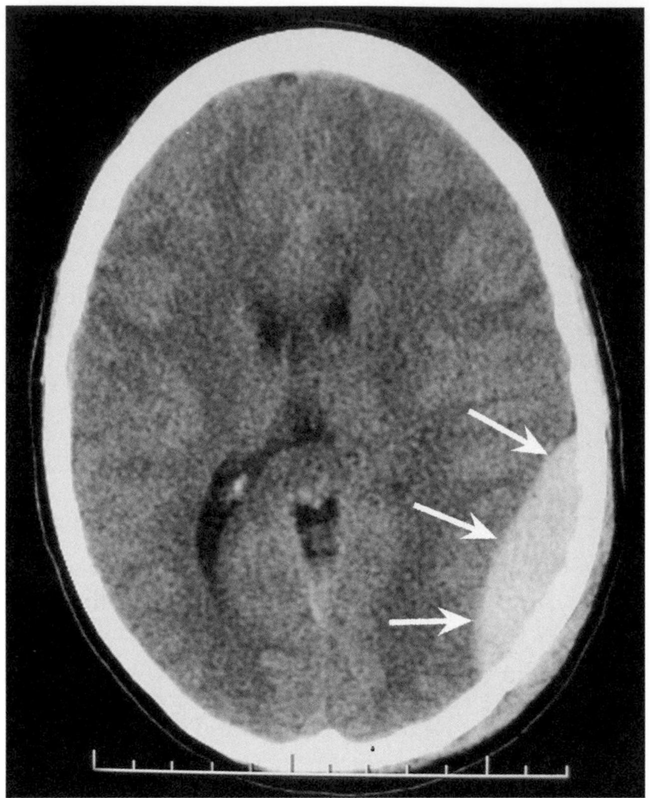

A

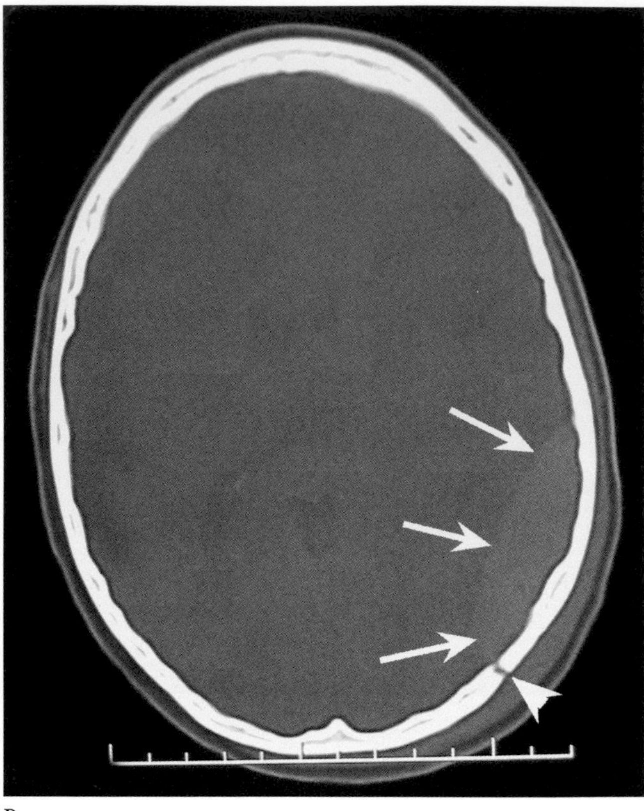

B

FIGURE 15-15. Typical biconvex epidural hematoma (*arrows*) with underlying skull fracture. **A.** Soft tissue window image. **B.** Bone window image. Skull fracture is depicted by arrowhead.

makes it highly susceptible to fractures by direct blows. The middle meningeal arterial and venous branches travel within the subperiosteal space through this region. These branches extend from the temporal to the frontal and parietal bones. Fractures through the bones commonly sever these vessels. Because epidural hematomas are usually bounded by sutures, the ability of the hemorrhage to disseminate is limited. Mass effect can progress extremely rapidly and is responsible for the classic clinical presentation. After a significant blow that produces temporary loss of consciousness, a patient regains consciousness during a "lucid interval" followed by a subsequent loss of consciousness often associated with a dilated pupil, typically indicating uncal herniation. This classic presentation is not, however, universal.[125,132,133] Identification of an epidural hematoma usually requires immediate evacuation. The resulting mass effect produces a dramatic decrease in cerebral profusion pressure, followed and exacerbated by increased tissue water content and, commonly, hydrocephalus.[134] The prognosis in the modern CT era has not been universally established.[131] However, it is age dependent, with outcomes that are better in the pediatric population.[132]

As in the case of SDHs, there are exceptions to the classic location, etiology, clinical presentation, and radiologic findings of epidural hematomas. The latter can occur at the vertex of the brain,[135,136] in the posterior fossa,[137–140] at the clivus,[141] or bilaterally.[142] The less common regions of epidural hematoma formation often involve tears of the dural sinuses or injury to diploic veins. In these cases, because bleeding is associated with the low-pressure venous system, it poses a less immediate threat of brain herniation. The hematomas are typically smaller, progress more slowly, and are less often biconvex than their counterparts of arterial origin (Figure 15-16). Because they are still subperiosteal, they do not cross sutures. They can present with delayed findings,[143] sometimes as chronic epidural hematomas.[144] They are a more common finding in the pediatric population.[145]

Although direct trauma is by far the most common cause of epidural hematomas, there are other etiologies.[146] These hematomas have been reported to occur opposite craniotomies,[147,148] after vacuum extraction in newborns,[149] after epidural anesthesia,[150] and as a consequence of hemophilia[151,152] after intraventricular shunting. Other unusual causes include metastatic small cell lung cancer[153] and Paget's disease.[154]

The majority of epidural hematomas require rapid surgery. It is not clear which cases can be treated medically. When initially undetected or treated conser-

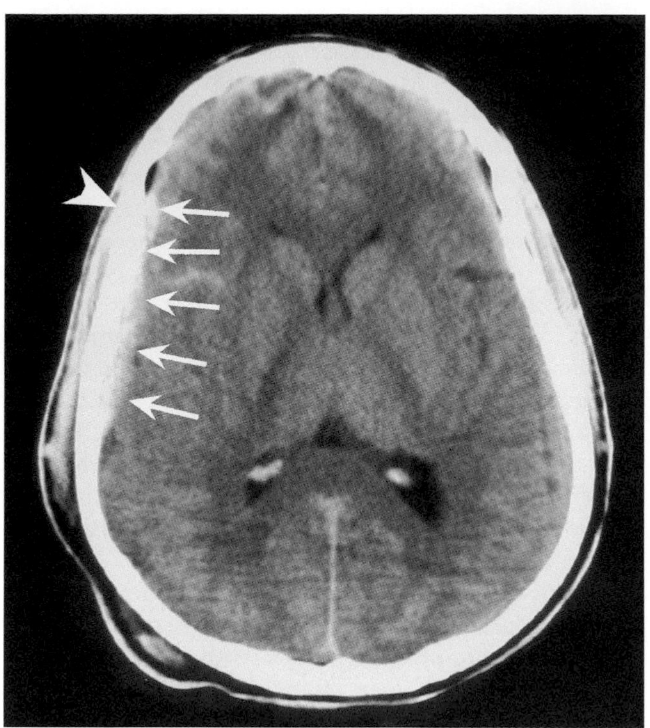
A

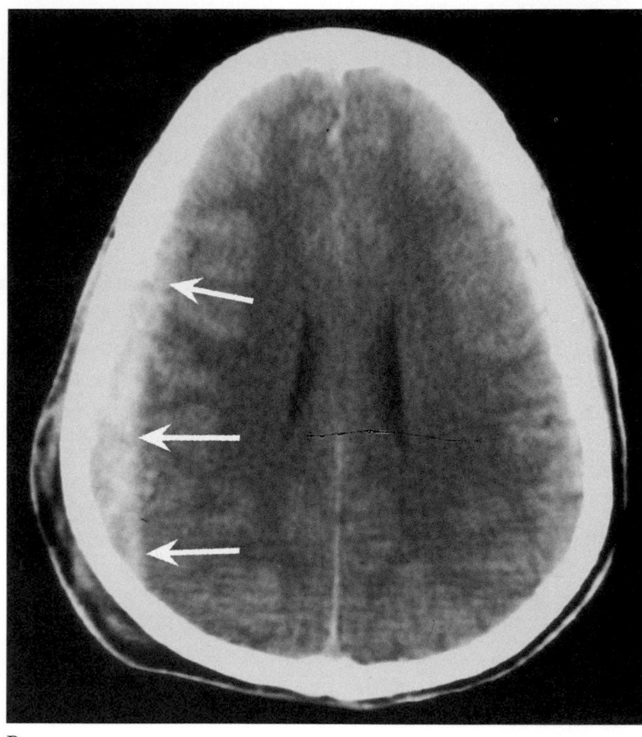
B

FIGURE 15-16. Epidural hematoma proven at surgery, with atypical features. **A.** More caudal image shows slightly convex shape (*arrows*) but apparently crosses the coronal suture (*arrowhead*). **B.** More cephalad image with the hematoma (*arrows*) has a crescentic appearance.

vatively,[135,155,156] these hematomas can resolve spontaneously,[157] evolve into chronic collections,[144] or ossify.[158]

IMAGING EPIDURAL HEMATOMAS

The CT imaging findings of epidural hematomas have been well characterized.[127,128,159] The typical rapid accumulation of hemorrhage usually results in a biconvex appearance by the time imaging is performed. In addition to this appearance, epidural hematomas (see Figure 15-15) are identified on imaging studies by their characteristic location adjacent to the temporal or parietal bones, their failure to cross suture lines, and an overlying associated fracture. In classic cases, these hematomas are easily distinguished from SDHs by these features. When atypical, however, it is not always easy to distinguish between the two entities. Figure 15-16 shows a slightly atypical hematoma that was found at surgery to be extradural. It was biconvex on only a single slice, although it had an overlying fracture. There is a suggestion that the hemorrhage in Figure 15-16A may cross the coronal suture. This can occasionally occur, especially in aging patients as the sutures fuse more completely or if there is a small subdural component to the hemorrhage. Furthermore, as previously discussed, SDHs can occasionally be biconvex. The latter can occur in the anterior middle cranial fossa. The location distinguishes these SDHs from typical epidural hematomas occurring at the squamous portion of the temporal bone. Venous hemorrhages, especially those seen in the pediatric population, are more likely to be concave than rapidly progressing arterial bleeds. Epidural hematomas that originate from sinus tears are often not associated with fractures.

As in SDHs, hyperacute blood is isodense to flowing blood on CT examinations. Clotting occurs rapidly in epidural hematomas because of the early activation of the coagulation cascade resulting from the bony injury. Hence, acute hemorrhage is typically hyperdense to gray matter and to flowing blood. The appearance of heterogeneous density within a suspected epidural hematoma may represent active bleeding, but lower hematocrit from aggressive fluid management or coagulopathy can also produce this finding. Occasionally, heterogeneity can also be seen within a chronic epidural hematoma. There is usually little confusion, however, when presentation and history are taken into account.

Because epidural hematomas are often evacuated, the typical evolution observed with SDHs is seen only in rare cases. When an epidural hematoma is not evacuated, the gradual reduction in density of the hemorrhage as the coagulated blood liquefies follows the pattern of SDHs.

SUMMARY

In acute traumatic CT examinations, a crescentic shape, absence of fracture, crossing suture lines, and layering along the falx or tentorium favor the diagnosis of SDH, whereas a biconvex shape, arrest at suture margins, and overlying fracture favor acute epidural hematoma. Low-density collections can represent chronic SDHs or hygromas.

In many, if not most, patients, subdural hygromas can be accurately differentiated from SDHs by MRI. MRI is significantly more sensitive than CT in detecting subacute and chronic SDHs and even vertex epidural hematomas. It is highly useful for staging hematomas and can be useful in determining rebleeding into chronic hematomas or hygromas.

REFERENCES

1. Stone JL, Rifai MH, Sugar O, et al. Subdural hematomas. I. Acute subdural hematoma: progress in definition, clinical pathology, and therapy. Surg Neurol 1983;19(3):216–231.

2. Rosenorn J, Gjerris F. Long-term follow-up review of patients with acute and subacute subdural hematomas. J Neurosurg 1978;48(3):345.

3. Shenkin HA. Acute subdural hematoma. Review of 39 consecutive cases with high incidence of cortical artery rupture. J Neurosurg 1982;57(2):254–257.

4. Wecht DA. A brief history of chronic subdural hematoma. Neurosurg Clin North Am 2000;11(3):395–398.

5. Schachenmayr A, Friede RL. The origin of subdural neomembranes. I. Fine structure of the dura-arachnoid interface in man. Am J Pathol 1978;92:53–68.

6. Killeffer JA, Killeffer FA, Schochet SS. The outer neomembrane of chronic subdural hematoma. Neurosurg Clin North Am 2000;11(3):407–412.

7. Yamashima T, Friede RL. Light and electron-microscopic studies on the subdural space, the subarachnoid space, and the arachnoid membrane. Neurol Med Chir (Tokyo) 1984;24:737–746.

8. Yamashima T. The inner membrane of chronic subdural hematomas: pathology and pathophysiology. Neurosurg Clin North Am 2000;11(3):413–424.

9. Nabeshima S, Reese TS, Landis DM, et al. Junctions in the meninges and marginal glia. J Comp Neurol 1975;164:127–170.

10. McKissock W, Richardson A, Bloom WH. Subdural haematoma. A review of 389 cases. Lancet 1960;1:1365–1369.

11. Rosenbluth PR, Arias B, Quartetti EV, et al. Current management of subdural hematoma. Analysis of 100 consecutive cases. JAMA 1962;179:253–258.

12. Gomori JM, Grossman RI, Steiner I. High-field magnetic resonance imaging of intracranial hematomas. Isr J Med Sci 1988;24(4–5):218–223.

13. Fobben ES, Grossman RI, Atlas SW, et al. MR characteristics of subdural hematomas and hygromas at 1.5T. AJNR Am J Neuroradiol 1989;10:687–693.

14. Gomori JM, Grossman RI, Hackney DB. Variable appearance of subacute intracranial hematomas on a high-field spin-echo MR. AJNR Am J Neuroradiol 1987;8:1109–1126.

15. Wilberger JE Jr, Harris M, Diamond DL. Acute subdural hematoma: morbidity, mortality, and operative timing. J Neurosurg 1991;74(2):212–218. Comment: J Neurosurg 1992;76(4):723.

16. Ishikawa E, Sugimoto K, Yanaka K, et al. Interhemispheric subdural hematoma caused by a ruptured internal carotid artery aneurysm: case report. Surg Neurol 2000;54(1):82–86.

17. Fukuhara T, Vorster SJ, Luciano MG. Critical shunt-induced subdural hematoma treated with combined pressure-programmable valve implantation and endoscopic third ventriculostomy. Pediatr Neurosurg 2000;33(1):37–42.

18. Maeda Y, Inamura T, Morioka T, et al. Hemorrhagic subdural effusion complicating an endoscopic III ventriculostomy. Childs Nerv Syst 2000;16(5):312–314.

19. Ito M, Miyajima T, Fujii T, Okuno T. Subdural hematoma during low-dose ACTH therapy in patients with west syndrome. Neurology 2000;54(12):2346–2347.

20. Kettaneh A, Biousse V, Bousser MG. [Neurological complications after roller coaster rides: an emerging new risk]? Presse Med 2000;29(4):175–180.

21. Dashti SR, Decker DD, Razzaq A, Cohen AR. Current patterns of inflicted head injury in children. Pediatr Neurosurg 1999;31(6):302–306.

22. Pullarkat VA, Kalapura T, Pincus M, Baskharoun R. Intraspinal hemorrhage complicating oral anticoagulant therapy: an unusual case of cervical hematomyelia and a review of the literature. Arch Intern Med 2000;160(2):237–240.

23. Fukutake T, Mine S, Yamakami I, et al. Roller coaster headache and subdural hematoma. Neurology 2000;54(1):264.

24. Mizushima H, Hanakawa K, Kobayashi N, et al. Acute subdural hematoma due to near-drowning—case report. Neurol Med Chir (Tokyo) 1999;39(11):752–755.

25. Huang D, Abe T, Kojima K, et al. Intracystic hemorrhage of the middle fossa arachnoid cyst and subdural hematoma caused by ruptured middle cerebral artery aneurysm. AJNR Am J Neuroradiol 1999;20(7):1284–1286.

26. Lavie F, Herve D, Le Ber I, et al. Bilateral intracranial subdural hematoma following lumbar

puncture: report of a case. Rev Neurol (Paris) 1998; 154(10):703–705.

27. Castillo M, Fordham LA. MR of neurologically symptomatic newborns after vacuum extraction delivery. AJNR Am J Neuroradiol 1995;16[Suppl 4]:816–818.

28. Gutierrez FA, McLone DG, Raimondi AJ. Physiopathology and a new treatment of chronic subdural hematoma in children. Childs Brain 1979;5(3): 216–232.

29. Yamashima T, Friede RL. Why do bridging veins rupture into the virtual subdural space? J Neurol Neurosurg Psychiatry 1984;47(2):121–127.

30. Lowenhielm P. Tolerance level for bridging vein disruption calculated with a mathematical model. J Bioeng 1978;2(6):501–507.

31. Huang HM, Lee MC, Chiu WT, et al. Three-dimensional finite element analysis of subdural hematoma. J Trauma 1999;47(3):538–544.

32. Gennarelli TA, Thibault LE. Biomechanics of acute subdural hematoma. J Trauma 1982;22(8):680–686.

33. Lee MC, Haut RC. Insensitivity of tensile failure properties of human bridging veins to strain rate: implications in biomechanics of subdural hematoma. J Biomech 1989;22(6–7):537–542.

34. Maxeiner H. Injuries of parasagittal bridging veins in fatally wounded victims of motor vehicle accidents [in German]. Unfallchirurg 2000;103(7):552–556.

35. Maxeiner H. Demonstration and interpretation of bridging vein ruptures in cases of infantile subdural bleedings. J Forensic Sci 2001;46(1):85–93.

36. Howard MA, Bell BA, Uttley D. The pathophysiology of infant subdural haematomas. Br J Neurosurg 1993;7(4):355–365.

37. Papasian NC, Frim DM. A theoretical model of benign external hydrocephalus that predicts a predisposition towards extra-axial hemorrhage after minor head trauma. Pediatr Neurosurg 2000;33(4):188–193.

38. Morinaga K, Matsumoto Y, Omiya N, et al. Subacute subdural hematoma—report of 4 cases and a review of the literature [in Japanese]. No To Shinkei 1990;42(2):131–136.

39. Imaizumi S, Onuma T, Kameyama M, Naganuma H. Organized chronic subdural hematoma requiring craniotomy—five case reports. Neurol Med Chir (Tokyo) 2001;41(1):19–24.

40. Iantosca MR, Simon RH. Chronic subdural hematoma in adult and elderly patients. Neurosurg Clin North Am 2000;11(3):447–454.

41. Chung SJ, Kim JS, Lee MC. Syndrome of cerebral spinal fluid hypovolemia: clinical and imaging features and outcome. Neurology 2000;55(9):1321–1327.

42. Murakami M, Morikawa K, Matsuno A, et al. Spontaneous intracranial hemorrhage associated with bilateral chronic subdural hematomas—case report. Neurol Med Chir (Tokyo) 2000;40(9):484–488.

43. Ueno M, Nakai E, Naka Y, et al. Acute subdural hematoma associated with vacuolated meningioma—case report. Neurol Med Chir (Tokyo) 1993; 33(1):36–39.

44. Chen JW, U HS, Grafe MR. Unsuspected meningioma presenting as a subdural haematoma. J Neurol Neurosurg Psychiatry 1992;55(2):167–168.

45. Sunada I, Nakabayashi H, Matsusaka Y, Yamamoto S. Meningioma associated with acute subdural hematoma—case report. Radiat Med 1998;16(6): 483–486.

46. Gotoh M, Tsuno K, Handa A, et al. Extraaxial primary malignant lymphoma associated with calcified chronic subdural hematoma: a case report [in Japanese]. No Shinkei Geka 2001;29(3):259–264.

47. Lafont M, Lamarque M, Daussac E. Favorable outcome of a subdural hematoma diagnosed in utero. Arch Pediatr 1999;6(9):962–965.

48. Kawabata I, Imai A, Tamaya T. Antenatal subdural hemorrhage causing fetal death before labor. Int J Gynaecol Obstet 1993;43(1):57–60.

49. McLaughlin MR, Jho HD, Kwon Y. Acute subdural hematoma caused by a ruptured giant intracavernous aneurysm: case report. Neurosurgery 1996; 38(2):388–392.

50. Sanchez R, Alfaro A, Perla C, et al. Subdural hemorrhage of aneurysmal origin. Neurologia 1994; 9(2):65–68.

51. Hiramatsu K, Miyazawa T, Katoh H, et al. Tiny aneurysms of cortical arteries presenting as an acute subdural hematoma: a case report [in Japanese]. No To Shinkei 2001;53(1):84–86.

52. Barami K, Ko K. Ruptured mycotic aneurysm presenting as an intraparenchymal hemorrhage and nonadjacent acute subdural hematoma: case report and review of the literature. Surg Neurol 1994;41(4):290–293.

53. Bandoh K, Sugimura J, Hosaka Y, Takagi S. Ruptured intracranial mycotic aneurysm associated with acute subdural hematoma—case report. Neurol Med Chir (Tokyo) 1987;27(1):56–59.

54. Wilberger JE. Pathophysiology of evolution and recurrence of chronic subdural hematoma. Neurosurg Clin North Am 2000;11(3):435–438.

55. Niikawa S, Sugimoto S, Hattori T, et al. Rapid resolution of acute subdural hematoma—report of four cases. Neurol Med Chir (Tokyo) 1989;29(9):820–824.

56. Sander HW, Haddad S, Masdeu JC. Spontaneous resolution of subdural hematoma. MRI findings. J Neuroimaging 1998;8(2):113–115.

57. Matsuyama T, Shimomura T, Okumura Y, Sakaki T. Rapid resolution of symptomatic acute subdural hematoma: case report. Surg Neurol 1997;48(2):193–196. Comment: Surg Neurol 1998;50(3):289.

58. Miller JD, Bullock R, Graham DI, et al. Ischemic brain damage in a model of acute subdural hematoma. Neurosurgery 1990;27(3):433–439.

59. Kuroda Y, Bullock R. Failure of cerebral blood flow-metabolism coupling after acute subdural hematoma in the rat. Neurosurgery 1992;31(6):1062–1071; discussion 1071.

60. Yamashima T, Yamamoto S. The origin of inner membranes in chronic subdural hematomas. Acta Neuropathol (Berl) 1985;67(3–4):219–225.

61. Munroe DMD. Surgical pathology of subdural hematoma. Based on a study of one hundred and five cases. Arch Neurol Psychology 1936;35:64–78.

62. Morinaga K, Matsumoto Y, Hayashi S, et al. Subacute subdural hematoma: findings in CT, MRI and operations and review of onset mechanism [in Japanese]. No Shinkei Geka 1995;23(3):213–216.

63. Morinaga K, Matsumoto Y, Hayashi S, et al. Subacute subdural hematoma—reexamination of mechanism by CT and MRI findings [in Japanese]. No To Shinkei 1993;45(10):969–972.

64. Nomura S, Orita T, Tsurutani T, Izumihara A. Subacute subdural hematoma: report of 3 cases [in Japanese]. Nippon Geka Hokan 1996;65(1):30–35.

65. Bergstrom M, Ericson K, Levander B, et al. Variation with time of the attenuation values of intracranial hematomas. J Comput Assist Tomogr 1977;1(1):57–63.

66. Bergstrom M, Ericson K, Levander B, Svendsen P. Computed tomography of cranial subdural and epidural hematomas: variation of attenuation related to time and clinical events such as rebleeding. J Comput Assist Tomogr 1977;1(4):449–455.

67. Barkovich AJ, Atlas SW. Magnetic resonance imaging of intracranial hemorrhage. Radiol Clin North Am 1988;26(4):801–820.

68. Park CK, Choi KH, Kim MC, et al. Spontaneous evolution of posttraumatic subdural hygroma into chronic subdural haematoma. Acta Neurochir (Wien) 1994;127(1–2):41–47.

69. Lee KS. The pathogenesis and clinical significance of traumatic subdural hygroma. Brain Inj 1998;12(7):595–603.

70. Lee KS, Bae WK, Bae HG, Yun IG. The fate of traumatic subdural hygroma in serial computed tomographic scans. J Korean Med Sci 2000;15(5):560–568.

71. Wippold FJ II. Definition and pathophysiology of subdural hygroma. AJR Am J Roentgenol 1996; 167(4):1061.

72. Parsch CS, Krauss J, Hofmann E, et al. Arachnoid cysts associated with subdural hematomas and hygromas: analysis of 16 cases, long-term follow-up, and review of the literature. Neurosurgery 1997;40(3):483–490.

73. Mayfrank L, Laborde G, Lippitz B, Reul J. Bilateral chronic subdural haematomas following traumatic cerebrospinal fluid leakage into the thoracic epidural space. Acta Neurochir (Wien) 1993;120(1–2):92–94.

74. Thomke F, Bredel-Geissler A, Mika-Gruttner A, et al. Spontaneous intracranial hypotension syndrome. Clinical, neuroradiological and cerebrospinal fluid findings [in German]. Nervenarzt 1999;70(10):909–915.

75. Watanabe S, Shimada H, Ishii S. Production of clinical form of chronic subdural hematoma in experimental animals. J Neurosurg 1972;37(5):552–561.

76. Watanabe S, Shimada H, Ishii S. Production of chronic subdural hematoma in the experimental animals [in Japanese]. Shinkei Kenkyu No Shimpo 1970;14(2):387–396.

77. Apfelbaum RI, Guthkelch AN, Shulman K. Experimental production of subdural hematomas. J Neurosurg 1974;40(3):336–346.

78. Kopp W. Pathogenesis of chronic subdural hematoma [in German]. Rofo Fortschr Geb Rontgenstr Neuen Bildgeb Verfahr 1990;152(2):200–205.

79. Scarrow AM, Segal R. Meningioma associated with chronic subdural hematoma. Acta Neurochir (Wien) 1998;140(12):1317–1318.

80. Popovic EA, Lyons MK, Scheithauer BW, Marsh WR. Mast cell–rich convexity meningioma presenting as chronic subdural hematoma: case report and review of the literature. Surg Neurol 1994;42(1):8–13.

81. Chen JC, Levy ML. Causes, epidemiology, and risk factors of chronic subdural hematoma. Neurosurg Clin North Am 2000;11(3):399–406.

82. Stoodley M, Weir B. Contents of chronic subdural hematoma. Neurosurg Clin North Am 2000;11(3): 425–434.

83. Weir B. Oncotic pressure of subdural fluids. J Neurosurg 1980;53(4):512–515.

84. Sato S, Suzuki J. Ultrastructural observations of the capsule of chronic subdural hematoma in various clinical stages. J Neurosurg 1975;43(5):569–578.

85. Mori K, Adachi K, Cho K, et al. Quantitative kinetic analysis of blood vessels in the outer membranes of chronic subdural hematomas. Neurol Med Chir (Tokyo) 1998;38(11):697–702; discussion 702–703.

86. Nagahori T, Nishijima M, Takaku A. Histological study of the outer membrane of chronic subdural hematoma: possible mechanism for expansion of hematoma cavity [in Japanese]. No Shinkei Geka 1993;21(8):697–701.

87. Ito H, Yamamoto S, Saito K, et al. Quantitative estimation of hemorrhage in chronic subdural hematoma using the ^{51}Cr erythrocyte labeling method. J Neurosurg 1987;66:862–864.

88. Weir B, Gordon P. Factors affecting coagulation: fibrinolysis in chronic subdural fluid collections. J Neurosurg 1983;58(2):242–245.

89. Kawakami Y, Chikama M, Tamiya T, Shimamura Y. Coagulation and fibrinolysis in chronic subdural hematoma. Neurosurgery 1989;25(1):25–29.

90. Giuffre R. Physiopathogenesis of chronic subdural hematomas: a new look to an old problem. Rev Neurol 1987;57(5):298–304.

91. Ernestus RI, Beldzinski P, Lanfermann H, Klug N. Chronic subdural hematoma: surgical treatment and outcome in 104 patients. Surg Neurol 1997;48(3):220–225.

92. El-Kadi H, Miele VJ, Kaufman HH. Prognosis of chronic subdural hematomas. Neurosurg Clin North Am 2000;11(3):553–567.

93. Okuyama T, Saito K, Fukuyama K, et al. Clinical study of cerebral blood flow in unilateral chronic subdural hematoma measured by 99mTc-HMPAO SPECT [in Japanese]. No To Shinkei 2000;52(2):141–147.

94. Okuyama T, Saito K, Fukuyama K, et al. Clinical study of cerebral blood flow in bilateral chronic subdural hematoma measured by 99mTc-HMPAO SPECT [in Japanese]. No To Shinkei 2000;52(8):709–714.

95. Kuwabara H. Regional cerebral blood flow and metabolism in chronic subdural hematoma. Neurosurg Clin North Am 2000;11(3):499–502.

96. Patel TR, Schielke GP, Hoff JT, et al. Comparison of cerebral blood flow and injury following intracerebral and subdural hematoma in the rat. Brain Res 1999;829(1–2):125–133.

97. Tanaka A, Kimura M, Yoshinaga S, et al. Quantitative electroencephalographic correlates of cerebral blood flow in patients with chronic subdural hematomas. Surg Neurol 1998;50(3):235–240.

98. Tanaka A, Nakayama Y, Yoshinaga S. Cerebral blood flow and intracranial pressure in chronic subdural hematomas. Surg Neurol 1997;47(4):346–351.

99. Ishikawa T, Kawamura S, Hadeishi H, et al. Cerebral blood flow and oxygen metabolism in hemiparetic patients with chronic subdural hematoma. Quantitative evaluation using positron emission tomography. Surg Neurol 1995;43(2):130–136; discussion 136–137.

100. Salvant JB Jr, Muizelaar JP. Changes in cerebral blood flow and metabolism related to the presence of subdural hematoma. Neurosurgery 1993;33(3):387–393; discussion 393.

101. Ogasawara K, Ogawa A, Okuguchi T, et al. Postoperative hyperperfusion syndrome in elderly patients with chronic subdural hematoma. Surg Neurol 2000;54(2):155–159.

102. Machulda MM, Haut MW. Clinical features of chronic subdural hematoma: neuropsychiatric and neuropsychologic changes in patients with chronic subdural hematoma. Neurosurg Clin North Am 2000;11(3):473–477.

103. Parlato C, Guarracino A, Moraci A. Spontaneous resolution of chronic subdural hematoma. Surg Neurol 2000;53(4):312–315; discussion 315–317.

104. Horikoshi T, Naganuma H, Fukasawa I, et al. Computed tomography characteristics suggestive of spontaneous resolution of chronic subdural hematoma. Neurol Med Chir (Tokyo) 1998;38(9):527–532; discussion 532–533.

105. Slater JP. Extramedullary hematopoiesis in a subdural hematoma. Case report. J Neurosurg 1966; 25(2):211–214.

106. Weissbach G, Hentsch R. Pachymeningosis hemorrhagica interna in early childhood. Padiatr Grenzgeb 1967;6(4):279–302.

107. Yan MJ, Lin KE, Lee ST, Tzaan WC. Calcified chronic subdural hematoma: case report. Changgeng Yi Xue Za Zhi 1998;21(4):521–525.

108. Donaldson JW, Edwards-Brown M, Luerssen TG. Arachnoid cyst rupture with concurrent subdural hygroma. Pediatr Neurosurg 2000;32(3):137–139.

109. Goldberg HI, Zimmerman RA, Bilaniuk LT. MR characteristics of subdural hematomas and hygromas at 1.5 T. AJR Am J Roentgenol 1989;153(3):589–595.

110. Lee KS, Bae WK, Bae HG, et al. The computed tomographic attenuation and the age of subdural hematomas. J Korean Med Sci 1997;12(4):353–359.

111. Curry TS 3d, Dowdey JE, Murry RC Jr. Computed Tomography. In TS Curry, JA Seibert (eds), Christensen's Physics of Diagnostic Radiology (4th ed). Philadelphia: Lea & Febiger, 1990;289–323.

112. Greenberg J, Cohen WA, Cooper PR. The "hyperacute" extraaxial intracranial hematoma: computed tomographic findings and clinical significance. Neurosurgery 1985;17(1):48–56.

113. Deb S, Bhaumik S, Pal H. Isodense acute subdural haematoma in anaemic patients. Neurol India 2000;48(3):298–299.

114. Kaufman HH, Singer JM, Sadhu VK, et al. Isodense acute subdural hematoma. J Comput Assist Tomogr 1980;4(4):557–559.

115. Asari S, Kunishio K, Suga M, et al. Coronal computerized angiotomography for the diagnosis of isodense chronic subdural hematoma. J Neurosurg 1984;61(4):729–732.

116. Boyko OB, Cooper DF, Grossman CB. Contrast-enhanced CT of acute isodense subdural hematoma. AJNR Am J Neuroradiol 1991;12(2):341–343.

117. Kostanian V, Choi JC, Liker MA, et al. Computed tomographic characteristics of chronic subdural hematomas. Neurosurg Clin North Am 2000;11(3):479–489.

118. Thulborn KR, Atlas SW. Intracranial Hemorrhage. In SW Atlas (ed), Magnetic Resonance Imaging of the Brain and Spine (2nd ed). New York: Lippincott–Raven, 1996;265–314.

119. Hosoda K, Tamaki N, Masumura M, et al. Magnetic resonance images of chronic subdural hematomas. J Neurosurg 1987;67(5):677–678.

120. Ashikaga R. Clinical utility of MR FLAIR imaging for head injuries. Nippon Igaku Hoshasen Gakkai Zasshi 1996;56(14):1045–1049.

121. Sui B. Image changes of hemoglobin in acute and hyperacute intracranial hematoma during hyperintensive magnetic resonance [in Chinese]. Zhonghua Yi Xue Za Zhi 1990;70(1):29–31.

122. Bradley WG Jr. Hemorrhage and hemorrhagic infections in the brain. Neuroimaging Clin North Am 1994;4(4):707–732.

123. Linfante I, Llinas RH, Caplan LR, Warach S. MRI features of intracerebral hemorrhage within 2 hours from symptom onset. Stroke 1999;30(11):2263–2267.

124. Zyed A, Hayman LA, Bryan RN. MR imaging of intracerebral blood: diversity in the temporal pattern at 0.5 and 1.0 T. AJNR Am J Neuroradiol 1991;12(3): 469–474.

125. Baykaner K, Alp H, Ceviker N, et al. Observation of 95 patients with extradural hematoma and review of the literature. Surg Neurol 1988;30(5):339–341.

126. Zulch KJ. Neuropathology of intracranial hemorrhage. Prog Brain Res 1968;30:151–165.

127. Tans JT. Computed tomography of extracerebral hematoma. Clin Neurol Neurosurg 1977;79(4): 296–306.

128. Zimmerman RA, Bilaniuk LT, Gennarelli T, et al. Cranial computed tomography in diagnosis and management of acute head trauma. AJR Am J Roentgenol 1978;131(1):27–34.

129. Spatz EL. Unconsciousness caused by neurosurgical lesions. Surg Clin North Am 1968;48(2):259–262.

130. Mendelow AD, Teasdale GM. Pathophysiology of head injuries. Br J Surg 1983;70(11):641–650.

131. Servadei F. Prognostic factors in severely head injured adult patients with epidural haematomas. Acta Neurochir (Wien) 1997;139(4):273–278.

132. Schutzman SA, Barnes PD, Mantello M, Scott RM. Epidural hematomas in children. Ann Emerg Med 1993;22(3):535–541.

133. Gurdjian ES. Recent advances in the study of the mechanism of impact injury of the head—a summary. Clin Neurosurg 1972;19:1–42.

134. Ganz JC, Thuomas KA, Vlajkovic S, et al. Changes in intracranial morphology, regional cerebral water content and vital physiological variables during epidural bleeding. An experimental MR study in dogs. Acta Radiol 1993;34(3):279–288.

135. Miller DJ, Steinmetz M, McCutcheon IE. Vertex epidural hematoma: surgical versus conservative management: two case reports and review of the literature. Neurosurgery 1999;45(3):621–624; discussion 624–625.

136. Song JH, Park JY, Lee HK. Vertex epidural hematomas: considerations in the MRI era. J Korean Med Sci 1996;11(3):278–281.

137. Bozbuga M, Izgi N, Polat G, Gurel I. Posterior fossa epidural hematomas: observations on a series of 73 cases. Neurosurg Rev 1999;22(1):34–40.

138. Roda JM, Gimenez D, Perez-Higueras A, et al. Posterior fossa epidural hematomas: a review and synthesis. Surg Neurol 1983;19(5):419–424.

139. Oliveira MA, Araujo JF, Balbo RJ. [Extradural hematoma of the posterior fossa. Report of 7 cases.] Arq Neuropsiquiatr 1993;51(2):243–246.

140. Holzschuh M, Schuknecht B. Traumatic epidural haematomas of the posterior fossa: 20 new cases and a review of the literature since 1961. Br J Neurosurg 1989;3(2):171–180.

141. Mizushima H, Kobayashi N, Sawabe Y, et al. Epidural hematoma of the clivus. Case report. J Neurosurg 1998;88(3):590–593.

142. Arienta C, Baiguini M, Granata G, Villani R. Acute bilateral epidural hematomas. Report of two cases and review of the literature. J Neurosurg Sci 1986;30(3):139–142.

143. Milo R, Razon N, Schiffer J. Delayed epidural hematoma. A review. Acta Neurochir (Wien) 1987; 84(1-2):13–23.

144. Tatagiba M, Sepehrnia A, el Azm M, Samii M. Chronic epidural hematoma—report on eight cases and review of the literature. Surg Neurol 1989;32(6):453–458.

145. Grossman RI, Yousem DM. Head Trauma. In RI Grossman, DM Yousem (eds), Neuroradiology: The Requisites. New York: Mosby, 1994;151–152.

146. Cabon I, Hladky JP, Lambilliotte A, et al. Uncommon etiology of extradural hematoma. Neurochirurgie 1997;43(3):173–176.

147. Sato M, Mori K. Postoperative epidural hematoma—five cases of epidural hematomas developed after supratentorial craniotomy on the contralateral side [in Japanese]. No Shinkei Geka 1981;9(11):1297–1302.

148. Yuki K, Kodama Y, Emoto K, et al. A case of epidural hematoma occurring on the opposite site of craniotomy after clipping surgery performed on internal carotid giant aneurysm. No Shinkei Geka 1990;18(6): 567–570.

149. Okuno T, Miyamoto M, Itakura T, et al. A case of epidural hematoma caused by a vacuum extraction without any skull fractures and accompanied by cephalohematoma [in Japanese]. No Shinkei Geka 1993;21(12):1137–1141.

150. Schmidt A, Nolte H. Subdural and epidural hematomas following epidural anesthesia. A literature review [German]. Anaesthesist 1992;41(5):276–284.

151. Fujimoto Y, Aguiar PH, Carneiro JD, et al. Spontaneous epidural hematoma following a shunt in an infant with congenital factor X deficiency. Case report and literature review. Neurosurg Rev 1999;22(4):226–229.

152. Mattle H, Kohler S, Huber P, et al. Anticoagulation-related intracranial extracerebral haemorrhage. J Neurol Neurosurg Psychiatry 1989;52(7):829–837.

153. Simmons NE, Elias WJ, Henson SL, Laws ER.

Small cell lung carcinoma causing epidural hematoma: case report. Surg Neurol 1999;51(1):56–59.

154. Drapkin AJ. Epidural hematoma complicating Paget's disease of the skull: a case report. Neurosurgery 1984;14(2):211–214.

155. Kolodziej W, Kita P, Podgorski D, et al. Acute post-traumatic epidural hematoma: report of 4 non-surgically treated cases. Neurol Neurochir Pol 1999;33(4):955–970.

156. Aoki N. Epidural haematoma in the newborn infants: therapeutic consequences from the correlation between haematoma content and computed tomography features. A review. Acta Neurochir (Wien) 1990;106(1–2):65–67.

157. Le Coz P, Corabianu O, Helias A, et al. Rapid spontaneous regression of epidural hematoma resulting from acute tetraplegia. Value of magnetic resonance imaging [in French]. Ann Med Interne (Paris) 1989; 140(6):527–529.

158. Kawata Y, Kunimoto M, Sako K, et al. Ossified epidural hematomas: report of two cases [in Japanese]. No Shinkei Geka 1994;22(1):51–54.

159. Zee CS, Go JL. CT of head trauma. Neuroimaging Clin North Am 1998;8(3):525–539.

CHAPTER

16

Hemorrhage Secondary to Cerebral Vascular Malformations

David T. Jeck and DeWitte T. Cross III

Four percent of the population harbors cerebral vascular malformations. Cerebral vascular malformations constitute a diverse group of lesions with a wide range of clinical manifestations. They may remain completely asymptomatic or present with severe intracranial hemorrhage. Cerebral vascular malformations represent the most common causes of nontraumatic intracerebral hemorrhage in patients between the ages of 15 and 45 years.[1–3] Current imaging techniques can differentiate between the different types of vascular malformations. This information guides the neurosurgeon, interventional neuroradiologist, and neurologist in deciding which lesions should be managed conservatively and which need aggressive treatment.

The different types of cerebral vascular malformations, with emphasis on those that present with intracranial hemorrhage, are reviewed. Cerebral vascular malformations are characterized by the presence or absence of arteriovenous shunting (Figure 16-1). They may be further divided into arterial, capillary, and venous etiologies.[4–6] Lesions with arteriovenous shunting are mainly of arterial origin. These include parenchymal arteriovenous malformations (AVMs), arteriovenous fistulas (AVFs), and dural arteriovenous malformations (DAVMs).

Nonshunting vascular malformations include lesions of arterial, capillary, and venous etiologies. Aneurysms and angioectasias that compromise the main nonshunting arterial malformations are traditionally considered as separate topics and are not discussed in this chapter. Capillary etiologies include the capillary malformation (capillary telangiectasia). Cavernous malformations (formerly called *cavernous angiomas* and *cavernomas*) are related to capillary malformations and likely are of capillary etiology. The main venous malformations include developmental venous anomalies (DVAs) (formerly called *venous angiomas*) and venous varices. Mixed vascular malformations, vein of Galen malformations, and malformations associated with syndromes are discussed separately.

IMAGING APPROACH TO VASCULAR MALFORMATIONS

A combination of computed tomography (CT), magnetic resonance imaging (MRI), and digital subtraction angiography (DSA) is used to optimally image cerebral vascular malformations. Noncontrast CT should be the initial diagnostic modality in the setting of an acute hemorrhage. CT is excellent at detecting acute hemorrhage associated with vascular malformations. However, the appearance of hemorrhage on CT is often nonspecific and other etiologies such as aneurysm, hypertension, venous thrombosis, neoplasm, sympathomimetic drugs, and amyloid angiopathy also need to be considered. Clinical information may help narrow the differential diagnosis, but further imaging is frequently necessary.

MRI and magnetic resonance angiography (MRA) often add further information regarding the underlying etiology of intracranial hemorrhage and frequently provide a definitive diagnosis. MRI is also more sensitive than CT for detecting subacute and chronic hemorrhage. In some cases of cavernous malformations, capil-

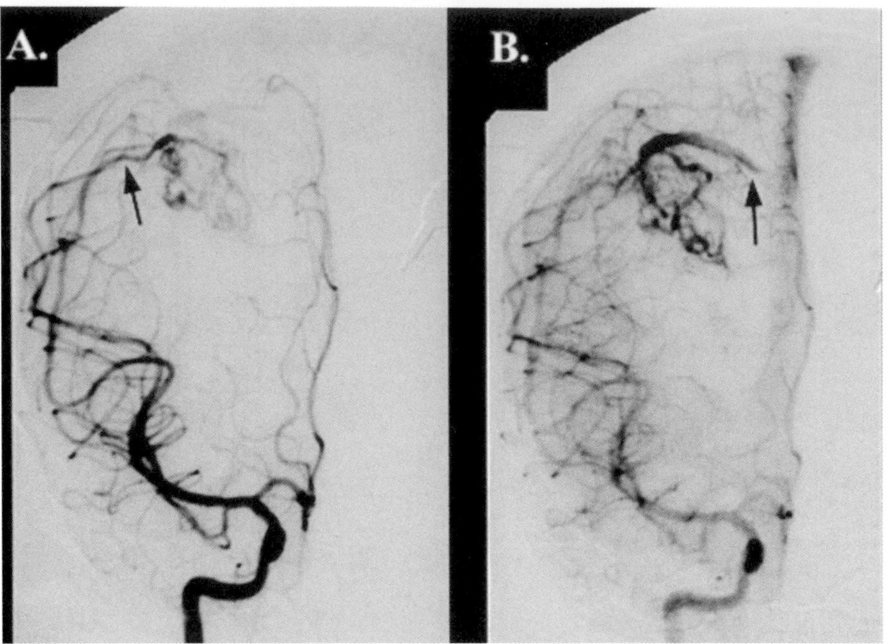

FIGURE 16-1. Arteriovenous shunting in a parenchymal arteriovenous malformation. The patient presented with spontaneous right frontal hemorrhage. **A.** Frontal carotid angiogram—early arterial phase. Typical features of an arteriovenous malformation with middle cerebral feeding artery (*arrow*) and nidus. **B.** Frontal carotid angiogram—late arterial phase. An early draining vein is present (*arrow*), which drains into the superior sagittal sinus. A stenosis is present near the entrance of the draining vein to the superior sagittal sinus. The early draining vein reflects decreased arteriovenous transit time characteristic of shunting vascular malformations.

lary malformations, and DVAs, no further imaging is usually necessary. MRI also adds important three-dimensional (3D) information for presurgical planning.

Angiography still plays a critical role in the evaluation of many vascular malformations. Angiography may be necessary to detect the cause of intracranial hemorrhage in cases in which a high clinical suspicion for a vascular malformation exists, and cross-sectional imaging is normal. This frequently occurs with small dural vascular malformations. Angiography is also necessary when cross-sectional imaging reveals a nonspecific abnormality, which frequently occurs in the presence of hemorrhage. Angiography has a very high diagnostic yield in patients younger than 45 years with spontaneous intracranial hemorrhage and no history of hypertension. The yield is even higher in these patients if the hemorrhage is in a lobar location. Patients of any age with isolated intraventricular hemorrhage also have a high diagnostic yield from angiography. The only patients with spontaneous intracranial hemorrhage who do not have a significant diagnostic yield from angiography are those with deep gray matter or posterior fossa hemorrhage and a history of hypertension.[7] In cases in which the presence of a vascular malformation has been established, angiography frequently complements MRI and CT, providing crucial information for surgical and endovascular interventions.

ARTERIOVENOUS MALFORMATIONS

Clinical Presentation

AVMs are classified in relation to their blood supply as parenchymal (pial), mixed pial-dural, or purely dural. Pure parenchymal AVMs receive their blood supply solely from cerebral and cerebellar arteries and are the most common type of AVM. Newton and Cronqvist reported that approximately 75% of supratentorial AVMs and 50% of infratentorial AVMs were purely parenchymal.[8] More recently, investigators have found that meningeal contribution to parenchymal AVMs is more common, occurring in as many as 50% of patients. Large AVMs recruit meningeal supply more often than small AVMs.[9]

Parenchymal AVMs are congenital lesions and are present in 0.1–0.8% of the population.[5,6,10,11] They are found equally in male and female patients. Eighty-five percent to 90% are supratentorial and 10–15% are infratentorial.[12–14] AVMs are usually solitary but may be multiple, particularly when associated with hereditary hemorrhagic telangiectasia (HHT) or Wyburn-Mason's syndrome.[12,15–20] Familial cases have also been reported.[18,21]

AVMs most commonly present with hemorrhage (30–50%) and seizures (25–40%).[12,14,22–26] Headache and neurologic deficits are other common presenting symptoms. Hydrocephalus may also be present. The mechanism of hydrocephalus may be secondary to venous hypertension, obstruction from mass effect, or prior episodes of bleeding. Intraparenchymal and subarachnoid hemorrhages are the most common patterns of intracranial hemorrhages reported with AVMs. Intraparenchymal hemorrhage is usually considered the most common type of hemorrhage from AVMs,[27] although in one series, the distribution of hemorrhage was 30% subarachnoid, 23% parenchymal, 16% intraventricular, and 31% combined.[28]

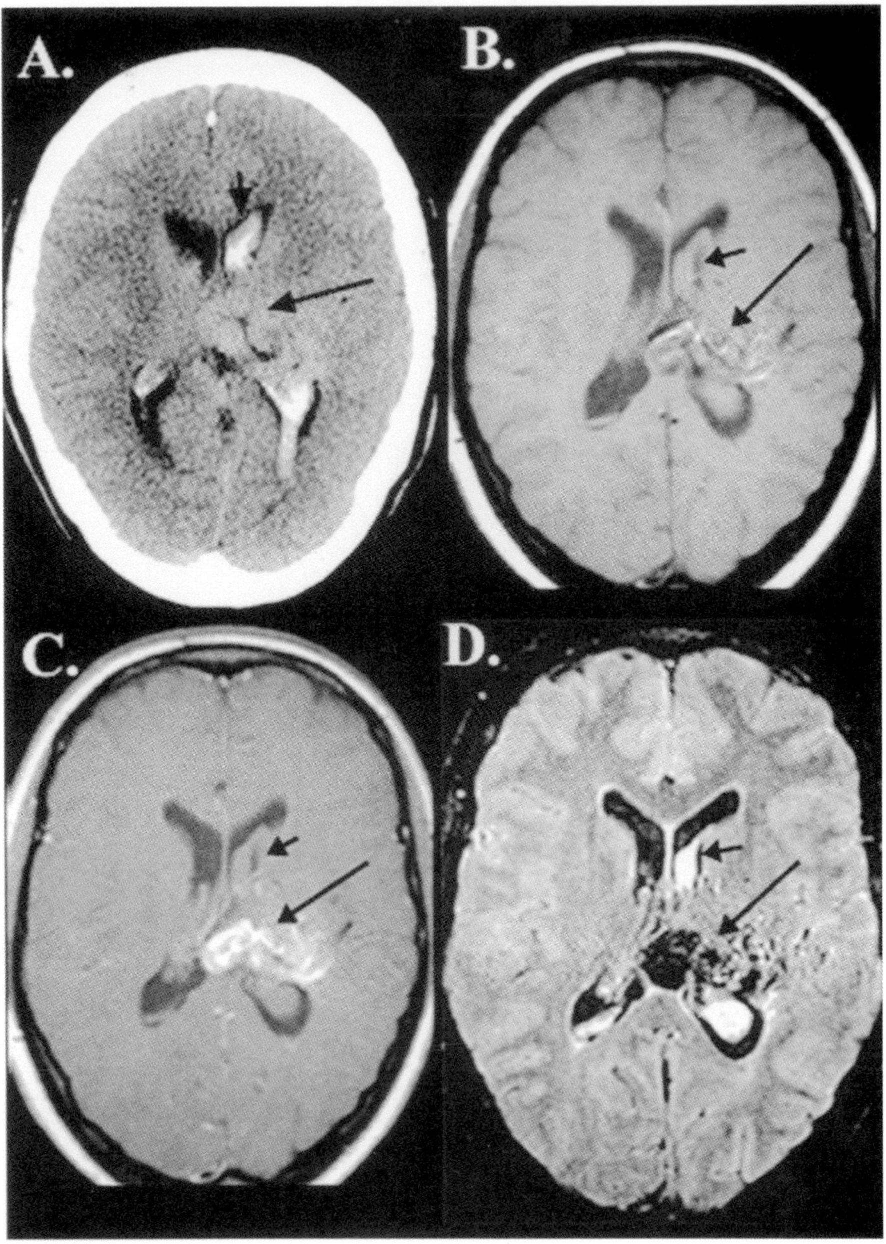

FIGURE 16-2. Thirty-three-year-old woman who presented with the worst headache of her life. Deep left periventricular arteriovenous malformation (AVM) with intraventricular hemorrhage. **A.** Computed tomography demonstrates typical, nonspecific features of an AVM with a lesion of increased attenuation centered in the left periventricular region (*arrow*). The left thalamus was also partially involved. Left lateral ventricular hemorrhage is also present. **B.** T1-weighted magnetic resonance image with areas of increased and decreased signal in the left periventricular AVM (*long arrow*), reflecting flow void and flow-related enhancement. Note the isodense left lateral ventricular hemorrhage (*short arrow*) and a tiny layering of blood product in the right lateral ventricle occipital horn. **C.** T1-weighted postgadolinium magnetic resonance image. The deep left periventricular AVM enhances (*long arrow*, compared with pregadolinium in **B**) with a large dilated central draining vein anterior to the splenium of the corpus callosum. The appearance of the intraventricular blood is the same as the noncontrast image (*short arrow*). **D.** Fluid-attenuated inversion recovery magnetic resonance image highlights the AVM (*long arrow*) and intraventricular blood product, which is bright compared to the dark cerebrospinal fluid (*short arrow*). Flow void is present in the dilated draining vein. Also, note the pulsation artifact in the phase (left to right) direction. Fluid-attenuated inversion recovery imaging is similar to T2-weighted imaging with cerebrospinal fluid signal suppressed.

Intraparenchymal hemorrhage is correlated with the most severe deficits.[28] AVMs are the second most common cause of subarachnoid hemorrhage, with saccular aneurysms being the most common cause. If only subarachnoid blood is present, then hemorrhage from an associated aneurysm should be considered. Deep AVMs and choroid plexus AVMs are the most prone to intraventricular hemorrhage (Figure 16-2). Subdural hemorrhage may also rarely occur. Sixty-four percent of AVMs present before the age of 40, and 20% of patients are symptomatic before age 15.[12,22,29] Hemorrhage reportedly occurs more frequently in children than adults and is associated with a higher mortality.[29]

The annual hemorrhage rate of AVMs is 2–4%, with an annual death rate of 1%.[12,14,26,30–34] AVMs account for 2% of all strokes.[22] The rate of rebleeding after initial presentation with hemorrhage is generally considered to be higher in the following year, ranging from 6% to 33%.[24,31,35,36] Some investigators have found that the rebleeding risk remains elevated if the initial presentation of the AVM was hemorrhage,[37] whereas others believe that the hemorrhage risk eventually returns to the baseline of 2–4% per year.[24,31,33,36] Hemorrhage is associated with a 10–15% mortality rate.[22,31] Significant morbidity is also associated with each hemorrhage, although recent studies have sug-

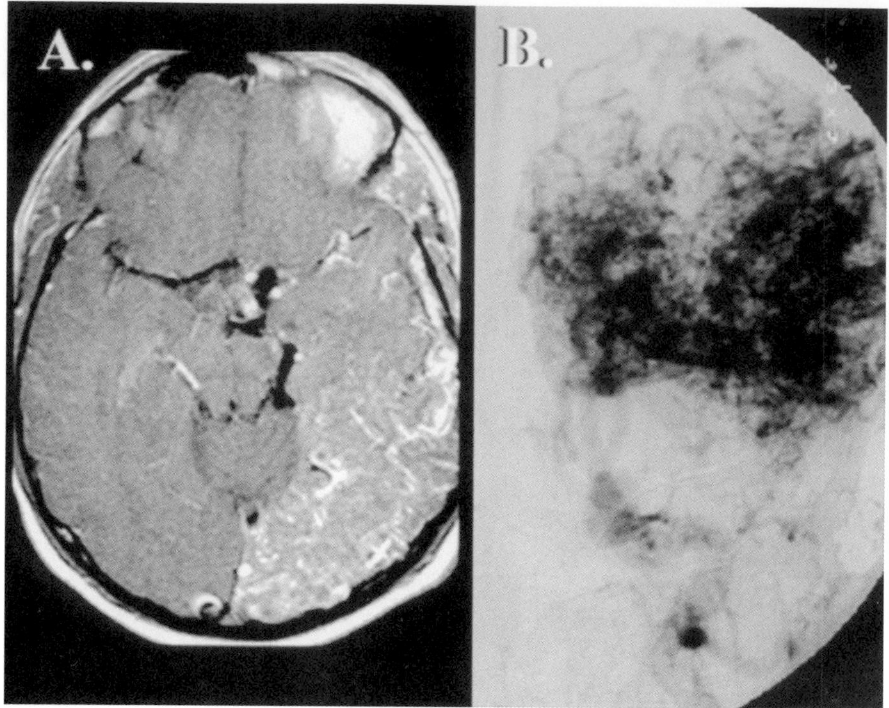

FIGURE 16-3. Diffuse type of arteriovenous malformation. Twenty-one-year-old man presented with 1 year of severe right-sided headaches. **A.** T1-weighted postgadolinium image with diffuse abnormal enhancement in the left temporoparieto-occipital lobes with significant amount of intervening parenchyma. Note the large flow voids in the circle of Willis and left perimesencephalic region, indicating flow in enlarged feeding vessels. **B.** Angiogram—late arterial phase. The nidus is diffuse and occupies a significant portion of the temporoparieto-occipital lobes with areas of intervening normal brain parenchyma. Arterial supply included branches of the posterior communicating, middle cerebral, posterior cerebral, and pericallosal branch of the anterior cerebral arteries. Several small flow-related aneurysms were present (not shown).

gested that the outcome is considerably better than aneurysms, with as many as 74% of patients having a good clinical outcome.[1,24,28] Posterior fossa hemorrhages, however, may have a worse prognosis than anterior cranial fossa hemorrhages.[36]

Pathology

Parenchymal AVMs are masses of tightly packed abnormal arteries and veins without a normal intervening capillary bed. They are functionally divided into feeding arteries, a central nidus, and draining veins. The nidus is the main functional unit of the AVM. Areas of intervening gliotic brain parenchyma, thrombosis with recanalization, dystrophic calcification, and amyloid deposition are often present. Overlying leptomeningeal thickening is often found. Rarely, intervening normal parenchyma is present. A large amount of normal intervening parenchyma may be present in atypical AVMs. These diffuse AVMs may occupy an entire lobe or hemisphere (Figure 16-3). Microscopic hemorrhage is frequently detected in AVMs, even in the absence of clinical hemorrhage. High-flow angiopathic changes affecting the arterial and venous components of AVMs are frequently present. Arterial angiopathic changes include regions of arterial ectasia, thinning, stenoses, and aneurysm formation. Arterial wall thinning is characterized by the segmental absence of media and elastica. Stenoses usually represent endothelial hyperplasia. Venous structures may be dilated with sacculations, varices, and stenoses. Varices occasionally may be huge. The vessels within the AVM often have intermediate features of both arteries and veins.[6,13,38]

Imaging

In addition to providing a diagnosis, imaging provides an abundance of clinically relevant information regarding management. The size, location, pattern of venous drainage, and the presence of arterial and venous abnormalities all affect the patient's prognosis and influence treatment decisions. For instance, small AVMs (less than 2–3 cm) frequently respond favorably to radiosurgery.[39] Size, location, and pattern of venous drainage also influence surgical risk. These criteria are often used to grade AVMs to help determine surgical risk.[40] Presurgical grading with the Spetzler-Martin system uses a five-point scale for AVMs according to their size (small, medium, or large), location (superficial or deep), and involvement of eloquent versus noneloquent brain. Higher-grade AVMs have an increased risk of major and minor neurologic deficits with surgery compared to lower-grade AVMs (Figure 16-4).[41,42] Other angioarchitectural features, such as the presence of aneurysms, size of the nidus, and pattern of venous drainage, help guide endovascular treatments, such as embolization with *N*-butylcyanoacrylate and endovascular coiling of associated aneurysms.

Computed Tomography

CT is the most useful imaging tool in diagnosing acute intracranial hemorrhage associated with AVMs. The

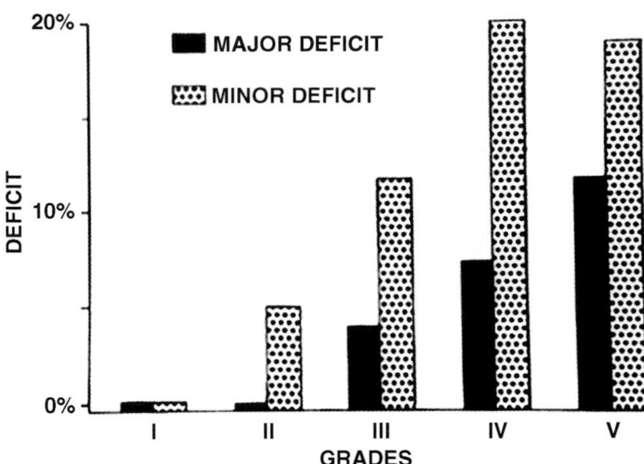

FIGURE 16-4. Increased incidence of minor and major neurologic deficits due to surgery occurs as the grade of the arteriovenous malformation increases. (Reprinted with permission from MG Hamilton, RF Spetzler. The prospective application of a grading system for arteriovenous malformations. Neurosurgery 1994;34[1]:2–6; discussion 6–7.)

presence of subarachnoid, intraparenchymal, subdural, or intraventricular hemorrhage may be identified. Associated hydrocephalus may also be detected. On noncontrast CT, the AVM nidus may appear isodense or hyperdense relative to brain parenchyma. Associated areas of infarcted brain may be hypodense. Noncontrast CT may be negative or nonspecific in the absence of hemorrhage. Calcification, usually located in the venous structures of the AVM, may be present in 25–30% of cases.[10] Dense enhancement is normally seen after the administration of intravenous contrast. A vermiform or tubular structure is frequently present, adjacent to the hematoma, which may occasionally allow a specific diagnosis (Figure 16-5).[43] Rarely, a thrombosed AVM may be present, making the diagnosis difficult. Thrombosed AVMs often are hyperdense on precontrast CT and may not demonstrate any enhancement following contrast administration.[44] Further imaging is necessary, but differentiation from other vascular malformations and neoplasm still may be difficult. Enhancement also may not be demonstrated in the setting of acute hemorrhage. Dedicated CT angiography may be used to evaluate the nidus size and identify the major feeding arteries and draining veins. CT angiography is faster than MRI and currently costs less.[45] It is particularly useful when patients have a contraindication to MRI, such as patients with a pacemaker. However, MRI is generally considered superior to CT for noninvasively demonstrating the relevant vascular architectural features of AVMs.[46]

Magnetic Resonance Imaging

MRI with and without intravenous gadolinium is an extremely useful modality for evaluating AVMs. MRI frequently provides a definitive diagnosis. AVMs are characteristically rounded or pyramidal-shaped lesions, with the base oriented toward the cortex and apex toward the ventricles. The overlying leptomeninges may be thickened. The mass effect from AVMs is often much less than expected given the size of the lesion, because AVMs tend to replace rather than displace parenchyma. Impressive mass effect may, however, be present in cases of acute hemorrhage or large venous varices. The vast majority of AVMs contains patent flow and will demonstrate serpentine, tightly packed flow voids on noncontrast T1- and T2-weighted images. Areas of internal high signal may also be seen where acute or subacute hemor-

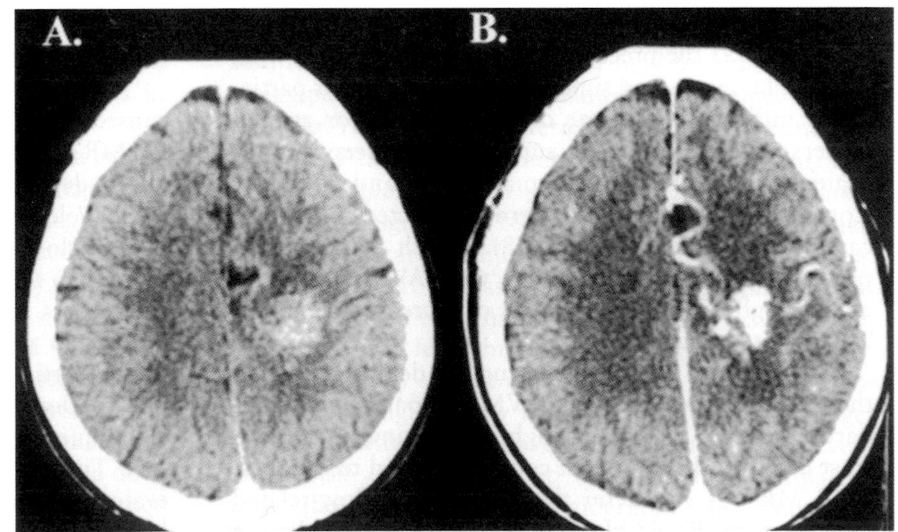

FIGURE 16-5. Characteristic computed tomography features of a parenchymal arteriovenous malformation. **A.** Computed tomography without contrast. A nonspecific round, high-attenuation lesion is present in the left frontoparietal lobe. **B.** After administration of intravenous contrast, enhancement of prominent serpentine vessels is present, indicating large feeding arteries and draining veins.

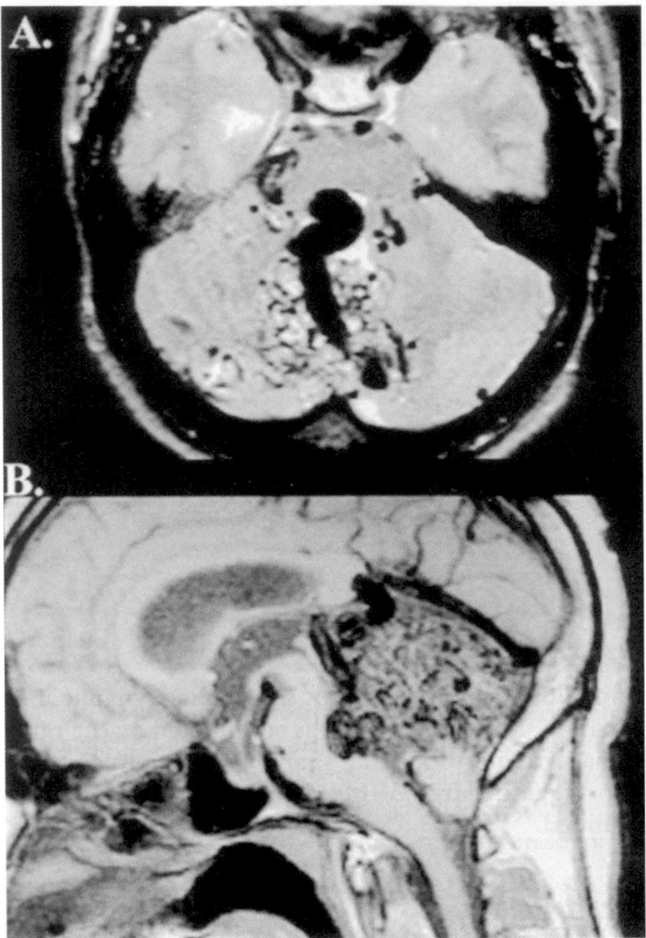

FIGURE 16-8. Forty-four-year-old man with fourth ventricular hemorrhage and cerebellar mass on computed tomography. This magnetic resonance image (MRI) demonstrates a posterior fossa arteriovenous malformation with deep venous drainage. **A.** Axial T2-weighted MRI with a large vermian arteriovenous malformation. A large, deep, draining vein is present. **B.** Sagittal T1-weighted image in the same patient. The MRI adds three-dimensional information regarding the arteriovenous malformation occupying the midline in the posterior fossa. Large draining veins are present, including a large vein of Galen draining into the straight sinus. An enlarged basilar artery is also present. Angiography confirmed the pattern of venous drainage (see Figure 16-11). MRI is excellent at defining the relationship to posterior fossa structures.

The angiographic evaluation involves close scrutiny of the angioarchitecture of the main components of the AVM, which include the arterial feeders, the AVM nidus, and the venous drainage (Figure 16-12).

Feeding Arteries

Pure parenchymal AVMs are supplied only by the cerebral and cerebellar arteries. Feeding arteries are usually uniformly enlarged due to the increased flow. Feeding arteries should be evaluated for changes of high-flow angiopathy, which is present in approximately 20% of AVMs.[11,58] Angiopathic changes include areas of stenosis, thrombosis, ectasia, and aneurysms. Feeding artery (pedicle) aneurysms should also be fully evaluated (Figure 16-13).

The type of arterial feeder may be characterized as terminal or en passage. Terminal feeding arteries may give off proximal branches to normal parenchyma but terminate in the nidus of the AVM. En passage feeders give rise to nonterminal branches that supply the AVM but continue to supply normal distal brain parenchyma.[58,59] The type of arterial supply has important implications for endovascular embolization and surgery. A terminal arterial feeder may be embolized or occluded distal to any normal branches, without risk of ischemia to normal brain parenchyma. However, extreme caution must be taken when embolizing an en passage feeder to avoid infarcting normal parenchyma. Superselective injection of sodium amytal, 20–50 mg, depending on flow within the vessel, may be helpful in determining whether a vessel to be embolized supplies normal brain function that will result in a neurologic deficit.[60] Feeding arteries may also be characterized as *direct* or *indirect*. *Direct feeders* are branches that supply the AVM and that originate in the vascular distribution of the AVM. *Indirect feeders* are collateral blood vessels to the nidus that originate outside the expected vascular territory of the AVM.

Angiomatous changes should also be evaluated. These represent collateral vessels supplying the AVM that do not directly arise from the vascular distribution of the arterial feeders. Rapid arteriovenous shunting should not be present. Angiomatous changes have been reported to be associated with a decreased risk of hemorrhage.[61] The brain parenchyma adjacent to the AVM should be examined for evidence of poor filling, possibly reflecting hypoperfusion secondary to venous hypertension. This may correlate clinically with ischemic symptoms.[62] Vasospasm in the feeding arteries is unusual with hemorrhage secondary to AVMs but may be seen, particularly in cases with associated aneurysmal bleeds.

Arteriovenous Malformation Nidus

The nidus is the functional unit of the AVM. The nidus must be evaluated with relation to size, location, flow characteristics, and presence of aneurysms. The nidus is usually compact but may be diffuse. The nidus may have fistulous and plexiform components. A fistulous nidus consists of a simple single arteriovenous connection, usually with high-flow characteristics. A plexiform nidus represents a very complex, compartmentalized collection of shunting units. Feeding arteries branch off to supply a variable number of arteriovenous units, each

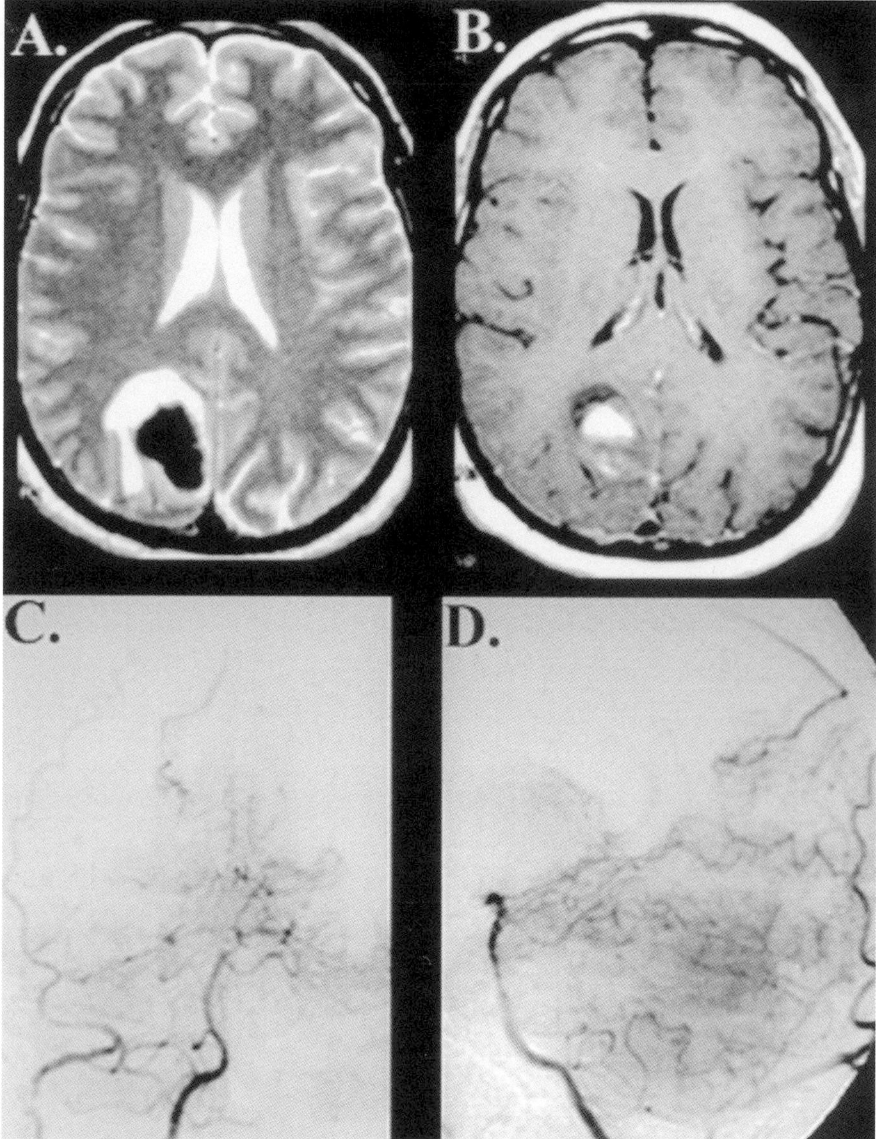

FIGURE 16-9. Thirty-three-year-old man with right occipital hemorrhage. **A.** T2-weighted magnetic resonance axial image with nonspecific, right parieto-occipital hemorrhagic lesion. **B.** T1-weighted postgadolinium image. Some enhancement is present in the lesion. The overall magnetic resonance imaging appearance is nonspecific. Hemorrhage from a neoplasm or vascular malformation would be the most likely possibilities. **C,D.** Frontal and lateral right vertebral angiograms—late arterial/capillary phase. Posterior cerebral artery feeders, a small nidus, and an early draining vein entering the superior sagittal sinus (best seen in **D**) allow diagnosis of arteriovenous malformation to be made. This example emphasizes the importance of angiography in cases of hemorrhage in young adults in whom arteriovenous malformation is a diagnostic possibility.

of which has its own draining vein. The draining veins may converge or leave the AVM separately. The units often have different features in terms of flow velocity, the presence of aneurysms, and the types of fistulous arteriovenous connections.[58]

Venous Drainage

Venous drainage must be evaluated with attention to the number of draining veins, the pattern of venous drainage, and the morphologic changes in the draining veins. The pattern of venous drainage should be identified as superficial or deep. Although this may frequently be predicted on the basis of the AVM location, some AVMs demonstrate unexpected drainage pattern. For instance, a superficial AVM may have a component of deep drainage. Venous morphology including stenoses and ectasias should also be identified. AVMs with deep venous drainage and venous stenosis or occlusion carry an increased risk of hemorrhage.[32,63–68] AVMs with a single draining vein have also been reported to have an increased incidence of hemorrhage.[32]

Superselective Angiography

Superselective angiography involves direct injection of the distal vessels supplying the AVM with flexible microcatheters. Microcatheters may be guidewire directed or flow directed. Superselective angiography further delineates components of the AVM by opacifying individual components of the AVM and decreasing overlap. Superselective angiography clearly identifies individual feeding arteries, identifies the compartments of the nidus supplied by these individual feeders, characterizes the various components of the nidus, and increases the detection of intranidal aneurysms. Identifying arterial

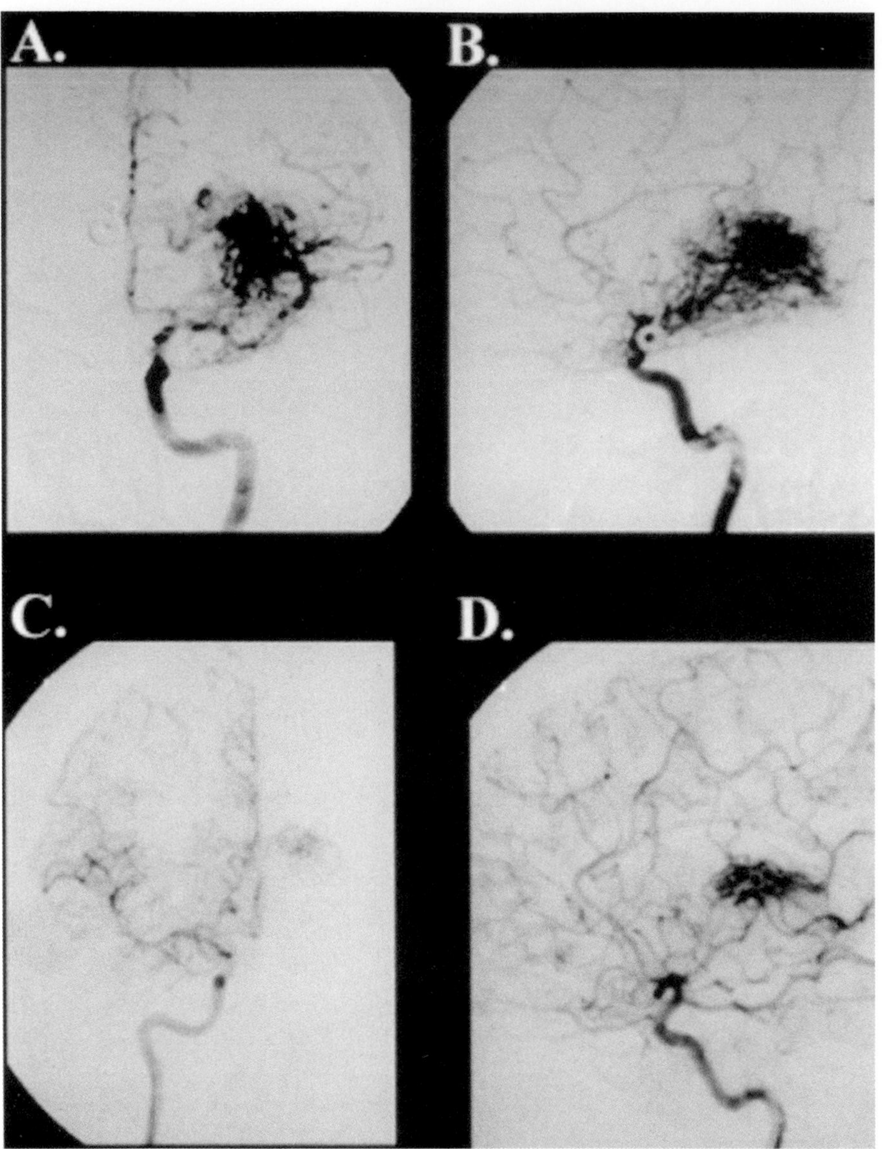

FIGURE 16-10. Left periventricular/thalamic arteriovenous malformation with bilateral carotid artery supply (same patient as in Figure 16-2). **A,B.** Frontal and lateral left carotid angiograms—arterial phase. Left middle cerebral artery perforators, lenticulostriate branches, and a small branch of the left anterior choroidal are all feeding the arteriovenous malformation nidus. Note the medially oriented early draining vein (**A**). Four-mm superior hypophyseal artery aneurysm was also present. **C,D.** Right frontal and lateral angiograms demonstrate right carotid artery contribution via the posterior communicating artery to thalamoperforating arteries.

feeders as terminal or en passage is often only possible with superselective angiography. This is crucial in planning and performing embolization.[69,70]

The angioarchitectural factors related to increased risk of hemorrhage have been extensively studied. Deep or periventricular location, deep venous drainage, venous stenoses and occlusion, and intranidal aneurysms are the commonly reported features of AVMs that increase the risk of hemorrhage.[24,61,63–68,71–73] Some investigators have also shown that a single draining vein and increased feeding arterial pressure increase the risk of hemorrhage.[32,63,66,72,74] Angiomatous changes and peripheral or mixed venous drainage are associated with a decreased risk of hemorrhage.[61]

Many investigators believe that small AVMs (<3 cm) hemorrhage more frequently than large AVMs, possibly secondary to increased arterial pressure.[24,72,74] Micro-AVMs, which are AVMs with an angiographically occult nidus or nidus less than 1 cm, have been reported to hemorrhage more frequently, cause larger hematomas than their larger counterparts, and present with significant neurologic deficits (Figure 16-14).[69,75,76] Other investigators have found that the hemorrhage rates of small and large AVMs are the same.[37] Hirai et al. found that large AVMs actually hemorrhage more often than small AVMs.[64] They argue that small AVMs only present more frequently with hemorrhage because they are less likely to present with seizures or headaches than large AVMs. Supporters of the latter argument note that in some series, the rate of rebleeding from small AVMs is not higher than that of larger AVMs.

Aneurysms and Arteriovenous Malformation

Increased prevalence of aneurysms with AVMs is well documented. The two types of aneurysms that are seen

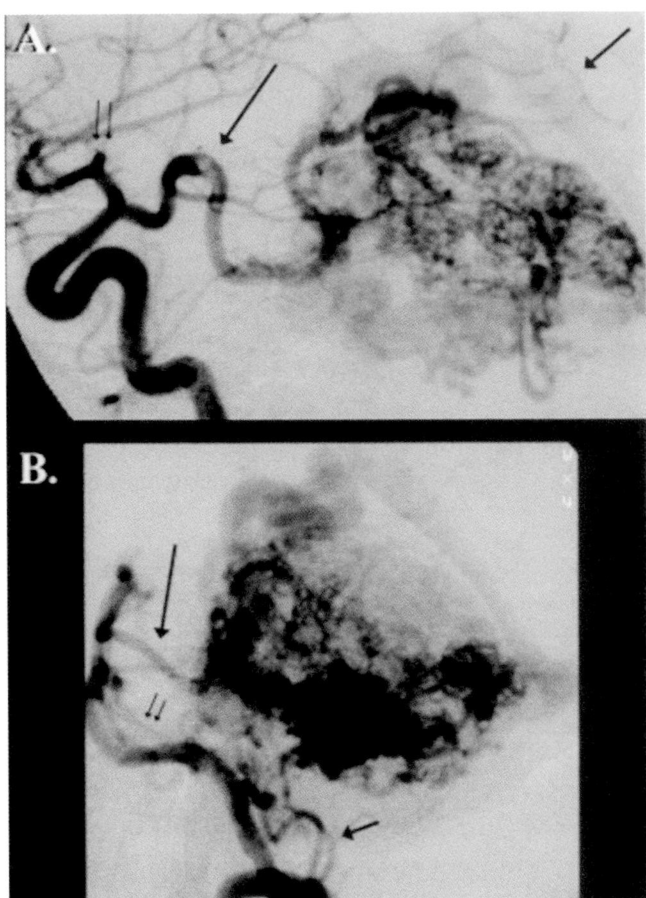

FIGURE 16-11. Large cerebellar arteriovenous malformation (same patient as in Figure 16-8). **A.** Lateral internal carotid angiogram—arterial phase. Large posterior communicating artery feeder is present (*long arrow*). Supply from the contralateral carotid artery is also present. The superior prominence arising from the supraclinoid carotid artery was confirmed to simply represent a looping vessel on other views (*double arrows*). Note the faint, early opacification of an enlarged vein of Galen and straight sinus despite still being in the arterial phase, indicative of early arteriovenous shunting (*short arrow*). **B.** Vertebral artery injection with superior cerebellar arteries (*long arrow*), anterior inferior cerebellar artery (*double arrows*), and posterior inferior cerebellar artery (*short arrow*) feeders. Venous and intranidal aneurysms are also present.

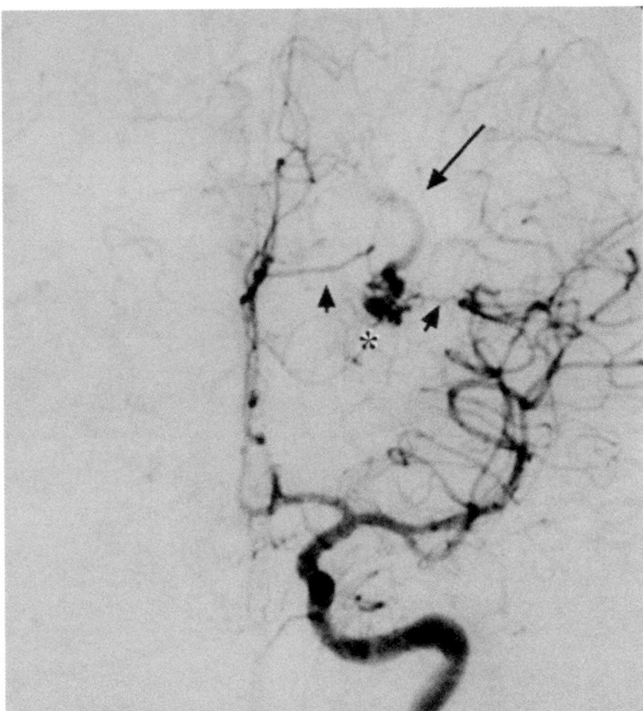

FIGURE 16-12. Typical angiographic features of a parenchymal arteriovenous malformation. Feeding branches from the anterior cerebral and middle cerebral arteries (*short arrows*), nidus (above *asterisk*), and early draining vein (*long arrow*) are demonstrated. The patient had received prior radiosurgery.

most frequently with AVMs are aneurysms on the feeding arteries and intranidal aneurysms. The reported incidence of aneurysms associated with AVMs varies between 3% and 58%,[61,67,70,77–79] but most investigators report associated arterial aneurysms in 10–20%.[80–82] These include saccular aneurysms not related to the feeding arteries of the AVM, pedicle aneurysms on the feeding arteries, and intranidal aneurysms (see Figure 16-13). The incidence of saccular aneurysms on vessels unrelated to the AVM is the same as in the general population.[81] The angiographic technique accounts for some of the differences in reported rates of associated intranidal aneurysms. Superselective angiography demonstrates a higher percentage of intranidal aneurysms.[67,70] Also, the presence of an intranidal aneurysm is subject to interpretation. Different readers may interpret similar findings as focal ectasia or an aneurysm. Irregular large aneurysms associated with hemorrhage may represent false aneurysms and should not be included in data representing true aneurysms. In fact, it is not clear whether many of the intranidal aneurysms represent true aneurysms or pseudoaneurysms. This distinction can even be difficult on pathologic examination.

The increased risk of hemorrhage in AVMs with associated aneurysms is controversial. The majority of investigators has shown an increased risk of hemorrhage with the presence of intranidal aneurysms, with annual hemorrhage rates of 7–10%, compared with the rate of 2–4% for AVMs without aneurysms.[25,64,67,68,70,80,81,83] However, several series have not found an increased risk of hemorrhage.[63,71,72,77] AVMs with associated intranidal aneurysms may also have an increased rate of rebleeding after the initial hemorrhage.[59] An increased risk of hemorrhage in AVMs with pedicle aneurysms (which are

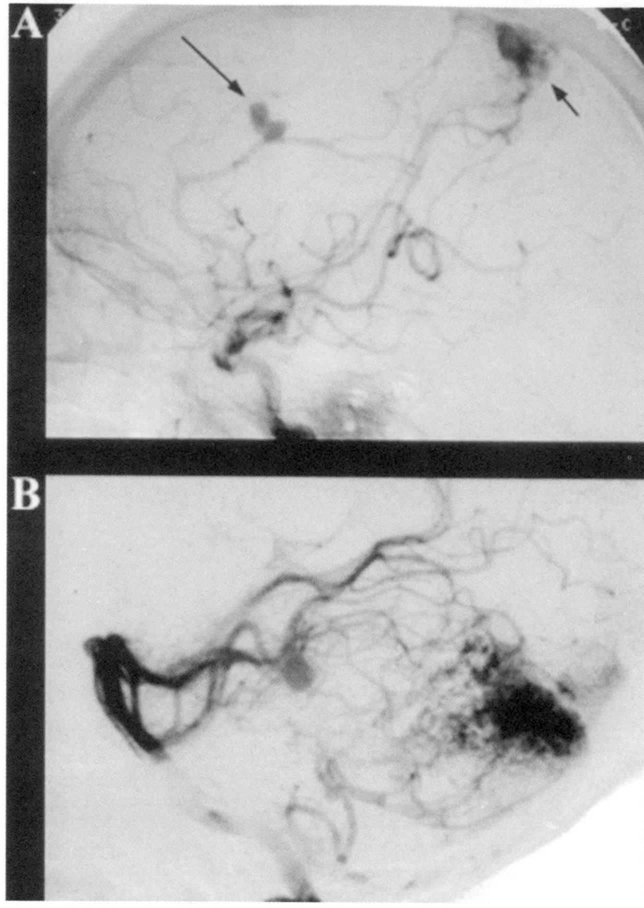

FIGURE 16-13. Pedicle arterial aneurysms. **A.** A lateral carotid angiogram with a large pericallosal artery pedicle aneurysm (*long arrow*) in this patient with an arteriovenous malformation nidus in the parietal lobe (*short arrow*). **B.** Lateral vertebral angiogram with an infratentorial arteriovenous malformation. A large aneurysm is present on a superior cerebellar artery pedicle. Also note the contribution of the posterior inferior cerebellar artery.

more common in infratentorial AVMs) has also been reported (see Figure 16-13B).[78,84]

The presence of aneurysms, regardless of their true impact on hemorrhage risk, needs to be carefully evaluated and considered in the treatment decisions.[82] Bleeding from aneurysms has a worse prognosis than AVM hemorrhage. It is uncertain whether this can be applied to intranidal aneurysms. In cases of hemorrhage, attention to whether the aneurysm or the AVM bled may dictate which lesion is treated first. Several investigators have reported that the aneurysm is the cause of hemorrhage in a higher percentage of cases when coexisting lesions are present.[32,79] This distinction may, of course, be difficult depending on the proximity of the lesions.

Differential Diagnosis

The hallmark of AVMs on angiography is the presence of early draining veins, reflecting arteriovenous shunting. Early draining veins, however, may also be seen with other entities, including acute ischemic infarct, hematoma, neoplasms, and abscess (Figure 16-15). Enlarged, tortuous feeding arteries, a nidus of closely packed entangled vessels, and large, tortuous draining veins are usually present to help identify a lesion as an AVM. Mass effect on adjacent vessels is usually not significant unless an associated hematoma is present (see Figure 16-9).

In some cases of small AVMs, or in the setting of a large hematoma, the distinction from a vascular neoplasm may be difficult. The vessels in a metastasis or neoplasm are often pathologic and separated by tissue, whereas the nidus of an AVM usually consists of tightly packed vessels. The feeders of AVMs are often very large compared to the normal size or slightly enlarged vessels supplying tumors. The terminal vessels supplying tumors often appear stretched and encircle the lesion, whereas the terminal vessels supplying an AVM remain dilated and directly enter the lesion. Draining veins are also usually much larger in AVMs than with neoplasms (Figure 16-16).[85] Differentiating an AVM from a hemangioblastoma or angioblastic meningioma is usually possible. Hemangioblastomas normally have a distinct appearance on cross-sectional imaging with a cystic component, and an enhancing mural nodule but may be solid. Angiographically, the cyst lacks tumor vascularity and displays mass effect (Figure 16-17). Angioblastic meningiomas normally have external carotid arterial supply, a disordered appearance, and a large amount of mass effect.[85] A thrombosed AVM may occasionally be present. These may be avascular or contain slow flow on angiography.[12]

Mixed Pial-Dural Arteriovenous Malformations

Mixed pial-dural AVMs have supply from meningeal arteries in addition to cerebral and cerebellar arteries. Larger AVMs tend to have meningeal contribution more frequently than smaller AVMs (Figure 16-18).[9] Newton and Cronqvist found that 15% of AVMs had mixed pial-dural supply.[8] Other investigators have noted meningeal contribution in a much higher percentage of AVMs.[9] The type of meningeal supply needs to be carefully evaluated. Transdural vessels may directly supply the AVM, anastomose with feeders that indirectly supply the AVM, or anastomose with feeders that supply brain parenchyma adjacent to the AVM. Arteries that directly supply the AVM are very conducive to embolization and may be safely occluded. Interfering with the meningeal

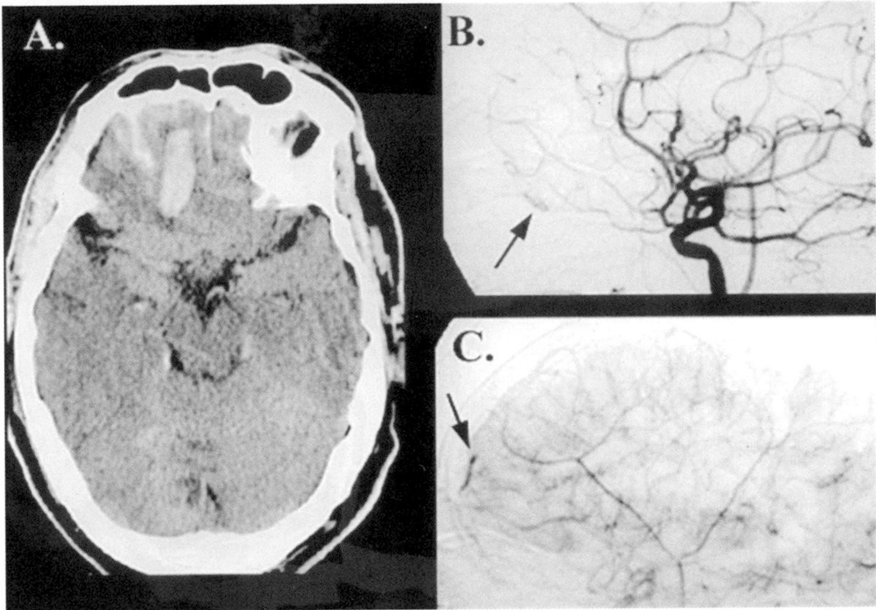

FIGURE 16-14. Spontaneous frontal hematoma in a 63-year-old patient. **A.** Noncontrast computed tomography with right frontal hematoma. **B.** Lateral right carotid angiogram—arterial phase. Small, less than 1-cm arteriovenous malformation nidus (*arrow*) is present, supplied from a frontal branch of the anterior cerebral artery. **C.** Lateral right carotid angiogram—late arterial/capillary phase. Early draining vein is noted (*arrow*) coursing superiorly to the superior sagittal sinus.

supply in which normal brain parenchyma is also supplied, however, should be avoided due to the risk of normal brain infarction.[86]

Dural Arteriovenous Malformations

Dural AVMs represent 10–15% of arteriovenous shunting intracranial vascular malformations. Thirty-five percent of infratentorial and 6% of supratentorial AVMs are purely dural. DAVMs have an annual hemorrhage rate of 1.8%.[87] Nonhemorrhagic clinical presentations include headache, bruit, tinnitus, hydrocephalus, and papilledema, depending on the location of the malformation. DAVMs may cause intraparenchymal, subarachnoid, or subdural hemorrhage. The mortality from bleeding is between 10% and 20%.

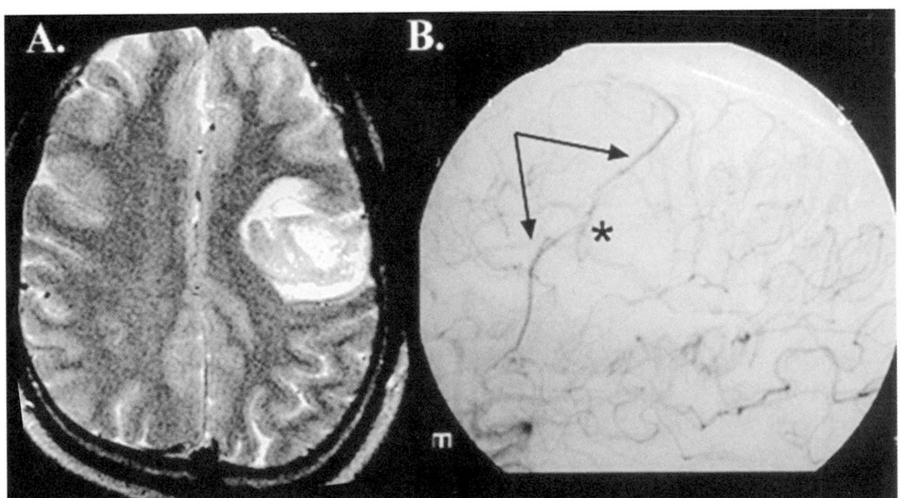

FIGURE 16-15. Patient presented with left parietal headache and acute onset of Broca's aphasia. **A.** This T2-weighted magnetic resonance image demonstrates a nonspecific left parietal hemorrhage, with the possibility of an underlying hemorrhagic lesion. Note the hematocrit level within the hematoma. Angiogram at presentation (not shown) demonstrated an avascular mass corresponding to the hematoma with no other abnormalities. **B.** Follow-up left lateral carotid angiogram 6 weeks later—late arterial phase. Early draining veins (*arrows*) are present in addition to the avascular mass (*asterisk*). These early draining veins resolved on the follow-up angiogram 2 months later. These findings are consistent with shunting from a hematoma, a potential mimic for an arteriovenous malformation. Follow-up angiography was crucial, in this case, to exclude an underlying arteriovenous malformation.

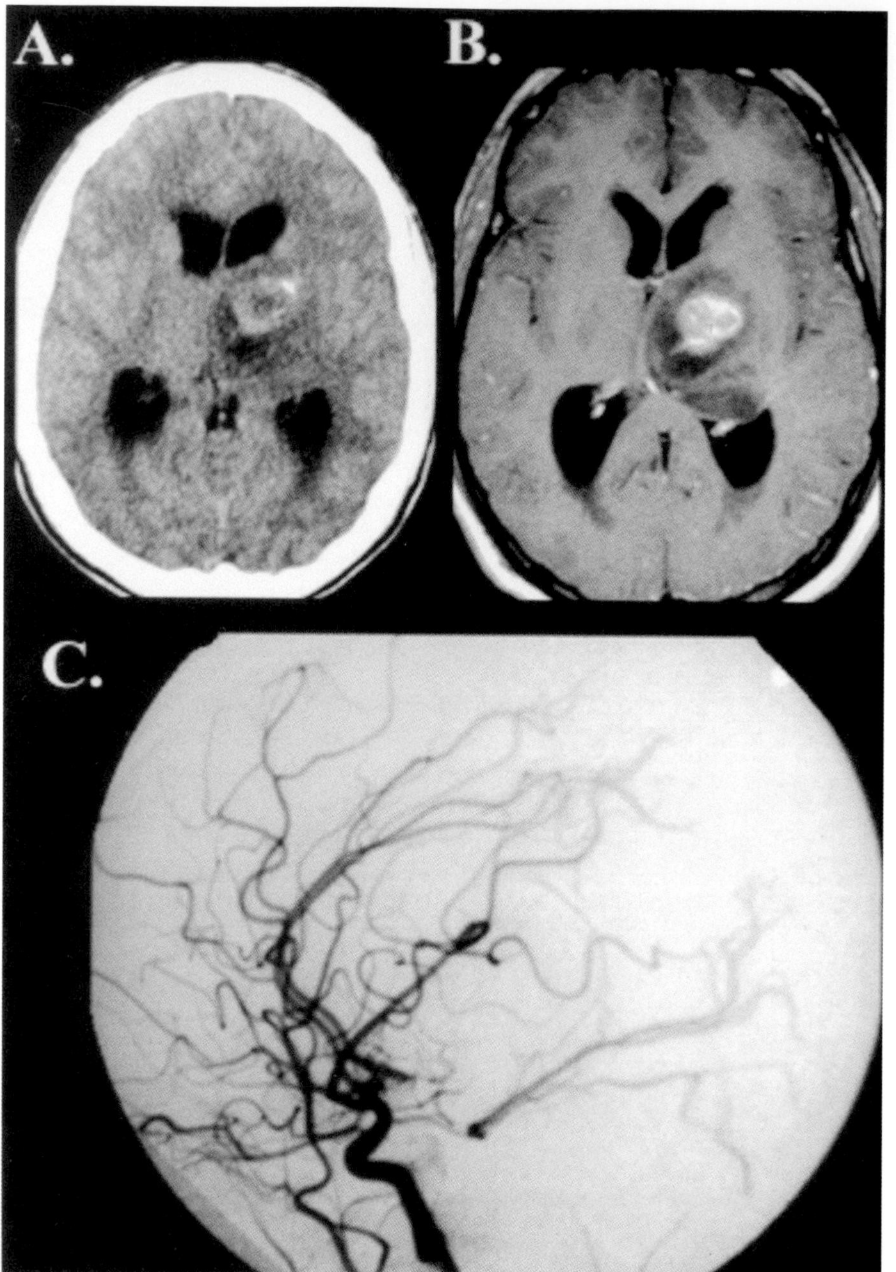

FIGURE 16-16. Hemorrhagic glioblastoma. **A.** Computed tomography without contrast demonstrates a nonspecific hemorrhagic lesion in the left thalamus. **B.** This T1-weighted magnetic resonance image with gadolinium is also nonspecific. A mass with areas of hemorrhage and enhancement is present. **C.** Left lateral carotid angiogram did not demonstrate evidence of enlarged feeding arteries or early draining veins to suggest an arteriovenous malformation. Subtle, abnormal enhancement (not well seen) in the left middle cerebral artery territory is present. Feeding arteries are not significantly enlarged. Biopsy demonstrated glioblastoma multiforme.

As opposed to parenchymal AVMs, these lesions receive blood only from dural branches of the external carotid artery, vertebral artery, or internal carotid artery (Figure 16-19). External carotid arterial supply is the most common. DAVMs tend to occur within or adjacent to the walls of the dural sinuses. The transverse, sigmoid, and cavernous sinuses are the most commonly involved.[88] DAVMs are generally considered to be acquired lesions. Dural sinus thrombosis is presumed to be the etiology in many cases. Occasionally, a history of trauma, craniotomy, sinus thrombosis, or infection is present. Congenital dural AVMs can also occur. These usually represent larger fistulas and present similarly to vein of Galen malformations.[89]

The likelihood of symptomatic life-threatening presentations (hemorrhage and neurologic deficits) has been correlated with the pattern of venous drainage. The most widely used classification system for DAVMs predicts the risk of hemorrhage and other aggressive behavior based on whether the drainage is into the dural sinuses or cortical veins, the direction of venous drainage (antegrade or retrograde), and the presence of venous varices.[90] DAVMs that drain antegrade into the dural sinuses have the lowest risk of hemorrhage. DAVMs that drain into cortical veins, particularly if associated with venous ectasia (>5 mm), have the highest risk of hemorrhage.[87,90–93] Also, drainage into the deep Galenic system is associ-

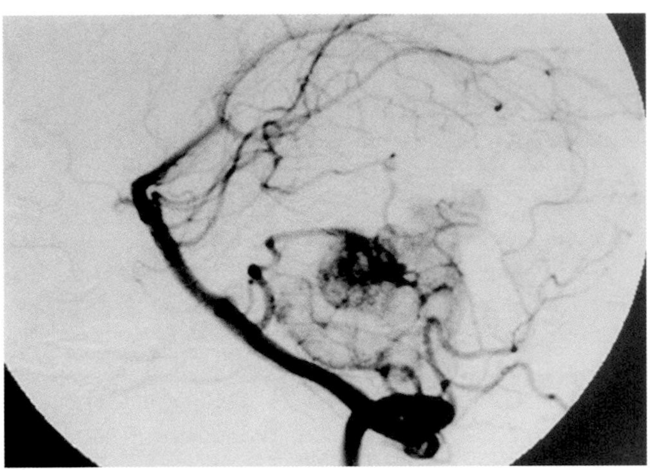

FIGURE 16-17. Twenty-seven-year-old woman with von Hippel-Lindau disease and multiple posterior fossa hemangioblastomas. Lateral vertebral angiogram demonstrates dense nodular enhancement with faint enhancement around the margin of the cyst. The main arterial supply is from an enlarged anterior inferior cerebellar artery. Contribution from branches of the posterior inferior cerebellar artery and vertebral artery are also present. No early draining veins were seen.

ated with a higher risk of hemorrhage, possibly due to increased stenoses in this system.[92]

CT may show subarachnoid, subdural, or intraparenchymal hemorrhage. Adjacent parenchymal edema, secondary to venous hypertension, may be present. After contrast administration, dural enhancement and enlarged cortical veins may be seen. CT scans are frequently normal.[86] On bone window settings, enlarged vascular grooves, secondary to enlarged feeding arteries, may be present.

MRI similarly may not detect a dural AVF, particularly if the DAVM drains into an unobstructed sinus. However, MRI is more sensitive to DAVMs than CT.[58,94,95] MRI may demonstrate dilated cortical vessels, especially if veno-occlusive disease is present. Edema, hemorrhage, and associated infarcts may also be seen. After gadolinium administration, small areas of dural enhancement or venous thrombosis may be apparent.[96–98] MRA may show an associated abnormality but is frequently negative.

Angiography remains the gold standard for the diagnosis of DAVMs. The internal carotid, external carotid, and vertebral arteries must all be separately evaluated. Like AVMs, the hallmark of DAVMs is arteriovenous shunting with an early draining vein. DAVMs are usually described by their location. Their location reflects the usual arterial supply and venous drainage as detailed below.[88]

Transverse and sigmoid sinus DAVMs are the most common. Typically, they present with bruit, tinnitus, focal pain, or headache. Occipital and ascending pharyngeal branches of the external carotid artery, the posterior branch of the middle meningeal artery, tentorial arteries, meningeal branches of the vertebral artery, and, rarely, posterior auricular branches most often supply these DAVMs. They usually drain into the sigmoid and transverse sinuses (see Figure 16-19). In high-grade stenotic lesions of the affected sinus or with sinus thrombosis, reflux into supratentorial and infratentorial cortical veins may occur.

Superior sagittal sinus DAVMs typically present with headache or hemorrhage.[58] Branches of the middle meningeal artery, transosseous branches of superficial

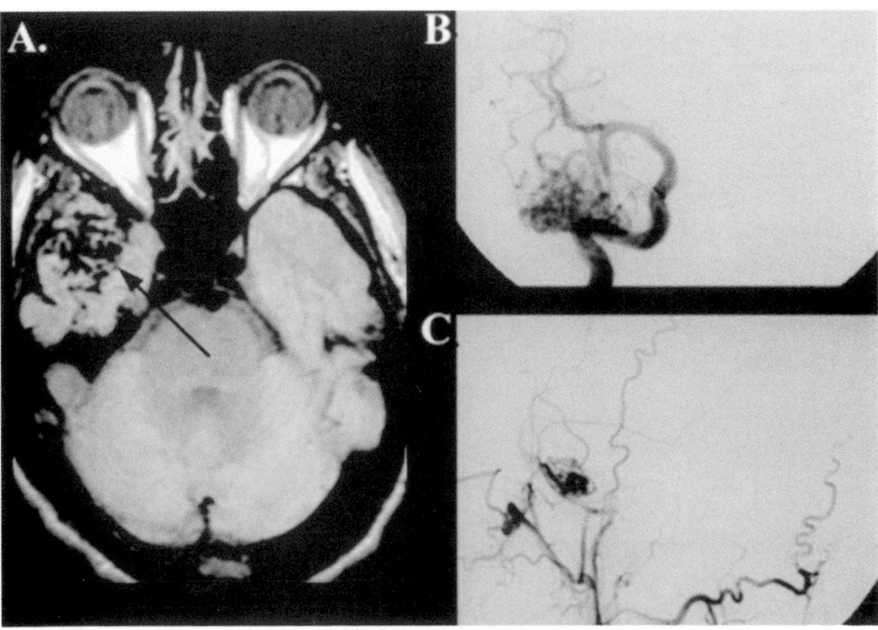

FIGURE 16-18. Right temporal mixed pial-dural arteriovenous malformation. **A.** This axial magnetic resonance image demonstrates characteristic flow voids in the right temporal arteriovenous malformation nidus (*arrow*). **B.** Frontal view of the right internal carotid artery. Enlarged right middle cerebral artery feeders are present, supplying the right temporal lobe arteriovenous malformation nidus. Posterior circulation supply was also present on the vertebral artery injection (not shown). **C.** Right lateral external carotid angiogram. External carotid supply via anterior middle meningeal branches is seen. Middle cerebral artery and external carotid artery branches were embolized.

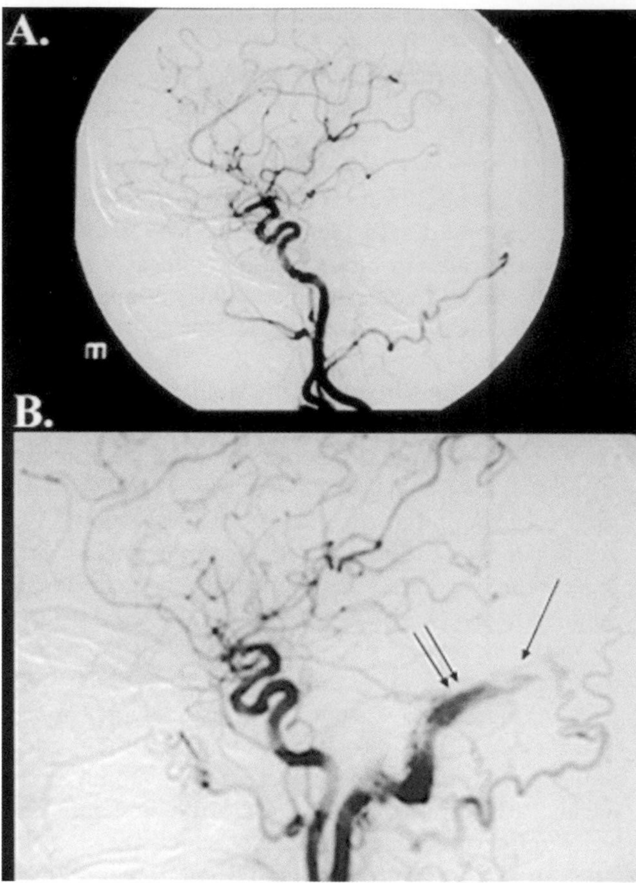

FIGURE 16-19. This patient heard a "whooshing" sound years after repair of a left cerebellar arteriovenous malformation. **A.** Left lateral common carotid artery injection—arterial phase. Prominent left occipital artery is present. **B.** Slightly later arterial phase demonstrates early antegrade filling of the left sigmoid sinus (*double arrows*) due to a left occipital dural arteriovenous malformation (*arrow*). This is near the site of the previous craniotomy. Antegrade flow into a major dural sinus and absence of reflux into cortical veins favor a nonaggressive type of dural fistula.

temporal artery, occipital artery, anterior falcine branch of the ophthalmic artery, and posterior meningeal branch from the vertebral artery constitute the most common supply of these DAVMs. They drain into the superior sagittal sinus with occasional pial venous drainage over the convexities.[58,88]

Anterior cranial fossa DAVMs frequently present with intracranial hemorrhage. They are usually supplied from ethmoidal dural branches of the ophthalmic artery or the sphenopalatine artery. Venous drainage is typically into pial veins in the frontal lobe.[58,88]

Tentorial DAVMs also frequently present initially with intracranial hemorrhage. The meningohypophyseal trunk from the internal carotid arteries, infratentorial branches from the posterior cerebral artery, and superior cerebellar arteries are the usual supply. Venous drainage is into the vein of Galen or straight sinus and may flow retrograde into the internal cerebral veins.[58,88]

Pial Arteriovenous Fistulas

Most pial AVFs are encountered as a component of an AVM nidus. Isolated pial AVFs are very uncommon.[11] Pial AVFs represent a direct, subpial communication between a single cerebral or cerebellar artery and a draining vein. They are seen most frequently in children. Congestive heart failure and seizures are the most common presenting symptoms in children. Hemorrhage may also occur. An acquired AVF has been reported but is extremely rare.[99]

NONSHUNTING VASCULAR MALFORMATIONS

Cavernous Malformations

Clinical Presentation

Cavernous malformations have an incidence of 0.4–1.0% in the general population and constitute 10–15% of all intracranial vascular malformations.[6,100–106] Sporadic and familial forms exist. The familial form may constitute as many as half of all cases.[104,107,108] Cases of the familial form have been mapped to several different loci, including two loci on chromosome 7 and one locus on chromosome 3.[105,109] Cavernous malformations are multiple in approximately 25% of patients. Multiple lesions are more common in the familial form.[104] With modern MR techniques, multiple lesions may be even more commonly diagnosed (Figure 16-20).[107]

In the brain, 80–90% of lesions are supratentorial and 10–20% are infratentorial.[6,100,103,105,110,111] Seizures are reported as the most common presenting symptom. Seizures occur in 25–50% of patients[100,105,111] with an annual new-onset seizure incidence of 2.4%.[101,112] Other patients may present with headaches, focal neurologic deficits, and hemorrhage. As many as 40% of patients remain asymptomatic. Hemorrhage occurs with an annual incidence between 0.25% and 3.10% per patient.[100,101,103,105,109,111,113–115] The incidence is higher in the familial form due to the increased number of lesions per patient. Patients who initially present with hemorrhage may be more likely to hemorrhage in the future,[114] although others have disputed this claim.[101] Female patients may hemorrhage from cavernous malformations more frequently than male patients.[103,114]

Pathology

Cavernous malformations are well-circumscribed lesions consisting of enlarged, sinusoidal vascular spaces with

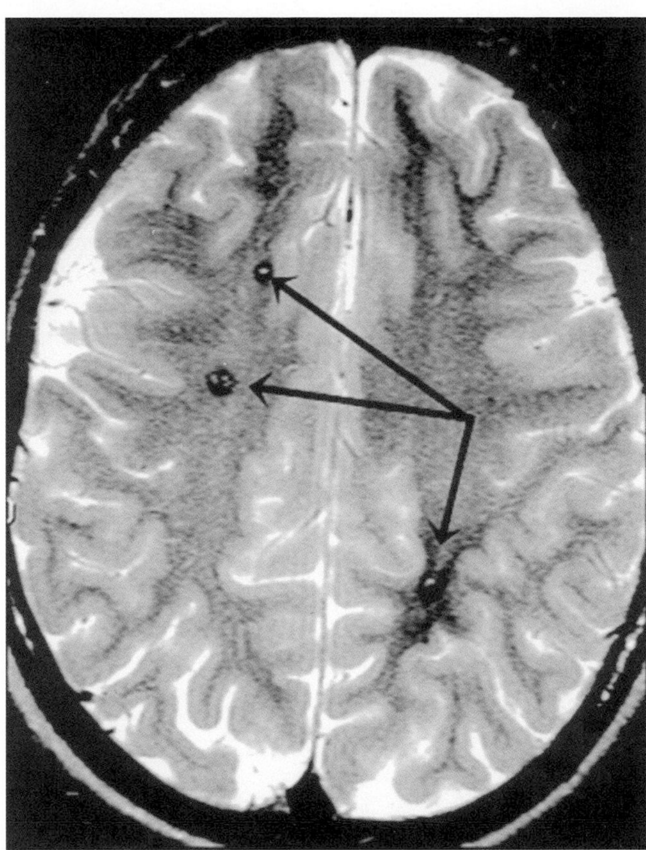

FIGURE 16-20. Patient with multiple cavernous malformations (*arrows*). This T2-weighted axial magnetic resonance image demonstrates typical dark hemosiderin rim and central increased signal.

little or no intervening brain parenchyma. The walls are lined by a single layer of vascular endothelium and do not contain elastin or smooth muscle. Focal areas of calcification may be present. Hemosiderin-laden macrophages are usually present. A rim of surrounding hemosiderin and ferritin is characteristic. Grossly, they appear as a lobulated purplish mass.[6,13,38,105,116] Cavernous malformations may be related to capillary malformations. Some investigators have suggested that these represent different ends of a spectrum of the same pathologic entity.[117] Cavernous malformations are dynamic lesions with changes in size secondary to repeated episodes of intralesional hemorrhage.[38,103,105,109,111] Although most lesions are congenital, de novo lesions have also been reported.[109,115,118,119]

Imaging

Computed Tomography Scans. CT scans of cavernous malformations demonstrate an irregular isodense or hyperdense lesion. Calcification may be present. Contrast enhancement is variable and may be absent. Associated hemorrhage may be present as well. Small AVMs and neoplasms occasionally have a similar appearance, particularly if hemorrhage is present. CT frequently misses lesions detected by MRI, which is a more sensitive test.[100,104,107,120,121]

Magnetic Resonance Scans. MRI is very sensitive and specific for detecting cavernous malformations.[100,101,105,107] Cavernous malformations frequently have a characteristic reticulated core of mixed but predominantly high signal intensity and a rim of low signal on T1- and T2-weighted images. The central signal represents blood products of different age and, occasionally, calcification. This reflects the dynamic nature of cavernous malformations with numerous, sometimes subclinical, episodes of hemorrhage. The rim of surrounding low signal, representing hemosiderin-laden macrophages and ferritin,[96,105] is more pronounced on T2- than T1-weighted images (see Figure 16-20; Figure 16-21). Smaller lesions may appear as punctate areas of low signal intensity on T2-weighted images. T1-weighted images are less sensitive than T2-weighted images. Variable enhancement, if any, may occur with gadolinium (Figure 16-22). Adjacent parenchymal gliosis also may be present, which appears as increased signal on T2-weighted images. A cavernous malformation may occasionally have surrounding edema or hemorrhage. Gradient echo sequences and high-resolution blood oxygenation level–dependent venography detect more lesions than conventional magnetic resonance sequences (Figure 16-23).[107,122–124]

Angiography

Angiography is frequently negative in patients with cavernous malformations.[96,104,105,125,126] Cavernous malformations constitute the most common causes of the so-called angiographic occult malformations. Occasionally, nonspecific findings, such as an avascular mass, a blush of contrast, or pooling of contrast may be seen. Enlarged arteries and early draining veins are not present (see Figure 16-22D). Presence of an enlarged venous structure raises the possibility of a coexistent developmental venous malformation (see Figure 16-22B and C). Angiography is frequently necessary to exclude the possibility of an AVM in cases in which an enlarged venous structure is present.

Differential Diagnosis

The magnetic resonance appearance of cavernous malformations is often diagnostic. However, in some cases, differentiation from hemorrhage of other causes, including malignancy, hypertension, and AVMs, may be difficult. The presence of an incomplete rim of hypointensity, a single blood product, and adjacent edema should make one consider other diagnoses, although these findings

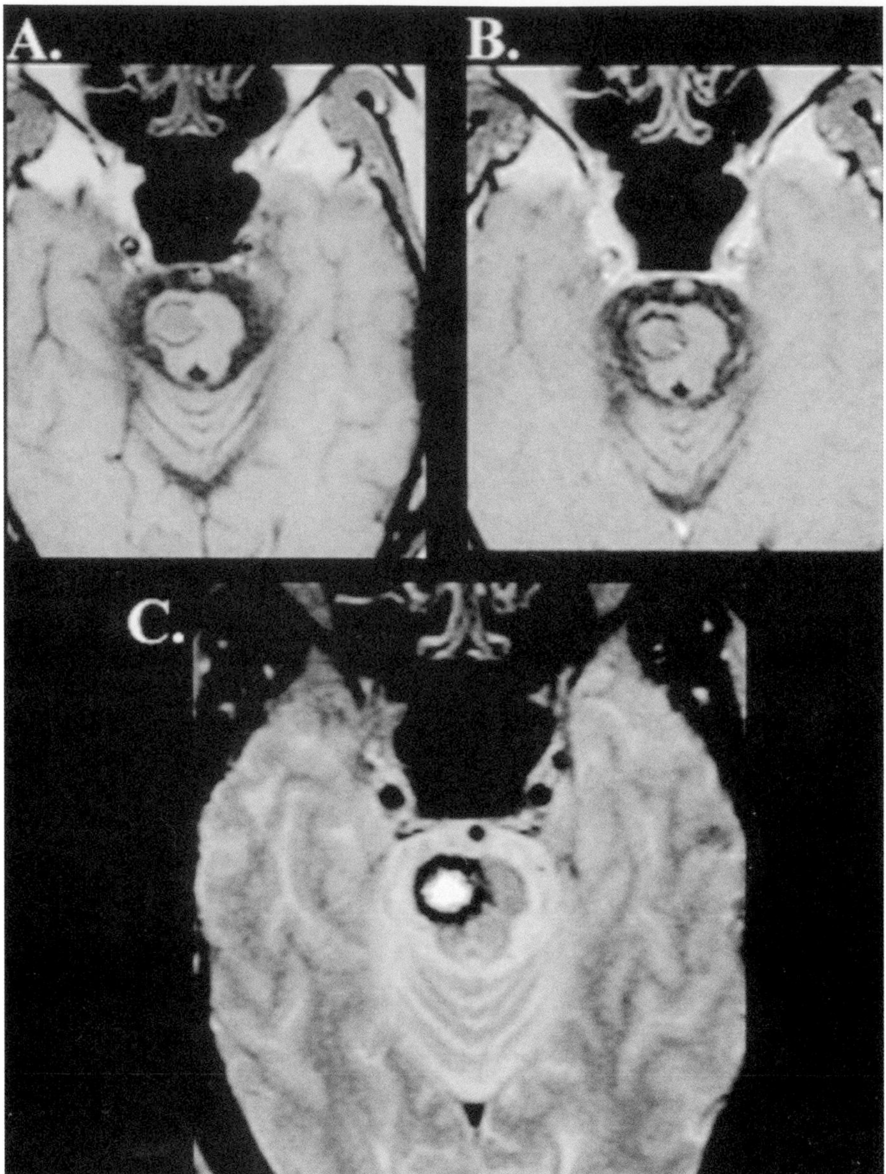

FIGURE 16-21. Classic cavernous malformation. **A.** T1-weighted magnetic resonance image with right pontine lesion. Low signal rim with central increased signal is present. **B.** T1-weighted postgadolinium image with very subtle enhancement. **C.** T2-weighted image with prominent rim of low signal due to hemosiderin and increased central signal. The rim of decreased signal is more prominent because T2-weighted images are affected more than T1-weighted images by the magnetic susceptibility effect of hemosiderin.

are occasionally seen with cavernous malformations as well (note the edema in Figure 16-22C).[127]

Capillary Malformations

Clinical Presentation

Capillary malformations are usually small, incidental lesions. They are seen most frequently in the pons but may also occur in the cerebral cortex and periventricular regions. Multiple lesions may be present. Hemorrhagic and symptomatic lesions are extremely rare but have been reported.

Pathology

Histologically, capillary malformations represent a collection of dilated, thin-walled vessels with normal intervening brain parenchyma. The walls of the vessels do not contain any muscle or elastica. The presence of normal, intervening brain parenchyma distinguishes capillary malformations from cavernous malformations.[38,105] Grossly, capillary malformations appear as a pinkish, discolored area.[5,38] Gliosis, mineralization, and hemorrhage are very rare but have been reported.[38,86] Hemosiderin is not present.[105] They are considered congenital lesions. Some consider capillary malformations to represent one end of the spectrum of the same pathologic entity as cavernous malformations.[117]

Imaging

On CT, capillary malformations may demonstrate subtle enhancement corresponding to a normal area on precontrast CT scans. MRI may demonstrate a discrete

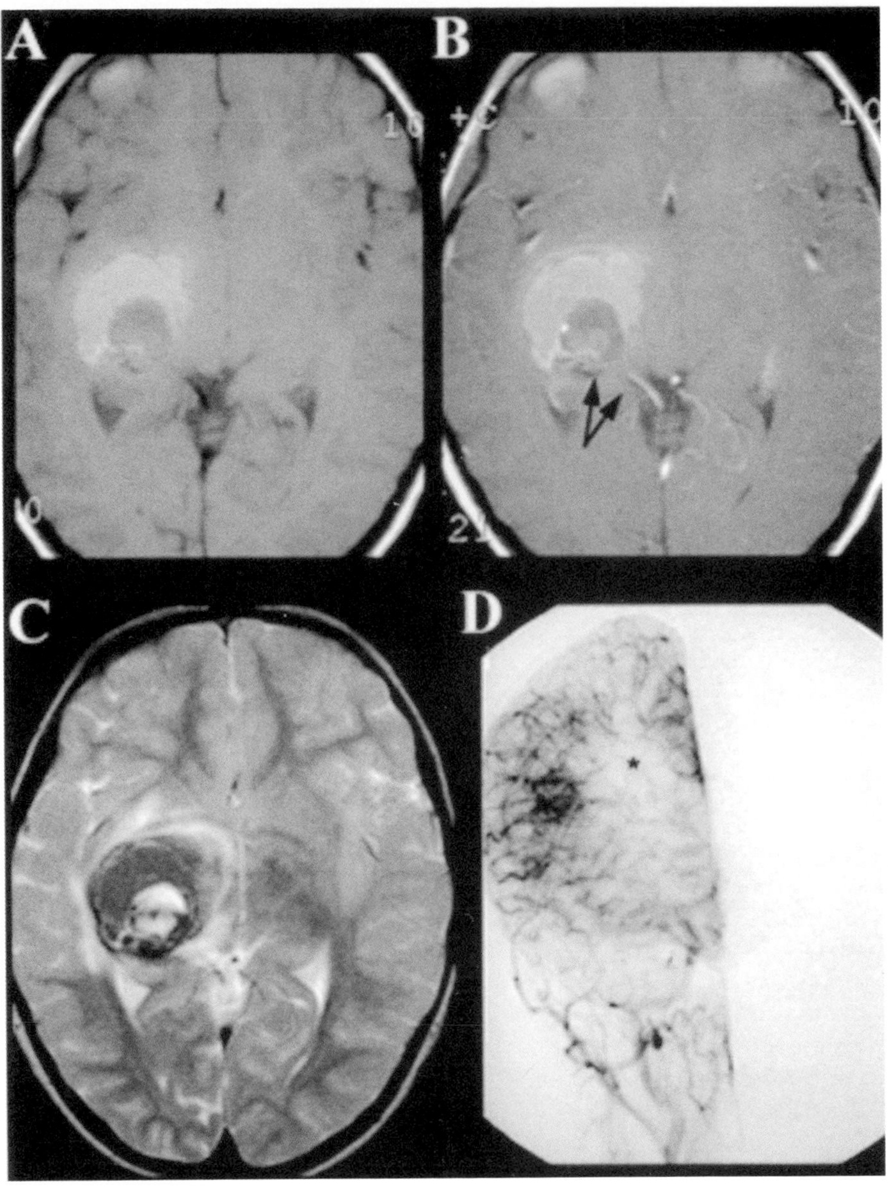

FIGURE 16-22. Five-year-old girl with new left-sided hemiparesis. Large hemorrhagic cavernous malformation with associated developmental venous anomaly. (Other images not shown here demonstrated multiple other cavernous malformations.) **A.** This T1-weighted magnetic resonance image demonstrates a large nonspecific, intraparenchymal hemorrhage in the right basal ganglia. **B.** This T1-weighted image with gadolinium demonstrates some nodular enhancement in the posterior aspect of the mass. Also, a linear component is present (*arrows*), likely representing an associated developmental venous anomaly. **C.** This T2-weighted image demonstrates the large hemorrhage with surrounding edema. (Note the faint flow void at the posterior aspect of the hemorrhage, corresponding with the linear enhancement in the developmental venous anomaly denoted by the *arrows* in **B.**) **D.** Right internal carotid angiogram—late arterial/capillary phase. The area corresponding to the hemorrhage is avascular (*asterisk*), with no early draining vein to suggest an arteriovenous malformation. The associated developmental venous anomaly seen in (**B**) and (**C**) is confirmed on the venous phase of the angiogram.

focus of enhancement without associated signal abnormality. A stippled or brush-like pattern of enhancement has been described.[58,105] No mass effect is present. Occasionally, a mild area of hypointensity on T1-weighted images and hyperintensity on T2-weighted images may be present. Gradient echo images frequently demonstrate low signal throughout the lesion, possibly due to susceptibility from deoxyhemoglobin in small vessels (Figure 16-24). Angiography is usually negative, although a subtle blush of contrast is occasionally seen.

Differential Diagnosis

The differential diagnosis includes gliomas, infarct, demyelination, central pontine myelinolysis, and infarct. Low signal on gradient echo images supports the diagnosis of a capillary malformation.

DEVELOPMENTAL VENOUS ANOMALIES

Clinical Presentation

DVAs represent the most common vascular malformation and are present in up to 3% of the population.[6,106] They represented 63% of vascular malformations in one large autopsy series.[106] They are also the most common vascular malformation seen on MRI brain scans.[128] The frontal lobe (40%) and posterior fossa (20%) are the most common locations. DVAs usually represent an incidental finding but may become symptomatic. The annual risk of symptomatic hemorrhage from DVAs has been reported to range from 0.22% to 0.34%. However, hemorrhage in the context of a venous malformation usually implies the presence of an underlying, undetected cavernous malformation.[96,129,130] Posterior fossa DVAs are symptomatic more frequently than other loca-

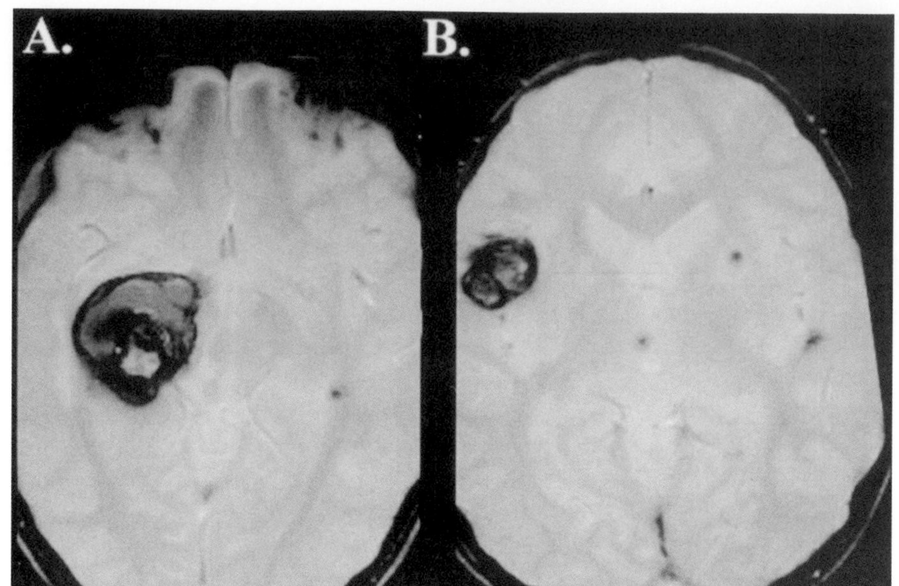

FIGURE 16-23. Same patient as in Figure 16-21. These gradient-echo axial images (**A**,**B**) demonstrate multiple cavernous malformations not seen well on the standard spin echo sequences (see Figure 16-21). Areas of signal loss are due to magnetic susceptibility from hemosiderin. This sequence is very sensitive for demonstrating cavernous malformations.

tions. Headache, diplopia, ataxia, numbness, dysphagia, trigeminal neuralgia, and hearing disturbances have all been reported in association with this lesion.[108,130–132]

Pathology

DVAs are abnormally enlarged venous structures separated by normal brain parenchyma. The vessels are arranged in a radial pattern and drain into a deep or superficial venous sinus.[38] The pattern of venous drainage cannot be accurately predicted based on the location of the DVA.[133] DVAs essentially represent normal venous structures in an abnormal location. Surgical removal may cause infarction of the territory drained by the DVA.

Imaging

Computed Tomography

On CT, DVAs most often appear as a subtle linear hyperdensity prior to contrast, with characteristic linear transcerebral enhancement entering a cortical vein, dural sinus, or deep vein after contrast administration. A characteristic *caput medusae*, representing the convergence of the medullary veins into a central draining vein, is frequently seen.[128,134] CT angiography may also demonstrate DVAs.[135] CT with contrast detects 86% of DVAs (Figure 16-25).[60]

Magnetic Resonance Imaging

On MRI, DVAs appear as a tubular hypointensity on T1-weighted images and are variable on T2-weighted images. A congruent hyperintensity may be seen adjacent to a hypointense vessel in oblique vessels on spin echo sequences secondary to slow flow.[89] Enhancement occurs after gadolinium administration, similar to the appearance on CT, with the characteristic caput medusae. Although diagnosis may be made with T2-weighted images, postgadolinium T1-weighted images optimally demonstrate DVAs (Figures 16-26 and 16-27A).[133] MRI often provides a specific diagnosis without the need for angiography.[136] Postcontrast MRA may be used to visualize these lesions,[96] although this is usually not necessary.

Angiography

Angiography may be needed in cases of large, atypical, or symptomatic DVAs to exclude arteriovenous shunting that could represent an AVM. Angiography demonstrates normal arterial and capillary phases in patients with DVAs. Characteristic dilated, radially oriented medullary veins are seen draining into the larger, transcerebral draining vein on the venous phase (see Figure 16-27B and C). The draining vein may enter a dural sinus, a cortical vein, a deep vein, or a subependymal vein. Arteriovenous shunting is not present. A focal stenosis at the site of drainage of the central draining vein into a dural sinus or superficial or deep vein is occasionally seen.[137]

MIXED VASCULAR MALFORMATIONS

AVMs, DVAs, cavernous malformations, and capillary malformations have all been reported to be associated with each other in various combinations.[12,138–140] DVAs and cavernous malformations are most commonly associated and the most easily recognized, because each

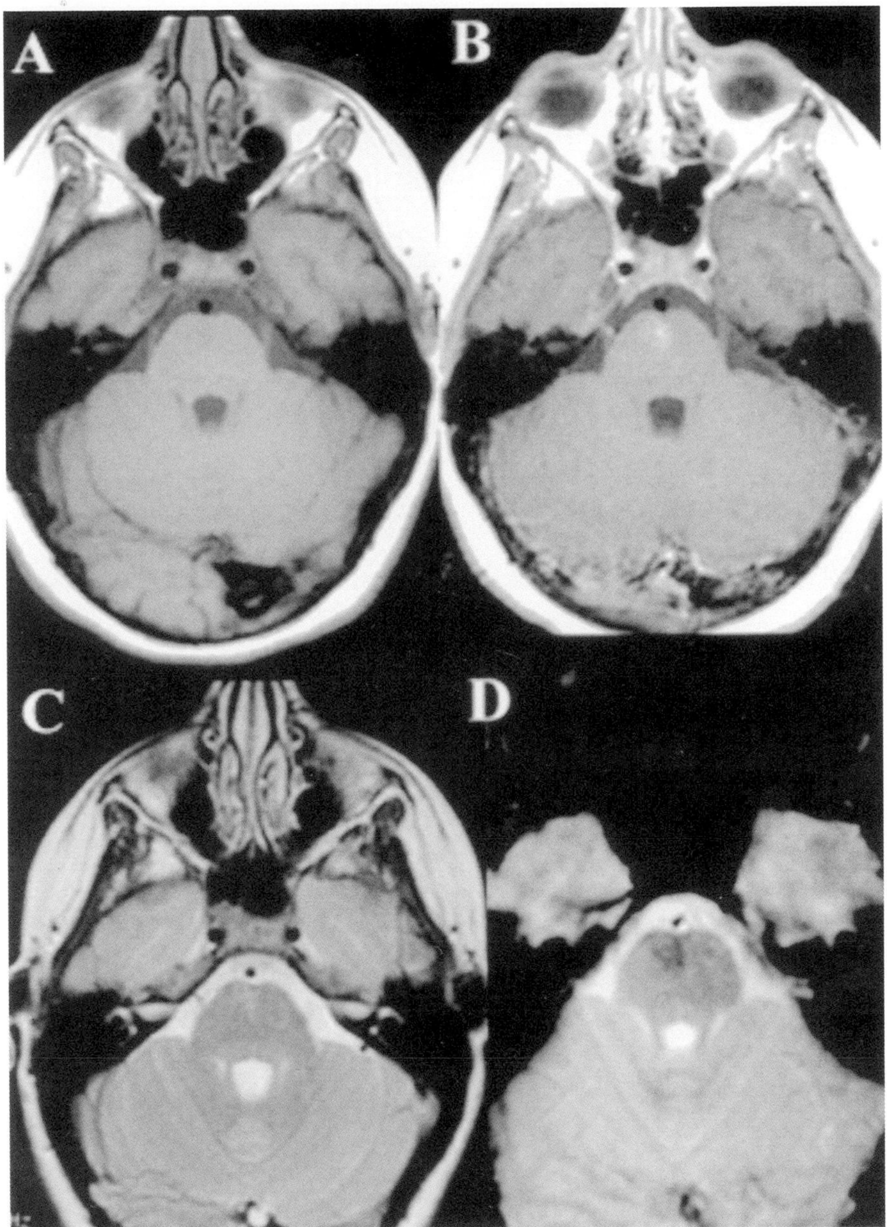

FIGURE 16-24. Capillary malformation. **A.** T1-weighted magnetic resonance image. Very subtle area of low signal intensity in the right pons. **B.** Postgadolinium T1-weighted image. Abnormal area of enhancement in right pons. No associated mass effect is present. **C.** T2-weighted image. The lesion has subtle increased signal. **D.** This gradient echo image demonstrates signal loss. This favors a capillary malformation. The lesion will be managed conservatively and followed with magnetic resonance imaging.

has a relatively distinct radiologic appearance (Figure 16-28). These two lesions coexist in 27–33% of cases.[131,141] AVMs occurring with cavernous malformations and DVAs may be more difficult to recognize. Angiography may be necessary in such cases to determine if arteriovenous shunting, the distinguishing feature of an AVM, is present.

VEIN OF GALEN MALFORMATIONS

Vein of Galen malformations include a complex set of abnormalities. These may be classified as vein of Galen aneurysmal malformations (VGAM) and vein of Galen dilatations.[11,12,142] VGAM are direct, fistulous communications between arteries and midline venous structures. The venous structures often represent persistence of primitive vascular structures. Vein of Galen dilatations simply represent shunting lesions draining into the normal vein of Galen. It may be difficult to distinguish between these types of entities.

VGAM include mural and choroidal types.[89] The more common choroidal type represents 90% of VGAM. These are characterized by numerous arteriovenous shunts in the velum interpositum and involve the anterior wall of the median prosencephalic vein.[11,89,142] The less common mural type represents a specific malformation, with fewer, larger dural AVFs within the wall of a venous sac that is located in the quadrigeminal cistern. The venous sac most likely represents the embryonic median prosencephalic vein and does not represent

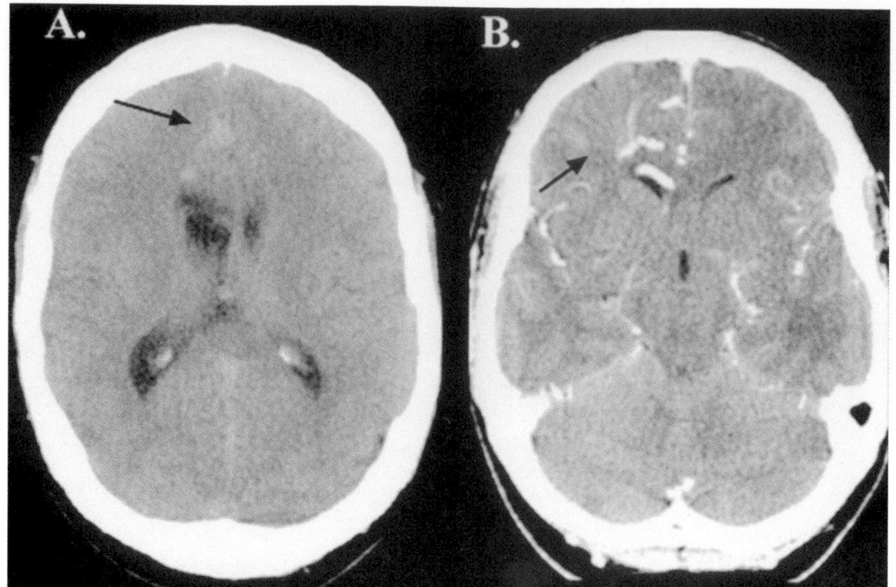

FIGURE 16-25. Thirty-eight-year-old man with headaches. Incidental developmental venous anomaly. **A.** Noncontrast computed tomography with slight hyperdensity in right frontal lobe (*arrow*). **B.** Postcontrast computed tomography with enhancing, dilated medullary veins (*arrow*) draining into a large, subependymal vein in the right frontal horn of the lateral ventricle. These are characteristic features of a developmental venous anomaly.

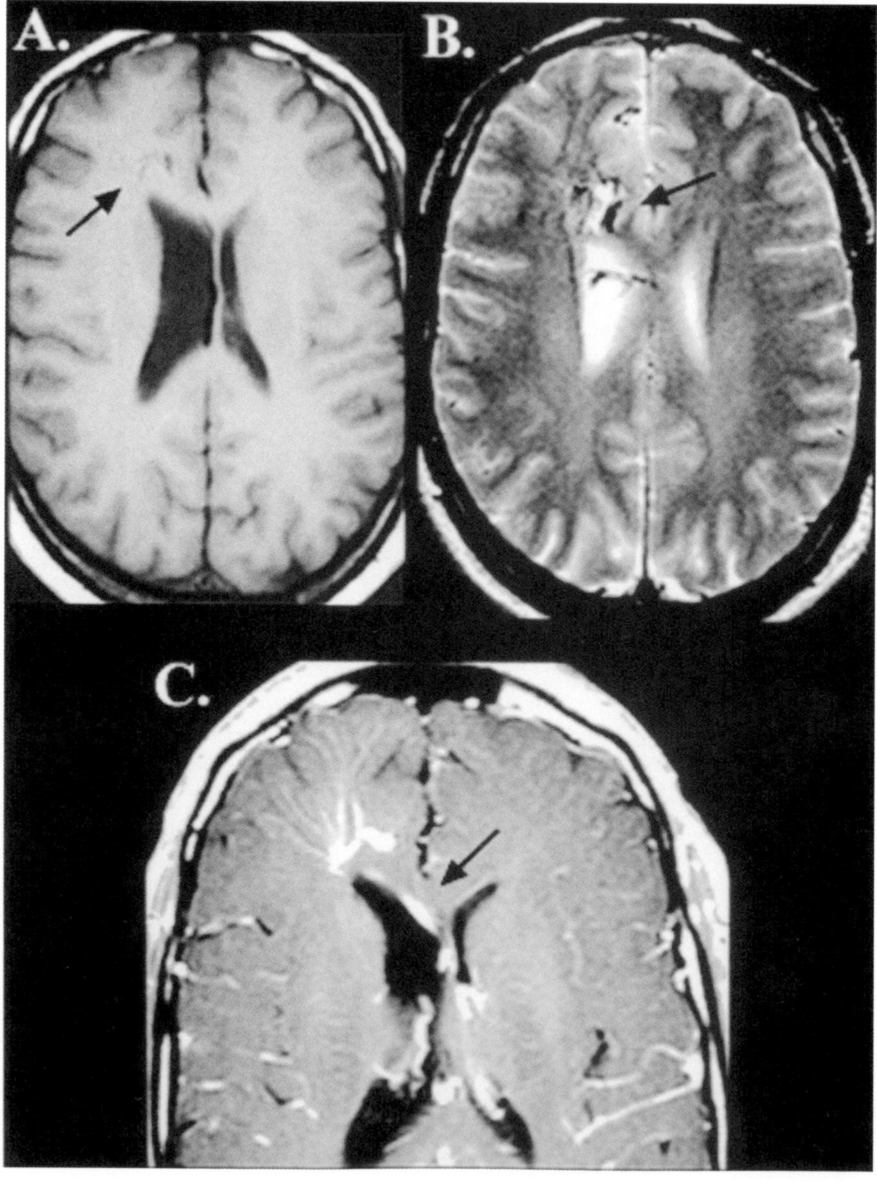

FIGURE 16-26. Developmental venous anomaly (same patient as in Figure 16-25). **A.** T1-weighted image with flow void (low signal) in the right frontal lobe demonstrates the developmental venous anomaly (*arrow*). **B.** T2-weighted image with flow void in the right frontal lobe also shows the developmental venous anomaly. The flow void in the draining subependymal vein in the right frontal horn is well demonstrated (*arrow*). **C.** T1-weighted postgadolinium image shows the characteristic pattern of enhancement of the right frontal lobe of the developmental venous anomaly. Enhancement is present in the enlarged, draining subependymal vein (*arrow*).

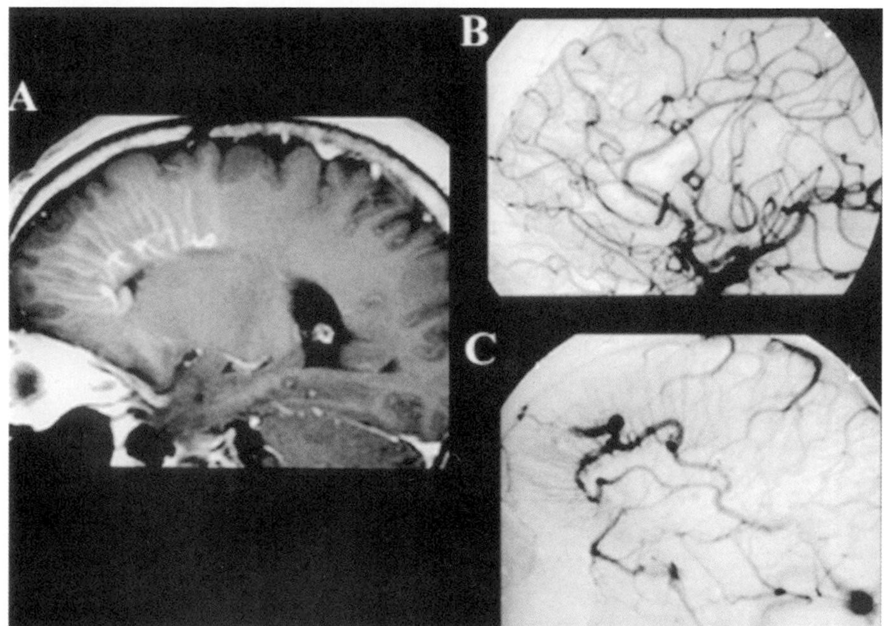

FIGURE 16-27. Developmental venous anomaly (same patient as in Figures 16-25 and 16-26). **A.** Sagittal T1-weighted postgadiolinium image shows the characteristic dilated medullary veins of a developmental venous anomaly. **B.** Lateral right carotid angiogram—arterial phase. No abnormality is present as expected. **C.** Lateral right carotid angiogram—venous phase. Characteristic dilated medullary veins draining into a large subependymal vein are present. The normal arterial phase and absence of early draining veins distinguish this from an arteriovenous malformation (although the magnetic resonance imaging is diagnostic in this case).

the true vein of Galen. This venous sac often drains into a persistent falcine sinus. The falcine sinus slopes upward in the anteroposterior direction as opposed to the downward slope of the normal straight sinus. The straight sinus may be present or absent. Often, features of both types are present.

The clinical symptoms of VGAM vary with the age of presentation.[143] Choroidal malformations usually present symptomatically during the neonate period or during early infancy. Congestive heart failure is the most common presentation. The condition is usually lethal without intervention. Prognosis is poor even with treatment. The mural form of VGAM typically presents later in infancy. Common presentations include hydrocephalus, macrocephaly, seizures, and developmental delay. Congestive heart failure is mild or absent.[89] Hydrocephalus may be secondary to aqueductal compression or venous hypertension, causing impaired cerebrospinal fluid resorption. Children older than 1 year of age may present with signs of venous obstruction from thrombosis of the straight or transverse sinus or jugular veins. Macrocephaly and huge facial and cervical veins may result. Stenosis and thrombosis of the venous drainage are frequent and

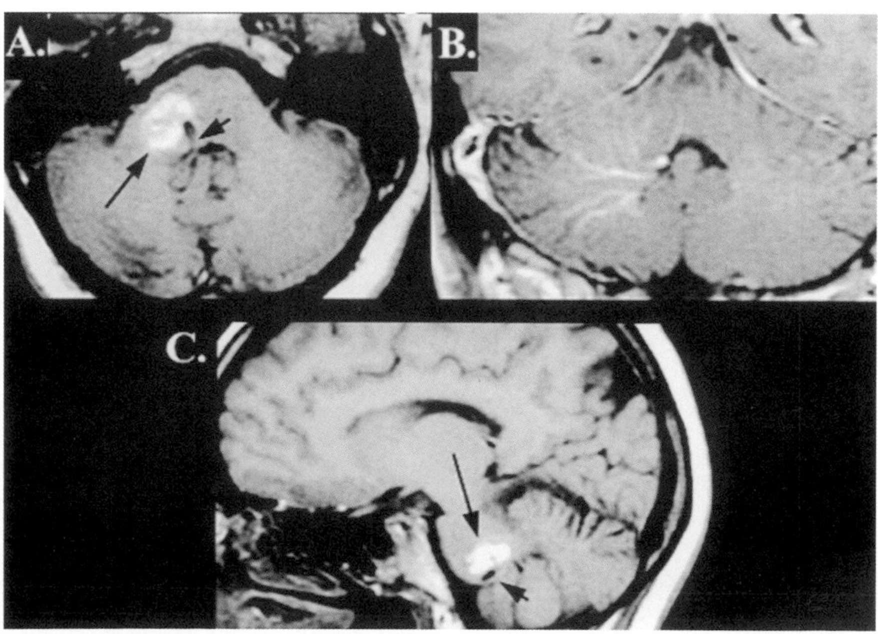

FIGURE 16-28. Associated cavernous malformation and developmental venous anomaly. **A.** T1-weighted image with bright signal intensity in a cavernous malformation in the right pons (*long arrow*). Note the flow void at the posterior aspect of the cavernous malformation (*short arrow*). **B.** T1-weighted postgadolinium magnetic resonance image with typical enhancement in the right cerebellum diagnostic of an associated developmental venous anomaly. This corresponds to the flow void in (**A**). **C.** Same patient with sagittal T1-weighted image with cavernous malformation (*long arrow*) and flow void in the associated developmental venous anomaly (*short arrow*).

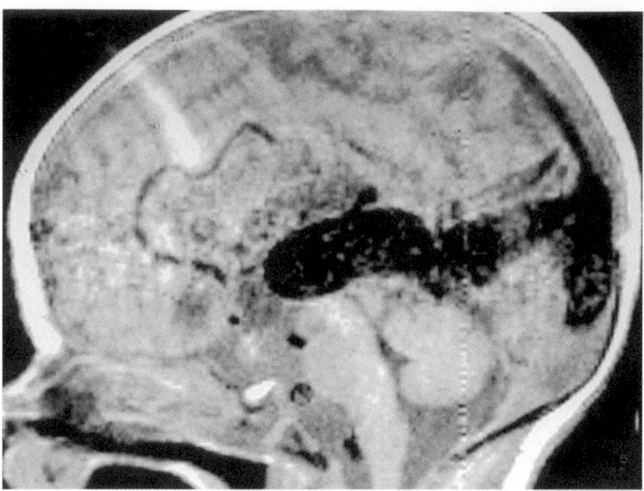

FIGURE 16-29. Neonate with congestive heart failure. This sagittal T1-weighted magnetic resonance image demonstrates the typical flow void in a large venous sac in the quadrigeminal cistern, consistent with a vein of Galen vascular malformation. Note the pulsation artifact in the anteroposterior direction.

lead to complications. Hemorrhage and neurologic deficits also may be presenting symptoms.[144]

The diagnosis of VGAM is frequently suggested on prenatal or neonatal ultrasound with identification of a large midline hypoechoic or anechoic structure. Color Doppler ultrasound scanning reveals a high-flow lesion. On CT scanning, an isodense or hyperdense midline structure in the expected location of the vein of Galen is present with dense contrast enhancement. MRI demonstrates a characteristic dilated venous structure in the quadrigeminal cistern with flow voids on spin echo sequences (Figure 16-29). The structure densely enhances with administration of contrast. Areas of thrombosis appear isointense on T1-weighted sequences and hypointense on T2-weighted sequences. Subacute thrombosis appears hyperintense on T1- and T2-weighted images.[89] MRA is also useful in demonstrating the abnormality. Venous drainage should be examined for either a stenosis or a thrombosis. Venous flow in the remainder of the brain is also frequently rerouted, with numerous other dilated venous structures present. Fast MRI sequences may be used to demonstrate the malformation prenatally (Figure 16-30).[145,146]

Angiography is normally not necessary for diagnosis but is usually performed, because endovascular treatment is the treatment modality of choice. Choroidal VGAM usually have bilateral supply from normal choroidal arteries, subfornical branches, pericallosal arteries, or thalamoperforating arteries (Figure 16-31).[11] Mural VGAM may have unilateral or bilateral supply. Posterior choroidal and collicular arteries are the most common feeders.

SYNDROMES

The most common syndromes associated with cerebral vascular malformations include hereditary hemorrhagic telangiectasia (HHT), Wyburn-Mason's syndrome, and Sturge-Weber syndrome. In HHT, a variety of cerebral vascular malformations may be found, including AVMs and capillary malformations.[15,17,147] Cerebral vascular malformations occur in 23% of patients with HHT.[15] Cerebral AVMs are found in 7%.[20] Skin lesions, mucous membrane vascular lesions, visceral telangiectasias, and pulmonary AVFs are other common manifestations. Pulmonary AVFs

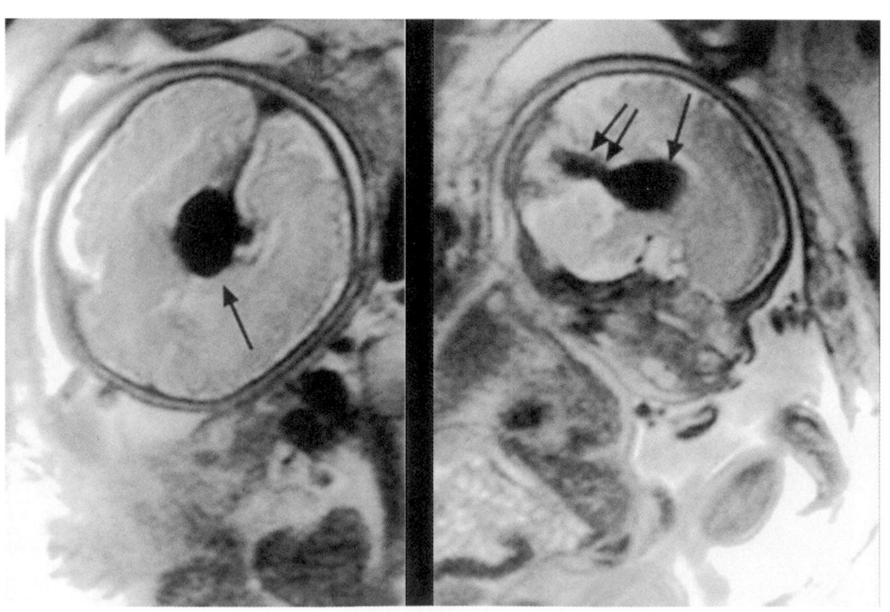

FIGURE 16-30. Prenatal ultrasound demonstrates a cystic midline mass suspicious for a vein of Galen malformation (**A**,**B**). The axial and sagittal in utero magnetic resonance imaging confirms the diagnosis of a vein of Galen malformation. Shown are the venous sac (*single arrow* in **A**,**B**) and persistent falcine sinus (*double arrows* in **B**).

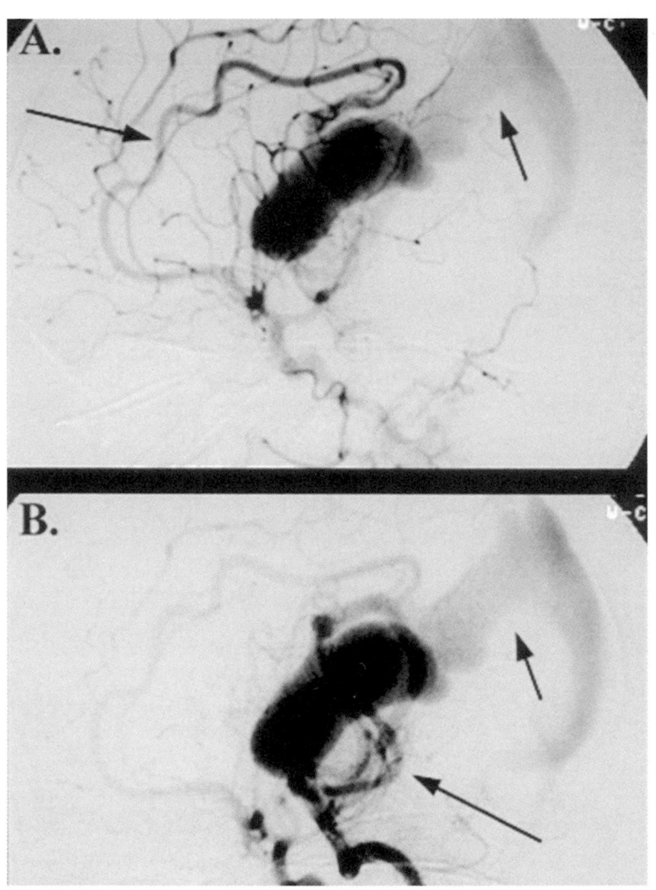

FIGURE 16-31. Same patient as in Figure 16-29. **A.** Lateral carotid angiogram before endovascular treatment. Large pericallosal branch arterial feeder from the anterior cerebral artery supplying the superior aspect (*long arrow*). Venous drainage is into the median vein of the prosencephalon and persistent falcine sinus. Note the superior and upward slant of the persistent falcine sinus (*short arrow*) as opposed to the inferior slant of a normal straight sinus. **B.** Lateral vertebral angiogram. Note the posterior choroidal feeders (*long arrow*) and venous drainage into the persistent falcine sinus (*short arrow*).

frequently lead to serious complications, including brain abscess and infarct. Wyburn-Mason's syndrome is a rare disorder with AVMs of the retina and mesencephalon. Associated facial nevi are present. HHT and Wyburn-Mason's syndrome account for a significant proportion of cases with multiple cerebral parenchymal AVMs.[15–17,147]

Sturge-Weber syndrome (encephalotrigeminal angiomatosis) is a neurocutaneous disorder characterized by nevus flameus of the skin and a leptomeningeal angiomatosis. Punctate calcifications are often seen in the underlying cortex and white matter. The malformation is most commonly seen in the occipital region, followed by the parietal and temporal lobes. Characteristic gyriform calcifications with a tram-track appearance may be present on CT. MRI frequently demonstrates diffuse leptomeningeal enhancement over the involved area. Decreased superficial cortical venous drainage and enlargement of the deep venous system may be seen on MRI and angiography (Figure 16-32). Hemangiomas of the choroid plexus may also be present. Hemorrhage is rare but may occur.[42,85]

SUMMARY

Parenchymal AVMs, dural AVMs, cavernous malformations, capillary malformations, and developmental venous anomalies are the most common types of cerebral vascular malformations. These vascular malformations are relatively common in the population and exhibit a wide range of clinical behavior. Parenchymal AVMs, DAVMs, and cavernous malformations are the most common vascular malformations that present with hemorrhage. Beside DAVMs, the different types of vascular malformations can usually be diagnosed with cross-sectional imaging, particularly MRI. CT is the preferred modality for detecting acute hemorrhage. Angiography may be necessary in cases for which the diagnosis remains unclear. This frequently occurs in the setting of

FIGURE 16-32. Sturge-Weber syndrome. **A.** T1-weighted postgadolinium image. Typical leptomeningeal enhancement with large subependymal draining vein. **B.** T2-weighted image with flow void in a large subependymal draining vein.

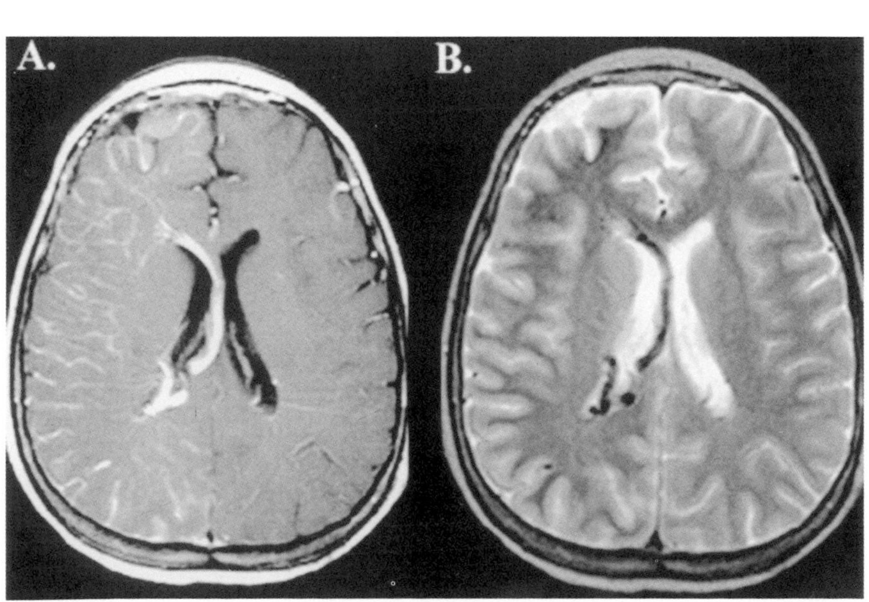

an acute hemorrhage. For parenchymal AVMs, DAVMs, and VGAM, angiography provides important information regarding treatment and is often performed as a precursor to endovascular therapy.

REFERENCES

1. Ruiz-Sandoval JL, Cantu C, Barinagarrementeria F. Intracerebral hemorrhage in young people: analysis of risk factors, location, causes, and prognosis. Stroke 1999;30(3):537–541.
2. Toffol GJ, Biller J, Adams HP Jr. Nontraumatic intracerebral hemorrhage in young adults. Arch Neurol 1987;44(5):483–485.
3. Schutz H, Bodeker RH, Damian M, et al. Age-related spontaneous intracerebral hematoma in a German community. Stroke 1990;21(10):1412–1418.
4. Chaloupka JC, Huddle DC. Classification of vascular malformations of the central nervous system. Neuroimaging Clin North Am 1998;8(2):295–321.
5. McCormick WF. The pathology of vascular ("arteriovenous") malformations. J Neurosurg 1966; 24(4):807–816.
6. McCormick WF. Pathology of Vascular Malformations of the Brain. In CB Wilson, BM Stein (eds), Intracranial Arteriovenous Malformations. Baltimore: Williams & Wilkins, 1984;44–63.
7. Zhu XL, Chan MS, Poon WS. Spontaneous intracranial hemorrhage: which patients need diagnostic cerebral angiography? A prospective study of 206 cases and review of the literature. Stroke 1997;28(7):1406–1409.
8. Newton TH, Cronqvist S. Involvement of dural arteries in intracranial arteriovenous malformations. Radiology 1969;93(5):1071–1078.
9. Miyachi S, Negoro M, Handa T, Sugita K. Contribution of meningeal arteries to cerebral arteriovenous malformations. Neuroradiology 1993;35(3):205–209.
10. Osborn AG. Diagnostic Neuroradiology. St. Louis: Mosby, 1994:936.
11. Lasjaunias PL, Berenstein A. Surgical Neuroangiography. Berlin: Springer, 1987.
12. Osborn AG, Jacobs JM. Diagnostic Cerebral Angiography (2nd ed). Philadelphia: Lippincott Williams & Wilkins, 1999;462.
13. Davis RL, Robertson DM. Textbook of Neuropathology (3rd ed). Baltimore: Williams & Wilkins, 1997;1409.
14. Luessenhop AJ. Natural History of Cerebral Arteriovenous Malformations. In CB Wilson, BM Stein (eds), Intracranial Arteriovenous Malformations. Baltimore: Williams & Wilkins, 1984;12–23.
15. Fulbright RK, Chaloupka JC, Putman CM, Sze GK, et al. MR of hereditary hemorrhagic telangiectasia: prevalence and spectrum of cerebrovascular malformations. AJNR Am J Neuroradiol 1998;19(3):477–484.
16. Willinsky RA, Lasjaunias P, Terbrugge K, Burrows P. Multiple cerebral arteriovenous malformations (AVMs). Review of our experience from 203 patients with cerebral vascular lesions. Neuroradiology 1990; 32(3):207–210.
17. Matsubara S, Mandzia JL, ter Brugge K, et al. Angiographic and clinical characteristics of patients with cerebral arteriovenous malformations associated with hereditary hemorrhagic telangiectasia. AJNR Am J Neuroradiol 2000;21(6):1016–1020.
18. Amin-Hanjani S, Robertson R, Arginteanu MS, Scott RM. Familial intracranial arteriovenous malformations. Case report and review of the literature. Pediatr Neurosurg 1998;29(4):208–213.
19. Nakayama Y, Tanaka A, Yoshinaga S, et al. Multiple intracerebral arteriovenous malformations: report of two cases. Neurosurgery 1989;25(2):281–286.
20. McDonald JE, Miller FJ, Hallam SE, et al. Clinical manifestations in a large hereditary hemorrhagic telangiectasia (HHT) type 2 kindred. Am J Med Genet 2000;93(4):320–327.
21. Kamiryo T, Nelson PK, Bose A, et al. Familial arteriovenous malformations in siblings. Surg Neurol 2000;53(3):255–259.
22. Perret G, Nishioka H. Report on the cooperative study of intracranial aneurysms and subarachnoid hemorrhage. Section VI. Arteriovenous malformations. An analysis of 545 cases of cranio-cerebral arteriovenous malformations and fistulae reported to the cooperative study. J Neurosurg 1966;25(4):467–490.
23. Hofmeister C, Stapf C, Hartmann A, et al. Demographic, morphological, and clinical characteristics of 1289 patients with brain arteriovenous malformation. Stroke 2000;31(6):1307–1310.
24. Itoyama Y, Uemura S, Ushio Y, et al. Natural course of unoperated intracranial arteriovenous malformations: study of 50 cases. J Neurosurg 1989;71(6): 805–809.
25. Stapf C, Mohr JP, Sciacca RR, et al. Incident hemorrhage risk of brain arteriovenous malformations located in the arterial borderzones. Stroke 2000;31(10): 2365–2368.
26. Wilkins RH. Natural History of Arteriovenous Malformations of the Brain. In DL Barrow (ed), Intracranial Vascular Malformations. Park Ridge, IL: American Association of Neurological Surgeons, 1990;31–44.
27. Shah MV, Heros RC. Intracerebral hemorrhage due to cerebral arteriovenous malformations. Neurosurg Clin North Am 1992;3(3):567–576.
28. Hartmann A, Mast H, Mohr JP, et al. Morbidity of intracranial hemorrhage in patients with cerebral arteriovenous malformation [see comments]. Stroke 1998;29(5):931–934.
29. Di Rocco C, Tamburrini G, Rollo M. Cerebral arteriovenous malformations in children. Acta Neurochir 2000;142(2):145–156.

30. Brown RD Jr, Wiebers DO, Forbes G, et al. The natural history of unruptured intracranial arteriovenous malformations. J Neurosurg 1988;68(3):352–357.

31. Graf CJ, Perret GE, Torner JC. Bleeding from cerebral arteriovenous malformations as part of their natural history. J Neurosurg 1983;58(3):331–337.

32. Pollock BE, Flickinger JC, Lunsford LD, et al. Factors that predict the bleeding risk of cerebral arteriovenous malformations. Stroke 1996;27(1):1–6.

33. Ondra SL, Troupp H, George ED, Schwab K. The natural history of symptomatic arteriovenous malformations of the brain: a 24-year follow-up assessment [see comments]. J Neurosurg 1990;73(3):387–391.

34. Woodard EJ, Barrow DJ. Clinical Presentation of Intracranial Arteriovenous Malformations. In DL Barrow (ed), Intracranial Vascular Malformations. Park Ridge, IL: American Association of Neurological Surgeons, 1990;53–62.

35. Arteriovenous malformations of the brain in adults. N Engl J Med 1999;340(23):1812–1818.

36. Fults D, Kelly DL Jr. Natural history of arteriovenous malformations of the brain: a clinical study. Neurosurgery 1984;15(5):658–662.

37. Mast H, Young WL, Koennecke HC, et al. Risk of spontaneous haemorrhage after diagnosis of cerebral arteriovenous malformation. Lancet 1997; 350(9084):1065–1068.

38. Zabramski JM, Henn JS, Coons S. Pathology of cerebral vascular malformations. Neurosurg Clin North Am 1999;10(3):395–410.

39. Meder JF, Oppenheim C, Blustajn J, et al. Cerebral arteriovenous malformations: the value of radiologic parameters in predicting response to radiosurgery. AJNR Am J Neuroradiol 1997;18(8):1473–1483.

40. Spetzler RF, Martin NA. A proposed grading system for arteriovenous malformations. J Neurosurg 1986;65(4):476–483.

41. Hamilton MG, Spetzler RF. The prospective application of a grading system for arteriovenous malformations. Neurosurgery 1994;34(1):2–6; discussion 6–7.

42. Martin N, Vinters H. Pathology and Grading of Intracranial Vascular Malformations. In DL Barrow (ed), Intracranial Vascular Malformations. Park Ridge, IL: American Association of Neurological Surgeons, 1990;1–30.

43. Norman D. Computerized Tomography of Cerebrovascular Malformations. In CB Wilson, BM Stein (eds), Intracranial Arteriovenous Malformations. Baltimore: Williams & Wilkins, 1984;105–120.

44. Mitnick JS, Pinto RS, Lin JP, et al. CT of thrombosed arteriovenous malformations in children. Radiology 1984;150(2):385–389.

45. Tanaka H, Numaguchi Y, Konno S, et al. Initial experience with helical CT and 3D reconstruction in therapeutic planning of cerebral AVMs: comparison with 3D time-of-flight MRA and digital subtraction angiography. J Comput Assist Tomogr 1997;21(5):811–817.

46. Chappell PM, Steinberg GK, Marks MP. Clinically documented hemorrhage in cerebral arteriovenous malformations: MR characteristics. Radiology 1992; 183(3):719–724.

47. Nussel F, Wegmuller H, Huber P. Comparison of magnetic resonance angiography, magnetic resonance imaging and conventional angiography in cerebral arteriovenous malformation. Neuroradiology 1991;33(1):56–61.

48. Noorbehesht B, Fabrikant JI, Enzmann DR. Size determination of supratentorial arteriovenous malformations by MR, CT and angio. Neuroradiology 1987;29(6):512–518.

49. Leblanc R, Levesque M, Comair Y, Ethier R. Magnetic resonance imaging of cerebral arteriovenous malformations. Neurosurgery 1987;21(1):15–20.

50. Dobson MJ, Hartley RW, Ashleigh R, et al. MR angiography and MR imaging of symptomatic vascular malformations. Clin Radiol 1997;52(8):595–602.

51. Huston J 3rd, Rufenacht DA, Ehman RL, Wiebers DO. Intracranial aneurysms and vascular malformations: comparison of time-of-flight and phase-contrast MR angiography. Radiology 1991;181(3):721–730.

52. Turski PA, Cordes D, Mock B, et al. Basic concepts of functional arteriovenous MR imaging malformations. Neuroimaging Clin North Am 1998;8(2):371–381.

53. Maldjian J, Atlas SW, Howard RS 2nd, et al. Functional magnetic resonance imaging of regional brain activity in patients with intracerebral arteriovenous malformations before surgical or endovascular therapy [see comments]. J Neurosurg 1996;84(3):477–483.

54. Leblanc E, Meyer E, Zatorre R, et al. Functional PET scanning in the preoperative assessment of cerebral arteriovenous malformations. Stereotact Funct Neurosurg 1995;65(1–4):60–64.

55. Tsuchiya K, Katase S, Yoshino A, Hachiya J. MR digital subtraction angiography of cerebral arteriovenous malformations. AJNR Am J Neuroradiol 2000;21(4):707–711.

56. Willinsky RA, Fitzgerald M, TerBrugge K. Delayed angiography in the investigation of intracerebral hematomas caused by small arteriovenous malformations. Neuroradiology 1993;35(4):307–311.

57. Cloft HJ, Joseph GJ, Dion JE. Risk of cerebral angiography in patients with subarachnoid hemorrhage, cerebral aneurysm, and arteriovenous malformation: a meta-analysis. Stroke 1999;30(2):317–320.

58. Jafar JJ, Awad IA, Rosenwasser RH. Vascular Malformations of the Central Nervous System. Philadelphia: Lippincott Williams & Wilkins, 1999;540.

59. Wallace RC, Bourekas EC. Brain arteriovenous malformations. Neuroimaging Clin North Am 1998;8(2):383–399.

60. Martin N, Dion JE. Imaging of Intracranial Vascular Malformations. In DJ Barrow (eds), Intracranial Vascular Malformations. Park Ridge, IL: American Association of Neurological Surgeons, 1990;63–90.

61. Marks MP, Lane B, Steinberg GK, Chang PJ. Hemorrhage in intracerebral arteriovenous malformations: angiographic determinants. Radiology 1990; 176(3):807–813.

62. Marks MP, Lane B, Steinberg GK, Chang PJ. Vascular characteristics of intracerebral arteriovenous malformations in patients with clinical steal. AJNR Am J Neuroradiol 1991;12(3):489–496.

63. Duong DH, Young WL, Vang MC, et al. Feeding artery pressure and venous drainage pattern are primary determinants of hemorrhage from cerebral arteriovenous malformations. Stroke 1998;29(6):1167–1176.

64. Hirai S, Mine S, Yamakami I, et al. Angioarchitecture related to hemorrhage in cerebral arteriovenous malformations. Neurol Med Chir (Tokyo) 1998;[Suppl 38]:165–170.

65. Kader A, Young WL, Pile-Spellman J, et al. The influence of hemodynamic and anatomic factors on hemorrhage from cerebral arteriovenous malformations. Neurosurgery 1994;34(5):801–807; discussion 807–808.

66. Miyasaka Y, Yada K, Ohwada T, et al. An analysis of the venous drainage system as a factor in hemorrhage from arteriovenous malformations [see comments]. J Neurosurg 1992;76(2):239–243.

67. Turjman F, Massoud TF, Vinuela F, et al. Correlation of the angioarchitectural features of cerebral arteriovenous malformations with clinical presentation of hemorrhage. Neurosurgery 1995;37(5):856–860; discussion 860–862.

68. Willinsky R, Lasjaunias P, Terbrugge K, et al. Brain arteriovenous malformations: analysis of the angio-architecture in relationship to hemorrhage (based on 152 patients explored and/or treated at the hospital de Bicetre between 1981 and 1986). J Neuroradiol 1988;15(3):225–237.

69. Willinsky R, TerBrugge K, Montanera W, et al. Micro-arteriovenous malformations of the brain: superselective angiography in diagnosis and treatment. AJNR Am J Neuroradiol 1992;13(1):325–330.

70. Turjman F, Massoud TF, Vinuela F, et al. Aneurysms related to cerebral arteriovenous malformations: superselective angiographic assessment in 58 patients. AJNR Am J Neuroradiol 1994;15(9):1601–1605.

71. Mansmann U, Meisel J, Brock M, et al. Factors associated with intracranial hemorrhage in cases of cerebral arteriovenous malformation. Neurosurgery 2000;46(2):272–279; discussion 279–281.

72. Langer DJ, Lasner TM, Hurst RW, et al. Hypertension, small size, and deep venous drainage are associated with risk of hemorrhagic presentation of cerebral arteriovenous malformations. Neurosurgery 1998;42(3):481–486; discussion 487–489.

73. Mine S, Hirai S, Ono J, Yamaura A. Risk factors for poor outcome of untreated arteriovenous malformation. J Clin Neurosci 2000;7(6):503–506.

74. Spetzler RF, Hargraves RW, McCormick PW, et al. Relationship of perfusion pressure and size to risk of hemorrhage from arteriovenous malformations [see comments]. J Neurosurg 1992;76(6):918–923.

75. Stiver SI. Microarteriovenous malformations. Neurosurg Clin North Am 1999;10(3):485–501.

76. Stiver SI, Ogilvy CS. Micro-arteriovenous malformations: significant hemorrhage from small arteriovenous shunts. Neurosurgery 2000;46(4):811–818; discussion 818–819.

77. Meisel HJ, Mansmann U, Alvarez H, et al. Cerebral arteriovenous malformations and associated aneurysms: analysis of 305 cases from a series of 662 patients. Neurosurgery 2000;46(4):793–800; discussion 800–802.

78. Perata HJ, Tomsick TA, Tew JM Jr. Feeding artery pedicle aneurysms: association with parenchymal hemorrhage and arteriovenous malformation in the brain. J Neurosurg 1994;80(4):631–634.

79. Cockroft KM, Thompson RC, Steinberg GK. Aneurysms and arteriovenous malformations. Neurosurg Clin North Am 1998;9(3):565–576.

80. Brown RD Jr, Wiebers DO, Forbes GS. Unruptured intracranial aneurysms and arteriovenous malformations: frequency of intracranial hemorrhage and relationship of lesions. J Neurosurg 1990;73(6):859–863.

81. Redekop G, TerBrugge K, Montanera W, Willinsky R. Arterial aneurysms associated with cerebral arteriovenous malformations: classification, incidence, and risk of hemorrhage. J Neurosurg 1998;89(4):539–546.

82. Liu Y, Zhu S, Jiao L, et al. Cerebral arteriovenous malformations associated with aneurysms—a report of 10 cases and literature review. J Clin Neurosci 2000;7(3):254–256.

83. Marks MP, Lane B, Steinberg GK, Snipes GJ. Intranidal aneurysms in cerebral arteriovenous malformations: evaluation and endovascular treatment. Radiology 1992;183(2):355–360.

84. Westphal M, Grzyska U. Clinical significance of pedicle aneurysms on feeding vessels, especially those located in infratentorial arteriovenous malformations. J Neurosurg 2000;92(6):995–1001.

85. Newton TH, Troost BT, Moseley I. Angiography of Arteriovenous Malformations and Fistulas. In CB Wilson, BM Stein (eds), Intracranial Vascular Malformations. Baltimore: Williams & Wilkins, 1984;64–104.

86. Barrow DL, AANS Publications Committee. Intracranial Vascular Malformations. Neurosurgical Topics. Park Ridge, IL: American Association of Neurological Surgeons, 1990;250.

87. Brown RD Jr, Wiebers DO, Nichols DA. Intracranial dural arteriovenous fistulae: angiographic predic-

tors of intracranial hemorrhage and clinical outcome in nonsurgical patients. J Neurosurg 1994;81(4):531–538.

88. Awad IA, Little JR. Dural Arteriovenous Malformations. In Barrow DJ (ed), Intracranial Vascular Malformations. Park Ridge, IL: American Association of Neurological Surgeons, 1990;219–226.

89. Barkovich AJ. Pediatric Neuroimaging (3rd ed). Philadelphia: Lippincott Williams & Wilkins, 2000;850.

90. Cognard C, Gobin YP, Pierot L. Cerebral dural arteriovenous fistulas: clinical and angiographic correlation with a revised classification of venous drainage. Radiology 1995;194(3):671–680.

91. Davies MA, TerBrugge K, Willinsky R, et al. The validity of classification for the clinical presentation of intracranial dural arteriovenous fistulas. J Neurosurg 1996;85(5):830–837.

92. Awad IA, Little JR, Akarawi WP, Ahl J. Intracranial dural arteriovenous malformations: factors predisposing to an aggressive neurological course. J Neurosurg 1990;72(6):839–850.

93. Duffau H, Lopes M, Janosevic V, et al. Early rebleeding from intracranial dural arteriovenous fistulas: report of 20 cases and review of the literature. J Neurosurg 1999;90(1):78–84.

94. Panasci DJ, Nelson PK. MR imaging and MR angiography in the diagnosis of dural arteriovenous fistulas. Magn Reson Imaging Clin North Am 1995;3(3): 493–508.

95. De Marco JK, Dillon WP, Halback VV. Dural arteriovenous fistulas: evaluation with MR imaging. Radiology 1990;175(1):193–199.

96. Kesava PP, Turski PA. Magnetic resonance angiography of vascular malformations. Magn Reson Imaging Clin North Am 1998;6(4):811–833.

97. Malek AM, Halbach VV, Dowd CF, Higashida RT. Diagnosis and treatment of dural arteriovenous fistulas. Neuroimaging Clin North Am 1998;8(2):445–468.

98. Willinsky R, Terbrugge K, Montanera W, et al. Venous congestion: an MR finding in dural arteriovenous malformations with cortical venous drainage. AJNR Am J Neuroradiol 1994;15(8):1501–1507.

99. Phatouros CC, Halbach VV, Dowd CF, et al. Acquired pial arteriovenous fistula following cerebral vein thrombosis. Stroke 1999;30(11):2487–2490.

100. Moriarity JL, Clatterbuck RE, Rigamonti D. The natural history of cavernous malformations. Neurosurg Clin North Am 1999;10(3):411–417.

101. Moriarity JL, Wetzel M, Clatterbuck RE, et al. The natural history of cavernous malformations: a prospective study of 68 patients [in process citation]. Neurosurgery 1999;44(6):1166–1171; discussion 1172–1173.

102. Otten P, Pizzolato GP, Rilliet B, Berney J. 131 cases of cavernous angioma (cavernomas) of the CNS, discovered by retrospective analysis of 24,535 autopsies [in French]. Neurochirurgie 1989;35(2):82–83.

103. Robinson JR Jr, Awad IA, Masaryk TJ, Estes ML. Pathological heterogeneity of angiographically occult vascular malformations of the brain. Neurosurgery 1993;33(4):547–554; discussion 554–555.

104. Rigamonti D, Rigamonti D, Hadley MN. Cerebral cavernous malformations. Incidence and familial occurrence. N Engl J Med 1988;319(6):343–347.

105. Hallam DK, Russell EJ. Imaging of angiographically occult cerebral vascular malformations. Neuroimaging Clin North Am 1998;8(2):323–347.

106. Sarwar M, McCormick WF. Intracerebral venous angioma. Case report and review. Arch Neurol 1978;35(5):323–325.

107. Rigamonti D, Drayer BP, Johnson PC, et al. The MRI appearance of cavernous malformations (angiomas). J Neurosurg 1987;67(4):518–524.

108. Rigamonti D. Natural History of Cavernous Malformations, Capillary Malformations (Telangiectasias), and Venous Malformations. In Barrow DJ (ed), Intracranial Vascular Malformations. Park Ridge, IL: American Association of Neurological Surgeons, 1990;45–52.

109. Labauge P, Labauge P, Brunereau L, et al. The natural history of familial cerebral cavernomas: a retrospective MRI study of 40 patients. Neuroradiology 2000;42(5):327–332.

110. Voigt K, Yasargil MG. Cerebral cavernous haemangiomas or cavernomas. Incidence, pathology, localization, diagnosis, clinical features and treatment. Review of the literature and report of an unusual case. Neurochirurgia (Stuttg) 1976;19(2):59–68.

111. Del Curling O Jr, Kelly DL Jr, Elster AD, Craven TE. An analysis of the natural history of cavernous angiomas. J Neurosurg 1991;75(5):702–708.

112. Imakita S, Nishimura T, Yamada N, et al. Cerebral vascular malformations: applications of magnetic resonance imaging to differential diagnosis. Neuroradiology 1989;31(4):320–325.

113. Porter PJ, Willinsky RA, Harper W, Wallace MC. Cerebral cavernous malformations: natural history and prognosis after clinical deterioration with or without hemorrhage. J Neurosurg 1997;87(2):190–197.

114. Aiba T, Tanaka R, Koike T, et al. Natural history of intracranial cavernous malformations. J Neurosurg 1995;83(1):56–59.

115. Zabramski JM, Wascher TM, Spetzler RF, et al. The natural history of familial cavernous malformations: results of an ongoing study. J Neurosurg 1994;80(3):422–432.

116. Rabinov JD. Diagnostic imaging of angiographically occult vascular malformations. Neurosurg Clin North Am 1999;10(3):419–432.

117. Rigamonti D, Johnson PC, Spetzler RF, et al. Cavernous malformations and capillary telangiectasia: a spectrum within a single pathological entity. Neurosurgery 1991;28(1):60–64.

118. Detwiler PW, Porter RW, Zabramski JM, Spetzler RF. De novo formation of a central nervous system cavernous malformation: implications for predicting risk of hemorrhage. Case report and review of the literature [see comments]. J Neurosurg 1997;87(4):629–632.

119. Brunereau L, Levy C, Laberge S, et al. De novo lesions in familial form of cerebral cavernous malformations: clinical and MR features in 29 non-Hispanic families. Surg Neurol 2000;53(5):475–482; discussion 482–483.

120. New PF, Ojemann RG, Davis KR, et al. MR and CT of occult vascular malformations of the brain. AJR Am J Roentgenol 1986;147(5):985–993.

121. Kucharczyk W, Lemme-Pleghos L, Uske A, et al. Intracranial vascular malformations: MR and CT imaging. Radiology 1985;156(2):383–389.

122. Atlas SW, Mark AS, Fram EK, Grossman RI. Vascular intracranial lesions: applications of gradient-echo MR imaging. Radiology 1988;169(2):455–461.

123. Lee BC, Vo KD, Kido DK, et al. MR high-resolution blood oxygenation level-dependent venography of occult (low-flow) vascular lesions. AJNR Am J Neuroradiol 1999;20(7):1239–1242.

124. Brunereau L, Labauge P, Tournier-Lasserve E, et al. Familial form of intracranial cavernous angioma: MR imaging findings in 51 families. French Society of Neurosurgery. Radiology 2000;214(1):209–216.

125. Ogilvy CS, Heros RC. Angiographically occult intracranial vascular malformations [letter]. J Neurosurg 1988;69(6):960–962.

126. Tomlinson FH, Houser OW, Scheithauer BW, et al. Angiographically occult vascular malformations: a correlative study of features on magnetic resonance imaging and histological examination. Neurosurgery 1994;34(5):792–799; discussion 799–800.

127. Vanefsky MA, Cheng ML, Chang SD, et al. Correlation of magnetic resonance characteristics and histopathological type of angiographically occult vascular malformations [in process citation]. Neurosurgery 1999;44(6):1174–1180; discussion 1180–1181.

128. Garner TB, Garner TB, Del Curling O Jr, et al. The natural history of intracranial venous angiomas. J Neurosurg 1991;75(5):715–722.

129. Pryor J, Setton A, Berenstein A. Venous anomalies and associated lesions. Neurosurg Clin North Am 1999;10(3):519–525.

130. McLaughlin MR, McLaughlin MR, Kondziolka D, et al. The prospective natural history of cerebral venous malformations. Neurosurgery 1998;43(2): 195–200; discussion 200–201.

131. Ostertun B, Solymosi L. Magnetic resonance angiography of cerebral developmental venous anomalies: its role in differential diagnosis. Neuroradiology 1993;35(2):97–104.

132. Kuker W, Mull M, Thron A. Developmental venous anomalies of the posterior fossa with transpontine drainage: report of 3 cases. Eur Radiol 1997; 7(6):913–917.

133. Lee C, Pennington MA, Kenney CM 3rd. MR evaluation of developmental venous anomalies: medullary venous anatomy of venous angiomas. AJNR Am J Neuroradiol 1996;17(1):61–70.

134. Rigamonti D, Spetzler RF, Drayer BP, et al. Appearance of venous malformations on magnetic resonance imaging. J Neurosurg 1988;69(4):535–539.

135. Peebles TR, Vieco PT. Intracranial developmental venous anomalies: diagnosis using CT angiography. J Comput Assist Tomogr 1997;21(4):582–586.

136. Fontaine S, de la Sayette V, Gianfelice D, et al. CT, MRI, and angiography of venous angiomas: a comparative study. Can Assoc Radiol J 1987;38(4):259–263.

137. Truwit CL. Venous angioma of the brain: history, significance, and imaging findings. AJR Am J Roentgenol 1992;159(6):1299–1307.

138. Rigamonti, D, Spetzler RF. The association of venous and cavernous malformations. Report of four cases and discussion of the pathophysiological, diagnostic, and therapeutic implications. Acta Neurochir 1988;92(1–4):100–105.

139. Awad IA, Robinson JR Jr, Mohanty S, Estes ML. Mixed vascular malformations of the brain: clinical and pathogenetic considerations. Neurosurgery 1993;33(2):179–188; discussion 188.

140. Chang SD, Steinberg GK, Rosario M, et al. Mixed arteriovenous malformation and capillary telangiectasia: a rare subset of mixed vascular malformations. Case report. J Neurosurg 1997;86(4):699–703.

141. Goulao A, Alvarez H, Garcia Monaco R, et al. Venous anomalies and abnormalities of the posterior fossa. Neuroradiology 1990;31(6):476–482.

142. Raybaud CA, Strother CM, Hald JK. Aneurysms of the vein of Galen: embryonic considerations and anatomical features relating to the pathogenesis of the malformation. Neuroradiology 1989;31(2):109–128.

143. Brunelle F. Arteriovenous malformation of the vein of Galen in children. Pediatr Radiol 1997; 27(6):501–513.

144. Meyers PM, Halbach VV, Phatouros CP, et al. Hemorrhagic complications in vein of Galen malformations. Ann Neurol 2000;47(6):748–755.

145. Campi A, Rodesch G, Scotti G, Lasjaunias P. Antenatal diagnosis of vein of Galen aneurysmal malformation: MR study of fetal brain and postnatal follow-up. Neuroradiology 1996;38(1):87–90.

146. Simon EM, Goldstein RB, Coakley FV, et al. Fast MR imaging of fetal CNS anomalies in utero [in process citation]. AJNR Am J Neuroradiol 2000;21(9): 1688–1698.

147. Willemse RB, Mager JJ, Westermann CJ, et al. Bleeding risk of cerebrovascular malformations in hereditary hemorrhagic telangiectasia. J Neurosurg 2000;92(5):779–784.

SECTION

V

Recent Developments

CHAPTER

17

Interventional Treatments in Ischemic Disease: Extracranial and Intracranial Angioplasty and Stenting

Peter J. Mitchell, Randall T. Higashida, Christopher F. Dowd, and Van Halbach

Cerebrovascular disease is the third leading cause of major morbidity and mortality in the United States, accounting for over 150,000–200,000 annual deaths.[1,2] The majority of strokes are due to cardiogenic thromboembolic disease and carotid atherosclerosis.[3–5] More than 170,000 cases of surgical carotid endarterectomy are performed annually for atherosclerotic carotid lesions,[6] with good evidence from prospective randomized trials that this is more effective than the best medical therapy alone in stroke prevention in both symptomatic[7] and asymptomatic[8] patients. Other diseases of the extracranial carotid artery include fibromuscular dysplasia, arterial dissection (traumatic, spontaneous, associated with other diseases), and arteritis. Carotid atherosclerosis remains the main indication for intervention, and most of the discussion that follows is directed at this pathology, with most of the technical aspects broadly applicable to other types of symptomatic diseases of the internal carotid artery presenting with ischemic symptoms.

In 1964, Dotter and Judkins first reported on the technique of percutaneous transluminal angioplasty (PTA) for treatment of high-grade atherosclerotic lesions of the peripheral arteries.[9] Angioplasty, either alone or stent supported, has been shown to be of unequivocal value in relieving ischemia to the coronary, renal, and peripheral vascular territories.[10–14] In the early 1980s, PTA for symptomatic vascular lesions involving the brachiocephalic arteries was initially reported.[15,16] PTA for cerebral vessels was delayed when compared to other regions of the body due to the more difficult technical problems of access and, more important, because of the perceived potential complications of inducing stroke by fragmentation of debris at the angioplasty site. As larger case series of cerebral angioplasty were reported, the safety, efficacy, and long-term success of the procedure were shown to be comparable in some cases to surgical alternatives. Successful results of cerebral PTA involving patients with atherosclerosis, fibromuscular dysplasia, radiation-induced fibrosis, acute dissection, vasculitis, and postsurgical restenosis from intimal hyperplasia have been described.[17–19]

The endovascular approach is currently providing greater therapeutic options for patients, particularly those at high risk for surgery, who are symptomatic despite maximal medical therapy. Such lesions include severe atherosclerosis in patients with significant comorbidity, tandem intracranial stenosis, distal lesions of the cervical carotid artery, contralateral carotid occlusion, and recurrent stenosis of vessels having previously undergone carotid endarterectomy. Increasingly, there are cases in which carotid endarterectomy is indicated, but in which carotid stent–assisted angioplasty is performed. Many factors contribute to this, but the results of multicenter randomized trials comparable to the trials of carotid endarterectomy are required for the necessary evidence on which to base such decisions.

CAROTID ANGIOPLASTY

In 1992, Theron reported 267 patients undergoing brachiocephalic PTA and an overall complication rate of 5.3% (1.9% permanent, 1.9% transient, 1.5% asymptomatic) with no deaths.[20] In 1996, Higashida et al.

TABLE 17-1. Selected Carotid Angioplasty and Stent-Assisted Angioplasty Series

Study	*Patients (n)*	*Technical success (%)*	*Deaths (%)*	*Major stroke (%)*	*Minor stroke (%)*
Roubin et al.[26]	146	99.0	0.6	1.3	4.6
Diethrich et al.[25]	110	99.1	1.8	2.0	4.5
Yadav et al.[28]	107	100.0	0.9	1.8	6.5
Theron et al.[29]	69	100.0	0.0	0.0	1.5
Wholey et al.[123]	108	95.0	1.9	1.8	1.8
Henry et al.[31]	163	99.0	0.0	1.8	1.2
Waigand et al.[124]	50	100.0	2.0	2.0	2.0
Teitelbaum et al.[125]	22	96.0	4.5	18.2	13.6

reported 325 cases; in the 292 cases of extracranial carotid angioplasty, there were 16 (5.5%) cases of transient cerebral ischemia, 7 (2.4%) strokes, and 21 (7.2%) cases of restenosis from 6 months to 7 years of follow-up and no deaths.[21]

In 1996, Kachel[22] summarized the cumulative literature up to 1995 of reported angioplasty cases involving the carotid, vertebral, subclavian, and innominate arteries and described 1,971 total cases with a technical success rate of 94.6%. The mortality rate varied by territory from 0.0% to 2.1%, with an overall permanent morbidity of 0.9% and minor technical complications of 0.0–6.3%.

A prospective analytic study of 29 patients having undergone carotid angioplasty for severe symptomatic ipsilateral carotid stenosis by the North American Symptomatic Carotid Endarterectomy Trial (NASCET) criteria was reported by Schoser et al. in 1998.[23] Neurologic and ultrasonographic follow-up (mean of 33 months) revealed that 78% of patients had no further neurologic sequelae, 10% experienced a single episode of ipsilateral transient ischemia or amaurosis fugax, and 7% experienced recurrent transient ischemic attack (TIA) episodes with no patient having a stroke. Fifty percent of treated vessels remained with normal ultrasound (<50% stenosis), 40% with mild stenosis (50–70%), and 10% with severe stenosis (>70%) after the angioplasty procedure.

Angioplasty alone can achieve reasonable long-term patency rates. Despite these results, there remain technical difficulties with periprocedural embolic events, arterial dissection, and, rarely, acute vessel closure of the carotid artery. The coronary artery experience has demonstrated greater primary patency rates and event-free survival when using stent-assisted angioplasty compared to simple balloon angioplasty alone. This has led to increasing use of stents in both the coronary as well as in the majority of peripheral arterial beds. Similarly, there has been a decline in the number of carotid arteries treated with simple balloon angioplasty alone and an increasing application of primary or secondary stent placement for carotid artery disease.

CAROTID ARTERY STENTING

Large individual series of patients who have undergone carotid artery stenting have been reported in the literature (Table 17-1). However, large randomized trials directly comparing endarterectomy versus carotid artery stenting have just started and require 3–5 years to complete. The results from some of these series are discussed and presented in Table 17-2 to indicate some aspects of the current literature on which clinical and trial decisions are based.

In 1996, Yadav et al. reported their experience in balloon angioplasty and stenting of carotid artery restenosis after endarterectomy in a series of 22 patients.[24] They were able to successfully decrease the stenosis by 79% with a reported minor morbidity rate of 4% and no restenosis at 6 months of follow-up.

In 1996, Diethrich et al.[25] reported on a study of 110 nonconsecutive patients, either symptomatic with stenoses of greater than 70% or asymptomatic with stenosis greater than 75%, treated with stenting. In 110 patients with 117 treated arteries, 109 (99.1%) were successfully treated. There were seven strokes (two major, five reversible) and five TIAs. Clinical success at 30 days was 89%, and over a mean 7.6-month follow-up, there were no new neurologic symptoms that developed.

In 1996, Roubin et al.[26] reported on the results of 146 carotid stent procedures in 74 patients, with only one technical failure. One in-hospital death occurred, and there were two major strokes and seven minor strokes. The restenosis rate at 6 months was less than 5%, and only one TIA was reported. No strokes or deaths occurred during the follow-up period.

In an updated series in 1999, Vitek et al. reported having treated a total of 445 vessels in 404 patients with carotid artery stenting.[27] Patients were pretreated with aspirin and ticlopidine. Their series included 40 patients with contralateral carotid occlusion and 70 patients with

TABLE 17-2. Selected Literature Reviews and Meta-Analyses of Brachiocephalic Angioplasty and Stent-Assisted Angioplasty

Author	*Patients (n)*	*Technical success (%)*	*Mortality (%)*	*All stroke (%)*	*Major stroke (%)*	*Transient ischemic attack/ minor complication (%)*
Kachel[22]	1,971	94.6	0.00	0.90	—	4.2
Kachel[22]	74	93.2	0.00	1.40	—	2.7
Higashida et al.[21]	325	100.0	1.20	5.20	—	7.1
Iyer et al.[126]	100	97.0	3.00	7.00	—	3.0
Wholey et al.[32]	2,048	98.6	1.37	1.32	—	3.1
Mathur et al.[30]	231	100.0	—	6.90	0.7	0.0
Jordan et al.[37]	107	100.0	1.10	8.60	—	4.1
Mathias et al.[33]	633	99.0	0.00	2.70	—	5.0

postendarterectomy restenosis. The overall technical success rate was 98.0%, with a 30-day combined mortality and morbidity rate of 1.9% (0.7% neurologic and 1.2% systemic) and a periprocedural complication rate of 0.7% risk for major stroke and 5.8% for minor stroke. They further demonstrated a steady decline in their minor stroke rate from 7.2% in 1994–1995 to 4.4% and 2.2% in each successive year. This decrease in complication rate over time illustrated that stent-assisted angioplasty was still early in its development and still appeared to have short-term risks comparable to those reported for carotid endarterectomy. The 6-month follow-up obtained in 80.0% of patients demonstrated a restenosis rate of greater than 50.0% in only 5.0% of patients in which 3.3% was the result of stent deformity of balloon expandable and compressible stents. Vitek et al., in a later report involving the same series, reported a clinical follow-up of 95% of patients and reported two neurologic deaths and one major and three minor strokes, with a freedom from any stroke risk of 92% and freedom from disabling stroke or death risk of 98% at 2 years.

The feasibility and safety of elective carotid artery stenting were evaluated prospectively in a consecutive series of 107 high-risk patients by Yadav et al. in 1997.[28] One hundred twenty-six carotid arteries with significant stenosis were treated. This series represented a high-risk subset that included patients with previous ipsilateral carotid endarterectomy and severe medical comorbidity. There were seven minor strokes, two major strokes, and one death during the initial hospitalization and within 30 days after the procedure. For the combined end point of all strokes and death, the incidence was 7.9% of vessels treated (9.3% of patients treated). For ipsilateral major stroke and death, the incidence was 1.6%. There were no strokes during the follow-up period. Of 81 asymptomatic patients in whom angiographic follow-up was available, four (4.9%) had restenoses managed with repeat angioplasty.

In 1996, Theron et al. reported angioplasty for carotid artery stenosis in 259 patients.[29] Cerebral protection with a triple coaxial catheter was used in 136 cases of atherosclerotic stenosis involving the carotid bifurcation or internal carotid artery. A stent was placed in 69 patients in vessels with arterial dissection or insufficient opening. No procedure-related complications occurred in the 71 cases of nonatherosclerotic stenosis and in 14 cases of proximal carotid artery or siphon atherosclerotic stenosis. Among the 38 patients who underwent angioplasty without cerebral protection, dissection occurred in two (5%) and embolic complication occurred in three (8%) during the procedure. Among 136 patients in whom cerebral protection was used, no embolic complications occurred during angioplasty, and two (1%) occurred during or after stent placement when protection was not possible. No residual dissection occurred after stenting, and the restenosis rate decreased from 16% to 4%.

In 1998, Mathur et al. reported their analysis of multiple factors that portend a higher risk of complication in stenting the carotid artery in 271 vessels in 231 patients.[30] Their patients constituted a high-risk subset suffering from coronary artery disease (71%), bilateral carotid disease (39%), and contralateral carotid occlusion (12%). The treated vessels had undergone previous endarterectomy (22%), contained ulcerated plaques (24%), or were calcified lesions (32%). Only 14% of these patients would have been eligible to undergo surgical carotid endarterectomy by NASCET criteria. The rate of minor stroke was 6.2%, and major stroke was 0.7% during the 30-day periprocedure period. The rate of any stroke for the NASCET-eligible subset was 2.7% for the same time interval. Multivariate analysis showed that advanced age and long or multiple stenoses were independent predictors of procedural-related stroke in their series.[30]

In 1998, Henry et al.[31] performed carotid angioplasty and stenting in 174 arteries in 163 patients, of whom there were 126 men with a mean age of 71 plus or minus 10 years and a range of 47 to 91 years of age. The majority (65%) of patients was asymptomatic.

Technical success was achieved in 173 of 174 patients (99.4%), and there were eight (4.6%) neurologic complications that occurred in the periprocedural period, consisting of three TIAs, two minor strokes, and three major strokes. Two major complications developed despite cerebral protection. There were no deaths or myocardial infarctions and only three cervical access site hematomas. Over a mean of a 12.7-month follow-up, there were no ipsilateral neurologic complications. There were four (2.3%) cases of restenoses for primary and secondary patency rates at 3 years of 96% and 99%, respectively.

A report in 1998, based on surveys and literature review, indicated the total number of endovascular carotid stent procedures performed worldwide included 2,048 cases, with a technical success rate of 98.6%.[32] Overall, there were 63 (3.08%) minor strokes, 27 (1.32%) major strokes, and 28 (1.37%) deaths within a 30-day postprocedure period.

In 1999, Mathias et al. reported their experience of angioplasty or stent placement for atherosclerotic internal carotid artery stenosis.[33] In 633 patients, 799 internal carotid artery lesions were treated, 70% symptomatic and 30% asymptomatic. In 99% of the patients, the stenoses were treated with a reduction of the degree of stenosis from 82% to 12%. Transient neurologic deficits occurred in 5.0%, and permanent deficits occurred in 2.7% of the patients, with a decreasing incidence of events over time. The 5-year patency rate was 91.6%.

In 1999, Al-Mubarak et al. reported 51 patients with severe coexisting carotid and symptomatic coronary artery occlusive disease who successfully underwent staged or simultaneous coronary angioplasty and carotid stenting.[34] One pericardial effusion and two minor strokes with full recovery occurred in the hospital; there were no major neurologic events, myocardial infarction, or deaths observed; no repeat revascularization was required within a 30-day follow-up.

These preliminary results are promising, with most early reports showing major stroke or death rates similar to those of carotid endarterectomy.[35,36] The risk of procedural stroke or death from endarterectomy using the NASCET[7] criteria is 5.8%; using the Asymptomatic Carotid Artery Surgery trial[8] criteria, it is 2.3%. In addition, the results also compare favorably to the retrospective analysis of 3,111 carotid endarterectomies performed by Sundt et al.,[35,36] given that a large proportion of the patients undergoing stent-assisted angioplasty constitute Sundt classes III and IV.[36] There are, however, some exceptions to this general trend. A 1998 comparison of carotid stenting in 107 patients versus surgical endarterectomy in 166 patients by Jordan et al.[37] reported an early minor stroke rate of 6.6% for stented patients and 0.6% for surgical patients, with a combined major stroke/death rate of 9.7% for stenting versus 0.9% for the surgical group. The authors concluded that angioplasty and stenting carry a higher neurologic risk and require more monitoring than carotid surgery for carotid artery stenosis. The proposed benefit for the use of stenting, which avoids general anesthesia, cannot be justified when compared with surgery that is performed with general anesthesia.

In 1998, Naylor et al. reported an attempted randomized study of 23 patients with symptomatic carotid artery stenosis greater than 70%. However, this resulted in a very high complication rate in the stented group, and this study was stopped. A criticism of this report was that the interventionist may have been inexperienced in basic carotid artery stenting techniques.[38] Only seven patients were treated by stenting, and five sustained a stroke. However, these two reports differ from other reports of acceptable complication rates associated with carotid artery stenting to date (see Table 17-2).

Extensive experience with carotid and cerebral angiography and with interventional procedures is a key requirement to achieve a low technical complication rate. In experienced hands, results from multiple centers (see Table 17-1) suggest that carotid stent-assisted angioplasty is currently an acceptable alternative to carotid endarterectomy in select patient subsets that are known to constitute very high risk for surgical complication.

Randomized controlled trials are clearly needed to further support this technique. Currently, the Carotid Revascularization Endarterectomy versus Stent Trial, a North American multicenter, randomized, controlled trial comparing the efficacy of surgical endarterectomy versus carotid stenting, has now started. The Carotid and Vertebral Transluminal Angioplasty Study—a large prospective, randomized, multicenter trial comparing carotid endarterectomy to carotid angioplasty—was recently completed.[39] Five hundred four patients were randomized between surgery and angioplasty. Although complication rates were higher in both groups compared to other controlled studies, the mortality and morbidity rates between the two procedures were *not* significantly different between carotid surgery versus angioplasty. A second Carotid and Vertebral Transluminal Angioplasty Study is now being planned.

Procedural Technique

The patient (Figure 17-1) should have a complete angiographic evaluation, including selective catheterization of both common carotid arteries and the dominant vertebral artery, using a high-quality digital subtraction unit to determine the location and severity of stenosis and the adequacy of collateral blood supply to the affected territory. A baseline activated clotting time (ACT) is performed, and an initial weight-based (70 U/kg) intravenous bolus of heparin is given to achieve an

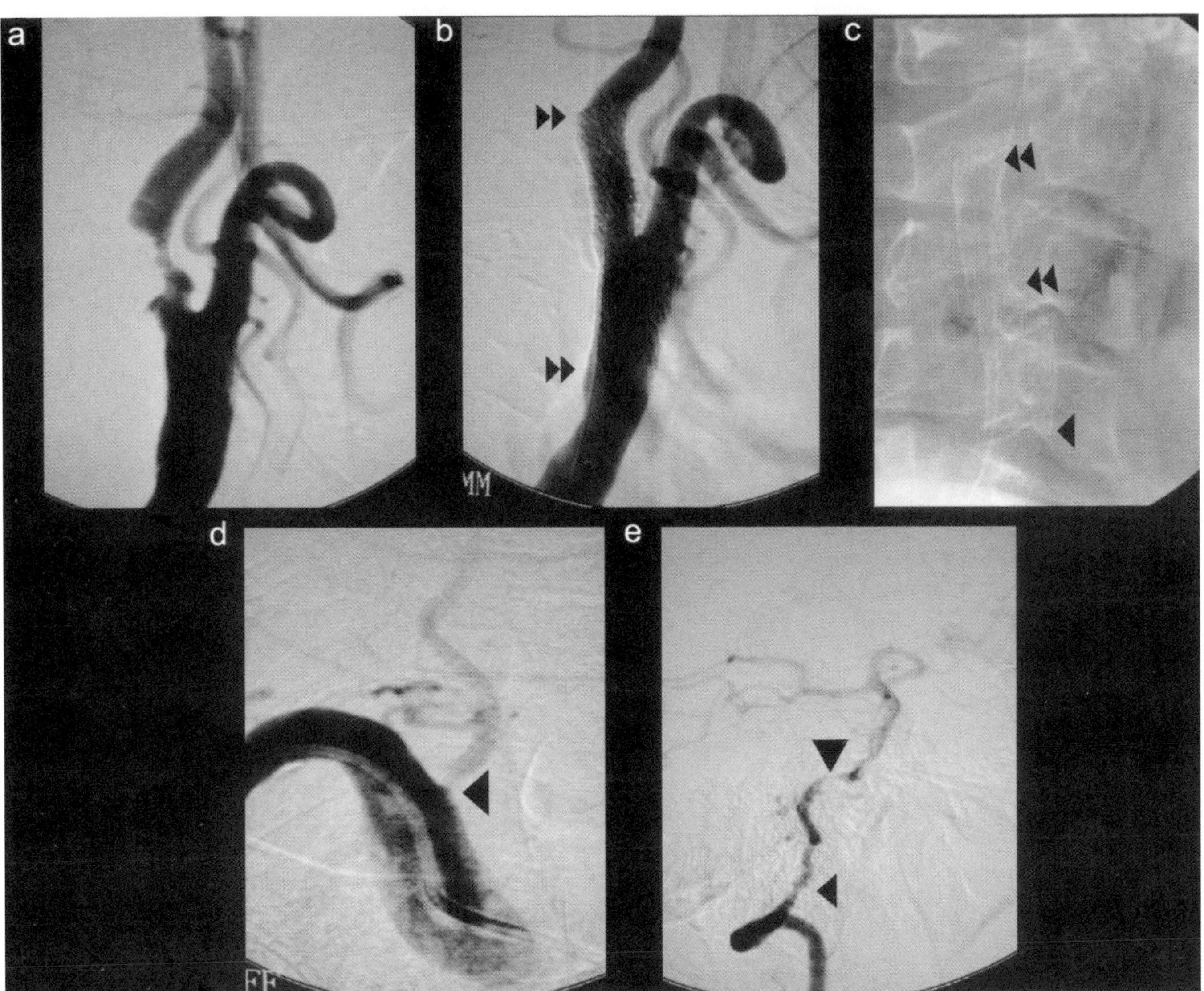

FIGURE 17-1. **A.** Eighty-three-year-old man presenting with repeated episodes of amaurosis fugax. The common carotid artery angiogram reveals an ulcerated and irregular stenosis of the proximal internal carotid artery of greater than 90% by the North American Symptomatic Carotid Endarterectomy Trial criteria. Due to multiple medical comorbidities and the presence of intracranial atherosclerotic disease, an endovascular approach to treatment was recommended. **B.** Postprimary placement of a nitinol carotid SMART stent (Cordis Endovascular, Miami, Florida) that was 10 mm in diameter and 4 cm long. The lateral digital subtraction angiography image shows wide patency and a normal caliber of the internal carotid artery after stent placement. The ends of the stent are indicated by the double arrowheads. **C.** Note that the self-expanding stent has excellent conformation to the diameter of the common carotid artery (*single arrowhead*) and tapers within the internal carotid artery (*double arrowheads*). **D.** This same patient also has severe vertebral artery origin stenosis (*arrowhead*). **E.** In addition, there is intracranial disease with a high-grade stenosis of the distal vertebral artery (*small arrowhead*) and origin of the basilar artery (*large arrowhead*), but these are currently asymptomatic and were not treated.

ACT value equal to or greater than 2.5 times the baseline value (>250 seconds). Patients are given enteric-coated aspirin (325 mg qd) and either ticlopidine (Ticlid, 250 mg bid) or clopidogrel (Plavix, 75 mg qd), starting at least 3 days before the procedure. After the procedure, the patient is kept on daily aspirin indefinitely and on ticlopidine or clopidogrel for 4–6 weeks. The role of glycoprotein IIb/IIIa inhibitors, which have been shown to decrease mortality and morbidity in a number of coronary artery stent studies,[40] remains to be defined in carotid and vertebral angioplasty and stenting.

External cutaneous pacing leads are placed, allowing constant monitoring by a transcutaneous pacer/defibrillator device in case of severe bradycardia or asystole from carotid body stimulation during the angioplasty procedure. Patients are administered atropine (0.5–1.0 mg intravenously) immediately before balloon dilatation of the carotid artery to blunt any parasympathetic discharge. The patients should be well hydrated during the procedure; this is tailored to the specific patient and his or her cardiac status, as the severity of any vasovagal episode is exacerbated by hypovolemia.

A femoral approach using a modified Seldinger technique is used almost exclusively, with brachial or direct carotid puncture occasionally being necessary. An infusion of heparinized saline (1 unit heparin/mL of normal saline) is used as a constant irrigation between the guide catheter and devices. The procedure consists of placing a 7- to 9-French (Fr) guiding catheter or a 6- to 7-Fr, 90-cm-long sheath in the common carotid artery, depending on the type of stent to be used. Most commonly, an 8- to 9-Fr guide catheter is used in the case of the WallStent (Schneider, Plymouth, Minnesota), SMART stent (Cordis Endovascular, Miami, Florida), Acculink stent (Guidant Corporation, Santa Clara, California), and an Arterial Vascular Engineering Carotid stent (Arterial Vascular Engineering/Medtronics, Santa Rosa, California).

In selected cases, smaller, more low-profile stents are used for distal high-cervical carotid disease, such as the S670 (Medtronics), Multi-Link (Guidant), BX-Velocity (Cordis Corporation), and Magic WallStent (Schneider). The guiding catheter or sheath is placed directly into the common carotid artery, with placement of a relatively stiff guidewire in the external carotid artery to facilitate guidance. In the case of a complex, severely stenosed lesion or in a high-cervical or intracranial location, a 2.3-Fr microcatheter (Rapid Transit [Cordis Neuro Vascular, Miami Lakes, Florida]) is used coaxially over a 0.014-in. microguidewire (Transend 14 [Boston Scientific, Boston, Massachusetts]). After crossing the lesion using a microcatheter, a 300-cm-long, 0.014-in. exchange microguidewire (Stabilizer [Cordis Endovascular], ACS Balance [Guidant]) is passed through the microcatheter and placed in the precavernous segment of the internal carotid artery; the microcatheter is then withdrawn.

With the exchange guidewire in place, primary or secondary stent-assisted angioplasty is then performed. In case of secondary stent placement, a low-profile angioplasty balloon (3.5–4.0 mm) is used to cross and predilate the lesion. Once the stenosis has been dilated, the stent is deployed, and a high-pressure noncompliant angioplasty balloon is then used to postdilate the stent to firmly embed it into the plaque.[32,41]

Stents, now being used for the carotid artery, are self-expandable and made of either nitinol or stainless steel, with significantly greater metal surface area coverage and finer and more numerous interstices than prior designs. Its compliant design and lower radial force can be a hindrance in severely calcified lesions; however, the benefits outweigh the limitations when contrasted with noncompliant balloon expandable stents that are deformable.

Potential Complications

Potential complications include abrupt or delayed vessel occlusion, perforation, dissection, vasospasm, thromboemboli, occlusion of adjacent vessels, transient ischemic episodes, and stroke.

ANGIOPLASTY-INDUCED PARTICULATE EMBOLIZATION

Angioplasty of atherosclerotic lesions has been reported to induce the release of multiple emboli, including atheroma, cholesterol crystals, thrombus, and platelet aggregates.[42–45] Embolization of microparticles has also been demonstrated during open surgical carotid endarterectomy and has been shown to correlate with complex plaque morphology[46] and with clinical postoperative cerebral ischemia.[47] Analysis of 28 patients undergoing percutaneous angioplasty versus endarterectomy with shunt placement revealed that endarterectomy resulted in significantly greater total occlusion time (337 seconds vs. 26 seconds) but a lower count of microembolic signals (52 events vs. 202 events) compared to angioplasty, although neither parameter was predictive of later neurologic events.[44]

It is unclear whether stent placement concomitant with balloon angioplasty may help decrease the number of microemboli by trapping them under the metal interstices or whether primary stenting would decrease emboli compared to secondary stenting. The problem of distal embolization during balloon dilatation of atherosclerotic stenoses has engendered interest in various methods of cerebral protection during the procedure. Distal protection using a specially designed triple-coaxial catheter has been described by Theron.[48] Distal embolic complications were found in three of 38 (8%) patients who had angioplasty without distal protection and in none of the 136 (0%) patients who underwent angioplasty with a distal protection device.[29] A number of carotid stent protection devices aimed at reducing the microembolic burden using filters, guidewire-attached balloons, and arteriovenous shunting methods are now undergoing investigation. The balloon protection and arteriovenous shunting methods have the disadvantage of temporary occlusion of carotid flow, whereas distal filter devices allow constant cerebral perfusion. All can increase the complexity, and potentially the duration, of the procedure, but their increasing popularity indicates the perceived need for such techniques to further decrease the morbidity associated with stent-assisted angioplasty.

Potential complications of this procedure include arterial access complications such as groin hematoma, retroperitoneal hemorrhage, pseudoaneurysm, arteriovenous fistula, arterial thrombosis, groin infection, contrast media allergic reaction, hypotension, and acute renal failure. In addition, angioplasty and stent placement complications including distal embolization, vessel dissection, rupture, pseudoaneurysm formation, and stent infection are also possible.[29] The rate of permanent neurologic complication from angiography alone was found to be very low at 0.07%.[49]

Current Indications

Angioplasty and stenting in the extracranial carotid artery have become viable alternatives to surgical carotid endarterectomy in certain subsets of very high-risk patients. Long-term clinical and angiographic follow-up, as well as randomized prospective trials, will help determine the precise role of percutaneous angioplasty with stenting in the treatment of carotid stenosis.

These high-risk cases include carotid artery dissection, which occurs as a result of trauma or may be spontaneous in onset. Associated disease may be present, including fibromuscular dysplasia and collagen-elastase abnormalities. Dissection is considered in the etiology of ischemic stroke, particularly in young patients, and includes symptoms of pain and Horner's syndrome. Extracranial carotid artery dissection may cause stroke, either from thromboemboli or hypoperfusion. When diagnosed, duplex carotid ultrasound, magnetic resonance imaging (MRI), magnetic resonance angiography, and catheter angiography can be diagnostic, and management is commonly with antiplatelet agents or anticoagulants. Most cases of localized dissection resolve; however, the degree of stenosis may progress, pseudoaneurysms may develop, and distal embolization with stroke may occur. Symptomatic dissection can be managed effectively with stent placement, correcting any stenosis, or covering the neck of a false aneurysm, allowing subsequent thrombosis or Guglielmi detachable coil placement to promote total occlusion (Figure 17-2). Patients who are symptomatic on conventional medical therapy, in whom there is a greater than 70% stenosis or a large pseudoaneurysm, should be treated.

EXTRACRANIAL VERTEBRAL ARTERY ANGIOPLASTY AND STENTING

The frequency and severity of atherosclerosis in the vertebral arteries is variably reported as equal to or some-

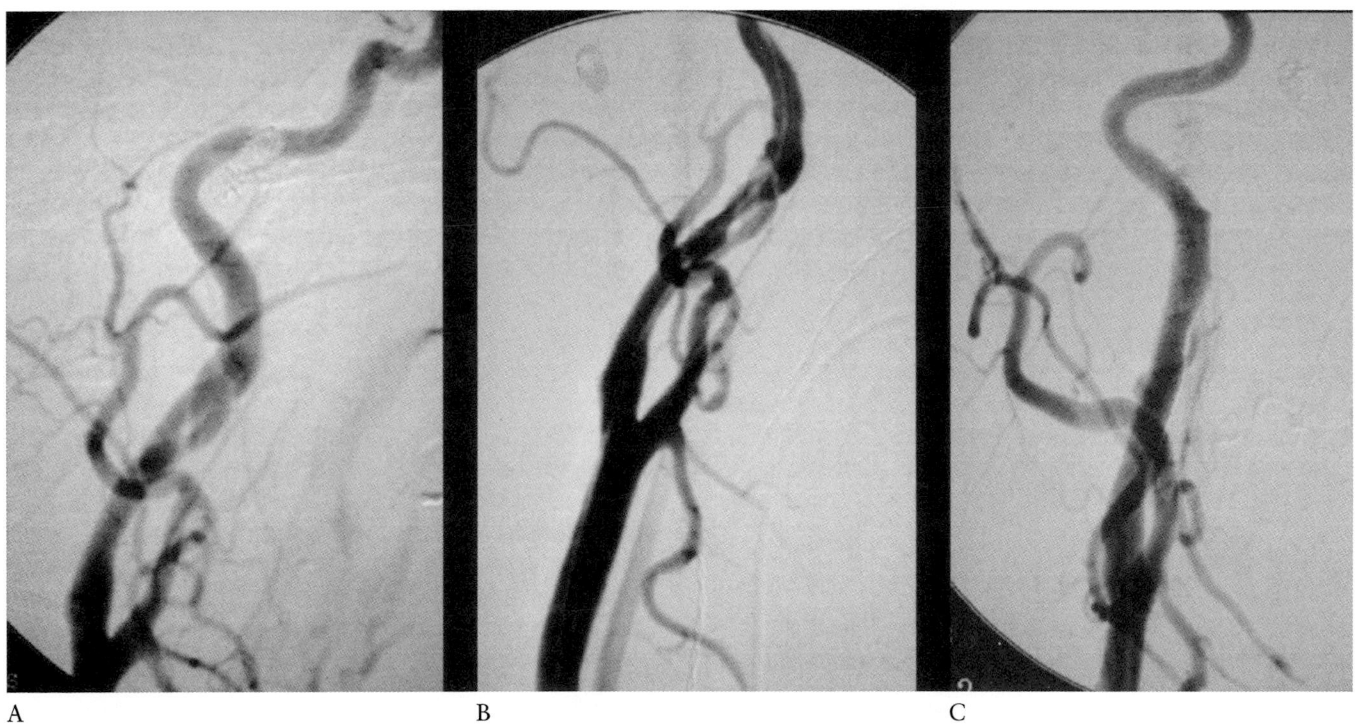

FIGURE 17-2. **A.** Fifty-four-year-old man who presented with fibromuscular dysplasia and had a known internal carotid artery dissection. He had no recovery over 12 months and presented with recurrent transient ischemic attacks referable to that hemisphere, despite antiplatelet and anticoagulant therapy. The common carotid artery angiogram shows a spiral dissection of the mid- to proximal one-third of the internal carotid artery. Note a prominent false lumen. **B.** After placing a guide catheter in the common carotid artery, a guidewire (0.035 in.) was placed across the dissection. **C.** After placement of a SMART stent (Cordis Endovascular, Miami, Florida), the spiral dissection flap has been held against the true wall, and the true lumen is now of normal caliber and of normal size.

what less than in the carotid arteries, and approximately equal to that of the intracerebral arteries. Most reports identify the origin or first segment of the vertebral artery to be the most frequent site of stenosis.[50] The morphologic and pathologic characteristics of atherosclerotic plaque of the vertebral artery differ from internal carotid artery disease, being more frequently annular and concentric, fibrous, and smooth, with a low incidence of ulceration or intramural hemorrhage.[51,52] Atherosclerotic plaque at the vertebral artery origin may also involve the adjacent subclavian artery. This has important implications for endovascular therapy, with particulate embolization during endovascular manipulations likely to be less frequent than with carotid plaque, but with increased vessel recoil, which may cause decreased long-term patency rates.

Natural History

There is no large prospective trial of treatment modalities stratified by degree of stenosis comparable to NASCET for vertebral artery stenosis. In general, intracranial vertebral artery disease probably has a worse prognosis than extracranial disease, and basilar artery stenosis is worse than vertebral artery stenosis. The exact pathophysiologic basis for stroke in this setting is often not determined and can include hypoperfusion, artery-to-artery embolization, and arterial thrombosis.

Moufarrij et al. reported 96 patients with greater than 50% unilateral vertebral artery stenosis after an average of 4.6 years.[50] None of the patients had definite vertebrobasilar TIAs, and only two patients (2%) who sustained a brain stem infarction had fatal strokes and were known to have both basilar and vertebral artery stenosis. They concluded that vertebral artery stenosis is most frequently located at the vertebral artery origin (93%) and is associated with a low incidence of brain stem infarction.

In a subsequent study, 44 patients with greater than 50% stenosis of a distal vertebral artery or basilar artery were followed up for an average of 6.1 years. Seven patients (16%) had definite and three patients had possible vertebrobasilar TIAs. Eight patients (18%) sustained a stroke, five of which were in the vertebrobasilar territory. The observed stroke rate was 17 times the expected rate for a matched normal population. Thus, distal vertebrobasilar occlusive disease appears to carry a higher risk for brain stem ischemia.[53]

In 1998, Wityk et al. reported on 80 patients with either occlusion or high-grade stenosis involving the V1 segment of the vertebral artery.[54] Hypertension, cigarette smoking, and coronary artery disease were common risk factors. Occlusive disease of the V1 segment was the primary mechanism of ischemia in 9% of patients, but in other cases, it was associated with severe intracranial occlusive disease of the posterior circulation, with evidence of artery-to-artery embolism and proximal vertebral arterial dissection.

In 1998, the Warfarin-Aspirin Symptomatic Intracranial Disease investigators[55] concluded that patients with symptomatic intracranial vertebral artery or basilar artery stenosis are at high risk for stroke, myocardial infarction, or sudden death. They reported on 68 patients with symptomatic stenosis of the intracranial posterior circulation of greater than or equal to 50% severity and treated with medical therapy. During the follow-up of over 12 months, 16% of patients had nonfatal strokes, and 6% of patients had fatal strokes.

Technique and Results

A guide catheter is positioned in the proximal subclavian artery; the stenosis is crossed using a microcatheter and a 0.014-in., soft-tipped microguidewire, and then an exchange wire (300-cm length, 0.014 in.) is left across the lesion (Figure 17-3). Appropriate monitoring of the position of the tip of the wire is necessary to ensure it does not move forward during the catheter exchange to minimize the chance of perforation or dissection.

Balloon angioplasty for the treatment of vertebral artery occlusive disease was first reported in 1981 by Motarjeme et al.[56] Over the following decade, numerous investigators reported favorable short-term results using angioplasty.[15,18,57–62] Higashida et al., in 1993, reported treating 34 proximal vertebral atherosclerotic lesions in 33 patients presenting with vertebrobasilar ischemic symptoms or stroke in whom medical therapy had failed. Technical success of less than 30% residual stenosis was achieved in all cases, with a 9% incidence of transient complications and no permanent complications. Follow-up revealed a 9% incidence of restenosis within 5 months but improved symptoms related to the site of stenosis in all patients.[63] In Kachel's review of the literature up to 1996, 268 vertebral balloon angioplasty procedures had been reported, with an overall technical success rate of 95.1%, a morbidity rate of 0.7%, a minor complication rate of 3.3%, and no procedure-related mortality.[22]

Endovascular therapy of extracranial vertebral artery lesions has evolved from simple balloon angioplasty to stent-supported angioplasty, principally to overcome the problems of elastic recoil and early restenosis.[64–66] Malek et al., in 1999, treated 21 patients with symptomatic occlusive subclavian (n = 13) or vertebral artery stenosis (n = 8) refractory to medical therapy using endovascular stents.[67] Technical success was achieved in all cases, with the mean degree of overall stenosis reduced from 75.0% to 4.5%. There were no periprocedural strokes, and only one patient experienced a periprocedural TIA. At a mean clinical follow-up of 21 months, 90.5% of surviv-

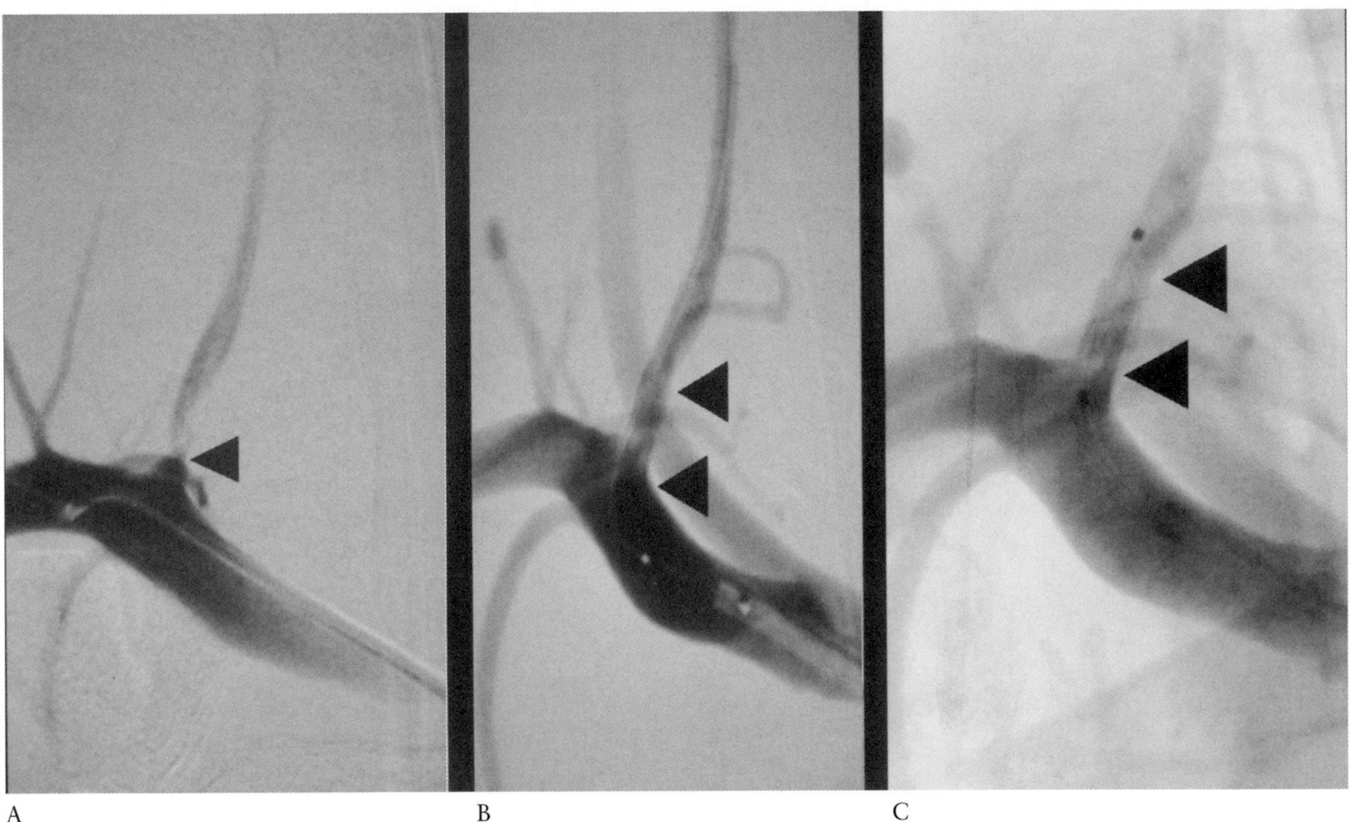

FIGURE 17-3. **A.** Right subclavian angiogram in a 41-year-old woman with vertebrobasilar transient ischemic attacks shows a high-grade stenosis of the vertebral artery origin (*arrowhead*). Note the concentric focal nature of this lesion without evidence of ulceration. **B.** The lesion has been primarily stented using a Palmaz P-104 stainless steel stent (*arrowheads*). The balloon remains across the lesion; the guidewire is positioned well distally within the distal vertebral artery. **C.** After withdrawal of the balloon catheter, a final angiogram is performed through the guide catheter. Note the close positioning of the guide catheter to the angioplasty site, which gives maximal mechanical advantage to crossing the often tortuous origin of the vertebral artery. More distal lesions can be treated with the catheter in this position, although placement of the catheter within the vertebral artery may be necessary in difficult cases. The stent is well positioned across the stenosis (*arrowheads*).

ing patients had experienced resolution or improvement of symptoms. One patient died from a carotid artery territory stroke.

Despite the limited published data, stent-supported angioplasty is emerging as a viable therapeutic option for medically refractive vertebral artery occlusive disease, offering improved rates of technical success and better long-term patency rates over balloon angioplasty alone. Our recommendation is for stent-assisted angioplasty, either primary or secondary, depending on the degree of stenosis.

SUBCLAVIAN AND INNOMINATE ARTERY ANGIOPLASTY AND STENTING

Less common sites of clinically significant atherosclerosis, with greater operative risk than carotid surgery and potentially lower risk of distal embolization from endovascular treatment, are the subclavian and innominate artery. Stent-assisted angioplasty is appropriate, associated with low morbidity, and, in short-term follow-up, appears effective.[68] The technical and procedural elements do not significantly differ from those discussed in the preceding sections.

INTRACRANIAL CEREBRAL VASCULAR DISEASE

In addition to the more common extracranial embolic etiologies of ischemic stroke, intracranial atherosclerotic stenoses can cause stroke from hypoperfusion or distal embolization. The estimated risk of stroke from intracranial stenosis varies widely from 10% to 46% per year, independent of medical therapy.[55,69–73] Intracranial arterial disease is an independent risk factor for subsequent stroke in medically treated patients with symptomatic extracranial carotid artery stenosis.[74]

Angioplasty

Angioplasty of the intracranial cerebral circulation was first reported in 1980 by Sundt et al.,[75] who described an operative approach to allow insertion of a coronary balloon angioplasty catheter and dilatation of a basilar artery stenosis. Since that time, numerous case reports and small series of intracranial angioplasty have been published.[21,76–85]

In 1996, Higashida et al. reported 325 cases of extracranial and intracranial lesions treated by balloon angioplasty, with a permanent complication rate of 17 strokes (5.2%) that included four deaths (1.2%). In the 33 cases of intracranial angioplasty, there were seven (21.2%) cases of transient cerebral ischemia and ten (30.3%) strokes that included four deaths. This contrasts markedly with the 292 cases of extracranial angioplasty, with 5.5% transient cerebral ischemia, 2.4% strokes, and no deaths. Intracranial angioplasty appeared to be inherently more difficult to perform safely. This was due to the smaller size of the vessels being treated, increased tortuosity of the intracranial vessels, presence of perforating side branches, and more difficult access to this region with the current balloon angioplasty systems. Patients treated since the initial series and with the use of stents had significant reduction in the overall complication rate.

In 1995, Clark et al. reported a series of 22 vessels in 17 patients with recurrent neurologic symptoms referable to the stenotic intracranial vessel despite optimal medical therapy who were treated with PTA.[76] PTA was successful in 82% of the vessels treated, with two strokes during angioplasty for a 30-day morbidity rate of 11.7%. The remaining patients were without further neurologic events. There was delayed improvement in the degree of residual stenosis.

In 1999, Connors and Wojack reported a retrospective analysis of balloon angioplasty in 70 patients with intracranial atherosclerotic stenosis.[84] They divided their experience into three distinct periods based on the technique used. In the middle period of 12 patients, the balloon size approximated the vessel size, but oversizing was permitted. Angioplasty was extremely rapid and brief. Angiographically visible dissection occurred in nine (75%) patients, necessitating urokinase (Abbott Laboratories, Chicago, Illinois) infusion in five (41.7%) cases and producing abrupt occlusion in one (8.3%), resulting in death. In the last period of 50 patients, the balloon was always undersized, inflation extremely slow (several minutes), and intravenous abciximab routinely administered. Dissection only occurred in seven (14%) patients. Overall results were a 4.2% stroke rate with none in the last 50 patients, 2.9% mortality rate, and 100% technical success rate, although with moderate residual stenosis. Conclusions reached from analysis of their 9-year experience were to minimize vessel trauma with deliberate undersizing of the balloon, slow inflation techniques, and use of abciximab to decrease the likelihood of platelet activation and aggregation at the angioplasty site. This technique sometimes yields suboptimal angiographic results but achieves the clinical goal safely.

There have been several reports of balloon angioplasty of the cerebral arteries for acute thromboembolic occlusion in the anterior and posterior cerebral circulations, which reported improved outcomes in cases of suboptimal cerebral thrombolysis.[86–88]

Stent-Assisted Angioplasty

Stenting for intracranial atherosclerosis has been used for patients who are symptomatic despite maximal medical therapy, have had complications from angioplasty, or were considered at increased chance of poor outcome from balloon angioplasty alone. Patient selection is in conjunction with a multidisciplinary team and requires a greater than 70% stenosis, with recurrent symptoms appropriate to the site of the disease despite "optimal" medical therapy. In the carotid artery territory, stent placement has been performed in the intracranial petrous, cavernous, proximal supraclinoid segments, and middle cerebral artery. In the posterior circulation, stents have been deployed in the intracranial V4 segment and in the mid- and distal segment of the basilar artery.[65,86,89,90] Compromise of perforating vessels supplying the brain stem remains a factor that may limit the use of stents in the basilar and middle cerebral artery.

Technique

Intracranial angioplasty and stent-assisted angioplasty carry significantly greater risk of complications than angioplasty at other sites. This is because of the delicate vascular structure with near lack of the media and muscular layers, more difficult access, subarachnoid site with fatal outcome from vessel rupture, and the likelihood of major disability from distal embolization. Typical complications may include intimal dissection, vessel rupture, acute vessel thrombosis, and reperfusion injury. Stent placement can be used for treatment of flow-limiting postangioplasty intimal dissection, but our preference is for primary stent placement, particularly for the intracranial vertebral and basilar arteries. Middle cerebral, posterior cerebral, and tortuous internal carotid sites are first subject to angioplasty alone (Figure 17-4).

The patient first undergoes a complete angiographic evaluation, including assessment of collateral circulation. The pharmacologic management is identical to that described previously, consisting of antiplatelet agents, procedural anticoagulation, and selective use of glycoprotein IIb/IIIa inhibitors.

The procedure consists of placing a 6- to 7-Fr guiding catheter (Envoy [Cordis Endovascular]) into the vertebral or internal carotid artery. A low-profile, balloon-mounted

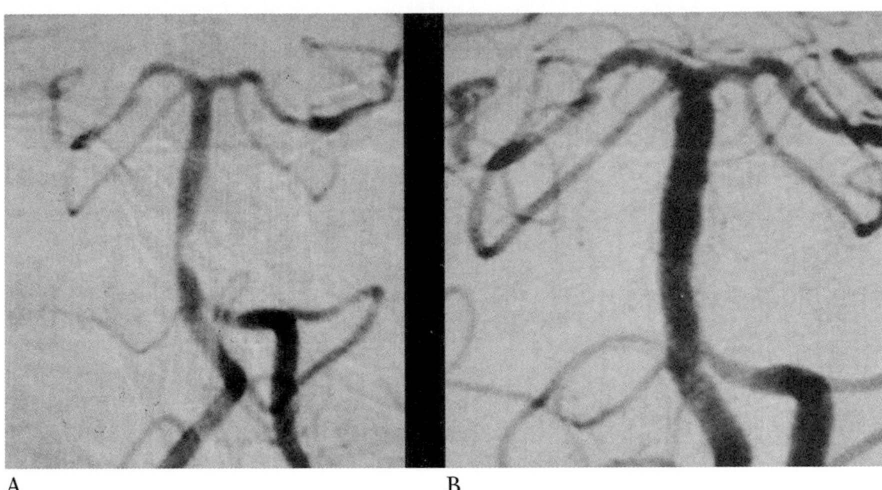

FIGURE 17-4. **A.** Elderly patient presented with recurrent dysarthria and ataxia while on coumadin and aspirin. The magnetic resonance angiography scan demonstrated a focal mid-basilar artery stenosis and no evidence of completed infarction. Cerebral angiography confirms the presence of a focal high-grade stenosis. The lesion was crossed with a microcatheter and guidewire, and primary stent placement was performed. **B.** After placement of a small microstent (GFX II, Arterial Vascular Engineering/Medtronics, Santa Rosa, California), reconstitution of a normal-caliber basilar artery is now demonstrated.

coronary stent such as the S670, INX neurovascular stent (Arterial Vascular Engineering/Medtronics), or BX-Velocity is usually used. A 2.3-Fr microcatheter (Rapid Transit) is used coaxially over a 0.014-in. microguidewire (Transend 14). After crossing the lesion using the microcatheter with meticulous care, a 300-cm-long, 0.014-in. exchange microguidewire (Stabilizer, ACS Balance) is then passed through the microcatheter and placed well beyond the site of stenosis; then, the microcatheter is withdrawn. With the exchange guidewire in place, primary or secondary stent-assisted angioplasty is performed (Figure 17-5). In the case of primary angioplasty, a low-profile balloon

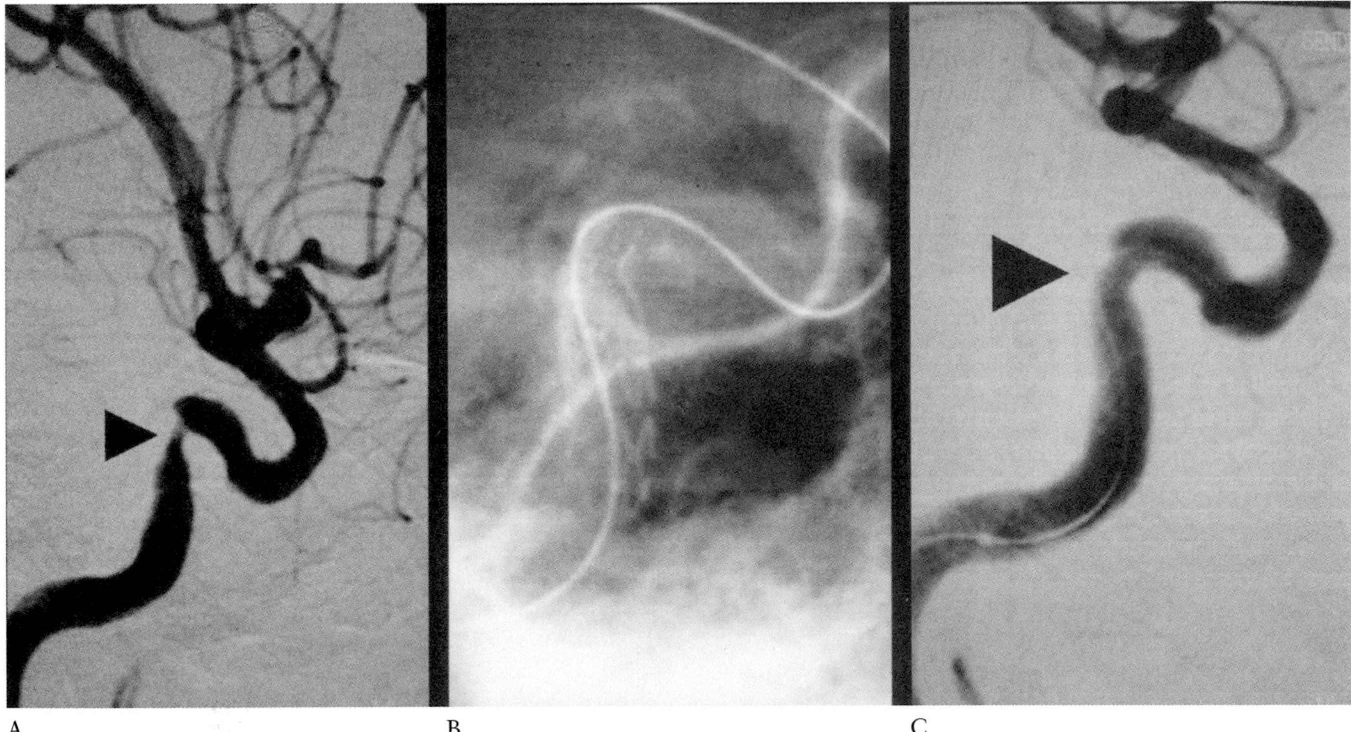

FIGURE 17-5. **A.** Sixty-eight-year-old woman who presented with recurrent transient cerebral ischemic symptoms. An angiographic study of both vertebral and carotid arteries demonstrated a focal 70% left cavernous internal carotid artery stenosis (*arrowhead*). **B.** The unsubtracted view demonstrates placement of a 3.5 mm × 18 mm GFX II stent (Arterial Vascular Engineering/Medtronics, Santa Rosa, California) across the stenosis. **C.** After balloon dilatation of the stent, there is now wide patency of the cavernous internal carotid artery (*arrowhead*).

catheter (Titan/Jupiter, Ninja [Cordis Corporation], Bandit NC Balloon, or Faststealth Balloon [Boston Scientific]) is used to cross and predilate the lesion. For intracranial vessels, balloon diameter size ranges from 2.0 to 4.5 mm. The balloon is inflated to the maximum rated burst pressure (10–21 atm) for 10–30 seconds. Some vessels require more than one dilatation to achieve a satisfactory result of less than 30% residual stenosis. Once the stenosis has been decreased, a stent can then be deployed.

Stent-assisted angioplasty is preferred for all focal high-grade and eccentric lesions to minimize the chance of acute vessel dissection or closure. Predilation may be performed, and the balloon and stent diameters are carefully chosen to be the same or 0.1–0.2 mm less than the diameter of the adjacent normal vessel. The stents currently used are second-generation, low-profile, balloon-premounted stents of 2.5–4.0 mm in diameter.

Connors and Wojack reported the routine use of glycoprotein IIb/IIIa inhibitor use,[84] with a very low incidence of ischemic stroke since adopting this protocol. The patient may be continued on heparin for 12–24 hours and transferred to the neurologic intensive care unit for close monitoring of blood pressure and neurologic status.

Improvements in balloon angioplasty devices, current stent technology, microguidewires, and high-resolution fluoroscopic equipment have dramatically decreased the complication rates associated with intracranial stenosis treatment. The development of current generation small vessel stents, such as those being used in the coronary arteries, has markedly improved access to the distal intracranial circulation and has decreased the incidence of acute vessel closure and associated periprocedural stroke. Currently, there are few low-risk surgical options available for symptomatic patients with intracranial stenosis who have failed medical therapy; therefore, endovascular approaches appear to offer a good opportunity for stroke prevention.

POST–SUBARACHNOID HEMORRHAGE AND VASOSPASM

Cerebral vasospasm after subarachnoid hemorrhage is the most important cause of death and disability for patients who present with a ruptured cerebral artery aneurysm.[91] It is estimated that 6,000–10,000 potential patients per year may benefit from revascularization therapy for arterial spasm.[92] The first reports of balloon angioplasty for cerebral arterial vasospasm were from Zubkov and Nikiforov in 1984.[93] They reported the successful treatment of 33 cases involving 105 vascular territories, with good clinical outcome in the majority of cases.

In 1992, Higashida et al. reported on 28 patients involving 99 vascular territories, in which 19 patients (66.7%) showed clinical and neurologic improvement after angioplasty.[94] In 1998, Eskridge et al. reported on 50 patients with clinical evidence of vasospasm-induced ischemia; 28 (61%) showed sustained neurologic improvement within 72 hours of angioplasty.[95]

Cerebral arterial vasospasm is due to direct endothelial damage, myointimal cellular proliferation, inflammatory changes, or a reduction in smooth muscle contractility within the vessel wall.[96] The mechanism of balloon dilatation is very different from that for atherosclerosis, with no evidence of disruption of the media and intima in animal studies that have used very soft silicone balloons at low pressures to dilate vasospastic blood vessels.[97]

The indications for using these techniques include patients who are clinically symptomatic, have failed maximal medical therapy, have angiographic stenosis correlating with their symptoms, and who do not have evidence of massive cerebral infarction or cerebral hemorrhage. Although acute subarachnoid hemorrhage, particularly with an unprotected aneurysm, is a relative contraindication, this must be weighed against the severity of the deficit caused by the vasospasm. The preference should be to treat the ruptured aneurysm with endovascular coiling or clipping before angioplasty if possible, to avoid revascularization involving an unprotected, acutely ruptured aneurysm.

Procedure

The angioplasty procedure for acute vasospasm is performed while the patient is anticoagulated, under general anesthesia, and with a specifically designed low-profile compliant balloon mounted on an atraumatic flexible microcatheter (Target Therapeutics Corporation, Fremont, California). In general, standard regimens of heparin, with an ACT of 250–300 seconds, can be safely tolerated in the immediate postoperative period and after endovascular treatment by endovascular coiling of the aneurysm.

The balloon catheter is deployed through a 6.0-Fr guide catheter positioned in the extracranial internal carotid or vertebral artery. The balloon is gently inflated for short durations to enable intermittent cerebral perfusion and is gently advanced, and the inflations are repeated (Figure 17-6). Vessels most commonly treated are the supraclinoid internal carotid artery, the M1 segment of the middle cerebral artery, and the vertebral and basilar arteries. There is a longer-lasting benefit with mechanical balloon angioplasty than with intraluminal infusion of vasodilatory drugs such as papaverine.[95,98]

Selective intra-arterial papaverine injection has been used via a microcatheter in symptomatic spastic vessels with doses of 300 mg in 100 mL of normal saline over 30 minutes at doses of 50–250 mg/vessel.[95,99,100] Although there are reports of transient elevation of intracranial pressure, transient monocular blindness, and significant systemic hypotension, this technique does offer radiographic improvement in acute vessel dilatation and appears somewhat efficacious in the treat-

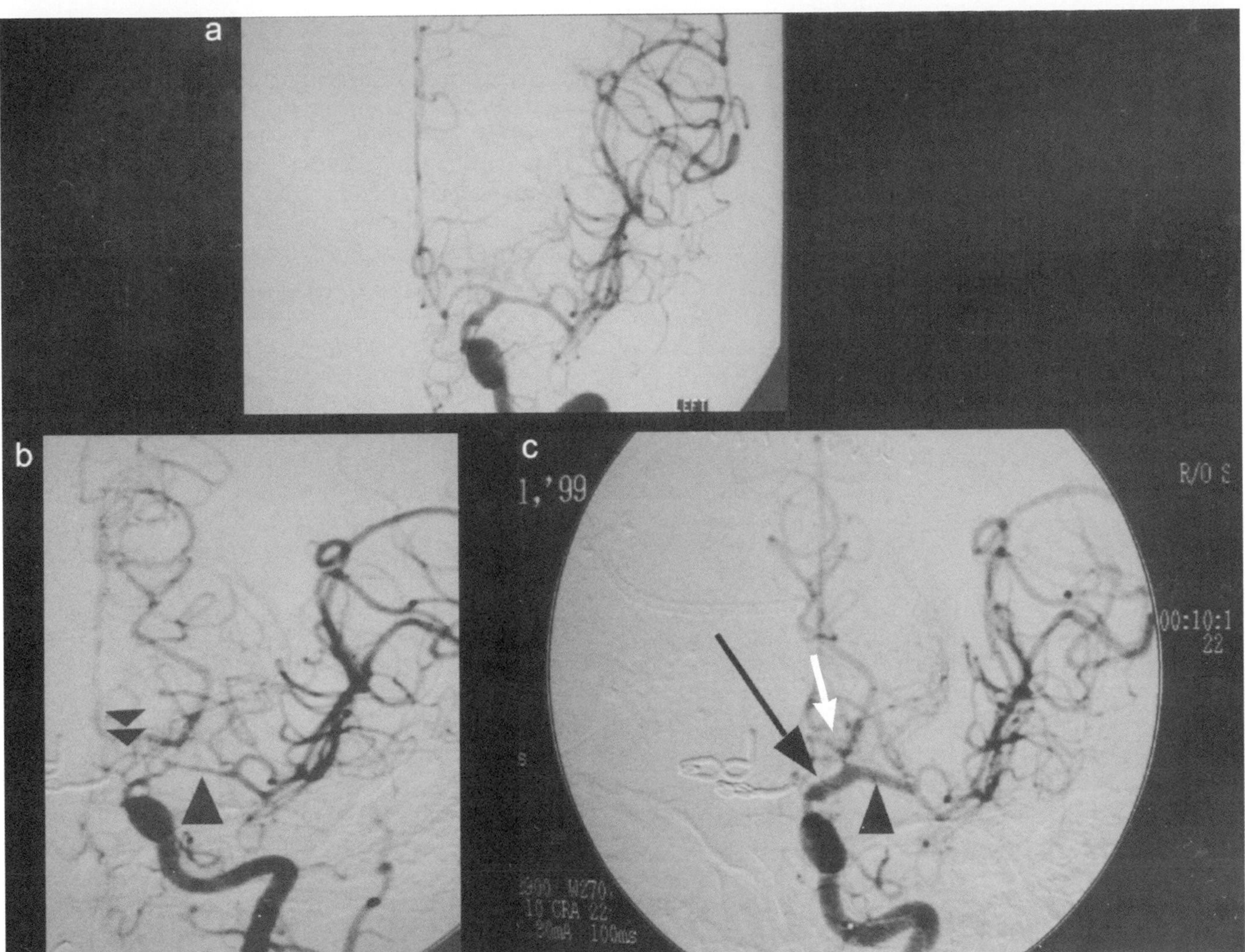

FIGURE 17-6. **A.** Cerebral angiogram on day 1 after a large subarachnoid hemorrhage from an anterior communicating artery aneurysm that filled from the right internal carotid artery. The left carotid angiogram shows the baseline caliber of the internal, middle cerebral, and anterior cerebral arteries. **B.** On day 7 after the bleed, the patient was obtunded with high velocities on transcranial Doppler ultrasound, which indicates severe vasospasm in all of the cerebral territories. A frontal view, left carotid angiogram reveals severe vasospasm of the middle cerebral artery (*single arrowhead*) and anterior cerebral artery (*double arrowhead*). The terminal internal carotid artery is also narrowed, which is typical in this setting. **C.** Frontal view angiogram after balloon angioplasty for vasospasm, with a compliant silicone balloon of the distal internal carotid artery and M1 segment of the middle cerebral artery. Note the reconstitution of the normal internal carotid (*black arrow*) and middle cerebral artery caliber (*arrowhead*). The A1 segment of the anterior cerebral artery (*white arrow*) is difficult to access after dilatation of the symptomatic middle cerebral artery, because the balloon catheter will tend to follow the high flow into the already dilated segments. Using over-the-wire balloons is possible, but there is concern about increased risk of vessel rupture or dissection. Percutaneous transluminal angioplasty was also performed in the basilar artery, and intra-arterial papaverine was infused into the anterior cerebral artery for treatment. The black arrow points to the supraclinoid carotid artery.

ment of early vasospasm. However, the effect of intra-arterial papaverine is short, lasting only several hours.

INTRA-ARTERIAL THROMBOLYTIC THERAPY FOR STROKE

The goal of emergency therapy for acute ischemic stroke is preservation of brain tissue that is not irreversibly damaged. Early recanalization correlates with improved outcome in acute stroke patients.[101] The recanalization rates with intra-arterial thrombolysis are superior to intravenous thrombolysis for major cerebrovascular large vessel occlusions.[102]

Several multicenter randomized trials evaluating intravenous administration of thrombolytic agents have been conducted,[103–108] and only the National Institute of

TABLE 17-3. Intra-Arterial Thrombolysis for Acute Ischemic Stroke: A Recent Series in Anterior, Posterior, and Combined Circulations

Author	*Mortality (%)*	*Recanalization (%)*
Barnwell et al.[127]	13	76.9
del Zoppo et al.[128]	20	90.0
Jahan et al.[129]	26	43.2
Jansen et al.[130]	16	12.5
Mori et al.[131]	22	90.0
Theron et al.[132]	12	100.0
Hacke et al.[114]	43	0.0
Mitchell et al.[113]	16	82.0
Becker et al.[115]	12	77.0
Higashida et al.[112]	27	82.2
Bockenheimer et al.[133]	18	0.0
Zeumer et al.[111]	31	93.5

Neurological Disorders and Stroke Tissue Plasminogen Activator Stroke Trial demonstrated an acceptably low rate of intracranial hemorrhage and significant efficacy.[103] In June 1996, tissue plasminogen activator received the U.S. Food and Drug Administration's approval for intravenous administration within 3 hours of onset of stroke symptoms.

The published series of intra-arterial thrombolysis in the carotid circulation (Table 17-3) has demonstrated good outcomes with mild increased rates of hemorrhage in similar proportions to those in the National Institute of Neurological Disorders and Stroke intravenous thrombolysis trial.

Randomized multicenter trials of local cerebral intra-arterial thrombolysis include the Prolyse for Acute Cerebral Thromboembolism (PROACT) I and II trials.[109] PROACT I demonstrated the safety of intra-arterial recombinant prourokinase, and the PROACT II trial showed a significant increase in the rate of reperfusion and a 60% relative neurologic improvement for prourokinase therapy with no significant increase in morbidity or mortality over the control group.[110]

Direct thrombolytic therapy in the vertebrobasilar territory has been associated with a markedly better outcome when compared to the natural history.[111–115] A wider therapeutic window is recognized in the vertebrobasilar territory, with good outcomes being reported up to 24 hours after symptom onset.[113]

Procedure

In the intravenous trials of thrombolytic therapy, case selection has been shown to be crucial to achieve good outcomes in acute ischemic stroke. A computed tomography scan or MRI brain scan with diffusion and perfusion imaging should be obtained before any therapy to exclude intracranial hemorrhage or large area of "completed" infarction and to exclude other pathologies such as tumor or demyelination. The presence of coma for several hours portends a poor prognosis, despite recanalization in patients presenting with vertebrobasilar thrombosis and stroke.[114,116]

A diagnostic catheter is placed into the high cervical segment of the vascular territory to be treated, followed by the introduction of a coaxial microcatheter and microguidewire system. The microcatheter is gently navigated through the intracranial circulation, using the road-map capability of a high-resolution fluoroscopy unit, until the tip is embedded within the central portion of the thrombus. For the majority of intra-arterial thrombolysis cases, a single end-hole microcatheter is used rather than the multiple side-hole infusion microcatheters used for pulse-spray thrombolysis. Angiography through the microcatheter is performed regularly to monitor the degree of clot lysis, allowing adjustment of the dose and volume of the thrombolytic agent.

Until recently, the preferred intra-arterial thrombolytic agent was urokinase in the dose range of 25,000–50,000 U, over 10-minute intervals, at the rate of 250,000–500,000 U per hour. Urokinase is available in the United States in 250,000-U vials and is mixed with 10 mL of sterile water, yielding a concentration of 25,000 U per mL. As the thrombus is dissolved, the catheter is directed into the more distal branches of the intracranial circulation so that the majority of the drug enters the occluded vessel. Currently, therapy is directed at treating patients within 4–6 hours of symptom onset. Treatment should not be denied to patients with vertebrobasilar thrombosis, even out to 24 hours, if other factors such as imaging scans not demonstrating large areas of completed infarction are favorable.

PROACT I[109] reported a 27% rate of symptomatic brain hemorrhage when a conventional heparin regimen (100 U/kg bolus, 1,000 U per hour for 4 hours) was used with intra-arterial recombinant prourokinase. Subsequently, a standard low-dose heparin regimen was used (2,000 U bolus, 500 U per hour for 4 hours), which reduced the symptomatic brain hemorrhage rate with intra-arterial recombinant prourokinase to 7% in PROACT I and 10% in PROACT II. Currently, the recommendations are for a low-dose regimen of heparinization in patients receiving thrombolysis.

The glycoprotein IIb/IIIa platelet inhibitor abciximab may be given as an intravenous bolus of 0.25 mg/kg followed by a continuous infusion of 10.00 μg per minute for 12 hours. This has been used successfully in patients undergoing acute or elective cerebrovascular interventions.[117] Coronary doses of abciximab appear to be safe in patients with acute ischemic stroke for up to

24 hours after onset in a preliminary phase I study.[118] However, until more studies are performed to demonstrate further safety and efficacy results, this treatment is still considered investigational.

Conclusion

Intra-arterial thrombolysis has become accepted as routine therapy for acute anterior circulation ischemic strokes and posterior circulation major vessel occlusive stroke. Patient selection and the therapeutic window will be refined by using perfusion-diffusion MRI, although there remains much work to be done. Early simplistic concepts of the ischemic penumbra correlating with the difference between the perfusion and diffusion abnormalities are being challenged, with "reversible" diffusion lesions and different patterns of infarct development. At this stage, there is no evidence to support absolute "triage" of patients entirely on the basis of MR data. Until this work is more advanced and access to the MR scanner and the results of the study are available within minutes, many patients must still be assessed using computed tomography and proceed to treatment based on the case series and trials that have been reported currently.

Ultimately, comprehensive management using all available therapies including intravenous thrombolysis, cytoprotective agents, and recanalization agents will be necessary to achieve improved patient outcomes. However, only when timely arrival of patients to emergency medical facilities occurs can treatment also be instituted appropriately. Mechanical clot removal, new catheter techniques, and new adjunctive antithrombotic agents should improve the degree, speed, and safety of intra-arterial recanalization.

Carotid territory stroke patients who arrive outside a 3-hour time window and, therefore, are outside the time window for intravenous thrombolysis may benefit from direct intra-arterial thrombolysis. Combined strategies such as commencing intravenous thrombolysis and neuroprotective agents at admission while organizing intra-arterial thrombolysis offer the potential advantages of both strategies in a more time-effective manner and warrant further assessment. In patients with the clinical syndrome of major vertebrobasilar stroke and with vertebral or basilar occlusion, intra-arterial thrombolysis has been associated with markedly improved outcomes compared against available natural history studies.

INTERVENTIONS FOR INTRACRANIAL VENOUS THROMBOSIS

Dural venous sinus occlusion can be asymptomatic, associated with minor symptoms of headache, vertigo, nausea, vomiting, and seizures, or present with focal neurologic deficits and a decreasing conscious state. The mortality and morbidity have been variably estimated and are difficult to predict. The outcome in the majority of cases of dural sinus thrombosis managed with anticoagulation or supportive measures has been excellent. Therefore, more aggressive therapy has been reserved for patients with clinical deterioration despite anticoagulation and medical therapy.

There remain cases of poor outcome despite these therapies, and one attempt to identify these patients has used MRI and direct dural sinus pressure measurements.[119] Patients have been identified with five distinct stages of brain parenchymal changes, and each stage is correlated with increasing intradural sinus pressure from 20 to 50 mm Hg. Brain parenchymal changes were reversible up to stage III if direct thrombolytic treatment was performed.

Excellent results of local, direct fibrinolytic therapy have been reported with no major complications.[119–121] Malek et al. have also reported on the successful technique of adjunctive stent placement within the dural sinuses to preserve patency, after extensive thrombosis of the dural sinuses had occurred with resultant neurologic deterioration.[122]

Procedure

Access is usually from femoral venous catheterization, after diagnostic evaluation with full cerebral angiography and study of the venous phase of the arterial injection. MR angiography has also been useful for the diagnosis of dural sinus thrombosis. Heparin is commenced before the interventional procedure and has also been used in the presence of small amounts of hemorrhage. If enlarging venous hemorrhages are demonstrated while the patient is on heparin, then a mechanical thrombectomy device for rapid recanalization should be considered.

Thrombolysis in the dural sinuses, either bolus or continuous infusions, can be used through a microcatheter at rates between 20,000 and 150,000 U of urokinase per hour. The catheter easily passes through recent acute and subacute thrombus despite occlusion on imaging.

Mechanical techniques include guidewire manipulation, balloon angioplasty catheters, and a rheolytic thrombectomy device (CF105 AngioJet, POSSIS Medical Inc., Minneapolis, Minnesota)—all of which have been reported for treatment of dural sinus thrombosis. The large volume of thrombus in the dural sinuses compared to arterial occlusions and the more frequent associated parenchymal hemorrhages are ideal situations for the use of mechanical clot disruption. The rheolytic thrombectomy device is effective in removing thrombus and, if efficacy is demonstrated in larger numbers, may become the preferred technique, especially in the presence of hemorrhage.

A significant proportion of patients with dural sinus thromboses experience major morbidity or die despite standard anticoagulant therapy. Patients who are at higher risk include those with extensive occlusion and with compromised blood flow in the remaining venous channels, major parenchymal changes on MRI, elevated pressure within the dural sinus at venography, and failed anticoagulant therapy. Combinations of chemical and mechanical thrombolysis are available and safe to use and should be used in these higher-risk patients.

CONCLUSION

Recent advances in neurointerventional therapy, including devices specifically designed for use in the extracranial and intracranial cerebral vasculature, have broadened the treatment of acute ischemic stroke. Carotid, vertebral, and subclavian angioplasty and stenting are now becoming established in selected high-risk patients as viable treatments for highly stenotic lesions. Intracranial balloon angioplasty for cerebral arterial vasospasm has become widely accepted for treatment in patients who have not responded to conventional medical therapy.

Intracranial angioplasty and stenting for symptomatic intracranial atherosclerosis are also gaining acceptance at many major medical centers. This is especially true for patients who have not responded to standard medical therapy with antiplatelet and anticoagulant treatment. Symptomatic patients with dural sinus thrombosis who do not respond to systemic anticoagulation are now being treated by interventional techniques by direct thrombolytic therapy and by mechanical revascularization techniques.

Acute ischemic stroke within 3 hours of acute symptom presentation is now widely treated with intravenous tissue plasminogen activator and within 3–6 hours by direct intra-arterial thrombolytic therapy.

Continued improvements in imaging strategies will also aid in patient selection for those candidates best suited for interventional neuroradiologic procedures to treat acute ischemic stroke patients. Future therapeutic strategies will make many of these procedures even more effective as these technologies continue to improve.

REFERENCES

1. The National Advisory Neurological Disorders and Stroke Council. Stroke and Cerebrovascular Disease. In Status Report: Decade of the Brain. National Institutes of Health Report, Public Health Services. Bethesda, MD: National Institutes of Health; 1992;26–27.

2. American Heart Association. 1993 Heart and Stroke Facts Statistics. Dallas, TX: American Heart Association, 1993.

3. Whisnant JP, Cartlidge NE, Elveback LR. Carotid and vertebral-basilar transient ischemic attacks: effect of anticoagulants, hypertension, and cardiac disorders on survival and stroke occurrence—a population study. Ann Neurol 1978;3(2):107–115.

4. Acheson J, Hutchinson EC. The natural history of "focal cerebral vascular disease." QJM 1971; 157:15–25.

5. Heros RC. Stroke: early pathophysiology and treatment. Summary of the Fifth Annual Decade of the Brain Symposium [see comments]. Stroke 1994;25(9): 1877–1881.

6. Strandness DE. Surgical Therapy for Extracranial Arterial Disease. In DE Strandness, A van Breda (eds), Vascular Diseases: Surgical and Interventional Therapy. New York: Churchill Livingstone, 1994;643–650.

7. Beneficial effect of carotid endarterectomy in symptomatic patients with high-grade carotid stenosis. North American Symptomatic Carotid Endarterectomy Trial Collaborators [see comments]. N Engl J Med 1991;325(7):445–453.

8. Executive Committee for the Asymptomatic Carotid Atherosclerosis Study. Endarterectomy for asymptomatic carotid artery stenosis [see comments]. JAMA 1995;273(18):1421–1428.

9. Dotter CT, Judkins MP. Transluminal treatment of arteriosclerotic obstruction: description of a new technique and preliminary report of its application. Circulation 1964;30:654–670.

10. Becker G, Katzen B, Dake M. Noncoronary angioplasty. Radiology 1989;170:921–940.

11. Gallino A, Mahler F, Probst P, Nachbur B. Percutaneous transluminal angioplasty of the arteries of the lower limbs: a 5 year follow-up. Circulation 1984; 70(4):619–623.

12. Klinge J, Mali WP, Puijlaert CB, et al. Percutaneous transluminal renal angioplasty: initial and long-term results. Radiology 1989;171(2):501–506.

13. Serruys PW, van Hout B, Bonnier H, et al. Randomised comparison of implantation of heparin-coated stents with balloon angioplasty in selected patients with coronary artery disease (Benestent II) [published erratum in Lancet 1998;352(9138):1478]. Lancet 1998;352(9129):673–681.

14. Macaya C, Serruys PW, Ruygrok P, et al. Continued benefit of coronary stenting versus balloon angioplasty: one-year clinical follow-up of Benestent trial. Benestent Study Group. J Am Coll Cardiol 1996;27(2):255–261.

15. Motarjeme A, Keifer JW, Zuska AJ. Percutaneous transluminal angioplasty of the brachiocephalic arteries. AJR Am J Roentgenol 1982;138(3):457–462.

16. Bockenheimer SA, Mathias K. Percutaneous transluminal angioplasty in arteriosclerotic internal carotid artery stenosis. AJNR Am J Neuroradiol 1983; 4(3):791–792.

17. Hodgins GW, Dutton JW. Subclavian and carotid angioplasties for Takayasu's arteritis. J Can Assoc Radiol 1982;33(3):205–207.

18. Courtheoux P, Tournade A, Theron J, et al. Transcutaneous angioplasty of vertebral artery atheromatous ostial stricture. Neuroradiology 1985;27(3): 259–264.

19. Tsai FY, Matovich V, Hieshima G, et al. Percutaneous transluminal angioplasty of the carotid artery. AJNR Am J Neuroradiol 1986;7(2):349–358.

20. Theron J. Angioplasty of Brachiocephalic Vessels. In V Vinuela, VV Halbach, JE Dion (eds), Interventional Neuroradiology: Endovascular Therapy of the Central Nervous System. New York: Raven Press, 1992;167–180.

21. Higashida RT, Tsai FY, Halbach VV, et al. Transluminal angioplasty, thrombolysis, and stenting for extracranial and intracranial cerebral vascular disease. J Interv Cardiol 1996;9(3):245–255.

22. Kachel R. Results of balloon angioplasty in the carotid arteries [see comments]. J Endovasc Surg 1996;3(1):22–30.

23. Schoser BG, Becker VU, Eckert B, et al. Clinical and ultrasonic long-term results of percutaneous transluminal carotid angioplasty. A prospective follow-up of 30 carotid angioplasties. Cerebrovasc Dis 1998;8(1):38–41.

24. Yadav JS, Roubin GS, King P, et al. Angioplasty and stenting for restenosis after carotid endarterectomy. Initial experience. Stroke 1996;27(11):2075–2079.

25. Diethrich EB, Ndiaye M, Reid DB. Stenting in the carotid artery: initial experience in 110 patients. J Endovasc Surg 1996;3(1):42–62.

26. Roubin GS, Yadav S, Iyer SS, Vitek J. Carotid stent supported angioplasty: a neurovascular intervention to prevent stroke. Am J Cardiol 1996;78:8–12.

27. Vitek J, Roubin G, Iyer S. Immediate and Late Outcome of Carotid Angioplasty with Stenting. Joint Section Meeting, AANS/CNS/ASITN, January 31–February 3, 1999; Nashville.

28. Yadav JS, Roubin GS, Iyer S, et al. Elective stenting of the extracranial carotid arteries [see comments]. Circulation 1997;95(2):376–381.

29. Theron JG, Payelle GG, Coskun O, et al. Carotid artery stenosis: treatment with protected balloon angioplasty and stent placement [see comments]. Radiology 1996;201(3):627–636.

30. Mathur A, Roubin GS, Iyer SS, et al. Predictors of stroke complicating carotid artery stenting. Circulation 1998;97(13):1239–1245.

31. Henry M, Amor M, Masson I, et al. Angioplasty and stenting of the extracranial carotid arteries. J Endovasc Surg 1998;5(4):293–304.

32. Wholey MH, Wholey M, Bergeron P, et al. Current global status of carotid artery stent placement [see comments]. Cathet Cardiovasc Diagn 1998; 44(1):1–6.

33. Mathias K, Jager H, Sahl H, et al. Interventional treatment of arteriosclerotic carotid stenosis [in German]. Radiologe 1999;39(2):125–134.

34. Al-Mubarak N, Roubin GS, Liu MW, et al. Early results of percutaneous intervention for severe coexisting carotid and coronary artery disease. Am J Cardiol 1999;84(5):600–602, A9.

35. Piepgras DG, Sundt TM, Marsh WR, et al. Recurrent carotid stenosis. Results and complications of 57 operations. Ann Surg 1986;203(2):205–213.

36. Sundt TMJ, Meyer FB, Piepgras DG, et al. Risk Factors and Operative Results. In FB Meyer (ed), Sundt's Occlusive Cerebrovascular Disease (2nd ed). Philadelphia: Saunders, 1994;241–247.

37. Jordan WD Jr, Voellinger DC, Fisher WS, et al. A comparison of carotid angioplasty with stenting versus endarterectomy with regional anesthesia [see comments]. J Vasc Surg 1998;28(3):397–402; discussion 3.

38. Naylor AR, Bolia A, Abbott RJ, et al. Randomized study of carotid angioplasty and stenting versus carotid endarterectomy: a stopped trial. J Vasc Surg 1998;28(2):326–334.

39. Sivaguru A, Venables GS, Beard JD, Gaines PA. European carotid angioplasty trial [see comments]. J Endovasc Surg 1996;3(1):16–20.

40. Tcheng JE. Glycoprotein IIb/IIIa receptor inhibitors: putting the EPIC, IMPACT II, RESTORE, and EPILOG trials into perspective. Am J Cardiol 1996;78(3A):35–40.

41. Mathur A, Dorros G, Iyer SS, et al. Palmaz stent compression in patients following carotid artery stenting. Cathet Cardiovasc Diagn 1997;41(2):137–140.

42. Theron J. Cerebral protection during carotid angioplasty [letter; comment]. J Endovasc Surg 1996; 3(4):484–486.

43. Muller M, Behnke S, Walter P, et al. Microembolic signals and intraoperative stroke in carotid endarterectomy. Acta Neurol Scand 1998;97(2):110–117.

44. Crawley F, Clifton A, Buckenham T, et al. Comparison of hemodynamic cerebral ischemia and microembolic signals detected during carotid endarterectomy and carotid angioplasty. Stroke 1997;28(12):2460–2464.

45. Bladin CF, Bingham L, Grigg L, et al. Transcranial Doppler detection of microemboli during percutaneous transluminal coronary angioplasty. Stroke 1998;29(11):2367–2370.

46. Gaunt ME, Brown L, Hartshorne T, et al. Unstable carotid plaques: preoperative identification and association with intraoperative embolisation detected by transcranial Doppler. Eur J Vasc Endovasc Surg 1996;11(1):78–82.

47. Levi CR, O'Malley HM, Fell G, et al. Transcranial Doppler detected cerebral microembolism fol-

lowing carotid endarterectomy. High microembolic signal loads predict postoperative cerebral ischaemia [see comments]. Brain 1997;120(4):621–629.

48. Theron J, Courtheoux P, Alachkar F, et al. New triple coaxial catheter system for carotid angioplasty with cerebral protection. AJNR Am J Neuroradiol 1990;11(5):869–874; discussion 75–77.

49. Cloft HJ, Joseph GJ, Dion JE. Risk of cerebral angiography in patients with subarachnoid hemorrhage, cerebral aneurysm, and arteriovenous malformation: a meta-analysis. Stroke 1999;30(2):317–320.

50. Moufarrij NA, Little JR, Furlan AJ, et al. Vertebral artery stenosis: long-term follow-up. Stroke 1984;15(2):260–263.

51. Imparato AM, Riles TS, Kim GE. Cervical vertebral angioplasty for brain stem ischemia. Surgery 1981;90(5):842–852.

52. Hass WK, Fields WS, North RR, et al. Joint study of extracranial arterial occlusion. II. Arteriography, techniques, sites, and complications. JAMA 1968;203(11):961–968.

53. Moufarrij NA, Little JR, Furlan AJ, et al. Basilar and distal vertebral artery stenosis: long-term follow-up. Stroke 1986;17(5):938–942.

54. Wityk RJ, Chang HM, Rosengart A, et al. Proximal extracranial vertebral artery disease in the New England Medical Center Posterior Circulation Registry. Arch Neurol 1998;55(4):470–478.

55. Prognosis of patients with symptomatic vertebral or basilar artery stenosis. The Warfarin-Aspirin Symptomatic Intracranial Disease (WASID) Study Group. Stroke 1998;29(7):1389–1392.

56. Motarjeme A, Keifer JW, Zuska AJ. Percutaneous transluminal angioplasty of the vertebral arteries. Radiology 1981;139(3):715–717.

57. Bruckmann H, Ringelstein EB, Buchner H, Zeumer H. Percutaneous transluminal angioplasty of the vertebral artery. A therapeutic alternative to operative reconstruction of proximal vertebral artery stenoses. J Neurol 1986;233(6):336–339.

58. Higashida RT, Hieshima GB, Tsai FY, et al. Percutaneous transluminal angioplasty of the subclavian and vertebral arteries. Acta Radiol Suppl 1986; 369:124–126.

59. Higashida RT, Hieshima GB, Tsai FY, et al. Transluminal angioplasty of the vertebral and basilar artery. AJNR Am J Neuroradiol 1987;8(5):745–749.

60. Kachel R, Endert G, Basche S, et al. Percutaneous transluminal angioplasty (dilatation) of carotid, vertebral, and innominate artery stenoses. Cardiovasc Interv Radiol 1987;10(3):142–146.

61. Theron J, Courtheoux P, Henriet JP, et al. Angioplasty of supraaortic arteries. J Neuroradiol 1984;11(3):187–200.

62. Tournade A, Zenglein JP, Braun JP, et al. Percutaneous transluminal angioplasty of the vertebral and subclavian arteries. An angiographic-velocimetry comparison. J Neuroradiol 1986;13(2):95–110.

63. Higashida RT, Tsai FY, Halbach VV, et al. Transluminal angioplasty for atherosclerotic disease of the vertebral and basilar arteries. J Neurosurg 1993;78(2):192–198.

64. Motarjeme A. Percutaneous transluminal angioplasty of supra-aortic vessels. J Endovasc Surg 1996;3(2):171–181.

65. Feldman RL, Trigg L, Gaudier J, Galat J. Use of coronary Palmaz-Schatz stent in the percutaneous treatment of an intracranial carotid artery stenosis. Cathet Cardiovasc Diagn 1996;38(3):316–319.

66. Storey GS, Marks MP, Dake M, et al. Vertebral artery stenting following percutaneous transluminal angioplasty. Technical note. J Neurosurg 1996;84(5):883–887.

67. Malek AM, Higashida RT, Phatouros CC, et al. Treatment of posterior circulation ischemia with extracranial percutaneous balloon angioplasty and stent placement. Stroke 1999;30(10):2073–2085.

68. Phatouros CC, Higashida RT, Malek AM, et al. Endovascular treatment of noncarotid extracranial cerebrovascular disease. Neurosurg Clin North Am 2000;11:331–350.

69. Chimowitz MI, Kokkinos J, Strong J, et al. The Warfarin-Aspirin Symptomatic Intracranial Disease Study. Neurology 1995;45(8):1488–1493.

70. Bogousslavsky J, Barnett HJ, Fox AJ, et al. Atherosclerotic disease of the middle cerebral artery. Stroke 1986;17(6):1112–1120.

71. Wechsler LR, Kistler JP, Davis KR, Kaminski MJ. The prognosis of carotid siphon stenosis. Stroke 1986;17(4):714–718.

72. Failure of extracranial-intracranial arterial bypass to reduce the risk of ischemic stroke. Results of an international randomized trial. The EC/IC Bypass Study Group. N Engl J Med 1985;313(19):1191–2000.

73. Marzewski DJ, Furlan AJ, St. Louis P, et al. Intracranial internal carotid artery stenosis: longterm prognosis. Stroke 1982;13(6):821–824.

74. Kappelle LJ, Eliasziw M, Fox AJ, et al. Importance of intracranial atherosclerotic disease in patients with symptomatic stenosis of the internal carotid artery. The North American Symptomatic Carotid Endarterectomy Trial. Stroke 1999;30(2):282–286.

75. Sundt TM Jr, Smith HC, Campbell JK, et al. Transluminal angioplasty for basilar artery stenosis. Mayo Clin Proc 1980;55(11):673–680.

76. Clark WM, Barnwell SL, Nesbit G, et al. Safety and efficacy of percutaneous transluminal angioplasty for intracranial atherosclerotic stenosis. Stroke 1995;26(7):1200–1204.

77. McKenzie JD, Wallace RC, Dean BL, et al. Preliminary results of intracranial angioplasty for vascular stenosis caused by atherosclerosis and vasculitis. AJNR Am J Neuroradiol 1996;17(2):263–268.

78. Mori T, Fukuoka M, Kazita K, Mori K. Follow-up study after intracranial percutaneous transluminal cerebral balloon angioplasty [see comments]. AJNR Am J Neuroradiol 1998;19(8):1525–1533.

79. Takis C, Kwan ES, Pessin MS, et al. Intracranial angioplasty: experience and complications. AJNR Am J Neuroradiol 1997;18(9):1661–1668.

80. Marks MP, Marcellus M, Norbash AM, et al. Outcome of angioplasty for atherosclerotic intracranial stenosis. Stroke 1999;30(5):1065–1069.

81. Eckard DA, Zarnow DM, McPherson CM, et al. Intracranial internal carotid artery angioplasty: technique with clinical and radiographic results and follow-up. AJR Am J Roentgenol 1999;172(3):703–707.

82. Terada T, Yokote H, Kinoshita Y, et al. Carotid endarterectomy and simultaneous percutaneous transluminal angioplasty for tandem internal carotid stenoses. Neuroradiology 1998;40(6):404–408.

83. Terada T, Higashida RT, Halbach VV, et al. Transluminal angioplasty for arteriosclerotic disease of the distal vertebral and basilar arteries. J Neurol Neurosurg Psychiatry 1996;60(4):377–381.

84. Connors JJ 3rd, Wojak JC. Percutaneous transluminal angioplasty for intracranial atherosclerotic lesions: evolution of technique and short-term results. J Neurosurg 1999;91(3):415–423.

85. Mitchell PJ. Interventional neuroradiology techniques in neurovascular disease. Br J Hosp Med 1997;58(1):8–14.

86. Phatouros CC, Higashida RT, Malek AM, et al. Endovascular stenting of an acutely thrombosed basilar artery: technical case report and review of the literature. Neurosurgery 1999;44(3):667–673.

87. Yokote H, Terada T, Ryujin K, et al. Percutaneous transluminal angioplasty for intracranial arteriosclerotic lesions. Neuroradiology 1998;40(9):590–596.

88. Nakayama T, Tanaka K, Kaneko M, et al. Thrombolysis and angioplasty for acute occlusion of intracranial vertebrobasilar arteries. Report of three cases. J Neurosurg 1998;88(5):919–922.

89. Mencken GS, Wholey MH, Eles GR. Use of coronary artery stents in the treatment of internal carotid artery stenosis at the base of the skull. Cathet Cardiovasc Diagn 1998;45(4):434–438.

90. Dorros G, Cohn JM, Palmer LE. Stent deployment resolves a petrous carotid artery angioplasty dissection. AJNR Am J Neuroradiol 1998;19(2):392–394.

91. Higashida RT, Halbach VV, Cahan LD, et al. Transluminal angioplasty for treatment of intracranial arterial vasospasm. J Neurosurg 1989;71(5 Pt 1):648–653.

92. Kassell NF, Sasaki T, Colohan AR, Nazar G. Cerebral vasospasm following aneurysmal subarachnoid hemorrhage. Stroke 1985;16(4):562–572.

93. Zubkov YN, Nikiforov BM, Shustin VA. Balloon catheter technique for dilatation of constricted cerebral arteries after aneurysmal SAH. Acta Neurochir 1984;70(1–2):65–79.

94. Higashida RT, Halbach VV, Dowd CF, et al. Intravascular balloon dilatation therapy for intracranial arterial vasospasm: patient selection, technique, and clinical results. Neurosurg Rev 1992;15(2):89–95.

95. Eskridge JM, McAuliffe W, Song JK, et al. Balloon angioplasty for the treatment of vasospasm: results of first 50 cases. Neurosurgery 1998;42(3):510–516; discussion 6–7.

96. Smith RR, Clower BR, Grotendorst GM, et al. Arterial wall changes in early human vasospasm. Neurosurgery 1985;16(2):171–176.

97. Higashida RT, Halbach VV, Tsai FY, et al. Interventional neurovascular techniques for cerebral revascularization in the treatment of stroke. AJR Am J Roentgenol 1994;163(4):793–800.

98. Elliott JP, Newell DW, Lam DJ, et al. Comparison of balloon angioplasty and papaverine infusion for the treatment of vasospasm following aneurysmal subarachnoid hemorrhage. J Neurosurg 1998;88(2):277–284.

99. Clouston JE, Numaguchi Y, Zoarski GH, et al. Intraarterial papaverine infusion for cerebral vasospasm after subarachnoid hemorrhage. AJNR Am J Neuroradiol 1995;16(1):27–38.

100. Morgan MK, Day MJ, Little N, et al. The use of intraarterial papaverine in the management of vasospasm complicating arteriovenous malformation resection. Report of two cases. J Neurosurg 1995;82(2): 296–299.

101. Wardlaw JM, Warlow CP. Thrombolysis in acute ischemic stroke: does it work? [see comments]. Stroke 1992;23(12):911–912.

102. Pessin M, del Zoppo GJ, Furlan AJ. Thrombolytic Treatment in Acute Stroke: Review and Update of Selective Topics. In MA Moskowitz, LR Caplan, (eds), Cerebrovascular Diseases. Nineteenth Princeton Stroke Conference. Boston: Butterworth–Heinemann, 1995;409–418.

103. Tissue plasminogen activator for acute ischemic stroke. The National Institute of Neurological Disorders and Stroke rt-PA Stroke Study Group [see comments]. N Engl J Med 1995;333(24):1581–1587.

104. Hacke W, Kaste M, Fieschi C, et al. Intravenous thrombolysis with recombinant tissue plasminogen activator for acute hemispheric stroke. The European Cooperative Acute Stroke Study (ECASS) [see comments]. JAMA 1995;274(13):1017–1025.

105. Thrombolytic Therapy with Streptokinase in Acute Ischemic Stroke. N Engl J Med 1996;335(3): 145–150.

106. Donnan GA, Hommel M, Davis SM, McNeil JJ. Streptokinase in acute ischaemic stroke. Steering Committees of the ASK and MAST-E trials. Australian Streptokinase Trial [letter; comment]. Lancet 1995; 346(8966):56.

107. Donnan GA, Davis SM, Chambers BR, et al. Trials of streptokinase in severe acute ischaemic stroke [letter; comment] [see comments]. Lancet 1995; 345(8949):578–579.

108. Donnan GA, Davis SM, Chambers BR, et al. Australian Streptokinase Trial (ASK). In GJ del Zoppo, E Mori, W Hacke (eds). Thrombolytic Therapy in Acute Ischemic Stroke II. Berlin: Springer, 1993;80–85.

109. del Zoppo GJ, Higashida RT, Furlan AJ, et al. PROACT: a phase II randomized trial of recombinant pro-urokinase by direct arterial delivery in acute middle cerebral artery stroke. PROACT Investigators. Prolyse in Acute Cerebral Thromboembolism [see comments]. Stroke 1998;29(1):4–11.

110. Furlan A, Higashida R, Wechsler L, et al. Intra-arterial prourokinase for acute ischemic stroke. The PROACT II study: a randomized controlled trial. Prolyse in Acute Cerebral Thromboembolism. JAMA 1999;282(21):2003–2011.

111. Zeumer H, Freitag HJ, Zanella F, et al. Local intra-arterial fibrinolytic therapy in patients with stroke: urokinase versus recombinant tissue plasminogen activator (r-TPA). Neuroradiology 1993;35(2):159–162.

112. Higashida RT, Halbach VV, Barnwell SL, et al. Thrombolytic therapy in acute stroke. J Endovasc Surg 1994;1:4–15.

113. Mitchell PJ, Gerraty RP, Donnan GA, et al. Thrombolysis in the vertebrobasilar circulation. The Australian Urokinase Stroke Trial (AUST) pilot study. Cerebrovasc Dis 1997;7:94–99.

114. Hacke W, Zeumer H, Ferbert A, et al. Intra-arterial thrombolytic therapy improves outcome in patients with acute vertebrobasilar occlusive disease. Stroke 1988;19(10):1216–1222.

115. Becker K, Monstein L, Ulatowski J, et al. Intraarterial thrombolysis in vertebrobasilar occlusion. AJNR Am J Neuroradiol 1996;17:255–262.

116. Brandt T, von Kummer R, Muller-Kuppers M, Hacke W. Thrombolytic therapy of acute basilar artery occlusion. Variables affecting recanalization and outcome. Stroke 1996;27(5):875–881.

117. Adams HP, Bogousslavsky J, Barnathan E, et al. Preliminary safety report of a randomized trial of abciximab (ReoProR) in acute ischemic stroke. Cerebrovasc Dis 1999;9(suppl 1):127–131.

118. Wallace RC, Furlan AJ, Moliterno DJ, et al. Basilar artery rethrombosis: successful treatment with platelet glycoprotein IIB/IIIA receptor inhibitor. AJNR Am J Neuroradiol 1997;18(7):1257–1260.

119. Tsai FY, Wang AM, Matovich VB, et al. MR staging of acute dural sinus thrombosis: correlation with venous pressure measurements and implications for treatment and prognosis. AJNR Am J Neuroradiol 1995;16(5):1021–1029.

120. Smith TP, Higashida RT, Barnwell SL, et al. Treatment of dural sinus thrombosis by urokinase infusion. AJNR Am J Neuroradiol 1994;15(5):801–807.

121. Tsai FY, Higashida RT, Matovich V, Alfieri K. Acute thrombosis of the intracranial dural sinus: direct thrombolytic treatment. AJNR Am J Neuroradiol 1992;13(4):1137–1141.

122. Malek AM, Higashida RT, Balousek PA, et al. Endovascular recanalization with balloon angioplasty and stenting of an occluded occipital sinus for treatment of intracranial venous hypertension: technical case report. Neurosurgery 1999;44(4):896–901.

123. Wholey MH, Jarmolowski CR, Eles G, et al. Endovascular stents for carotid artery occlusive disease. J Endovasc Surg 1997;4:326–338.

124. Waigand J, Gross CM, Uhlich F, et al. Elective stenting of carotid artery stenosis in patients with severe coronary artery disease. Eur Heart J 1998;19:1365–1370.

125. Teitelbaum GP, Lefkowitz MA, Giannotta SL. Carotid angioplasty and stenting in high-risk patients. Surg Neurol 1998;50(4):300–311; discussion 11–12.

126. Iyer SS, Roubin GS, Yadav S, et al. Elective Carotid Stenting. J Endovasc Surg 1996;3:42–62.

127. Barnwell SL, Clark WM, Nguyen TT, et al. Safety and efficacy of delayed intraarterial urokinase therapy with mechanical clot disruption for thromboembolic stroke. AJNR Am J Neuroradiol 1994; 15(10):1817–1822.

128. del Zoppo GJ, Ferbert A, Otis S, et al. Local intra-arterial fibrinolytic therapy in acute carotid territory stroke. A pilot study. Stroke 1988;19(3):307–313.

129. Jahan R, Duckwiler GR, Kidwell CS, et al. Intraarterial thrombolysis for treatment of acute stroke: experience in 26 patients with long-term follow-up [see comments]. AJNR Am J Neuroradiol 1999;20(7): 1291–1299.

130. Jansen O, von Kummer R, Forsting M, et al. Thrombolytic therapy in acute occlusion of the intracranial internal carotid artery bifurcation [see comments]. AJNR Am J Neuroradiol 1995;16(10):1977–1986.

131. Mori E, Tabuchi M, Yoshida T, Yamadori A. Intracarotid urokinase with thromboembolic occlusion of the middle cerebral artery. Stroke 1988;19(7):802–812.

132. Theron J, Courtheoux P, Casasco A, et al. Local intraarterial fibrinolysis in the carotid territory. AJNR Am J Neuroradiol 1989;10:753–765.

133. Bockenheimer S, Reinhuber F, Mohs C. Intraarterial thrombolysis of vessels supplying the brain [in German]. Radiologe 1991;31(4):210–215.

CHAPTER

18

Endovascular Treatment of Aneurysms and Arteriovenous Malformations

John D. Barr and Bohdan W. Chopko

Aneurysms and arteriovenous malformations (AVMs) of the brain represent some of the most significant lesions that may be detected and evaluated by radiologic imaging techniques. Left undetected or untreated, they also represent potentially fatal lesions. When an aneurysm or an AVM has been detected, it is important to know which tests should be ordered to fully evaluate the lesion with regard to potential treatment. Current imaging modalities are often complementary; typically, the most complete diagnostic picture is a fusion of multiple imaging modalities, including computed tomography (CT), magnetic resonance imaging (MRI), magnetic resonance angiography (MRA), and catheter-based angiography. After obtaining the necessary anatomic and clinical information, the involved physicians may then formulate an appropriate treatment plan.

Whether to treat an aneurysm or AVM depends on a variety of pertinent issues. All treatments carry some risk of stroke or death. The patient's clinical presentation, age, other medical risk factors, and estimated risks associated with potential treatments must all be considered. These factors must be balanced against the natural history of the untreated aneurysm or AVM. The final treatment plan requires integration of a host of information and often includes the input from multiple physicians from different specialties. Current therapy of aneurysms and AVMs may include open neurosurgical procedures, endovascular procedures, stereotactic radiosurgery (for AVMs), or a combination of these strategies.

ANEURYSMS

The natural history of patients presenting with an acute subarachnoid hemorrhage (SAH) from a ruptured aneurysm is quite poor. Although estimates vary widely and the true incidence may never be known, approximately one-half of all patients die almost immediately after aneurysmal rupture. Of the survivors, approximately one-half have a "good" neurologic recovery. However, only a relatively small fraction of patients experience complete or nearly complete recovery that allows them to resume all of their previous activities.[1,2]

The most important factor to consider in the treatment of a cerebral aneurysm is the patient's clinical presentation. Patients presenting with acute SAH from a ruptured aneurysm are at very high risk for rebleeding, which usually results in a poor or fatal outcome. The risk of rebleeding is highest within the first 24 hours after the initial hemorrhage. The incidence of rebleeding is estimated to be 20–50% within 2 weeks after the initial hemorrhage.[2–5] In general, unless the patient is too ill to undergo treatment or the anatomy of the aneurysm predicts a very high risk from treatment, patients with ruptured aneurysms should be treated either by endovascular coiling or surgical clipping.

For patients with asymptomatic unruptured aneurysms, the size of the aneurysm and the age of the patient are very important factors to consider in the decision of how to treat. Patients with small (<5–10 mm) unruptured aneurysms may have only a low risk of hemorrhage that does not justify intervention. Younger patients with longer life expectancies, however, have a greater cumulative risk of aneurysm rupture. Whether small unruptured aneurysms should be treated is the subject of much debate. The International Study of Unruptured Intracranial Aneurysms reported by Wiebers et al. in 1998 suggests a very benign natural history for small unruptured aneurysms (defined as <10 mm in maximum dimension).[6] They concluded that the annualized risk of rupture was only 0.05% for these small aneurysms. There are two significant criticisms of this study. First, the patients studied did not represent a consecutive group presenting with unruptured aneurysms. Perhaps more important, their conclusion that small aneurysms rarely rupture contradicts the predominance of small aneurysms among patients presenting with SAH. In the authors' personal experiences at multiple institutions, these small aneurysms are responsible for a large majority of the patients admitted with SAH. Our opinion is shared by many others. Throughout the neurosurgical and neurointerventional community, it is more commonly believed that 3–5 mm is the appropriate threshold size for treatment versus observation of an unruptured aneurysm. Because the estimated risk of treatment, and thus the relative benefit of treatment, depends on the location and morphology of the aneurysm, these factors must also be considered in the decision to treat.

Approximately 20% of patients harbor multiple intracranial aneurysms.[7,8] Not surprisingly, they represent a special challenge for treatment. Particularly in the acute setting, it is not always possible to treat each aneurysm. Treatment, however, should be directed at the aneurysm thought to be the cause of the SAH. The pattern of hemorrhage on the CT scan may provide useful clues as to which of the multiple aneurysms has ruptured.[9,10] For example, hemorrhage into the septum pellucidum is a very reliable indicator of bleeding from an anterior communicating artery aneurysm. Hemorrhage predominating in one sylvian fissure suggests bleeding from an ipsilateral middle cerebral artery aneurysm. In many cases, however, there is diffuse SAH that does not help to identify which aneurysm has ruptured. Lacking evidence to the contrary, the largest aneurysm or the most irregular aneurysm present is then assumed to be the source of hemorrhage.

Pretreatment Imaging

For a ruptured aneurysm presenting with SAH, the first imaging study obtained is usually a noncontrast CT scan that reveals the presence of SAH but rarely depicts the aneurysm itself. In rare cases, a relatively large aneurysm may be identified as a less dense mass within a focal area of SAH. When SAH is confirmed, complete diagnostic cerebral angiography is indicated. Although the recently developed techniques of MRA and CT angiography provide useful noninvasive information, neither has developed into a true substitute for traditional catheter-based angiography. For patients who present with an incidental aneurysm identified on a CT or magnetic resonance scan, further evaluation with MRA or CT angiography may be useful. Preliminary decisions about treatment may be made from these studies. If endovascular treatment appears to be an appropriate treatment option, complete catheter-based cerebral angiography should then be performed with endovascular treatment immediately after, if the diagnostic arteriogram confirms that the aneurysm may be treated effectively by endovascular techniques. Catheter-based angiography is currently performed using filmless, digital image acquisition. It is important to note that this technique is very sensitive to patient motion, which may lead to severe image degradation. Obtaining a high-quality study is important, especially if no aneurysm is detected. For patients who cannot reliably follow commands, the use of general anesthesia is recommended. Conscious sedation may be attempted, but this does not yield consistent good results. The latest development in catheter-based angiography is three-dimensional angiography obtained by rapidly acquiring images from multiple angles as the imaging equipment is rotated about the patient. These three-dimensional images provide new insight into the anatomy of an aneurysm and its relationships to the adjacent vessels.

Treatment Options

Optimal treatment for an aneurysm includes (1) exclusion of the aneurysm from the circulation, (2) preservation of the parent and branch arteries, and (3) relief of mass effect caused by the aneurysm. However, it is not always possible to achieve these goals with acceptable treatment morbidity. Open surgical clip ligation with preservation of the artery from which the aneurysm arises has a proven history of success and durability. Depending on the location of the aneurysm, the skill of the surgical team, and the condition of the patient at the time of surgery, the morbidity associated with aneurysm clipping varies widely. In certain cases, occlusion of both the aneurysm and the parent artery may need to be performed when the anatomy and morphology of the aneurysm make direct surgical clipping impossible. Large aneurysms, aneurysms with wide necks, and fusiform aneurysms arising from the internal carotid artery are frequently treated in this manner. Sacrifice of the parent artery requires the presence of an adequate collateral blood supply that limits the applicability of this technique. Temporary occlusion of the artery using a small balloon catheter is usually performed to assess the patient's tolerance for permanent arterial occlusion.[11]

For many years, occlusion of the parent artery was performed by direct surgical ligation. For the past two decades, less invasive endovascular occlusion of the parent artery using small detachable balloons or platinum embolization coils has become commonplace and is now the treatment of choice.[12–14] Direct endovascular treatment of aneurysms with sparing of the parent artery by placing small detachable balloons within the aneurysm was attempted with rather limited success.[15,16] This technique has since been abandoned. In the past decade, direct endovascular aneurysm occlusion using platinum microcoils has become a minimally invasive alternative to surgical clip ligation.[17,18]

Surgical Clipping of Aneurysms

A thorough review of the techniques of open microneurosurgical aneurysm clip ligation is beyond the scope of this text. However, a few important points must be summarized to contrast this technique with the newer minimally invasive therapies that are discussed in more detail. Clip ligation requires a craniotomy in a location appropriate to the target aneurysm. Unless they are in close anatomic proximity, clip ligation of multiple aneurysms, therefore, requires multiple craniotomies. Surgical exposure and access to certain anatomic regions such as the basilar artery apex are difficult and limited. In general, surgery for aneurysms within the posterior fossa is much more difficult and carries greater surgical risks of complications. Surgical exposure of an aneurysm requires retraction of important nerves, blood vessels, and brain tissue—all of which may be subject to temporary or permanent injury. The postoperative recovery phase after craniotomy is prolonged relative to a minimally invasive catheter-based procedure. These are the potential negative features of surgical clip ligation. On the positive side, if the clip or clips are placed successfully, the aneurysm has a low incidence of recurrence or rupture.

The true incidence of morbidity and mortality for direct surgical aneurysm clip ligation remains unknown. Reported mortality rates range from 0% to 7% and morbidity from 4% to 15%.[6,19–25] The analysis of 2,460 patients reported by Raaymakers et al. described a mortality rate of 2.6% and morbidity of 10.9%, giving a cumulative surgical morbidity rate of 13.5%.[20] For the 798 treated patients without a history of SAH from another aneurysm, the International Study of Unruptured Intracranial Aneurysms reported a mortality rate of 2.3% at 30 days and a 12.0% incidence of neurologic disability at one year. Neurologic disability reported in this study included major cognitive impairment. This kind of neuropsychiatric dysfunction has not been assessed or reported in any other large study.

Endovascular Coiling of Cerebral Aneurysms

Treatments are performed with the patient under general anesthesia to restrict patient motion. Particularly when treating small aneurysms, patient motion must be eliminated to be able to work safely. Endovascular aneurysm treatment is usually performed from a femoral artery approach using a 2-mm-diameter catheter to access the cervical portion of the carotid or vertebral artery proximal to the target aneurysm. A microcatheter measuring 0.5–1.0 mm in diameter is then advanced through the larger guiding catheter and into the cerebral vasculature under direct fluoroscopic visualization. A steerable 0.010- to 0.016-in. microguidewire is placed through the lumen of the microcatheter. To safely guide microcatheter placement within the aneurysm, digital angiograms of the cerebral arteries are obtained and superimposed on the live x-ray fluoroscopy images of the microcatheter and microguidewire, a technique referred to as *road-mapping*. The road-mapping technique is shown in case 1 (Figure 18-1). The microcatheter and microguidewire are then carefully navigated into the target aneurysm.

Soft platinum microcoils are then placed directly into the aneurysm. The first such device was approved by the U.S. Food and Drug Administration (FDA) for endovascular aneurysm treatment in 1995 (Guglielmi detachable coil [GDC] system [Target Therapeutics, Natick, Massachusetts]). Two different types of GDCs are shown in Figure 18-2. Four other similar coil systems for treating cerebral aneurysms have recently been approved by the FDA. The majority of patients has been treated with the GDC system. Almost all published reports and all long-term follow-up studies are based on use of the GDC system. The GDCs are available in a wide range of sizes and shapes. The coils are attached to microguidewires that allow the coils to be removed or repositioned if desired. After each coil is advanced into the aneurysm, its size and shape may be assessed. If the coil is too large to fit entirely within the aneurysm or too small to stay within the aneurysm, it can be removed. If the coil appears to be satisfactorily positioned, it is detached by application of a small electrical current applied to the microguidewire. The largest coils are placed first, with progressively smaller coils filling the center of the coil mass. Coils must be placed within the aneurysm so that there is minimal impingement on the adjacent parent artery. The most favorable aneurysms for endovascular coil treatment have necks smaller than the fundus of the aneurysm. Coil placement becomes much more difficult as the size of the neck approaches that of the fundus of the aneurysm.

Coils are sequentially placed within the aneurysm until the aneurysm lumen has been filled. Cerebral arteriograms are repeated frequently as the coils are placed to demonstrate progressive occlusion of the aneurysm. When no injected x-ray contrast fills the aneurysm, or placement of additional coils becomes difficult, treatment is complete. The microcatheter is gently removed from within the aneurysm. When adequately filled with coils, blood no longer flows within the aneurysm, and thrombosis of the aneurysm lumen occurs. Recent developments in endovascular techniques have enabled the use of coils to occlude even very broad-necked aneurysms without causing occlusion of the parent artery.

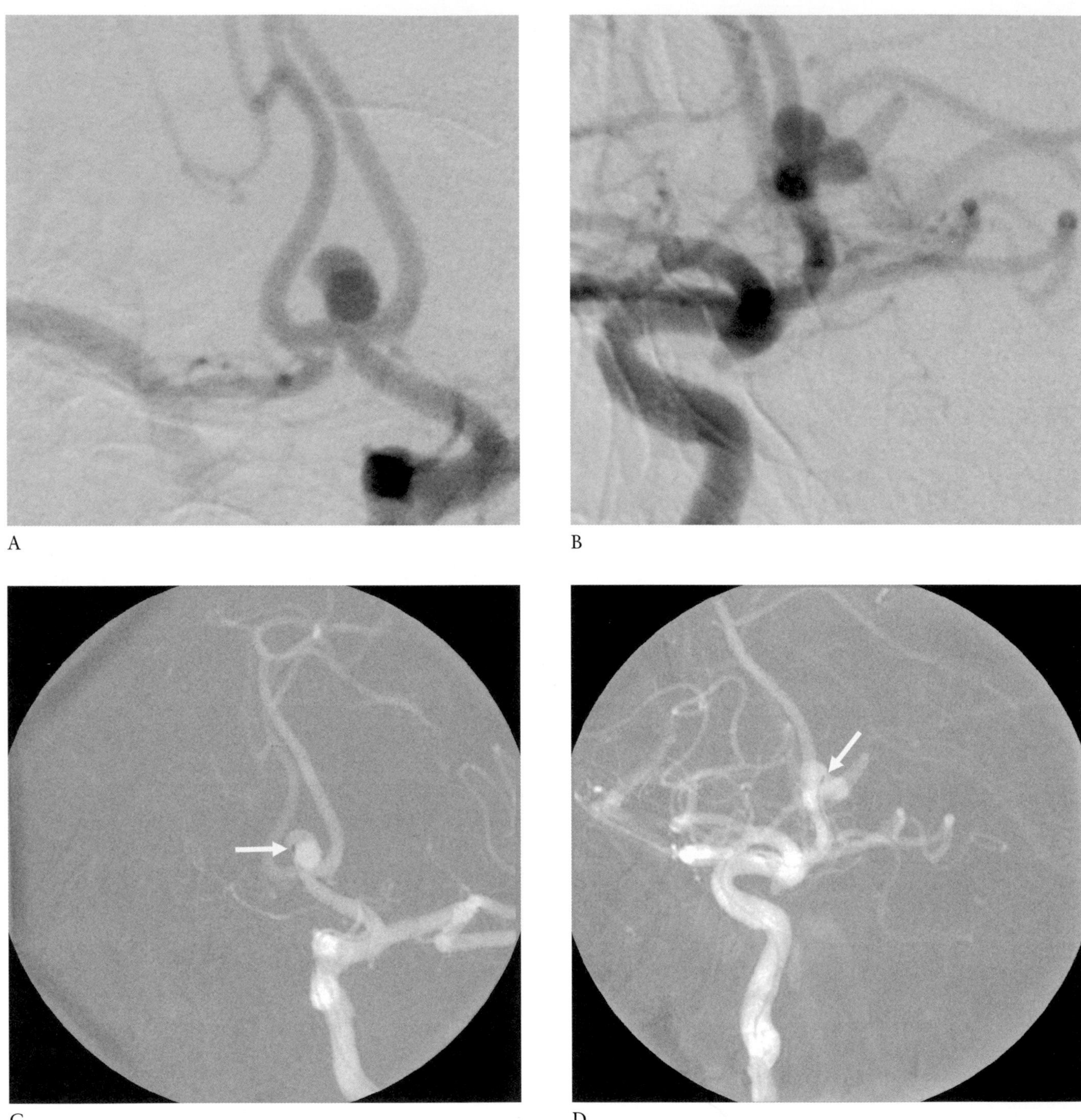

FIGURE 18-1. Fifty-five-year-old woman who presented with acute subarachnoid hemorrhage. Diagnostic angiography revealed a 9-mm bilobed anterior communicating artery aneurysm (**A,B**). **A.** Left anterior oblique (LAO) view. **B.** Ninety-degree orthogonal right anterior oblique (RAO) view. A larger 16-mm right carotid-ophthalmic artery aneurysm was also identified (not shown). A computed tomography scan (not shown) showed focal hemorrhage into the septum pellucidum, indicating that the smaller anterior communicating artery aneurysm was the source of the patient's hemorrhage. Although the anatomy of the aneurysm is complex, the LAO view (**A**) shows a relatively narrow neck with a clear delineation between the aneurysm and the anterior communicating artery. Note that the neck of the aneurysm is very difficult to appreciate in the RAO view (**B**). Safe endovascular treatment is possible using biplane fluoroscopic guidance with road-mapping. A road map is obtained by injecting radiographic contrast material into the artery to define the contours of the artery. This saved image is subtracted from the live fluoroscopic images to yield a road map of the cerebral vasculature. This technique allows for safe intravascular navigation with greatly reduced risk of arterial perforation or injury. The road-mapping technique is a cornerstone of neuroendovascular therapy. **C.** LAO view. **D.** RAO view. Biplane road-map images show the tip of a microcatheter (*arrow* in **C,D**) has been successfully positioned into the posterior lobe of the aneurysm. *(continued)*

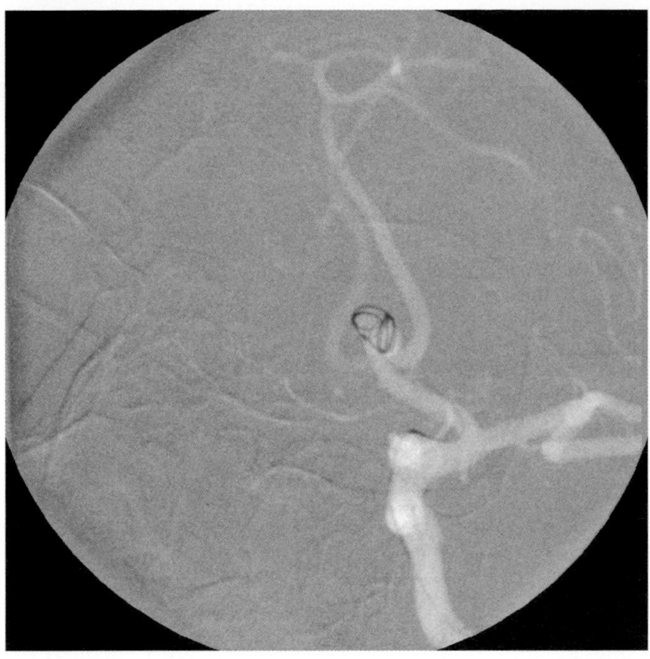

E

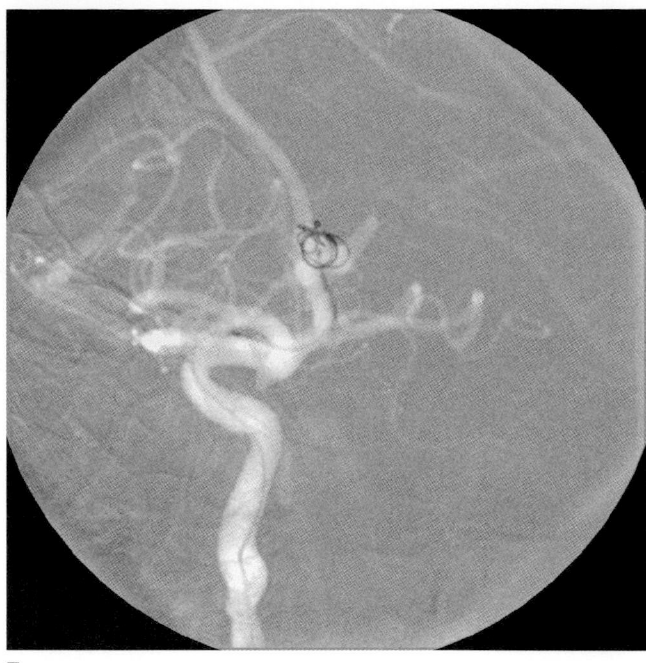

F

FIGURE 18-1. *Continued.* Corresponding images show the satisfactory position of the first Guglielmi detachable coil placed within the aneurysm before its detachment (**E,F**). Seven Guglielmi detachable coils were eventually placed within the aneurysm to achieve complete filling. The patient recovered well from her subarachnoid hemorrhage. Successful endovascular treatment of her right carotid-ophthalmic artery aneurysm was later performed.

Temporary placement of a small balloon catheter adjacent to the aneurysm during coil placement or permanent implantation of a stent is now a widely used technique to protect the parent artery.[26–28] These techniques are illustrated in Figures 18-3 and 18-4. A typical stent used for such procedures is shown in Figure 18-5. Intravascular stents specific to the intracranial circulation are now being developed to treat complex and large aneurysms.

The principal benefits of coil embolization include markedly decreased invasiveness and correspondingly brief recovery time. Patients are often discharged within 24 hours after coil embolization of unruptured aneurysms. Aneurysms located in areas that are difficult to access surgically, such as the basilar apex, are often good candidates for endovascular therapy and require intravascular access. Injury to adjacent structures is decreased with an intravascular approach. The current generation of microcatheter and microguidewire technology has allowed access to most all types of cerebral aneurysms. A disadvantage of coil embolization is the difficulty in achieving complete occlusion of the aneurysm, including the critical neck area in some cases. Failure to adequately pack an aneurysm with an adequate mass of coils may allow continued blood flow and eventual regrowth of the aneurysm, both of which mean that the risk of aneurysm rupture has not been completely eliminated. Additional shapes and sizes of coils and softer coils that allow for more complete packing of the aneurysm have therefore been developed to address these shortcomings. For large and giant aneurysms that may cause mass effect on adjacent structures, the lack of reduction of the aneurysm mass after coiling may be a negative aspect of endovascular treatment. Thrombosis of the aneurysm does decrease or eliminate pulsatility, which may, however, contribute to the decrease in mass effect symptoms.

The earliest reports of clinical application of the GDC system indicated favorable results for treatment of aneurysms that were felt to have high surgical risk. In 1999, Brilstra and colleagues reported a meta-analysis of 1,383 patients treated with the GDC system.[29] Treatment-related morbidity of 3.7% and mortality of 1.0% were lower than those associated with surgical clipping. However, complete aneurysm obliteration was present in only 54% of treated cases. Most of these cases with subtotal occlusion had very small persistent neck remnants after coiling. The long-term effects of these very small (mostly 1 mm or less) persistent neck remnants remain uncertain. Some long-term follow-up data are available from the initial patients treated with the GDC system. Malisch et al. reported on 100 consecutive patients with a mean follow-up period of 3.5 years.[30] The incidences of rebleeding were 4% for large aneurysms (15–25 mm maximum diameter) and 33% for giant aneurysms (>25 mm maximum diameter). Delayed

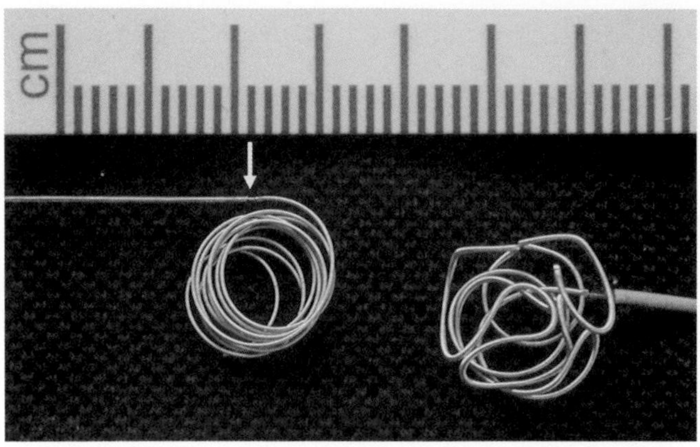

FIGURE 18-2. Two different types of Guglielmi detachable aneurysm embolization coils are shown. An 8-mm-diameter × 20-cm-long standard helical coil is shown on the left. An arrow marks the junction between the soft platinum coil and the stainless steel guidewire to which the coil is attached. After the coil is placed within the aneurysm, its position is evaluated by angiography. If the coil position or size is unsatisfactory, it is removed by retracting the attached guidewire. Otherwise, the coil is detached within the aneurysm by applying a small current to the guidewire, which results in rapid electrolysis of the joint between the platinum and stainless steel wires. A three-dimensional 6-mm-diameter × 15-cm-long coil is shown on the right. The three-dimensional coil is seen exiting from an 0.8-mm-diameter microcatheter (RapidTransit, Cordis Neurovascular, Miami Lakes, Florida). The three-dimensional coil has omega-shaped loops rather than the simple helical design of the other coil. The introduction of the three-dimensional coils has facilitated treatment of aneurysms with relatively larger necks, without the need for adjunctive temporary balloon placement or permanent stent implantation. Detachable coils are available in a wide range of sizes and shapes that allows treatment of almost all aneurysms.

hemorrhage was not found in patients with small aneurysms (<15 mm maximum diameter). It is important to note that the earliest patients treated with the GDC system underwent treatment with first-generation devices. The first GDCs were available in only a very limited number of shapes and sizes. There are now three-dimensional shaped coils and softer "filler" coils in use.

MRA may be used as a noninvasive means of monitoring the status of an incompletely occluded aneurysm.[31–33] Significant recurrence or growth of an aneurysm remnant exceeding 3 mm in size may be readily detected by this method. Malisch and colleagues' report indicates that such monitoring may be especially useful after treatment of giant aneurysms that are prone to delayed rupture. The presumed mechanism of such delayed ruptures is compaction of the coils due to very high shear stresses and, in some cases, persistent aneurysm growth at the incompletely occluded neck. Retreatment may be performed with additional coils placed when there is a significant residual or recurrent aneurysm lumen detected. This should help to decrease the incidence of delayed hemorrhages.

Surgical versus Endovascular Treatment: Clinical Results

The debate between endovascular and open surgical aneurysm treatment is still ongoing. No randomized, controlled trial of surgical versus endovascular treatment has yet been performed to thoroughly assess the relative merits of each technique. Currently available data support that short-term complications are significantly reduced by endovascular treatment compared to surgery.[34–36] The long-term prevention of aneurysmal hemorrhage after endovascular aneurysm treatment appears to be slightly less than surgical clipping. Delayed hemorrhage after aneurysm coiling is more likely with treatment of larger and broad-necked aneurysms. However, these types of aneurysms also have substantially higher-than-average risks associated with surgical clipping. The total risk of endovascular treatment, including both the procedure-related risks and the risk that the aneurysm may still rupture due to ineffective treatment, appears to be lower than that associated with surgical clipping. Particularly for relatively small, unruptured aneurysms that may have a low risk of rupture if not treated, endovascular therapy appears to be the treatment of choice. There is also some preliminary evidence that endovascular therapy may be associated with a decreased incidence of clinically significant vasospasm after SAH.[37]

As the current generation of endovascular devices is replaced by improved technology that allows for more complete aneurysm occlusion, the advantages of endovascular therapy will continue to grow. Whether endovascular therapy at present has evolved to an equal or better alternative to surgical clipping is still in discussion. However, given the rapid and continuing technological advances, there seems to be little doubt that endovascular therapy may become accepted as the preferred treatment for aneurysms in the near future.

ARTERIOVENOUS MALFORMATIONS

AVMs appear to be more prone to hemorrhage than cerebral aneurysms. However, the clinical effects of hemorrhage are usually much less severe. The largest study of untreated AVMs was reported by Ondra et al. in 1990.[38] They reported a 4% annual incidence of hemorrhage from a freshly diagnosed AVM. After an initial hemorrhage, the risk of a second hemorrhage is increased. The risk of a repeat hemorrhage is estimated to be between 6% and 34% in the following year.[39–42] The risk of a repeat hemorrhage diminishes with time, eventually returning to the baseline risk of approxi-

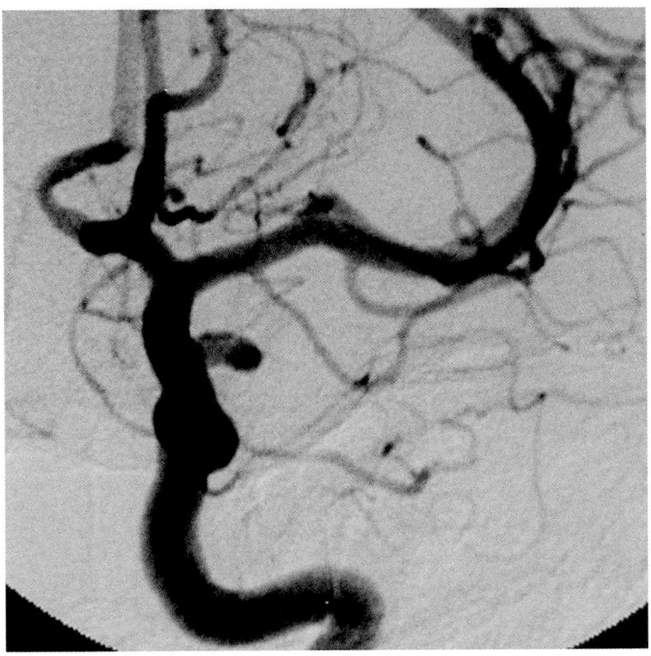

A

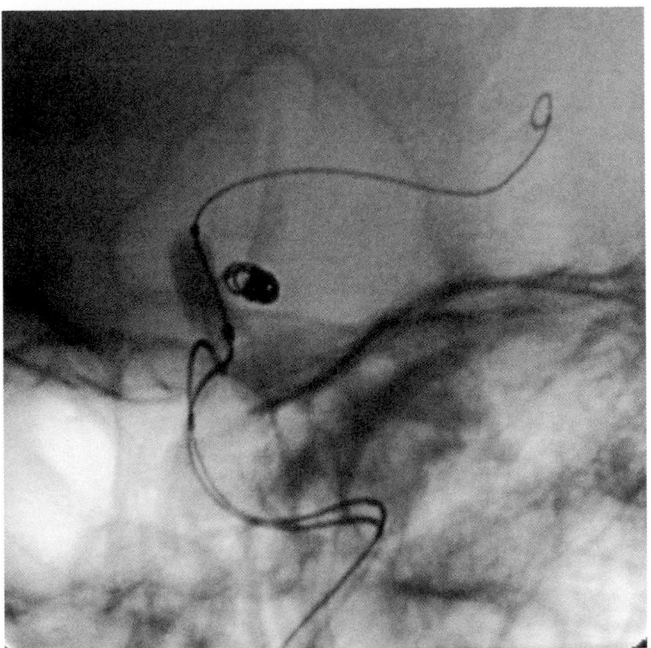

B

FIGURE 18-3. Sixty-one-year-old woman who presented with an incidental, unruptured 5-mm left superior hypophyseal artery aneurysm (**A**). The aneurysm had been identified on a magnetic resonance imaging study performed for evaluation of a right hemisphere transient ischemic attack. Although the aneurysm is small, the neck is wide relative to the body of the aneurysm. Placement of a temporary occlusion balloon across the neck of the aneurysm during coil placement was thought to be necessary to allow dense packing of the aneurysm without leaving a significant neck remnant. **B.** A nonsubtracted image shows the inflated balloon positioned across the neck of the aneurysm as the first detachable coil is placed. **C.** Angiography after placement of three coils shows that the aneurysm has been completely occluded with no neck remnant or encroachment on the internal carotid artery.

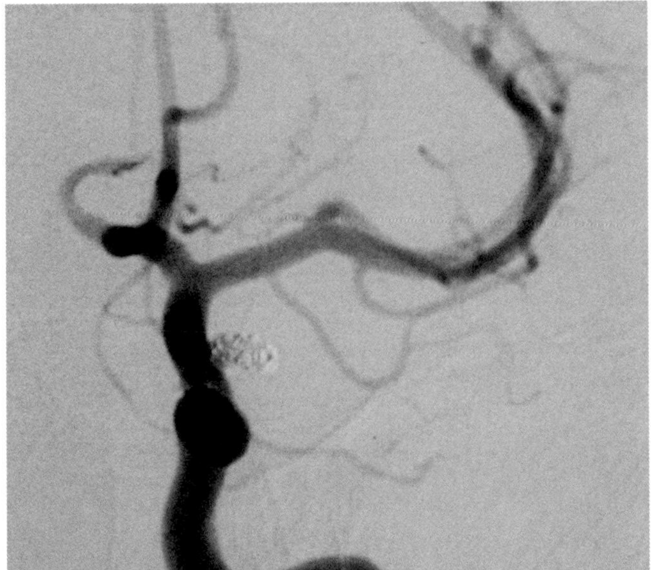

C

mately 4% per year. The risk of death approximates 10% with a first hemorrhage. Most patients recover well from an initial hemorrhage, with much less morbidity than that associated with aneurysmal SAH.

AVMs may be located anywhere within the brain. The size of an AVM may range from a few millimeters to several centimeters. Unlike aneurysms, there is no evidence that larger AVMs are more likely to hemorrhage. It is a common misconception that a small, asymptomatic AVM is a relatively benign lesion. Many AVMs present as incidental findings on CT or MRI scans obtained for unrelated symptoms. AVMs may also present due to symptoms of cerebral ischemia (caused by the AVM stealing blood from the surrounding normal brain), seizures, pulsatile tinnitus, and bruit.

The nidus of the AVM represents an abnormal collection of vessels with arteriovenous shunting. These

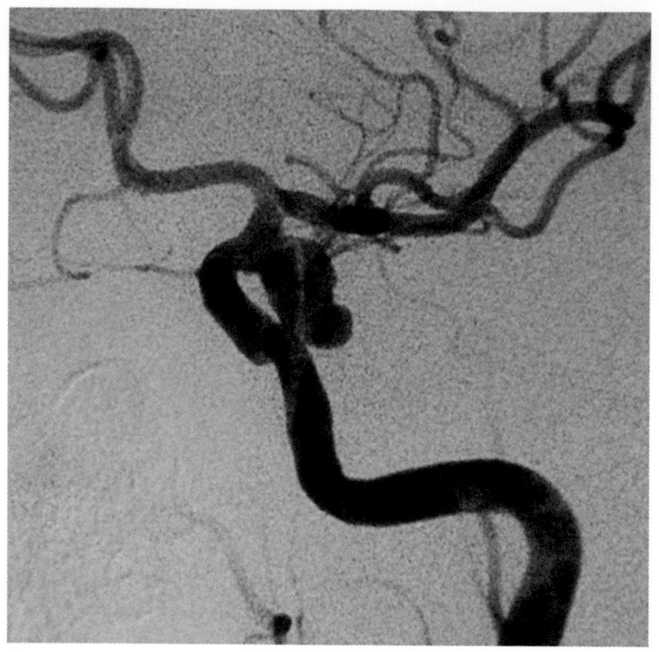

A

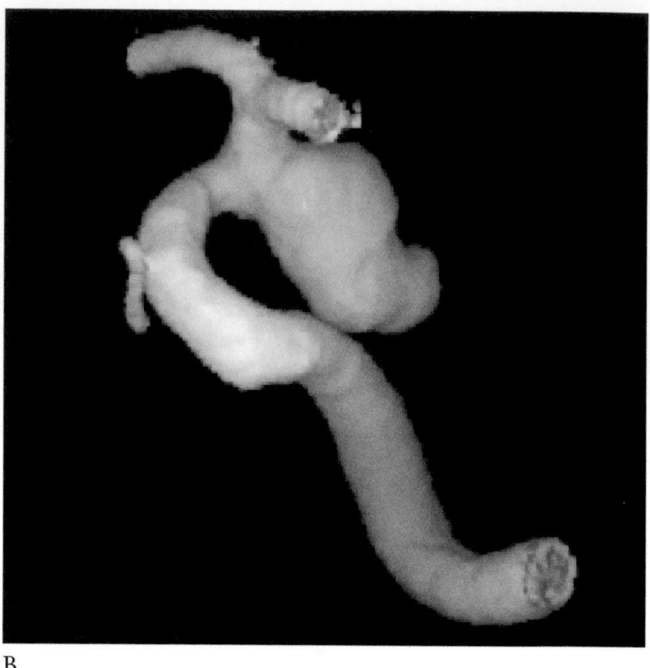

B

FIGURE 18-4. Forty-seven-year-old woman who presented with an acute subarachnoid hemorrhage. Diagnostic angiography revealed a 13-mm left posterior communicating artery aneurysm and a 4-mm right posterior communicating artery aneurysm. The larger aneurysm was presumed to be the source of hemorrhage. Both conventional digital subtraction angiography and rotational angiography with three-dimensional reconstructed images showed that the aneurysm had a large neck (**A,B**). Even though the neck of the aneurysm is large, Guglielmi detachable coils (GDCs) would be retained within the aneurysm because the neck of the aneurysm is much smaller than the body of the aneurysm. However, the curved surface of the coils would protrude from the neck of the aneurysm, causing significant encroachment on the internal carotid artery (ICA). An embolic stroke or even occlusion of the ICA could result. To preserve the integrity of the ICA, a 3.5-mm-diameter, balloon-expandable coronary stent was placed across the neck of the aneurysm. (*continued*)

fragile vessels often possess histologic characteristics of both arteries and veins.[43] There is usually no normal brain tissue within the nidus of the AVM. Aneurysms are found on the feeding arteries or within the nidus in approximately 20% of patients with AVMs.[44–46] An example of a particularly large intranidal aneurysm is shown in Figure 18-6. These aneurysms probably develop due to the abnormally high flow within the vessels. They are rarely found in association with small, low-flow AVMs. Intranidal aneurysms are felt to have a particularly high risk of rupture.

The majority of AVMs may be cured by surgical resection or stereotactic radiosurgery. In many cases, and particularly for large, high-flow AVMs, endovascular embolization is used as an adjunct to both surgical resection and radiosurgery. Total elimination of the AVM is necessary to provide protection from hemorrhage. Partial resection or subtotal obliteration of the AVM nidus with radiosurgery does not reduce the risk of hemorrhage. Endovascular or surgical treatment of associated aneurysms is widely thought to reduce the risk of hemorrhage. However, this remains unproven. Although uncommon, embolization alone may completely occlude the AVM as judged by angiographic follow-up. In such cases, continued angiographic surveillance may be advisable unless the AVM is resected.

Pretreatment Imaging

Imaging studies are essential to assess for hemorrhage and to determine the size, location, and unique arterial supply and venous drainage of a brain AVM. CT remains a mainstay to assess for acute hemorrhage, although the presence of dystrophic calcifications within the lesion may at times confound the diagnosis of small amounts of acute hemorrhage. Due to the high-flow characteristics of AVMs, artifacts within and around the AVM nidus sometimes make detection of small amounts of acute or chronic hemorrhage difficult on MRI scans.

MRI is, however, a very accurate means to determine the precise size and location of the nidus of the AVM. Its multiplanar capability makes it superior to CT for this purpose. Multidetector helical CT scanners have become available recently. Like MRI, these new CT scanners also produce high-resolution multiplanar

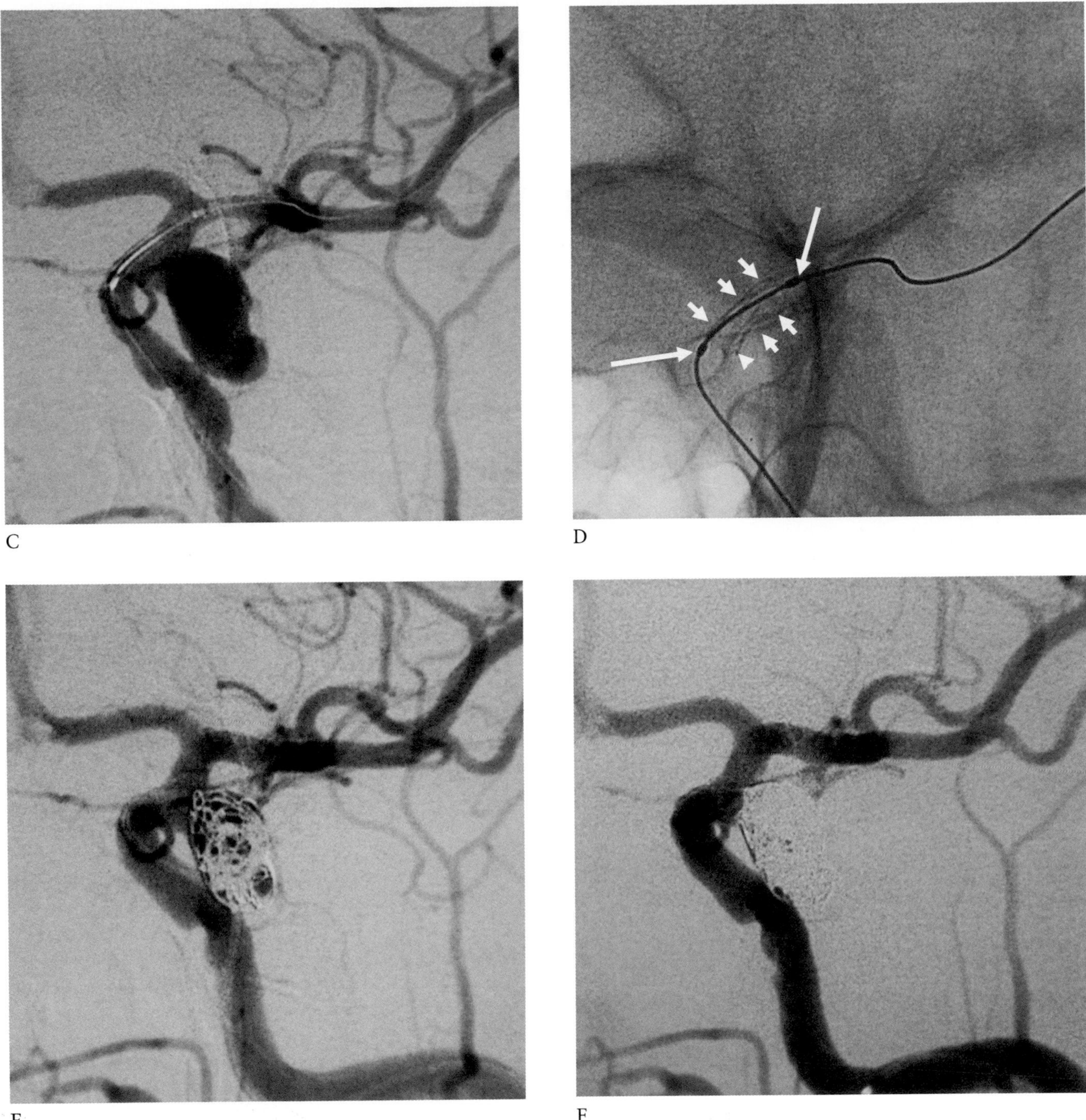

FIGURE 18-4. *Continued.* **C.** The unexpanded stent positioned across the neck of the aneurysm is readily visible on an angiogram obtained immediately before balloon inflation. **D.** A nonsubtracted image shows the faintly visible expanded stent (*short arrows*). The stent is made of stainless steel, whereas the much more radiopaque guidewire, used to position the stent delivery system, has a platinum tip. Radiopacity is strongly dependent on the atomic number of the element being imaged. Stainless steel (largely composed of iron) has an effective atomic number of approximately 26, whereas platinum has an atomic number of 78. Not surprisingly, many endovascular devices incorporate platinum elements to aid fluoroscopic visualization. The stent delivery system has two small platinum markers (*long arrows*) to delineate the proximal and distal margins of the stent. **E.** After placing the stent, a microcatheter was advanced into the aneurysm through the interstices of the stent. Eighteen GDCs were then placed into the aneurysm. **F.** An immediate post-treatment angiogram shows that the aneurysm has been densely packed with coils and that the ICA remains widely patent. The patient recovered completely with no neurologic deficit. The smaller right side aneurysm was treated successfully with GDCs 1 month later.

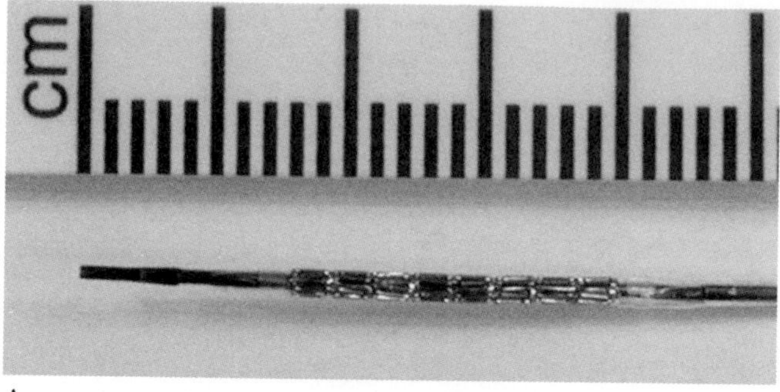

A

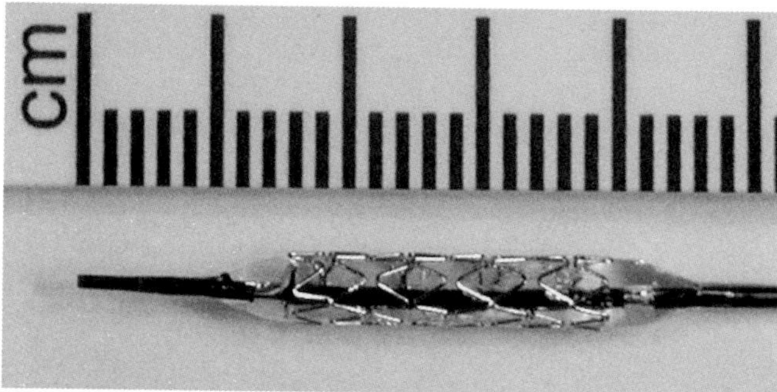

B

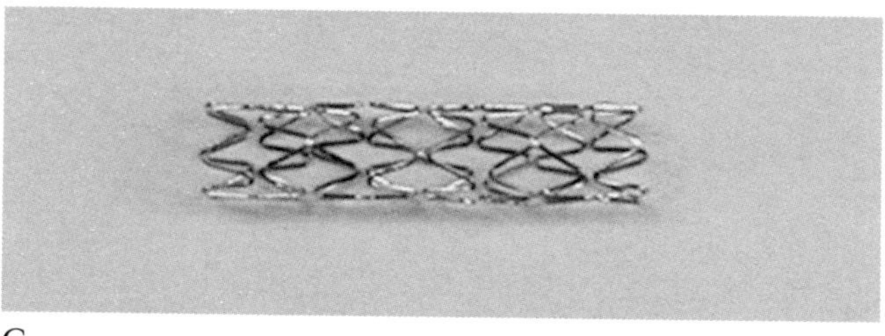

C

FIGURE 18-5. **A.** A 2.5-mm-diameter × 12-mm-long coronary stent (S660, Arterial Vascular Engineering/Medtronics, Santa Rosa, California) is shown mounted on a 0.9-mm-diameter delivery catheter. **B.** The stent is expanded and embedded into the vessel wall by inflating the balloon integrated into the delivery catheter. The balloon is then deflated and the catheter withdrawn, leaving the fully expanded stent in place (**C**). The stent shown is very similar to that used in Figure 18-4.

images. MRI continues to provide superior soft tissue contrast and delineation of gray and white matter structures. A widely used classification of brain AVM features, predictive of the risk of surgical resection was developed by Spetzler et al. (Table 18-1).[47] The size of the AVM nidus is important because of the increasing risk of surgical resection of larger lesions. The size of the nidus is even more critical with regard to treatment with radiosurgery. Imaging helps to determine the location of the nidus with regard to eloquent and critical brain functions. It is important to understand that concept, because the AVM itself contains no normal brain tissue, and functional areas may be significantly displaced around the nidus. Optimal treatment planning may therefore require elaborate functional imaging to determine the precise location of important structures such as the motor strip. Determination of the location of critical functional areas is used to direct the surgical approach, minimize the risk of neurologic deficit, and, in some cases, decide that radiosurgery rather than surgical resection may be the lower-risk treatment option.

Determination of the unique vascular characteristics of the AVM is also essential for treatment strategy. MRA, magnetic resonance venography, and, to a lesser extent, CT angiography provide very useful noninvasive means to predict the vasculature. However, as with aneurysms, catheter angiography remains the gold standard for vascular evaluation. Noninvasive imaging does provide useful information that helps to streamline the treatment process. Noninvasive imaging is usually able to identify the presence of deep versus superficial venous drainage, which is an important consideration for surgical resection. Endovascular therapy may often be planned to immediately follow diagnostic angiography, based on the vascular characteristics predicted by noninvasive imaging.

Stereotactic Radiosurgery

A thorough review of the principles and techniques of stereotactic radiosurgery is beyond the scope of this text. However, several important details are pertinent, as they apply to the combined use of endovascular interventional therapy and radiosurgery for AVM treatment. Radiosurgery induces vascular injury within the nidus of the AVM,

FIGURE 18-6. ▶ Twenty-two-year-old man who presented with a Spetzler-Martin grade 5, right temporal, parietal, and occipital lobe arteriovenous malformation (AVM). The patient had a long history of poorly controlled seizures and severe headaches. The AVM had been declared untreatable many years previously. **A.** A pretreatment magnetic resonance imaging scan shows the enhancing AVM within the occipital and posterior temporal lobes. A large enhancing vascular structure (*arrow*) was thought to represent a dilated draining vein. **B,C.** A right internal carotid artery arteriogram performed immediately before embolization (anterior-posterior view—early [**B**] and later [**C**] phases) revealed that the vascular structure seen on the magnetic resonance imaging scan was, in fact, a very large intranidal aneurysm (**D**, *arrow*). The feeding artery from which the intranidal aneurysm arose was effectively occluded using cyanoacrylate tissue adhesive. The aneurysm was treated first to prevent it from rupturing as embolization altered the hemodynamics of the AVM. Five stages of embolization were performed, with extensive devascularization of the AVM achieved. The AVM was then completely resected with only brief hemisensory dysesthesia resulting.

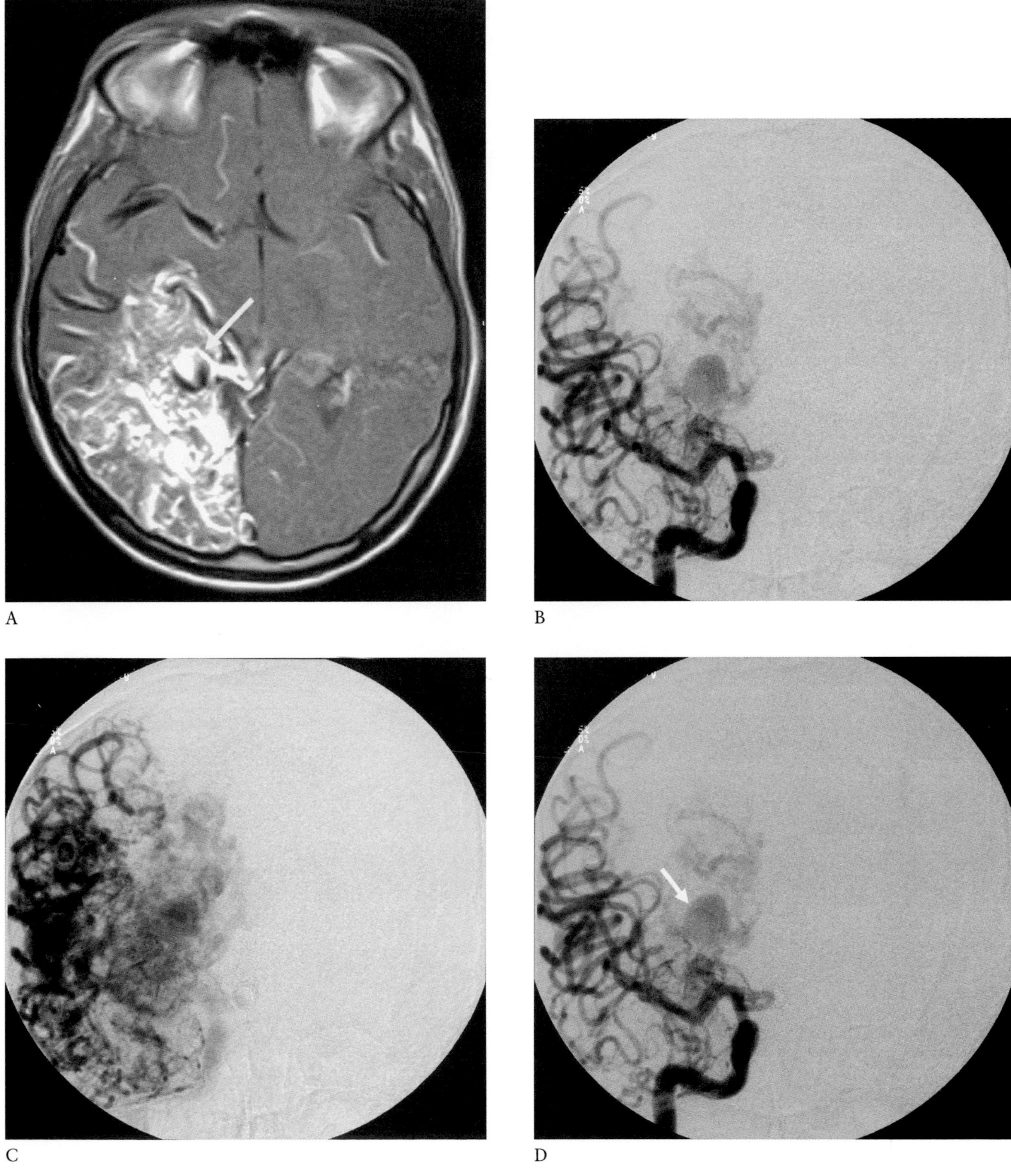
A
B
C
D

TABLE 18-1. Spetzler-Martin Grading Scale for Brain Arteriovenous Malformations

Feature	*Point value*
Size	
<3 cm	1
3–6 cm	2
>6 cm	3
Eloquence of adjacent tissue	
Noneloquent	0
Eloquent	1
Venous drainage pattern	
Superficial	0
Deep	1

Source: Adapted from RF Spetzler, NA Martin, LP Carter, et al. Surgical management of large AVMs by staged embolization and operative excision. J Neurosurg 1987;67(1):17–28.

leading to obliteration of most treated AVMs within 12–36 months.[48–50] However, until the AVM has been obliterated completely, there is no protection against hemorrhage. Thus, the patient remains at risk for hemorrhage during the period between radiosurgery and AVM obliteration. This risk must be balanced against the risk of surgical resection that, if successful, results in immediate elimination of the bleeding potential. Smaller AVMs have a higher rate of obliteration, because higher doses of radiation may be delivered to the nidus without excessive risk of injury to the surrounding normal brain. Larger AVMs are more difficult to cure. When the maximum dimension of the AVM exceeds 3.5–4.0 cm, delivery of an adequate radiation dose to the AVM, to effectively cure the lesion, is impaired by the increasing dose to the surrounding normal tissue.

Treatment of AVMs that are too large for radiosurgery may be performed after embolization has obliterated part of the nidus, with the remaining nidus reduced to a size suitable for radiosurgery.[51,52] However, the effects of embolization are unpredictable with regard to reduction of the overall size of the nidus. Embolization to reduce the size of the nidus to allow for radiosurgery is illustrated in Figure 18-7. Embolization

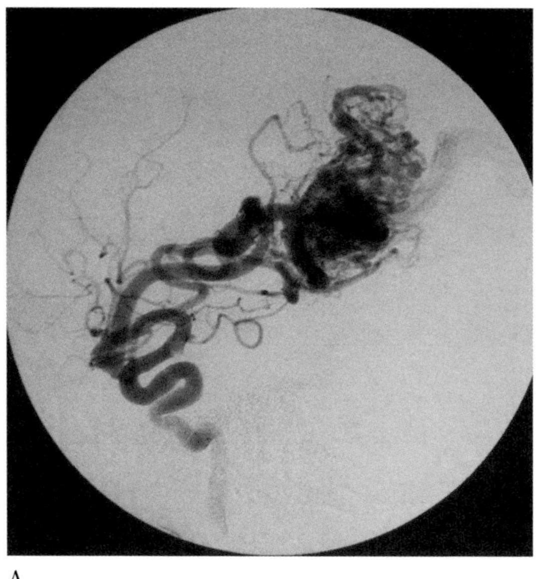

A

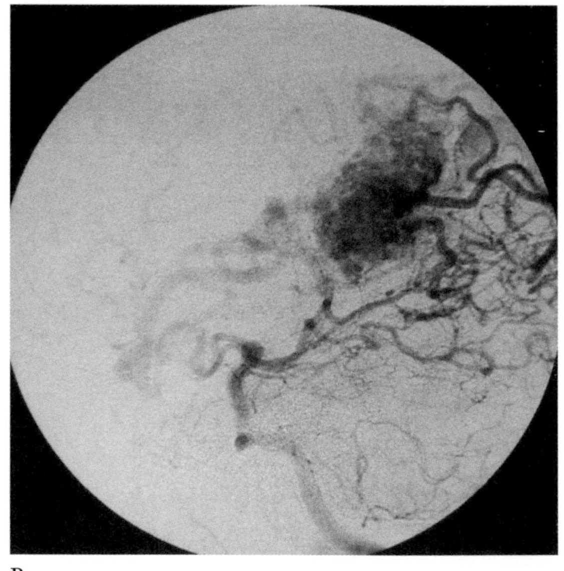

B

FIGURE 18-7. Forty-seven-year-old woman who presented with a severe acute headache. A computed tomography scan (not shown) revealed a large right parietal arteriovenous malformation (AVM) with a small amount of acute hemorrhage. Angiography revealed a high-flow AVM with supply from branches of the anterior, middle, and posterior cerebral arteries (**A,B**). **A.** Right internal carotid artery lateral view. **B.** Left vertebral artery lateral view. Both deep and superficial venous drainage were present. The Spetzler-Martin grade 5 AVM was thought to have significant risk associated with surgical resection. Embolization using cyanoacrylate "tissue adhesive" was planned, so that the nidus could be reduced to a size amenable to treatment by radiosurgery. Embolization was performed with the patient awake to allow provocative pharmacologic testing. **C.** A super-selective angiogram of a right middle cerebral artery branch shows supply to a portion of the AVM. On this subtracted image, a cast of cyanoacrylate "tissue adhesive" is faintly seen within a portion of the nidus immediately cranial (*arrow*). Two embolization procedures were performed with extensive reduction in the size of the AVM nidus. Anterior-posterior (**D**) and lateral (**E**) nonsubtracted images of the skull show the radiopaque cyanoacrylate "liquid adhesive" filling much of the AVM nidus. **F,G.** A post-treatment, right internal carotid artery angiogram (lateral view—early [F] and late [G] phases) revealed a small residual nidus (F, *arrow*) with much slower venous outflow. The remaining nidus was well below the maximum size limit to allow stereotactic radiosurgery.

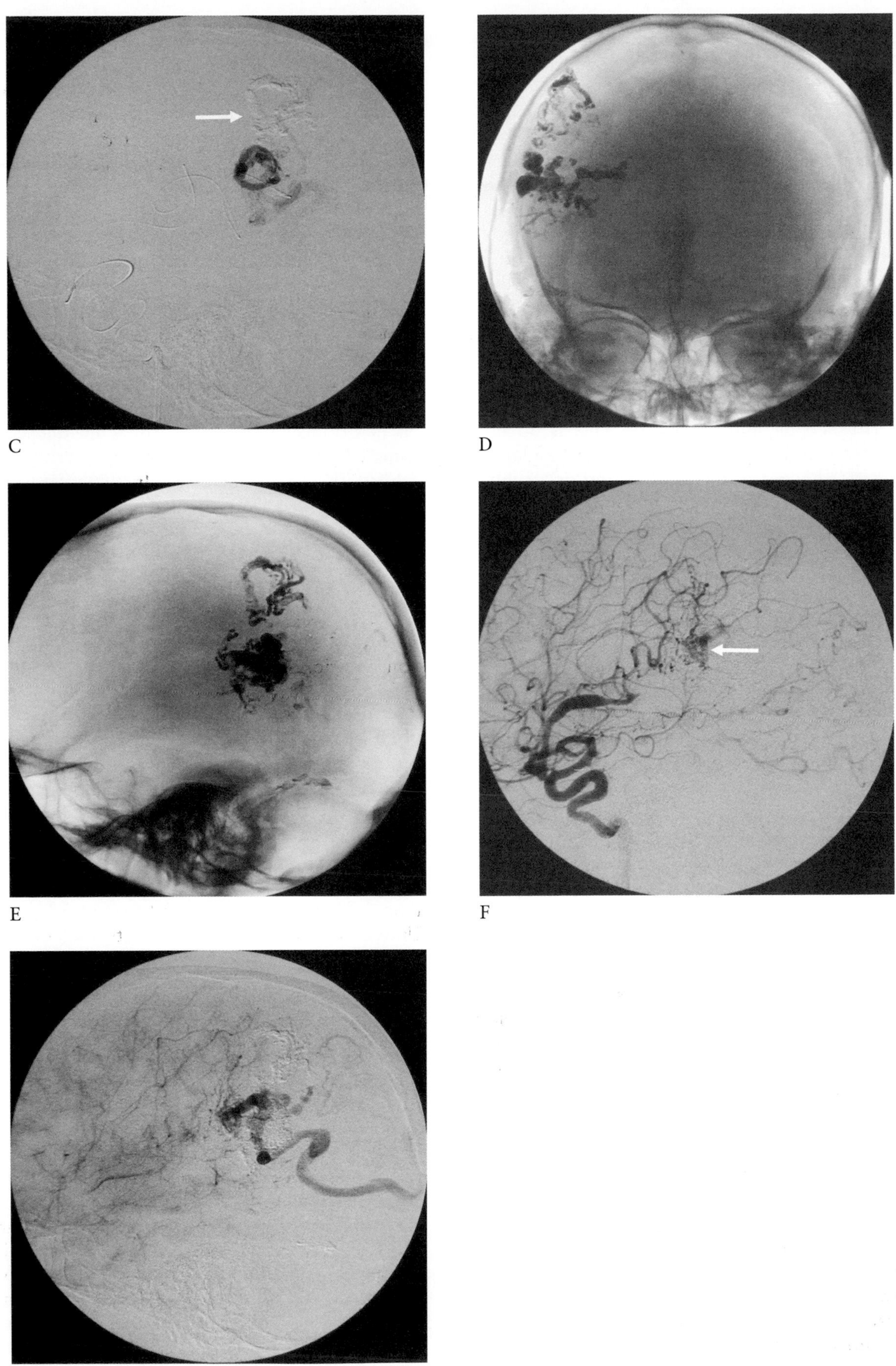
C D E F G

will reduce the number of vessels within the nidus, leading to a substantial reduction in blood flow. Substantial portions of the nidus may be completely obliterated by embolization. Alternatively, many small areas scattered throughout the nidus may be occluded. The latter result may produce no significant decrease in the overall dimensions of the nidus, which does not facilitate radiosurgery. Particularly with very large AVMs, one may not be certain that technically successful embolization will reduce the remaining nidus to a treatable size. In addition, there is a small risk of delayed recanalization of the embolized AVM, which may not have been irradiated. In some cases, large AVMs may be treated by multiple modalities including embolization, partial resection, and radiosurgery of the remaining nidus.

For treatment of large AVMs, embolization is often performed in multiple stages. This is done to allow the surrounding normal vasculature to adapt to the dramatic changes in blood flow that occur when the AVM is eliminated. Because of the very high flow into the AVM, the surrounding normal arteries will have become maximally dilated to attempt to maintain normal perfusion. Their autoregulatory curve has been markedly shifted to compensate for chronic hypoperfusion. These arteries may be incapable of rapid constriction to accommodate normal perfusion pressure, if an adjacent large AVM is suddenly removed or flow is diverted to the normal arteries by extensive embolization of the AVM. Intracranial hemorrhage due to the arterial pressure exceeding the limits of autoregulation may occur in this circumstance. This is referred to as the *normal pressure perfusion breakthrough phenomenon*.[53] Progressive, staged embolization of an AVM allows the surrounding arteries to slowly adapt to a normal autoregulatory curve, which markedly diminishes the risk of hemorrhage. There is widespread variation in the timing of staged embolizations. Some physicians wait only 24–48 hours between stages, whereas others advocate waiting 4–6 weeks between stages. The patient's blood pressure may be maintained slightly below baseline for 24–48 hours after embolization and subsequent surgical resection to help prevent a postprocedural hemorrhage.

Goals of Embolization

An overall treatment plan should be developed for each individual case. The location of the AVM may suggest the very high probability of a specific neurologic deficit as a result of treatment. For example, treatment of an AVM within the occipital lobe carries a high risk for development of a visual field deficit. The potential effect of this on the patient's lifestyle and occupation should be discussed and considered in the treatment plan. The surgeons who may resect or radiate the AVM should discuss the anticipated surgical approach or radiosurgery plan with the interventionist who will perform the embolization. In many cases, feeding arteries that are expected to be difficult to occlude during the surgical exposure will be targeted for endovascular occlusion. Conversely, embolization may be deemed unnecessary for superficial arteries that will be directly and immediately accessible after the craniotomy has been performed. Specific areas of the nidus may be targeted for embolization to allow radiosurgery to be performed. Because there are risks associated with preoperative embolization, embolization should be limited to the extent that it is necessary to allow the AVM to be treated. A very close working relationship between the surgeon, radiosurgeon, and interventionist is essential to achieving good outcomes. Embolization must always be tailored to help achieve the treatment goals. In some cases, the final decision to resect or radiate the AVM must await the results of embolization with regard to reduction of the size of the nidus.

Risks of Embolization

Embolization of brain AVMs carries a small but not insignificant risk of stroke and even death. It is important to understand the risks of embolization as a part of an integrated treatment plan. The risk of a significant complication occurring during one or more embolization procedures is difficult to estimate. The treatment's goal, AVM characteristics, embolization technique, and devices vary greatly among reported case series. Tomsick and colleagues conducted the only randomized, controlled trial of brain AVM embolization.[54] This study was performed at 13 sites in the United States by interventionists experienced with brain AVM embolization. One hundred two patients underwent preoperative brain AVM embolization with either polyvinyl alcohol (PVA) particles or normo butyl cyanoacrylate liquid tissue adhesive (NBCA glue). Intracerebral hemorrhage occurred in four patients during embolization and seven patients after embolization but before resection. Most intracerebral hemorrhages were small and well tolerated. Strokes occurred in five patients. Two deaths occurred before surgery. Seizures occurred in 10 patients. This study represents the best available data from which a realistic estimate of the complications associated with brain AVM embolization may be made. The potential complications of embolization must always be balanced against the perceived benefits. The risks of embolization should not exceed the potential benefits of resection of a less vascular lesion and the decreased potential for normal perfusion pressure breakthrough hemorrhage.

Embolization Technique

AVM embolization is usually performed from a femoral artery approach using a 2-mm-diameter catheter to access the carotid or vertebral artery. A 0.5- to 1.0-mm-diameter microcatheter is then advanced through the guiding catheter into the intracranial vasculature. The microcatheter must be advanced very distally, so that the microcatheter tip lies beyond all of the arterial branches that supply normal brain tissue. In most cases, the terminal branches within an arterial branch supply the AVM alone. In some cases, multiple small side branches supply the AVM, with the terminal arterial branches supplying normal brain tissue. This type of arterial supply to an AVM is referred to as *en passage vessels*. Successful embolization of en passage feeding arteries may be impossible unless each feeding artery is large enough to access individually with the microcatheter.

As with endovascular treatment of aneurysms, road-mapping is used to navigate the cerebral arterial system. Control of patient motion is important to allow such navigation. Treatment of a conscious patient requires that he or she be highly cooperative. The high-flow characteristics of some AVMs allow the use of flow-directed microcatheters that are carried to the AVM by the rapid blood flow. The advantage of using such catheters is that the risk of arterial injury is reduced when a microguidewire is not used to direct and support the catheter. In many cases, wire-guided microcatheters similar or identical to those used for aneurysm treatment are necessary to access the desired arterial branch. Careful and gentle manipulation of the microcatheter and microguidewire is necessary to prevent perforation or dissection of the artery.

Embolization of brain AVMs may be performed with the patient conscious, heavily sedated, or under general anesthesia. The different approaches are linked to the use of provocative pharmacologic testing (PPT) by some practitioners. PPT involves the injection of small amounts of barbiturates distal to the microcatheter into the vasculature.[55] Based on the anatomic principle that brain AVMs do not contain normal neural tissue, the barbiturate should produce no detectable neurologic changes if the microcatheter is positioned within an arterial branch that supplies only the AVM. Thus, it should be safe to embolize the tested arterial branch without producing infarction of normal tissue. Clinical and neurologic evaluation of a conscious and cooperative patient is used to detect possible neurologic changes after injection of the barbiturate. Neurophysiologic monitoring, including electroencephalography and somatosensory evoked potentials, may also be used with PPT. Although evaluation of electroencephalography and somatosensory evoked potential changes does not require that the patient be conscious or cooperative, the utility of such testing is less than that of a clinical neurologic evaluation.

The counterpoint to such PPT is that careful evaluation of the super-selective angiogram obtained by injection of contrast material through the microcatheter should suffice to detect any normal vessels present. Therefore, many consider it unnecessary to conduct such testing. Additionally, there are many areas of the brain that control such complex functions that the limited neurologic examination, possible during the embolization procedure, cannot be expected to detect all potential neurologic changes induced by an injected barbiturate. If PPT will not be used, total control of patient motion is possible by performing the procedure with the patient under general anesthesia. Elimination of undesired patient motion improves imaging so that navigation of the intracranial arteries is made safer. Many practitioners feel that this is the safer approach to AVM embolization and treatment.

The use of PPT is a controversial topic. Valid arguments have been made by expert physicians to support brain AVM embolization either with or without PPT. As with most techniques, it is important to understand the validity of both approaches. The authors were trained by some of the innovators of PPT. Not surprisingly, we use PPT frequently and believe that it helps to minimize complications. However, it is important to recognize the limitations of PPT. The potential benefits of PPT are lost if uncontrolled patient motion increases the risk of arterial injury and stroke; we treat uncooperative patients under general anesthesia without PPT.

Embolic Devices

A wide variety of devices are available to occlude the desired arterial branches that supply a brain AVM. Typically used devices include an FDA-approved NBCA glue (TrueFill NBCA, Cordis Neurovascular Inc.), absolute ethanol, plastic foam sponge particles of PVA (True Fill PVA Particles, Cordis Neurovascular Inc.), and platinum microcoils. Platinum embolization coils, PVA foam particles, often referred to as *PVA particles*, and detachable balloons used to occlude vessels are illustrated in Figure 18-8. The vessel anatomy, physician preference, and the reason for which embolization is being performed determine the devices used. When embolization is performed to reduce the size of the AVM nidus before radiosurgery, permanent nidus occlusion is desired. Embolization performed before surgical resection may require only temporary occlusion of the feed-

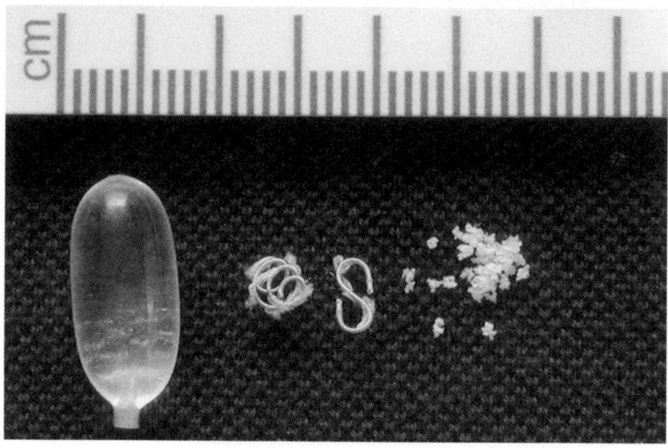

FIGURE 18-8. From left to right, an 8-mm-maximum-diameter detachable balloon (shown inflated) (Detachable Silicone Balloon, Target Therapeutics Corporation, Fremont, California); 3-mm-diameter spiral-shaped platinum embolization coil (Diamond Vortex, Target Therapeutics Corporation); 2-mm × 5-mm S-shaped platinum embolization coil (Complex Helical Fibered Platinum Embolization Coil, Target Therapeutics Corporation); and several 500- to 710-μm-diameter polyvinyl alcohol foam (PVA) particles (Contour Embolization Particles, Target Therapeutics). Balloons, coils, and PVA particles are available in a wide range of sizes. Each of these devices may be used to occlude vessels of an appropriate diameter. A deflated balloon is mounted on the tip of a 0.7- to 1.0-mm-diameter microcatheter to allow it to be advanced into the appropriate position. The inflated balloon is then detached by gently retracting the microcatheter. Friction between the vessel wall and the balloon holds the balloon in place as the microcatheter is withdrawn. A self-sealing valve at the base of the balloon closes as the microcatheter is removed. The spiral- and S-shaped coils may be either pushed through the lumen of a microcatheter with a blunt-tipped guidewire or delivered into the vessel by a forceful injection of saline. The PVA particles are injected through the microcatheter. The PVA particles themselves are not radiopaque. Therefore, it is necessary to suspend the particles in radiographic contrast material and then inject the radiographically visible mixture into the vessel.

ing arteries, without deep penetration of the embolic material into the AVM nidus.

Cyanoacrylates are liquid tissue adhesive agents that may be injected through even the very smallest microcatheters. The use of cyanoacrylate adhesives for brain AVM embolization was first reported by Kerber in 1976. Cyanoacrylates polymerize almost instantaneously on contact with anions, including those in the bloodstream. Their very rapid transition from a liquid to a solid state allows effective occlusion of large arteries with very high blood flow. Because of their rapid polymerization and adhesive nature, cyanoacrylates are among the most difficult devices to use. Cyanoacrylates are usually mixed with ethiodized oil that both slightly decreases polymerization time and renders the mixture radiopaque.[56] The addition of ethiodized oil also decreases the adhesiveness of the cyanoacrylate. Cyanoacrylates are generally considered to be permanent embolic devices, although vessel recanalization has been reported. Cyanoacrylates became widely accepted as the preferred embolic device for AVM treatment after Kerber's initial report in 1976, and in September 2000, the FDA approved the first cyanoacrylate for AVM embolization (TruFill nBCA, Cordis Neurovascular Inc.).

PVA particles are tiny plastic sponges that may be injected through microcatheters. PVA particles are available in sizes ranging from 45 to 2,000 μm in diameter. Neurovascular embolization with PVA particles was first used in 1978.[57] Delivery of sufficiently large particles through a microcatheter to occlude high-flow AVMs may be difficult. Larger, wire-guided microcatheters are often necessary when PVA is used.[58] The nidus of the AVM is not as well penetrated with the PVA particles as with liquid tissue adhesive. The permanence of occlusion with PVA particles also appears to be less than that achieved with cyanoacrylates. Although the occlusive characteristics of PVA particles seem to be inferior to those of cyanoacrylates, this must be balanced against the greater ease of use of PVA particles.

Ethanol

Absolute ethanol has been used in selected cases as an embolic agent for brain AVMs.[59] Ethanol induces very severe endothelial injury, which leads to delayed arterial occlusion. Ethanol may be the most toxic and difficult embolic agent to use. It is also probably the most permanent agent available. Curative treatment of large AVMs may be facilitated by embolization with ethanol alone or as an adjunct to surgery or radiosurgery. The delayed effects of ethanol embolization make it difficult to use as a preresection embolization agent, unless resection may be delayed for several weeks. Few interventionists have chosen to use ethanol as a primary embolic agent. Many believe that the difficulty in using ethanol and the associated complications outweigh the potential benefits.

Coils

Platinum coils similar to those used for treatment of cerebral aneurysms may also be used to occlude arteries associated with an AVM. The coils used for AVM embolization are usually pushed through the catheter with a blunt-tipped guidewire or injected through the catheter with a bolus of saline. The coils are released into the artery without the possibility of retrieval or repositioning. This is safe because coil position is not as critical as it is during aneurysm treatment. The primary advantage in using these freely released coils is decreased cost. A secondary advantage is that coil placement is much faster. Coils are frequently used to occlude large direct arteriovenous shunts within an AVM that would be difficult to close using smaller PVA particles or that might allow a liquid embolic agent to penetrate into the venous outflow. Coils are also used frequently to obtain complete occlusion of a feeding artery after injection of PVA particles has markedly slowed blood flow.

SUMMARY

Endovascular intervention for aneurysms and brain AVMs is a rapidly evolving field. Technological advances will continue to improve on the safety and efficacy of the techniques described. Conventional open surgical aneurysm treatment will progressively yield to less invasive endovascular techniques. However, surgical resection of small, readily accessible brain AVMs is likely to persist as the preferred treatment. Treatment of larger AVMs will become less invasive and safer as improved embolic devices and delivery systems are developed.

REFERENCES

1. Johnston SC, Selvin S, Gress DR. The burden, trends, and demographics of mortality from subarachnoid hemorrhage. Neurology 1998;50:1413–1418.

2. Jane JA, Kassell NF, Torner JC, Winn HR. The natural history of aneurysms and arteriovenous malformations. J Neurosurg 1985;62:321–323.

3. Drake CG. Management of cerebral aneurysms. Stroke 1981;1:273–283.

4. Hunt WE, Hess RM. Surgical risk as related to the time of intervention in the repair of intracranial aneurysms. J Neurosurg 1968;28:14–20.

5. Brott T, Mandybur TI. Case-controlled study of clinical outcome after aneurysmal subarachnoid hemorrhage. Neurosurgery 1986;19:891–895.

6. International Study of Unruptured Intracranial Aneurysms Investigators. Unruptured intracranial aneurysms: risks of rupture and risks of surgical intervention. N Engl J Med 1998;339:1725–1733.

7. Vajda J. Multiple intracranial aneurysms: a high risk condition. Acta Neurochir (Wien) 1992;118: 59–75.

8. Stone JL, Crowell RM, Gandi YN, Jafar JJ. Multiple intracranial aneurysms: magnetic resonance imaging for determination of site of rupture. Neurosurgery 1988;23:97–100.

9. Watanabe AT, Mackey JK, Lufkin RB. Imaging diagnosis and temporal appearance of subarachnoid hemorrhage. Neuroimaging Clin North Am 1992;2:53–59.

10. Osborne AG. Intracranial Hemorrhage. In Diagnostic Neuroradiology. St. Louis: Mosby, 1994;154.

11. Barr JD. Temporary and permanent occlusion of cerebral arteries: indications and techniques. Neurosurg Clin North Am 2000;11(1):27–38.

12. Serbinenko FA. Balloon catheterization and occlusion of major cerebral vessels. J Neurosurg 1974;41:125–145.

13. Barr JD, Lemley TJ. Endovascular arterial occlusion using microcoils deployed both with and without proximal flow arrest: results in 19 patients. AJNR Am J Neuroradiol 1999;20(8):1452–1456.

14. Graves VB, Perl J, Strother CM, et al. Endovascular occlusion of the carotid or vertebral artery with temporary proximal flow arrest and microcoils: clinical results. AJNR Am J Neuroradiol 1997;18: 1201–1206.

15. Romodanov AP, Shcheglov VI. Endovascular method of excluding from the circulation saccular cerebral arterial aneurysms, leaving intact vessels patent. Acta Neurochir Suppl 1979;28:312–315.

16. Higashida RT, Halbach VV, Dowd C, et al. Endovascular detachable balloon embolization therapy of cavernous carotid artery aneurysms: results in 87 cases. J Neurosurg 1990;72:857–863.

17. Guglielmi G, Vinuela F, Sepetka I, et al. Electrothrombosis of saccular aneurysms via endovascular approach. Part 1: electrochemical basis, technique, and experimental results. J Neurosurg 1991;75:1–7.

18. Guglielmi G, Vinuela F, Dion J, et al. Electrothrombosis of saccular aneurysms via endovascular approach. Part 2: Preliminary clinical experience. J Neurosurg 1991;75:8–14.

19. King JT Jr, Berlin JA, Flamm ES. Morbidity and mortality from elective surgery for asymptomatic, unruptured, intracranial aneurysms: a meta-analysis. J Neurosurg 1994;81:837–842.

20. Raaymakers TW, Rinkel GJ, Limburg M, et al. Mortality and morbidity of surgery for unruptured intracranial aneurysms: a meta-analysis. Stroke 1985; 16:48–52.

21. Nishimoto A, Ueta K, Onbe H, et al. Nationwide cooperative study of intracranial aneurysm surgery in Japan. Stroke 1985;16:48–52.

22. Sundt TM Jr, Kobayashi S, Fode NC, et al. Results and complications of surgical management of 809 intracranial aneurysms in 722 cases: related and unrelated to grade of patient, type of aneurysm, and timing of surgery. J Neurosurg 1982;56:753–765.

23. Wirth FP, Laws ER Jr, Piepgras D, et al. Surgical treatment of intracranial aneurysms. Neurosurgery 1983;12:507–511.

24. Solomon RA, Fink ME, Pile-Spellman J. Surgical management of unruptured intracranial aneurysms. J Neurosurg 1994;80:440–446.

25. Rice BJ, Peerless SJ, Drake CG. Surgical treatment of unruptured aneurysms of the posterior circulation. J Neurosurg 1990;73:165–173.

26. Moret J, Cognard C, Weill A, et al. Reconstruction technic in the treatment of wide-neck intracranial aneurysms. Long-term angiographic and clinical results. Apropos of 56 cases. J Neuroradiol 1997;24: 30–44.

27. Moret J, Ross IB, Weill A, et al. The retrograde approach: a consideration for the endovascular treatment of aneurysms. AJNR Am J Neuroradiol 2000;21:262–268.

28. Higashida RT, Smith W, Gress D, et al. Intravascular stent and endovascular coil placement for a ruptured fusiform aneurysm of the basilar artery. Case report and review of the literature. J Neurosurg 1997;87:944–949.

29. Brilstra EH, Rinkel GJE, van der Graff Y, et al. Treatment of intracranial aneurysms by embolization with coils: a systematic review. Stroke 1999;30:470–476.

30. Malisch TW, Guglielmi G, Vinuela F, et al. Intracranial aneurysms treated with the Guglielmi detachable coil: midterm clinical results in a consecutive series of 100 patients. J Neurosurg 1997;87:176–183.

31. Atlas SW, Listerud J, Chung W, et al. Intracranial aneurysms: depiction on MR angiograms with a multi-feature extraction, ray-tracing postprocessing algorithm. Radiology 1992;183:379–389.

32. Ross JS, Masaryk TJ, Modic MT, et al. Intracranial aneurysms: evaluation by MR angiography. AJR Am J Roentgenol 1990;155:159–165.

33. Derdeyn CP, Graves VB, Turski PA, et al. MR angiography of saccular aneurysms after treatment with Guglielmi detachable coils: preliminary experience. AJNR Am J Neuroradiol 1997;18(2):279–286.

34. Johnston SC, Dudley RA, Gress DR, et al. Surgical and endovascular treatment of unruptured cerebral aneurysms at university hospitals. Neurology 199;52:1799–1805.

35. Johnston SC. Effect of endovascular services and hospital volume on cerebral aneurysm treatment outcomes. Stroke 2000;31:111–117.

36. Johnston SC, Wilson CB, Halbach VV, et al. Endovascular and surgical treatment of unruptured cerebral aneurysms: comparison of risks. Ann Neurol 2000;48:11–19.

37. Yalamanchili K, Rosenwasser RH, Thomas JE, et al. Frequency of cerebral vasospasm in patients treated with endovascular occlusion of intracranial aneurysms. AJNR Am J Neuroradiol 1998;19(3):553–558.

38. Ondra S, Troupp H, George ED, et al. The natural history of symptomatic arteriovenous malformations of the brain: a 24-year follow-up assessment. J Neurosurg 1990;73:387–391.

39. Wilkins RH. Natural history of intracranial vascular malformations: a review. Neurosurgery 1985;16:421–430.

40. Svien HJ, Olive I, Angulo-Rivero P. The fate of patients who have cerebral arteriovenous anomalies without definitive surgical treatments. J Neurosurg 1956;13:381–387.

41. Perret G, Nishioka H. Report on the cooperative study of intracranial aneurysms and subarachnoid hemorrhage. Section VI: Arteriovenous malformations: an analysis of 545 cases of cranio-cerebral arteriovenous malformations and fistulae reported to the cooperative study. J Neurosurg 1966;25:467–490.

42. Brown RD, Wiebers DO, Forbes G, et al. The natural history of unruptured intracranial arteriovenous malformations. J Neurosurg 1988;68:352–357.

43. McCormickWF. Pathology of vascular arteriovenous malformations. J Neurosurg 1966;24:807–816.

44. Batjer H, Suss RA, Samson D. Intracranial arteriovenous malformations associated with aneurysms. Neurosurgery 1986;18:29–35.

45. Brown RD, Wiebers DO, Forbes GS. Unruptured intracranial aneurysms and arteriovenous malformations: frequency of intracranial hemorrhage and relationship of lesions. J Neurosurg 1990;73:859–863.

46. Cunha E, Sa MJ, Stein BM, et al. The treatment of associated intracranial aneurysms and arteriovenous malformations. J Neurosurg 1992;77:853–859.

47. Spetzler RF, Martin NA, Carter LP, et al. Surgical management of large AVMs by staged embolization and operative excision. J Neurosurg 1987;67(1): 17–28.

48. Schneider BF, Eberhard DA, Steiner LE. Histopathology of arteriovenous malformations after gamma knife radiosurgery. J Neurosurg 1997;87(3):352–357.

49. Karlsson B, Lindquist C, Steiner L. Prediction of obliteration after gamma knife surgery for cerebral arteriovenous malformations. Neurosurgery 1997; 40(3):425–430.

50. Lindquist M, Steiner L, Blomgren H, et al. Stereotactic radiation therapy of intracranial arteriovenous malformations. Acta Radiol Suppl 1986;369:610–613.

51. Gobin YP, Laurent A, Merienne L, et al. Treatment of brain arteriovenous malformations by embolization and radiosurgery. J Neurosurg 1996;85(1):19–28.

52. Mathis JA, Barr JD, Horton JA, et al. The efficacy of particulate embolization combined with stereotactic radiosurgery for treatment of large arteriovenous malformations of the brain. AJNR Am J Neuroradiol 1995;16(2):299–306.

53. Spetzler RF, Wilson CB, Weinstein P. Normal perfusion pressure breakthrough theory. Clin Neurosurg 1978;25;651–672.

54. N-butyl cyanoacrylate embolization of cerebral arteriovenous malformations: results of a prospective, randomized, multi-center trial. The n-BCA Trial Investigators. AJNR Am J Neuroradiol 2002;23(5): 748–755.

55. Barr JD, Mathis JM, Horton JA. Provocative Pharmacologic Testing. In RJ Maciunas (ed), AANS Topics in Neurosurgery: Endovascular Neurologic Intervention. Park Ridge, IL: The American Association of Neurological Surgeons, 1995;75–89.

56. Cromwell LD, Kerber CW. Modification of cyanoacrylate for therapeutic embolization: preliminary experience. AJR Am J Roentgenol 1979;132:799–802.

57. Kerber CW, Bank WO, Horton JA. Polyvinyl alcohol foam: prepackaged emboli for therapeutic embolization. AJR Am J Roentgenol 1978;130:1193–1194.

58. Barr JD, Lemley TJ, Petrochko CN. Polyvinyl alcohol foam particle sizes and concentrations injectable through microcatheters. J Vasc Interv Radiol 1998;9:113–118.

59. Yakes WF, Krauth L, Ecklund J, et al. Ethanol endovascular management of brain arteriovenous malformations: initial results. Neurosurgery 1997;40: 1145–1152.

CHAPTER

19

Imaging as a Surrogate Marker in Clinical Trials

Marc Fisher

The development of acute stroke therapies has proved to be a complex and difficult process with a plethora of unsuccessful clinical trials and a few studies that have been successful. The reasons why so many acute stroke trials have been unsuccessful are myriad, but the assessment tools used in these trials may have contributed to difficulties in determining treatment effects or lack thereof. The presumed goal of therapy is to preserve function by salvaging ischemic tissue that is not irreversibly injured when therapy is initiated.[1] This concept is widely used in experimental stroke models to evaluate the potential efficacy of purported acute therapies, typically by measuring infarct volume histologically 1–7 days after stroke onset.[2] Tissue salvage in noncritically hypoperfused regions is the direct target of neuroprotective therapy, whereas thrombolytic therapy salvages ischemic tissue by restoring blood flow. Both of these approaches lend themselves to the possibility of assessing treatment effects by using a substitute, biologically meaningful response that should be ultimately related to clinical benefits (i.e., surrogate markers of therapeutic efficacy).[3] For thrombolytic therapy, recanalization of previously occluded blood vessels or reperfusion of the microcirculation is a relevant biologic effect of the intervention, and measuring these effects can serve as a surrogate marker of drug activity. Successful thrombolytic therapy should lead to tissue salvage, and this effect can serve as an additional marker of therapeutic activity. With neuroprotective therapy, salvage of ischemic tissue can serve as a marker of therapeutic efficacy. This chapter reviews the current status of acute stroke therapy trials and methods of end point assessment, animal studies demonstrating the utility of imaging techniques as surrogate markers, initial attempts to use imaging techniques as surrogate markers in clinical stroke trials, and potential applications of these imaging surrogates in future trials.

LESSONS FROM PRIOR STROKE TRIALS

Currently, only three acute stroke trials have demonstrated a statistically significant treatment effect on the primary outcome measure chosen.[4–6] The National Institute of Neurological Disorders and Stroke (NINDS) intravenous recombinant tissue plasminogen activator (rt-PA) trial is the only study that led to the regulatory approval of a drug evaluated in an acute stroke trial. The end points chosen in these three positive trials were clinical ones that evaluated functional and neurologic outcomes 90 days after stroke onset. In both the NINDS rt-PA trial and the Stroke Treatment with Ancrod Trial, the time window for enrollment was up to 3 hours, and in the Prolyse for Acute Cerebral Thromboembolism (PROACT)-II study of intra-arterial prourokinase, the time window was 6 hours. In the NINDS rt-PA trial, half of the patients were randomized within 90 minutes of stroke onset. This early randomization of patients is likely one of the predominant reasons for the treatment effect observed, because a recent reanalysis of the data relating time to initiation of treatment to outcome demonstrated that in patients treated beyond 160 minutes after stroke onset, the confidence intervals no longer assured a significant treatment effect. The PROACT-II study differed from the other two positive studies in several important design features. The time window for enrollment was longer, but patients were selected for inclusion based on angiographic documentation of a proximal middle cerebral artery occlusion (MCAO). Therefore, a more homogeneous group of patients was included, and a significantly greater percentage of treated patients demonstrated a favorable outcome, defined as a Rankin score of 2 or less. This benefit occurred despite the inclusion of a very severely affected group of stroke patients at baseline (National Institutes of Health Stroke Scale [NIHSS] median score of 17). Three other intravenous rt-PA studies that either enrolled most patients beyond the 3-hour window (European Cooperative Acute Stroke Study [ECASS]-I and II) or were limited to a 3–5 hour window (Acute Noninterventional Therapy in Ischemic Stroke) did not demonstrate a significant treatment effect.[7–9] In the two ECASS trials, however, there was a suggestion of efficacy in subset analyses. None of these three trials used neuroimaging studies to select patients more likely to respond to therapy. In the ECASS trials, computed tomography (CT) scanning was used to identify patients at increased risk for hemorrhage. An attempt was made to exclude patients with early involvement of more than one-third of the MCA territory.[10] In ECASS-I, patients who violated this exclusion had a much greater risk for cerebral hemorrhage and death than those without this finding. In ECASS-II, the investigators did a better job at excluding patients with extensive early CT changes, but this was associated with the inclusion of a less severely affected stroke population at baseline and a better-than-anticipated outcome in the placebo group.

A large number of neuroprotective drugs (Table 19-1) has been studied in clinical trials, and so far none has demonstrated unequivocal efficacy.[11] A variety of reasons have been postulated for these negative results, as outlined in Table 19-2. Some of the neuroprotective drugs had either a limited benefit or a very short time window of efficacy. Such data in preclinical assessment would make it unlikely that efficacy could be demonstrated in stroke patients. Other neuroprotective drugs demonstrated substantial side effects such as hypotension, psychomimetic activity, sedation, and drug–drug interactions in animals or early human studies. These side effects precluded the achievement of drug plasma concentrations necessary to salvage ischemic tissue. In some cases, drug concentrations were limited by the side effect profile, and therefore any chance to induce a reasonable amount of ischemic tissue salvage was lost. Other potential explanations for unsuccessful neuroprotective trials come from an analysis of the trial designs used in some studies. Almost all neuroprotective studies have used a 6-hour or longer time window as an inclusion criterion. Current experimental and clinical imaging data support the concept that as time passes after stroke onset, less potentially salvageable ischemic tissue exists.[12] The maxim "time is brain" exemplifies this concept and suggests that the longer the delay to initiating any treatment, the less likely that the treatment will be beneficial. It is quite plausible that one or more of the previously tested neuroprotective drugs could be beneficial, if they were studied again in a clinical trial with a very short time window for patient enrollment. A second lesson from acute stroke trials is that baseline severity is an important predictor of outcome.[13] In trials that included a high percentage of patients with a mild baseline deficit, a potential treatment effect could be lost because of a large placebo response rate. Conversely, patients with severe baseline deficits have little chance to improve, and treatment effects could be obscured because they are too modest. A third lesson relates to stroke subtyping, which is important in clinical trial design. Patients with isolated white matter lesions that typify lacunar infarcts may be inappropriate targets for drugs that have little or no effect on white matter

TABLE 19-1. Neuroprotective Drug Platforms

N-methyl-D-aspartate antagonists: MK-801, dextrorphan, selfotel, Cerestat
Other *N*-methyl-D-aspartate antagonists: elprodil, GV150526, ACEA 1021
4-Aminophenylmercuric acetate antagonists
Presynaptic modulators of glutamate release: BW619C89, fos-phenytoin
Free radical scavengers: tirilazad
Nitric oxide synthase inhibition: lubeluzole
Glycinergic and gamma-aminobutyric acid agonists: clomethiazole
Maxi-K channel agonists: BMS204352
Serotonin agonists: Bay-3702
Antiadhesion molecules
Growth factors: basic fibroblast growth factor

TABLE 19-2. Potential Reasons for Neuroprotective Drug Trial Failures

Inadequate demonstration of neuroprotective effects in animal models
Inadequate time window for efficacy
Inability to achieve neuroprotective doses in clinical trials secondary to toxicity
Inclusion of patients in clinical trials not likely to respond to the mechanism of action of the drug tested
Inclusion of too many mildly or severely affected patients in the trial
Inadequate end point to assess drug efficacy

ischemic injury, a process that appears to be mechanistically different from gray matter ischemic injury.[14] Additionally, the natural history of lacunar infarcts is much more favorable than that of cortical infarcts, and this may enhance the placebo response rate.

The choice of the primary end point for an acute stroke trial is critical. One primary end point must be chosen with a small number of secondary end points to support the observed treatment effects. Typical end points for acute stroke trials have included measures of handicap, impairment, and neurologic deficits. Commonly used scales include the NIHSS, the Rankin Scale, and the Barthel Index.[15] Each type of deficit and scoring scale has inherent advantages and disadvantages. It remains uncertain what the best assessment scale is to reliably capture the treatment effects. One interesting index used in the NINDS rt-PA trial was a global statistic. The latter does not rely on a single outcome measure but simultaneously evaluates multiple, predefined outcome measures such as the three scales mentioned previously.[16] This combined assessment may provide a more accurate evaluation of drug treatment effect than reliance on one measure alone. However, choosing one primary outcome measure or using the global statistic requires a large sample size with 300–600 patients per treatment arm to ensure adequate power to avoid type 1 and 2 errors. Such large trials are time consuming and expensive. Demonstration of clinical efficacy is certainly necessary for providing convincing evidence that a drug effectively improves outcome after ischemic stroke, leading to regulatory approval and physician acceptance. However, in the drug development process, the use of clinical assessment measures in the earlier phases may not be valuable or cost-effective. Phase 2 trials of acute stroke drugs typically include 100 or perhaps 200 patients per treatment group and are marginally powered to even detect a trend of efficacy with a clinical end point. Phase 2 trials are primarily safety trials. Yet, after a phase 2 trial, a decision must be made whether to proceed with the large phase 3 trial. Including a surrogate marker of drug activity in the phase 2 trial programs could enhance the development program for new acute stroke therapies. Open questions remain regarding which surrogate measure to use and how best to evaluate treatment efficacy with the measure chosen.

CLINICAL AND TRIAL UTILITY OF DIFFUSION AND PERFUSION MAGNETIC RESONANCE IMAGING

The new magnetic resonance imaging (MRI) techniques of diffusion-weighted imaging (DWI) and perfusion-weighted imaging (PWI) afford many potential opportunities for the evaluation of acute stroke patients.[17] They may also be useful in the development of acute stroke therapies. DWI can identify ischemic brain tissue within minutes after the onset of focal brain ischemia in experimental models and in less than 1 hour after stroke onset in patients.[18,19] The hyperintense abnormalities associated with acute ischemic stroke are conspicuous and can easily be used to derive a volumetric analysis of the ischemic lesion. The regions of hyperintensity observed on DWI represent tissue changes associated with the failure of high-energy metabolism and the rapid accumulation of cytotoxic edema.

TABLE 19-3. Clinical Utility of Diffusion Magnetic Resonance Imaging

Demonstrate ischemic lesions and their location rapidly after stroke onset
Differentiate between acute and chronic ischemic lesions
Identify multiple acute ischemic lesions
Provide evidence to aid in stroke subtyping
Identify potentially salvageable ischemic tissue
Guide acute stroke therapy
Provide a surrogate marker of efficacy for new stroke therapies

The clinical utility of DWI is readily apparent (Table 19-3) and has been documented by an expanding number of published studies. An obvious application of DWI is accurate stroke localization (Figure 19-1). Subcortical and posterior circulation ischemic lesions can readily be distinguished from cortical events.[20] Such distinctions are important for both diagnostic and prognostic reasons. For stroke therapy trials, the exclusion of subcortical and posterior circulation ischemic events is typically done because the outcome measures used to assess treatment effects may be relatively insensitive, and the drugs being studied may not be as effective as in cortical strokes. DWI can therefore be used to ensure that the target population is actually included in the trial. Several DWI studies reported that multiple acute lesions are present in 20–25% of the ischemic stroke population, whereas the clinical evaluation suggested only involvement in one vascular territory.[21] The detection of multiple acute ischemic lesions, especially in more than one vascular territory, strongly suggests a cardioembolic source. In a small percentage of patients, the initial DWI study may be negative.[22] Such a finding with an obvious PWI abnormality implies that ischemic tissue injury is currently minimal and that the patient may be a good candidate for acute intervention. In a patient without DWI and PWI abnormalities, a resolving ischemic deficit is likely or an alternative and nonischemic diagnosis should be considered (e.g., postictal state, resolving migraine aura). An important differential diagnostic consideration is the exclusion of intracranial hemorrhage. Currently, CT scanning is the gold standard for the diagnosis of intracranial hemorrhage. There is, however, increasing evidence that susceptibility-weighted

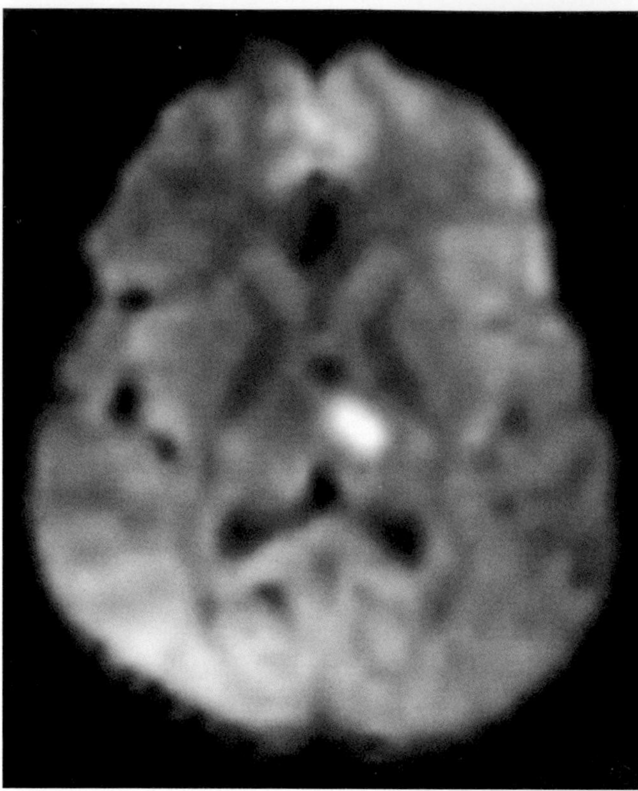

FIGURE 19-1. Diffusion imaging demonstrates an acute thalamic infarction.

MRI can reliably detect acute intracerebral hemorrhage.[23,24] This technique presumably will be validated soon and then included in the MRI assessment of acute stroke patients, obviating the need for a CT scan in addition to the MRI battery.

PWI is currently performed with a bolus tracking technique, using the injection of contrast agents that have susceptibility effects and impede the acquisition of T2* signal.[25] Multiple repetitive images are rapidly obtained, leading to the generation of a signal washout curve. A variety of measures can be derived from this signal intensity curve, including mean transit time and cerebral blood volume.[26] The relationship of these two parameters can be used to derive an index of cerebral blood flow that is not absolute, unless the arterial input function is known and deconvolution techniques are used. In clinical practice, perfusion maps based on the mean transit time or time to peak of the signal washout curve are typically used, and the region of perfusion abnormality is hypointense on these maps. PWI studies are used to document the presence of a region of reduced tissue perfusion consistent with reduced blood flow.[17] This finding confirms that a region of ischemia is present and may help to identify the vascular territory involved, especially when combined with findings on magnetic resonance angiography (MRA).

Combining the information obtained from DWI and PWI studies along with MRA of acute stroke patients appears to provide a powerful and timely way to assess tissue and vascular status individually. Current information from acute stroke patients studied within 6 hours of onset suggests that approximately 70% will have a PWI lesion volume that is at least 20% greater than the DWI lesion volume.[27,28] This difference in volume is called the *diffusion-perfusion mismatch* (Figure 19-2). The territory of perfusion abnormality without a DWI abnormality suggests a region of mild to moderate ischemia that may progress to more severe ischemic injury without rapid intervention. This region of mismatch may therefore roughly approximate the ischemic penumbra and identify a potential target for therapy in individual patients. Other DWI/PWI patterns are seen in acute stroke patients that may also be relevant for individual treatment decisions and clinical trial design. In approximately 20% of patients studied within the first 6 hours, the DWI and PWI lesion volumes are of almost the same size, whereas in 10% of patients, the DWI lesion volume is substantially larger than the PWI lesion,

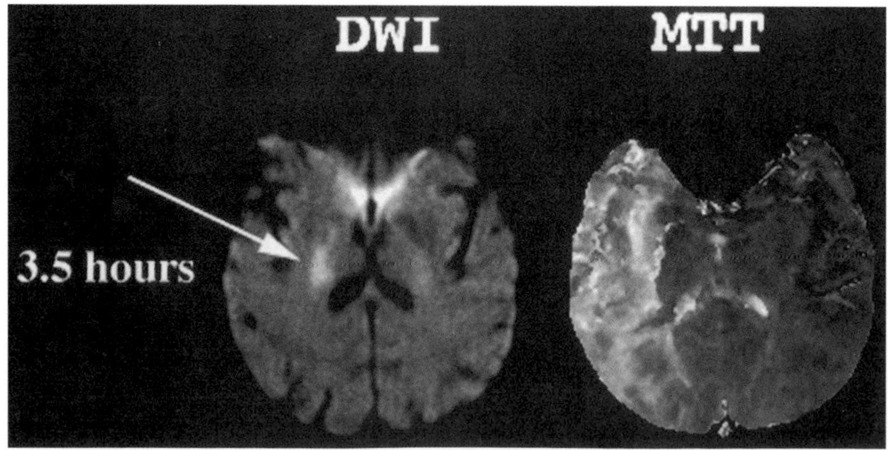

FIGURE 19-2. A diffusion-perfusion magnetic resonance image study obtained 3.5 hours after stroke onset demonstrating a much larger region of perfusion abnormality on the mean transit time (MTT) map than on the diffusion-weighted image (DWI). Arrow indicates region of diffusion abnormality. (Courtesy of Dr. Steven Warach.)

or there is no obvious PWI abnormality. Several preliminary studies suggest that these acute DWI/PWI patterns may be useful in choosing patients for intravenous thrombolytic therapy and evaluating treatment effects. In a small study in which the MRI battery was obtained shortly after the start of intravenous t-PA, initial PWI volumes were smaller than DWI volumes in five of the six patients who received t-PA and in only one of the five patients who did not receive it, implying that thrombolytic therapy had early reperfusion effects.[29] In another preliminary study, DWI, PWI, and MRA were performed in 24 patients who received intravenous tPA within 6 hours of stroke onset.[30] The MRI studies were done in 16 of the 24 patients before the start of therapy. Vessel occlusion was confirmed in 20 of the patients. Of these 20, 19 had a PWI/DWI mismatch of more than 20%. In eleven of the 20 patients, subsequent recanalization of the occluded vessel was confirmed, whereas in the other nine patients, it was not. Clinical outcome was better in the group that recanalized than in the nonrecanalized group. These preliminary studies suggest that DWI/PWI may be useful in both clinical practice and the development of drugs for acute ischemic stroke.

ANIMAL EXPERIENCE WITH DIFFUSION-PERFUSION MAGNETIC RESONANCE IMAGING AS A MARKER OF DRUG EFFICACY

The traditional method used to assess drug efficacy in animal stroke models is to compare infarct volumes, corrected for edema, in the actively treated group versus the placebo group.[2] The goal of therapy in animal stroke models is to salvage ischemic tissue as the proof of principle that the drug under evaluation has activity. Concomitant effects on behavioral outcome are also assessed in some instances. Assessment of infarct volume provides a late evaluation of drug activity but does not evaluate how therapeutic intervention affects the dynamic evolution of the ischemic lesion. Shortly after the initial observations that DWI could image experimental stroke rapidly after onset, the technique was applied to drug treatment experiments. An initial experiment with RS-87476, a sodium–calcium channel ion modulator, demonstrated that DWI could detect in vivo treatment effect.[31] DWI was also used to evaluate the treatment effects of a nitrogen *N*-methyl-D-aspartate antagonist, Cerestat, in both permanent and temporary occlusion models.[32] A highly significant effect of Cerestat on early in vivo ischemic lesion development was observed, and it correlated well with histologically confirmed infarct size at 24 hours. There was some increase in lesion size from last imaging time point to histologic evaluation time point, implying that Cerestat treatment should have been continued for a longer time. This type of information about the best duration of therapy would be difficult to obtain with postmortem infarct data alone.

Another potentially important contribution of DWI is to evaluate when a therapy begins to have its effect. Two groups studied the glycine antagonist, ZD9379, initiated either immediately or 30 minutes after MCAO. In the first study, no significant difference between the treated and placebo groups was observed on DWI 2.5 hours after stroke onset, but at 6 hours the lesion size was 41% smaller in the treated group.[33] In the second study, therapy was initiated 30 minutes after stroke onset, and no difference in lesion volume was detected between the treated and placebo groups during the first 3 hours after stroke onset.[34] At 3.5 hours, the lesion size demonstrated a trend toward reduction in the group of treated animals; however, imaging was stopped at this point (Figure 19-3). At postmortem examination 24 hours after permanent MCAO, the treated group had a greater than 40% reduction of histologically confirmed infarct size. Interestingly, the delayed salvage of ischemic tissue associated with treatment occurred primarily in the borderzone between the middle and anterior cerebral arteries, a region of modestly reduced blood flow that would meet criteria for the ischemic penumbra. Results from the two studies suggest this glycine antagonist has a delayed treatment effect that is clearly different from the temporal profile observed with Cerestat. The glycine antagonist might have a broader therapeutic time window. Such informa-

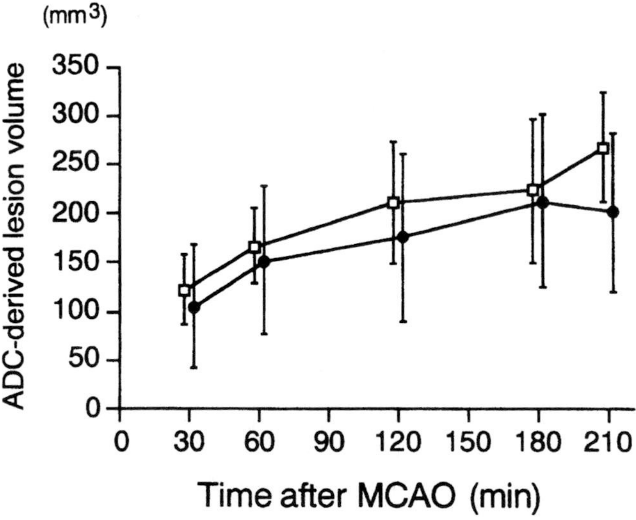

FIGURE 19-3. Evolution of ischemic lesion volume in the ZD9379 and placebo groups showing a late divergence. (ADC = apparent diffusion coefficient; MCAO = middle cerebral artery occlusion.) (Reprinted with permission from K Takano, T Tatlisumak, JE Formato, et al. Glycine site antagonist attenuates infarct size in experimental focal ischemia. Postmortem and diffusion mapping studies. Stroke 1997;28[6]:1255–1262; discussion 1263.)

tion would be difficult to obtain without in vivo evaluation of treatment effects provided by DWI.

PWI has also been used to evaluate the effects of mechanical reperfusion and thrombolytic therapy on ischemic lesion evolution assessed by DWI. The suture occlusion stroke model in rats is readily amenable to mechanical reperfusion by withdrawing the suture occluder. Using this technique, Muller et al. used PWI to confirm successful reperfusion and DWI to evaluate the effect of this reperfusion on lesion size.[35] They observed that lesion size was reduced by two-thirds 45 minutes after the onset of ischemia. However, at 120 minutes, reperfusion was associated with a small increase in ischemic lesion size.

Jiang et al. used DWI and PWI to evaluate the therapeutic effects of rt-PA in a rat embolic stroke model.[36] rt-PA, injected 1 hour after embolization, improved blood flow and reduced the number of abnormal pixels as determined by a combined DWI and T2 analysis. The individual animal responses to rt-PA treatment varied, but imaging readily detected responders and nonresponders. Prourokinase was also evaluated in a rat embolic model using PWI/DWI.[37] It was infused either intravenously or intra-arterially 30 minutes after embolization. Both types of treatments were associated with a significant reduction in the volume of hypoperfused tissue, with slightly better results from intra-arterial therapy. The reperfusion effect was associated with a significant reduction in ischemic lesion volume on DWI for the intra-arterial therapy group and no increase over time in the intravenous group. The placebo group demonstrated a noticeable increase over time. These studies exemplify how DWI/PWI can provide a sophisticated evaluation of group and individual therapeutic responses in experiments evaluating the efficacy of therapies designed to promote reperfusion. PWI can also be combined with DWI in neuroprotective drug experiments, especially with temporary occlusion models.[38]

PWI and DWI evaluated simultaneously in animals can be used to follow the evolution of the diffusion-perfusion mismatch. Recently, Omae et al. used these MRI techniques in rats undergoing permanent and temporary arterial occlusion with the suture model.[39] They observed a large diffusion-perfusion mismatch 30 minutes after MCAO. By 90 minutes after MCAO, there was no significant difference in the PWI and DWI lesion volumes, and at 120 minutes and beyond, the two volumes were almost identical. Interestingly, the PWI lesion volume stayed essentially the same over the entire 4-hour imaging protocol and was highly correlated with postmortem infarct volume. This observation supports the hypothesis that hypoperfusion will lead to infarction if left untreated.

Several recent studies with diffusion-perfusion MRI in rat temporary occlusion models have confirmed the hypothesis of reperfusion injury. Li et al. observed that reperfusion after very brief periods of focal temporary ischemia (8–30 minutes) is associated with the complete disappearance of initial DWI lesions within 60–90 minutes (Figure 19-4).[40] However, despite the apparent reversal of DWI lesions, postmortem studies 3 days later demonstrated variable degrees of ischemic injury. The severity of these pathologically demonstrated ischemic lesions was directly correlated to the degree of initial blood flow decline and the length of time over which the decline persisted. In two follow-up studies, the same research group characterized the temporal and spatial characteristics of these secondary DWI lesions.[41,42] They observed that secondary DWI ischemic lesions began to reappear 3–4 hours after reperfusion, and that by 12 hours, the secondary ischemic lesions were approximately 50% of the volume detected during arterial occlusion. From 24 to 72 hours after reperfusion, the DWI volumes approximated those seen during occlusion and were highly correlated with the histologically determined volume at 72 hours. The longer the time until reperfusion, the less likely that initial DWI lesion will

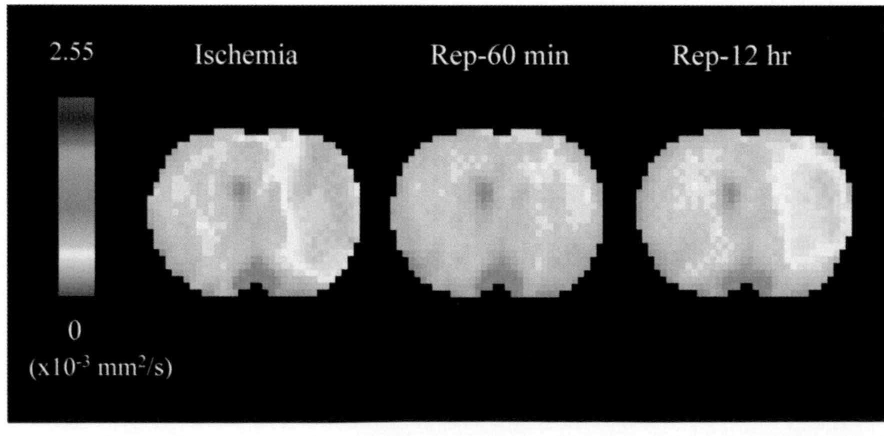

FIGURE 19-4. Color-coded diffusion imaging demonstrating a region of low apparent diffusion coefficient values during occlusion that disappears almost entirely 60 minutes after reperfusion (Rep) and then reappears at 12 hours.

occur. With 2.0–2.5 hours of temporary occlusion, little if any reversal is detectable. The pathophysiologic mechanisms that induce the secondary DWI lesions after reperfusion remain to be definitively established, but secondary energy failure and mitochondrial function deterioration are the most likely contributors. Apoptosis may contribute to secondary ischemic injury, especially in the peripheral aspects of the initial lesion where blood flow declines are modest. Secondary DWI abnormalities have now also been observed in patients undergoing successful intra-arterial thrombolysis. Kidwell et al. performed serial DWI and PWI studies in seven patients who were successfully reperfused with intra-arterial thrombolytic therapy.[43] They observed that the initial DWI lesion volume markedly diminished several hours after thrombolysis-induced reperfusion. However, on day 7 of MRI studies, 50% of patients had a substantial secondary increase in DWI ischemic lesion volume, also detectable on T2 imaging (Figure 19-5). The clinical relevance of these secondary MRI-detected lesions remains uncertain. As the mechanisms associated with reperfusion-related injury become apparent, interventions will likely be directed at them. DWI and PWI studies will assume an important role for investigating the effects of these therapies.

CLINICAL TRIAL EXPERIENCE WITH SURROGATE MARKERS

Currently, there is limited experience with the use of imaging techniques as surrogate markers in stroke drug development. In the phase 2 study of prourokinase, PROACT-I, the overall early recanalization rate on standard angiography was 58% in the treated group and 14% in the placebo group.[44] A higher rate of recanalization was seen with the concomitant use of high-dose heparin in comparison to low-dose heparin. This recanalization effect of prourokinase was accompanied by a

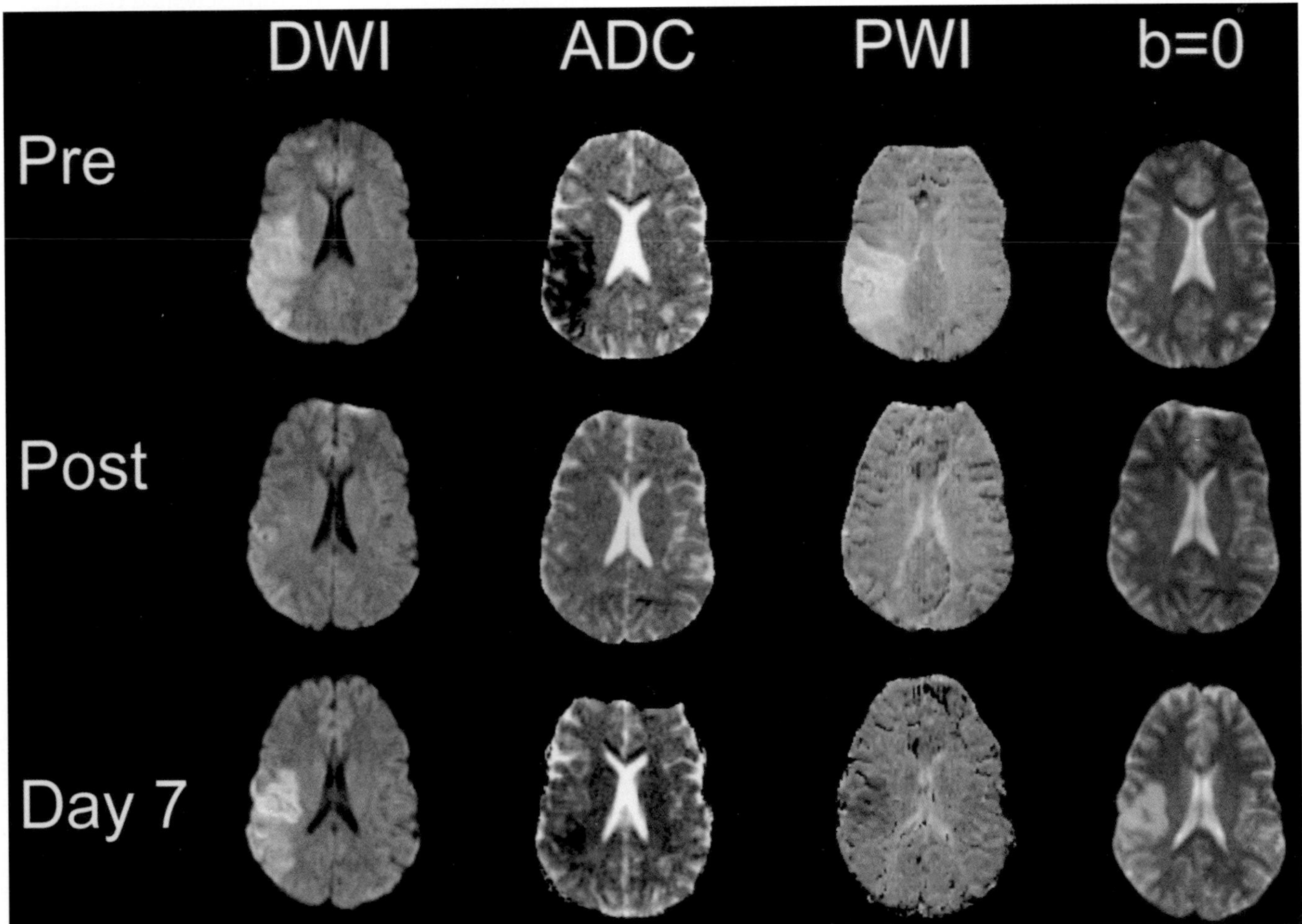

FIGURE 19-5. An early lesion is observed on diffusion imaging. The patient was treated with intra-arterial thrombolysis, and the diffusion lesion resolved, only to reappear at 7 days. (ADC = apparent diffusion coefficient; b=0 = there is no diffusion weighting; DWI = diffusion-weighted imaging; PWI = perfusion-weighted imaging.) (Courtesy of Dr. Chelsea S. Kidwell.)

trend toward more favorable clinical outcome. In the larger PROACT-II trial, the recanalization rate was 66% in the treated group and 18% in the placebo group.[5] This treatment effect on the target of thrombolysis was associated with a significantly favorable effect on the prespecified outcome measure. The prourokinase trials demonstrate that thrombolytic therapy can be effective with a median time to treat of 5.3 hours after stroke onset in a targeted and homogeneous group of stroke patients with a high degree of baseline impairment. They support the surrogate marker concept for stroke drug development, because the drug effect on reperfusion did relate to clinical benefit. Other imaging methods that evaluate the blood vessels or brain perfusion, such as MRA, CT angiography, xenon CT, and transcranial Doppler ultrasound, may be useful in future thrombolytic trials.

Imaging of the brain parenchyma with CT or MRI is another way to evaluate treatment effects on the target organ. In the NINDS rt-PA trial, the effect of treatment on the CT-documented infarct volume was assessed.[45] There was a nonsignificant trend toward smaller volumes in the rt-PA–treated group. The use of infarct volume on CT or MRI days after stroke onset as a measure of the effect of treatment on ischemic lesion volume has many inherent difficulties. The primary problem is that the sizes of lesions are quite variable, and the variance markedly reduces the power of the statistical evaluation.

One approach to this variability is to assess treatment effects on the evolution of ischemic lesion volume from a baseline value to the ultimate infarct size. This can be accomplished with DWI, because an initial lesion can be detected in most cases when the patient presents for evaluation before treatment assignment is done. Several preliminary acute stroke therapy trials have used this approach. In a pilot study of 12 patients randomized to treatment with citicoline or placebo, Warach et al. demonstrated that ischemic lesion volume increased in three of four placebo-treated patients and became smaller in seven of eight treated patients.[46] This led to a moderately sized MRI-based citicoline trial.[47] Patients were randomized to citicoline or placebo within 24 hours of stroke onset, and they had to demonstrate a baseline DWI lesion volume of 1–120 cc involving cerebral gray matter. Patients were treated for 6 weeks and had a follow-up MRI and clinical evaluation at 12 weeks. The primary MRI assessment was the change in ischemic lesion volume from the baseline DWI study to the week-12 T2 study. One hundred patients were entered into the study, and 81 completed the final evaluation. The mean increase in lesion volume was 180% in the placebo group and 34% in the citicoline group. This was not statistically significant because of the large variability. Secondary analyses demonstrated a significant reduction in lesion volume from the week-1 to week-12 scan in the treated group when compared to placebo. Interestingly, in both treated and placebo patients who achieved the primary clinical end point of a seven-point or greater improvement in the NIHSS, a significantly larger reduction in lesion volume occurred in comparison to patients not achieving this clinical improvement. Patients treated within 12 hours of stroke onset were more likely to show an effect on lesion evolution. This study provides many important and valuable lessons. It was underpowered and would have been statistically significant with a larger sample size. Patients with small subcortical lesions were difficult to assess. In addition, the drug used and the time window to enrollment were not optimal to demonstrate a treatment effect on MRI.

A second MRI-based study, the Glycine Antagonist in Neuroprotection study with the glycine antagonist, GV150526, was also reported. In this study, patients were randomly and blindly assigned to placebo or active drug within 6 hours of stroke onset with a baseline DWI, PWI, and T2-battery performed before randomization.[48] Inclusion criteria included a baseline DWI lesion diameter of greater than 1.5 cm or volume of greater than 5 cc. One hundred six of 181 patients screened by MRI met the inclusion criteria, and 75 of 106 patients had the final scan performed at week 12. The absolute change in lesion size from baseline to week 12 was 10 cc in the placebo group and 3 cc in the treated group. The percentage change was 23% in the placebo group and 2% in the treated group, with a large variance in both groups. These differences were not significant because of the large variance. The results in the MRI substudy were concordant with the overall lack of efficacy of GV150526 in two large clinical trials.[49] The study does provide valuable information about the feasibility of doing a large multicenter MRI-based trial within the typical 6-hour window of current acute stroke treatment trials. The results of another large multicenter MRI substudy with the maxi-K channel antagonist, BMS-204352, also did not demonstrate any difference between the treated and placebo groups.

FUTURE DIRECTIONS

The use of surrogate markers in the stroke drug development process is just beginning. With prourokinase, the demonstration of reperfusion efficacy on standard angiography was useful, because it confirmed the thrombolytic efficacy of the drug and helped lead to a larger trial that demonstrated clinical efficacy. Standard angiography is time consuming and somewhat risky to perform, although necessary for intra-arterial drug delivery. In future intravenous thrombolytic trials, other modalities previously mentioned can be used for assessment of response to treatment. Several trials of intravenous thrombolytic drugs now use PWI and MRA as the basis for including appropriate patients and to assess the reperfusion efficacy of the thrombolytic agent. For example, vascular occlusion on MRA, or a minimum lesion volume in a particular vascular territory on PWI, can be required for inclusion. A follow-up study in several hours can then be done to evaluate the effect of treatment. This approach in a phase 2 study can be used to demonstrate whether a given dose of the thrombolytic agent induces an appropriate response in the vasculature. The dose producing the most favorable vascular response can then be tested for clinical efficacy in a larger sample size. Additionally, a requirement for a DWI/PWI mismatch can be included in the inclusion criteria, and the effect of treatment on lesion evolution over 30–90 days assessed. This approach will likely ensure enrollment of patients with the greatest possibility of responding to treatment and provide an assessment of the effect of the thrombolytic treatment on ischemic tissue salvage, the ultimate target of the intervention. A similar phase 2 trial could be envisioned with CT angiography and CT-perfusion imaging as the imaging modalities used to assess the reperfusion effects of the thrombolytic agent. Disadvantages of a CT-based study include the lack of a marker of ischemic penumbra and the difficulty of evaluating tissue salvage. With xenon CT, some estimation of the ischemic penumbra may be available from determinations of the level of blood-flow decline.

Neuroprotective drug trials will also expand the use of surrogate markers in the near future. The use of DWI/PWI in phase 2 neuroprotective trials is attractive, because with a relatively small sample size, such as 60–100 patients per treatment arm, it should be possible to detect significant effects on ischemic lesion volume evolution by comparing the percent change from the baseline lesion volume on DWI to the day 30–90 volume on T2-weighted imaging. Focusing on patients with a DWI/PWI mismatch should enhance the homogeneity of the treatment population and provide additional power to such an MRI-based study. Demonstrating an effect on lesion evolution will then provide encouragement to proceed to a large phase 3 trial sufficiently powered to detect a beneficial effect on an appropriate clinical end point. Hopefully, the combination of significant imaging and clinical benefit will provide sufficient evidence of efficacy to allow for drug registration without a second large clinical trial, as is currently done. Thus, using DWI/PWI in phase 2 will presumably eliminate further development of molecules that are not promising and enhance the timely and cost-effective development of drugs with therapeutic efficacy. Currently, several new neuroprotective drugs are being assessed with DWI/PWI in phase 2 trials. The decision to proceed to phase 3 or abandon these drugs will likely be made based on the outcome of the phase 2 trials. The future of drug development of combination therapy for acute ischemic stroke will also likely use surrogate markers such as DWI/PWI to determine how to best put together existing and novel therapies in the most effective manner.

REFERENCES

1. Fisher M. Characterizing the target of acute stroke therapy. Stroke 1997;28:866–872.
2. Li F, Irie K, Anwer U, Fisher M. Delayed triphenyltetrazolium chloride staining remains useful for evaluating cerebral infarct volume in a rat stroke model. J Cereb Blood Flow Metab 1997;12:1132–1135.
3. Johnston KC. What are surrogate outcome measures and why do they fail in clinical research? Neuroepidemiology 1999;18:167–173.
4. The National Institute of Neurological Disorders and Stroke rt-PA Stroke Study Group. Tissue plasminogen activator for acute ischemic stroke. N Engl J Med 1995;333:1581–1587.
5. Furlan AJ, Higashida R, Wechsler L, et al. Intra-arterial prourokinase for acute ischemic stroke. The PROACT-II study: a randomized controlled trial. Prolyse in Acute Cerebral Thromboembolism. JAMA 1999;282:2003–2011.
6. Sherman DG, Atkinson RP, Chippendale T, et al. Intravenous ancrod for treatment of acute ischemic stroke: the STAT study: a randomized controlled trial. Stroke Treatment with Ancrod Trial. JAMA 2000;283:2395–2403.
7. Hacke W, Kaste M, Fieschi C, et al. Intravenous thrombolysis with recombinant tissue plasminogen activator for acute hemispheric stroke. The European Cooperative Acute Stroke Study (ECASS). JAMA 1995;274:1017–1025.
8. Hacke W, Kaste M, Fieschi C, et al. Randomized double-blind placebo-controlled trial of thrombolytic therapy with intravenous alteplase in acute ischaemic stroke (ECASS II). Second European-Australasian Acute Stroke Study Investigators. Lancet 1998;352:1245–1251.
9. Clark WM, Wissman S, Albers GW, et al. Recombinant tissue-type plasminogen activator (alteplase) for ischemic stroke 3 to 5 hours after symptom onset. The ATLANTIS trial: a randomized controlled trial. Alteplase Thrombolysis for Acute Noninterventional Therapy in Ischemic Stroke. JAMA 1999;282:2019–2026.
10. von Kummer R, Allen K, Helle R, et al. Acute stroke: usefulness of early CT findings before thrombolytic therapy. Radiology 1997;205:327–333.
11. Fisher M. Neuroprotection of acute ischemic stroke: where are we? Neuroscientist 1999;6:392–401.
12. Fisher M, Garcia J. Evolving stroke and the ischemic penumbra. Neurology 1996;47(4):884–888.
13. Adams HP, Davis PH, Leira EC, et al. Baseline NIH stroke scale score strongly predicts outcome after

stroke: a report of the Trial of Org 10172 in Acute Stroke Treatment (TOAST). Neurology 1999;53:126–131.

14. Stys PK. Anoxic and ischemic injury of myelinated axons in CNS white matter: from mechanistic concepts to therapeutics. J Cereb Blood Flow 1998;18: 2–25.

15. Duncan PW, Jorgensen HS, Wade DT. Outcome measures in acute stroke trials. Stroke 2000;31: 1429–1438.

16. Tilley BC, Marler J, Geller NC, et al. Use of a global test for multiple outcomes in stroke trials with application to the National Institute of Neurological Disorders and Stroke t-PA stroke trial. Stroke 1996;27:2136–2142.

17. Neumann-Haefelin T, Moseley ME, Albers GW, et al. New magnetic resonance imaging methods for cerebrovascular disease: emerging clinical applications. Ann Neurol 2000;31:559–570.

18. Moseley ME, Cohen Y, Mintorovitch J, et al. Early detection of regional cerebral ischemia in cats: comparison of diffusion and T2 weighted MRI and spectroscopy. Magn Reson Med 1990;14:330–336.

19. Yoneda Y, Tokui K, Hanihara T, et al. Diffusion-weighted magnetic resonance imaging: detection of ischemic injury 39 minutes after onset in a stroke patient. Ann Neurol 1999;45:794–797.

20. Albers G, Lansberg MG, Norbash AM, et al. Yield of diffusion-weighted MRI for detection of potentially relevant findings in stroke patients. Neurology 2000;54:1562–1567.

21. Roh KJ, Kang DW, Lee SH, et al. Significance of acute multiple brain infarctions on diffusion-weighted imaging. Stroke 2000;31:688–694.

22. Ay H, Rordorf G, Buonanno FS, et al. Normal diffusion-weighted MRI during stroke like deficits. Neurology 1999;52:1784–1792.

23. Patel MR, Edelman RR, Warach S. Detection of hyperacute primary intraparenchymal hemorrhage by magnetic resonance imaging. Stroke 1996;27:2321–2324.

24. Schellinger PD, Jansen O, Fiebach JB, et al. A standardized MRI stroke protocol: comparison with CT in hyperacute intracerebral hemorrhage. Stroke 1999;30:765–768.

25. Rosen BR, Belliveau JW, Vevea JM, Brady TJ. Perfusion imaging with NMR contrast agents. Magn Reson Med 1990;14:249–265.

26. Sorensen AG, Copen WA, Ostergaard L, et al. Hyperacute stroke: simultaneous measurement of relative cerebral blood volume, relative cerebral blood flow, and mean tissue transit time. Radiology 1999;212:519–527.

27. Neuman-Hacflin T, Wittsack H-J, Wenerski F, et al. Diffusion and perfusion-weighted MRI: the DWI/PWI mismatch region in acute stroke. Stroke 1999;30:1591–1597.

28. Beaulieu C, de Crespigny AJ, Tong DC, et al. Longitudinal magnetic resonance imaging study of perfusion and diffusion in stroke: evolution of lesion volume and correlation with clinical outcome. Ann Neurol 1999;46:568–578.

29. Marks MP, Tong DC, Beaulieu C, et al. Evaluation of early reperfusion and IV-tPA therapy using diffusion- and perfusion-weighted MRI. Neurology 1999;52:1792–1798.

30. Schellinger FD, Jansen O, Fiebach JB, et al. Monitoring intravenous recombinant tissue plasminogen activator thrombolysis for acute ischemic stroke with diffusion and perfusion MRI. Stroke 2000;31: 1318–1328.

31. Kucharczyk KJ, Mintorovitch J, Moseley ME, et al. Ischemic brain damage: reduction by sodium-calcium ion channel modulator RS-87476. Radiology 1991;179:221–227.

32. Minematsu K, Fisher M, Li L, et al. Effects of a novel NMDA antagonist on experimental stroke rapidly and quantitatively assessed by diffusion-weighted MRI. Neurology 1993;42:397–403.

33. Qiu H, Hedlund CW, Gewalt SL, et al. Progression of a focal ischemic lesion in a rat brain during treatment with a novel glycine NMDA antagonist. J Magn Reson Imaging 1997;7:793–744.

34. Takano K, Tatlisumak T, Formato J, et al. A glycine site antagonist attenuates infarct size in experimental focal ischemia: postmortem and diffusion mapping studies. Stroke 1997;28:1255–1263.

35. Muller TB, Haraldseth D, Jones RA, et al. Combined perfusion and diffusion-weighted magnetic resonance imaging in a rat model of reversible middle cerebral artery occlusion. Stroke 1995;26:451–458.

36. Jiang Q, Zhang RL, Zhan GZ, et al. Diffusion T2 and perfusion-weighted nuclear magnetic resonance imaging of middle cerebral artery embolic stroke and recombinant tissue plasminogen activator intervention in the rat. J Cereb Blood Flow Metab 1998;18:758–767.

37. Takano K, Carano RAD, Tatlisumak T, et al. The efficacy of intraarterial and intravenous prourokinase in an embolic stroke model evaluated by diffusion-perfusion magnetic resonance imaging. Neurology 1998;50:870–875.

38. Tatlisumak T, Carano RAD, Takano K, et al. A novel endothelin antagonist, A-127722, attenuates ischemic lesion size in rats with temporary middle cerebral artery occlusion. Stroke 1998;29:850–858.

39. Omae T, Silva M, Mayzel O, et al. Temporal evolution of diffusion-perfusion mismatch in a rat stroke model. Stroke 2001;32:352.

40. Li F, Haw S, Tatlisumak T, et al. Reversal of acute apparent diffusion coefficient abnormalities and delayed neuronal death following transient focal cerebral ischemia in rats. Ann Neurol 1999;46:333–342.

41. Li F, Silva MD, Sotak CH, Fisher M. Temporal evolution of ischemic injury evaluated with diffusion, perfusion and T2-weighted MRI. Neurology 2000;54:689–696.

42. Li F, Liu KF, Silva MD, et al. Secondary decline in apparent diffusion coefficient and neurological outcome after a short period of focal brain ischemia in rats. Ann Neurol 2000;48:236–244.

43. Kidwell CS, Saver JL, Mattiello J, et al. Thrombolytic reversal of acute human cerebral ischemic injury shown by diffusion/perfusion magnetic resonance imaging. Ann Neurol 2000;47:462–469.

44. del Zoppo GJ, Higashida RT, Furlan AJ, et al. PROACT: a phase II randomized trial of recombinant pro-urokinase by direct arterial delivery in acute middle cerebral artery stroke. Stroke 1998;29:4–11.

45. The NINDS rt-PA Stroke Study Group. The effect of intravenous rt-PA on ischemic lesion volume as measured by computed tomography. Stroke 2000;31:2912–2919.

46. Warach S, Benfield A, Schlaug G, et al. Reduction of lesion volume in human stroke by citicoline detected by diffusion-weighted magnetic resonance imaging. Ann Neurol 1996;39:527.

47. Warach S, Pettigrew LC, Dashe JF, et al. Effect of citicoline on ischemic lesions as measured by diffusion-weighted MRI. Ann Neurol 2000;48:713–772.

48. Warach S, Kaste M, Fisher M. The effect of GV150526 on ischemic lesion volume: the GAIN Americas and GAIN International MRI Substudy. Neurology 2000;54(Suppl 3):A87–A88.

49. Lees KR, Asplund K, Carolie A, et al. Glycine antagonist (gavestinel) in neuroprotection (GAIN International) in patients with acute stroke: a randomised controlled trial. GAIN International Investigators. Lancet 2000;355:1949–1954.

CHAPTER

20

New Techniques in Ultrasound

Erwin P. Stolz and Manfred Kaps

Ultrasound techniques play an important role in the diagnosis and follow-up of patients with cerebrovascular disorders. The clear advantages of neurosonologic techniques include their noninvasiveness and bedside capability. The clinical applications of neurologic ultrasound are reviewed in Chapter 1.

Despite their effectiveness, however, neurosonologic examinations have certain limitations secondary to physical principles underlying the technique. One of these problems is the detection of ultrasound signals in the setting of a low signal to noise ratio,[1,2] in which only backscattered signals from a few erythrocytes cross the detection threshold of the ultrasound system. Further problems arise due to the attenuation of ultrasound signals in transcranial ultrasound examinations. Only 10–20% of the emitted ultrasound energy reaches the intracranial compartment due to attenuation of the ultrasound beam by the skull bone. The backscattered signal is subject to attenuation as well, so that eventually only a small fraction of the initial ultrasound signal can be used for diagnostic purposes.[3]

One approach to overcome these limitations is the use of echo-contrast–enhancing agents (ECEAs) that are based on stabilized gaseous microbubbles. ECEAs significantly improve the signal to noise ratio, thereby increasing the diagnostic yield in the assessment of extracranial and intracranial brain arteries. ECEAs have found their place in routine clinical ultrasound examination and have also enabled new, experimental ultrasound imaging techniques.

Because ECEAs are the most important new development in diagnostic ultrasound in recent years, this chapter focuses on their clinical and experimental applications in neurologic ultrasound. Furthermore, it discusses recent developments specific to either transcranial color-coded duplex sonography (TCCS) or transcranial Doppler sonography (TCD).

NEW TECHNIQUES IN DUPLEX SONOGRAPHY

Echo-Contrast–Enhancing Agents

Physical Principles

Ultrasound propagation into tissue is subject to reflection, dispersion, refraction, and attenuation. Important parameters for this ultrasound-tissue interaction consist of acoustic impedance, sound velocity (v) within the tissue, and the ultrasound reflection coefficient. Compared to water (v = 1,500 m per second), acoustic impedance, sound velocity, and reflection coefficient of soft tissues lie in a very close range and do not differ substantially between different soft tissue types (v = 1,476 – 1,521 m per second).[4] The relatively small reflection coefficient of soft tissues (<5%) will let most of the emitted ultrasound pass on to deeper tissue segments. Based on the propagation time in tissue and the backscattered ultrasound intensity, two-dimensional ultrasound images can be generated by the ultrasound system.

Color mode imaging as well as pulse wave Doppler generate parameter images that are dependent on the Doppler frequency shift generated by moving backscat-

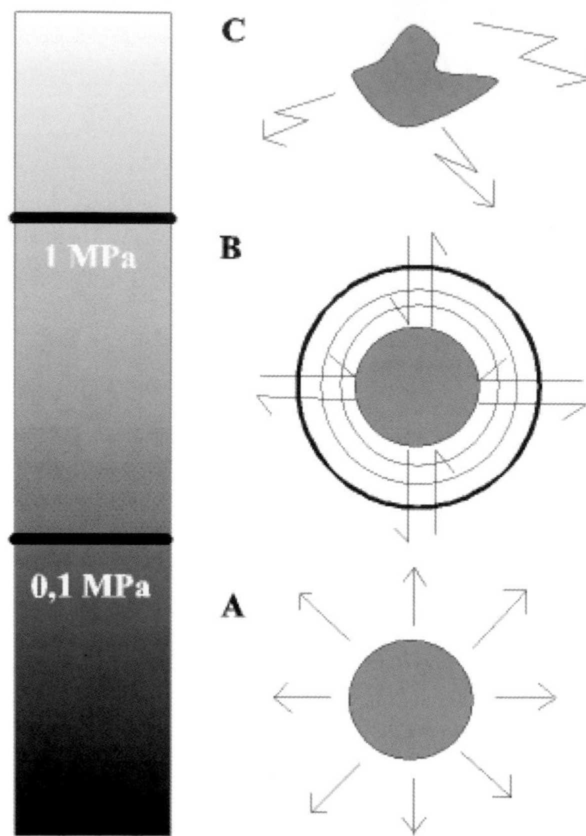

FIGURE 20-1. Microbubble physics. **A.** Linear backscatter. **B.** Harmonic resonance. **C.** Stimulated acoustic emission. (MPa = mega Pascal.)

terers. In case of flowing blood, moving erythrocytes act as reflectors. Because their reflection coefficient is low, a large number of flowing erythrocytes and a high flow velocity are necessary to cause a sufficiently high Doppler shift frequency to cross the detection threshold of the ultrasound system. Increasing the reflection coefficient of moving blood facilitates vascular ultrasound in low-flow settings (i.e., tight stenoses, veins, capillaries) or in conditions characterized by high ultrasound attenuation (i.e., transcranial Doppler or color-coded duplex sonography).

Gas bubbles fulfill this condition. Their acoustic properties differ significantly from those of soft tissues as they nearly totally reflect emitted ultrasound. The backscatter properties of gas bubbles depend on their concentration per volume unit and the bubble radius.[5] Naturally, for biologic applications, these bubbles have to be small (≈5 μm diameter), and the concentration in flowing blood has to be low. Compared to solid particles, gas bubbles begin to vibrate in an acoustic field. This vibration makes them act as if they have an increased diameter by a factor of 10^{14}.[6] Despite the low concentration and small size of gas bubbles, their properties of passive backscatter become effective for diagnostic ultrasound. If the energy of the emitted ultrasound is low, gas bubbles react as passive, yet very effective, backscatterers. Because the energy of the backscattered signal increases proportionally to the emitted ultrasound energy, this behavior is called *linear.*

When the emitted ultrasound energy is increased (100–500 mW/cm^2), gas microbubbles start to resonate (i.e., they vibrate and emit the fundamental frequency and, in addition, multiples of this fundamental).[7] This is because the microbubble is forced into volume pulsation when the ultrasound wavelength is much longer than the bubble size. The size of the bubble decreases during the positive half cycle of the ultrasound wave and expands during the negative half cycle. With increasing acoustic pressure, nonlinearities occur in the vibration, because it becomes progressively harder to compress the gas bubble than to relax it, so that compression is generally retarded relative to the expansion.[8] Therefore, nonlinear vibration is frequency dependent and shows a clear maximum at a specific frequency, the so-called resonance frequency. This process can be compared to a swinging violin string emitting harmonic frequencies. The resonance phenomenon is important, because the bubble behaves as a moving ultrasound source emitting harmonic frequencies besides the fundamental, rather than a passive reflector.[9] Furthermore, the process is nonlinear, as the ultrasound energy emitted by bubbles is no longer proportional to the acoustic pressure applied by the fundamental ultrasound pulse. The resonance frequency is dependent on the fundamental frequency, the composition of the gas filling the bubbles, the bubble diameter, and the bubble stability. This effect is used in second harmonic imaging and wide-band harmonic imaging.

A further increase in emitted energy (>500 mW/cm^2) destroys the microbubbles, causing them to emit a short, highly energetic ultrasound pulse that is interpreted by the ultrasound system as a Doppler signal originating from moving erythrocytes (pseudo-Doppler).[8,10] Using frequency- and direction-sensitive color modes results in colorful images with a wide band of encoded colors and directions, which no longer display flowing blood in terms of direction and velocity. The process of ultrasound-induced destruction of microbubbles is referred to as *stimulated acoustic emission* (SAE). The older terms, *flash echo imaging* or *sono-scintigraphy*, refer to the images generated by the ultrasound system.[11] The interaction of emitted ultrasound and microbubbles is summarized in Figure 20-1.

For clinical purposes, microbubbles have to fulfill important criteria when administered as an intravenous injection. They have to be small enough (approximately

TABLE 20-1. Echo-Contrast–Enhancing Agents in Use or in Development

Agent	*Shell*	*Gas*
Levovist (Schering AG, Berlin, Germany)	Palmitinic acid adsorbed on galactose microcrystals	Air
Optison (Mallinckrodt Inc., St. Louis, Missouri)	Albumin	Perfluoropropane
BY963	Phospholipids	Air
Albunex (Molecular Biosystems Inc., San Diego, California)	Albumin	Air
MRX-115	Phospholipids	Air
BR1	Phospholipids	Sulfurhexafluoride
F20	Phospholipids	Perfluoro-octylbromide
Imagent (Alliance Pharmaceutical Corp., San Diego, California)	Phospholipids	Perfluorocarbon
ImaRx	Phospholipids	Nitrogen
EchoGen (Sonus Pharmaceuticals, Bothell, Washington)	Phase-shift	Dodecafluoropentane
QW7437	Phase-shift	Dodecafluoropentane
Quantison (Quadrant, Nottingham, United Kingdom)	Albumin	Air

5 μm diameter) to pass through the capillary bed of the lungs and stable enough to survive the left ventricular pressure.[12] Contrast-enhancing agents consist of gas bubbles (either air or lipophilic gases) encapsulated by a shell (i.e., phospholipids, albumin). The shell stabilizes the microbubble and prevents premature diffusion and physical solution of the gas in blood. In most cases, the gas is responsible for the acoustic and pharmacokinetic properties of an ECEA, whereas the shell determines most of the side effects.[13–16] There are two exceptions to this rule: Levovist (Schering AG, Berlin, Germany) is a galactose-based ECEA. The galactose microcrystals are covered by a thin film of palmitinic acid. When microcrystals are dissolved in water and the aqueous solution is shaken, air microbubbles adhere to them. The size of the microcrystals determines the size of the adhering air bubbles that are eventually covered by the palmitinic acid film and thereby stabilized.[17] The second exception is phase-shift ECEAs. They are liquids with a low boiling point. When injected intravenously, body temperature induces them to evaporate. Table 20-1 gives a selection of ECEAs currently in use or under development.

Clinical Applications of Echo-Contrast–Enhancing Agents

Of all the ECEAs, Levovist has been used most extensively in clinical studies, in large part because of its low side effect profile. Therefore, if not indicated otherwise, the studies mentioned in this section used Levovist as the echo-contrast enhancer. Several studies evaluated ECEAs in carotid artery disease.[1,1–23] ECEAs are capable of improving the depiction of the anatomic course of tortuous or stenosed vessels; they facilitate the imaging of accelerated flow in carotid stenoses and identify the point of maximum stenosis. A typical problem in the evaluation of the Doppler frequency spectrum in very tight stenoses is the systolic "fading" of the spectrum that prevents the correct identification of the peak systolic frequency or velocity. This is due to the fact that only a few very fast erythrocytes move in the highest velocity band. Although the Doppler shift frequency produced by these erythrocytes is high, their total signal intensity is not high enough to be detected beyond the detection threshold of the ultrasound system. This problem can be solved by echo-contrast enhancers[21] that increase the signal by approximately 20 dB (Figure 20-2).

Shadowing artifacts and preventing a sonographic evaluation of stenoses are frequently encountered. Although ECEAs cannot overcome this problem, flow signals of neighboring regions can be raised above the detection threshold of the system.[18]

The differentiation between internal carotid artery occlusion and pseudo-occlusion has practical clinical relevance, as carotid endarterectomy is possible only when pseudo-occlusion is present. Conventional duplex sonography is able to differentiate occlusion and pseudo-occlusion with a sensitivity of 88% and a specificity of 99%.[23] In an angiographically controlled study,

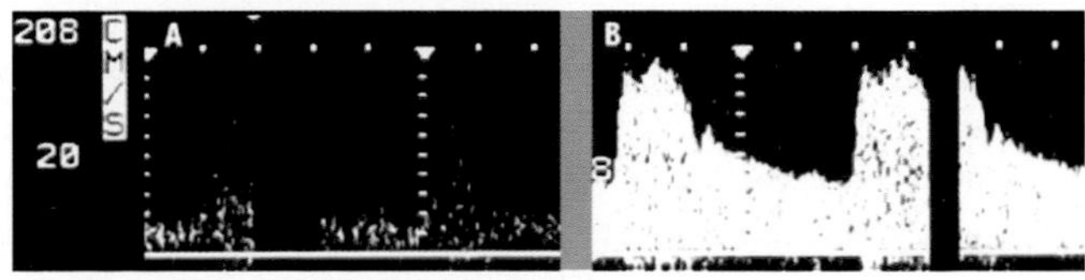

FIGURE 20-2. Enhancement of the Doppler frequency spectrum by an echo-contrast–enhancing agent. Before (**A**) and after (**B**) application of Levovist (Schering AG, Berlin, Germany).

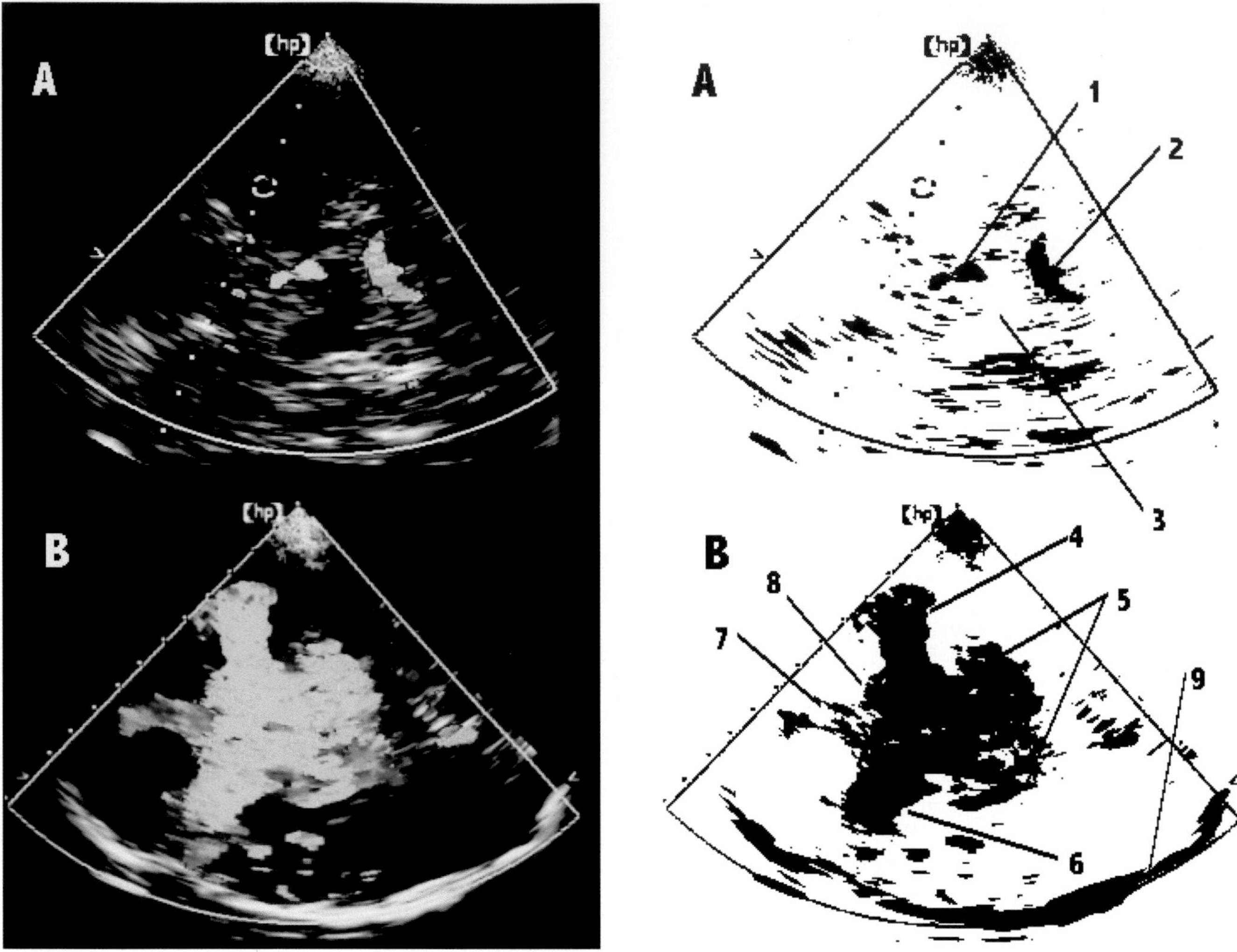

FIGURE 20-3. Signal enhancement in a patient with an inadequate acoustic bone window. **A.** Unenhanced transcranial color-coded duplex sonography examination. **B.** Echo-contrast–enhanced examination in the phase of "blooming." *1.* P1 segment of the posterior cerebral artery. *2.* P2 segment of the posterior cerebral artery. *3.* Mesencephalon. *4.* M1 segment of the middle cerebellar artery. *5.* Posterior cerebral artery. *6.* Contralateral M1 segment of the middle cerebellar artery. *7.* A2 segment of the anterior cerebral artery. *8.* A1 segment of the anterior cerebral artery. *9.* Skull.

ECEAs increased the sensitivity to 92% and the specificity to 83%. Echo-contrast–enhanced power angio mode (see the section Power Doppler) increased the sensitivity of duplex sonography to 94% and its specificity to 100%.[1]

Sonographic examination of the extracranial vertebral arteries is often more difficult than evaluation of the anterior circulation arteries. Compared to the carotid arteries, the vertebral arteries have lower flow velocities, usually require a deeper examination window, and are frequently subject to anatomic variants. Echo-contrast enhancement facilitates the identification of the vertebral arteries and their anatomic course and increases the diagnostic yield.[24] The so-called blooming artifact[25] (Figure 20-3B) is specific for ECEAs and arises from amplifier overload and beam line errors. It can hamper the examination of the origin of the vertebral artery from the subclavian artery. Reduction of the color gain or the administration of contrast enhancers via continuous intravenous infusion usually attenuates the artifact.

Due to the massive signal attenuation by the skull, transcranial Doppler and duplex sonography impose high demands on the ultrasound system. Approximately 20% of patients cannot be examined by TCD or TCCS because of insufficient acoustic cranial windows. This is a substantial limitation, especially during the evaluation of acute stroke patients. Several studies have shown that ECEAs can solve this problem at least partially, and they considerably increase diagnostic confidence.

ECEAs significantly improve the depiction of intracranial vessels in patients with inadequate acoustic bone windows.[26–32] An example is presented in Figure 20-3. Approximately 80% of patients, in whom a diag-

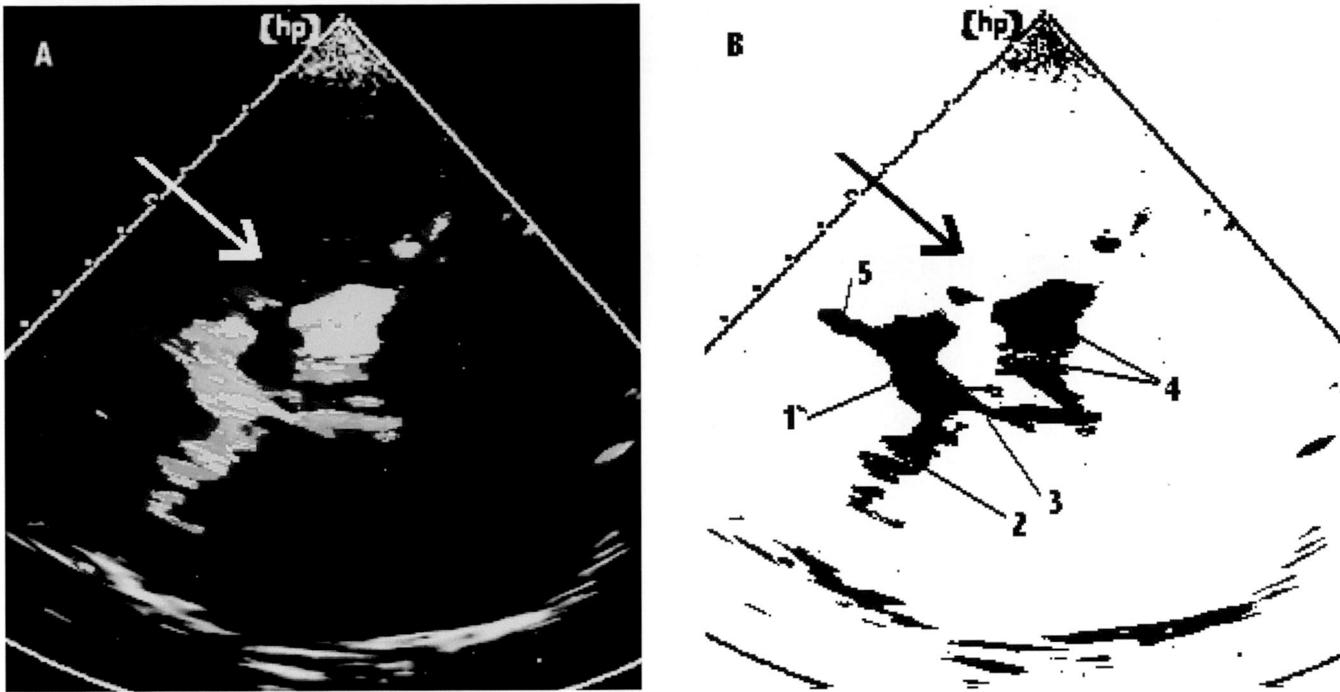

FIGURE 20-4. **A,B.** Diagnosis of middle cerebral artery mainstem occlusion after echo-contrast–enhancing agent administration. *1.* Contralateral A1 segment of the anterior cerebral artery. 2. Contralateral M1 segment of the middle cerebral artery. *3.* Contralateral posterior communicating artery. *4.* Ipsilateral and contralateral P1 segments of the posterior communicating arteries. *5.* A2 segment of the anterior cerebral artery. The arrow marks the missing M1 segment of the ipsilateral middle cerebral artery.

nostic confidence is not reached by native TCCS, can be sufficiently examined with the help of ECEAs (see Figure 20-3).[26,30,32] Intracranial vessel occlusions and stenoses are diagnosed with a high diagnostic precision. In patients with inadequate acoustic bone windows, the positive and negative predictive value for diagnosis of a middle cerebral artery (MCA) occlusion or stenosis is 86% and 100%, respectively, when ECEAs are used.[30]

In our experience, ECEAs should not only be applied in suboptimal insonation conditions, but they should also be used in all cases of suspected intracranial arterial occlusions (Figure 20-4). Although generally undesirable, the blooming artifact of echo-contrast enhancers facilitates the diagnosis of vessel occlusion (see Figure 20-3B). Further advantages of ECEAs include the shortening of the examination time and the applicability of the method even in agitated patients who need sedation to complete computed tomography (CT) or magnetic resonance angiography testing.

Since the early 1990s, a number of large, randomized, placebo-controlled trials have been performed to evaluate the benefit of thrombolytic therapy in acute stroke. The results are controversial and have been intensively debated. Although the National Institute of Neurological Disorders and Stroke (NINDS) study[33] demonstrated a functional improvement after intravenous thrombolysis compared to placebo, the European Cooperative Acute Stroke Study (ECASS) trials[34,35] did not show a clear benefit from this therapy. Arterial patency was verified angiographically in Prolyse for Acute Cerebral Thromboembolism (PROACT) II,[36] but none of the large intravenous thrombolytic studies tested patients for the presence of vessel occlusion before therapy, even though their goal was to recanalize occluded arteries. It is likely that a number of patients had been referred to intravenous thrombolysis despite a normal cerebrovascular status and, therefore, could not benefit from this particular therapy. Furthermore, those trials did not provide any information regarding recanalization after thrombolysis.

In this setting, sonographic methods may have a place not only in future stroke trials but also in effective patient management. In one multicenter study,[37] consecutive patients with acute ischemic stroke were examined with TCCS within 6 hours after stroke onset. There was a 100% agreement with reference arterial imaging examinations (digital subtraction, magnetic resonance, or CT angiography) regarding patency, stenosis, or occlusion of the symptomatic MCA. Two hours after start of the treatment, a 50% recanalization rate for the MCA M1 segment and the internal carotid siphon was observed in the thrombolysis group, whereas no recanalization could be observed in the remaining patients. These results highlight two points. First, intravenous thrombolysis is effective in restoring

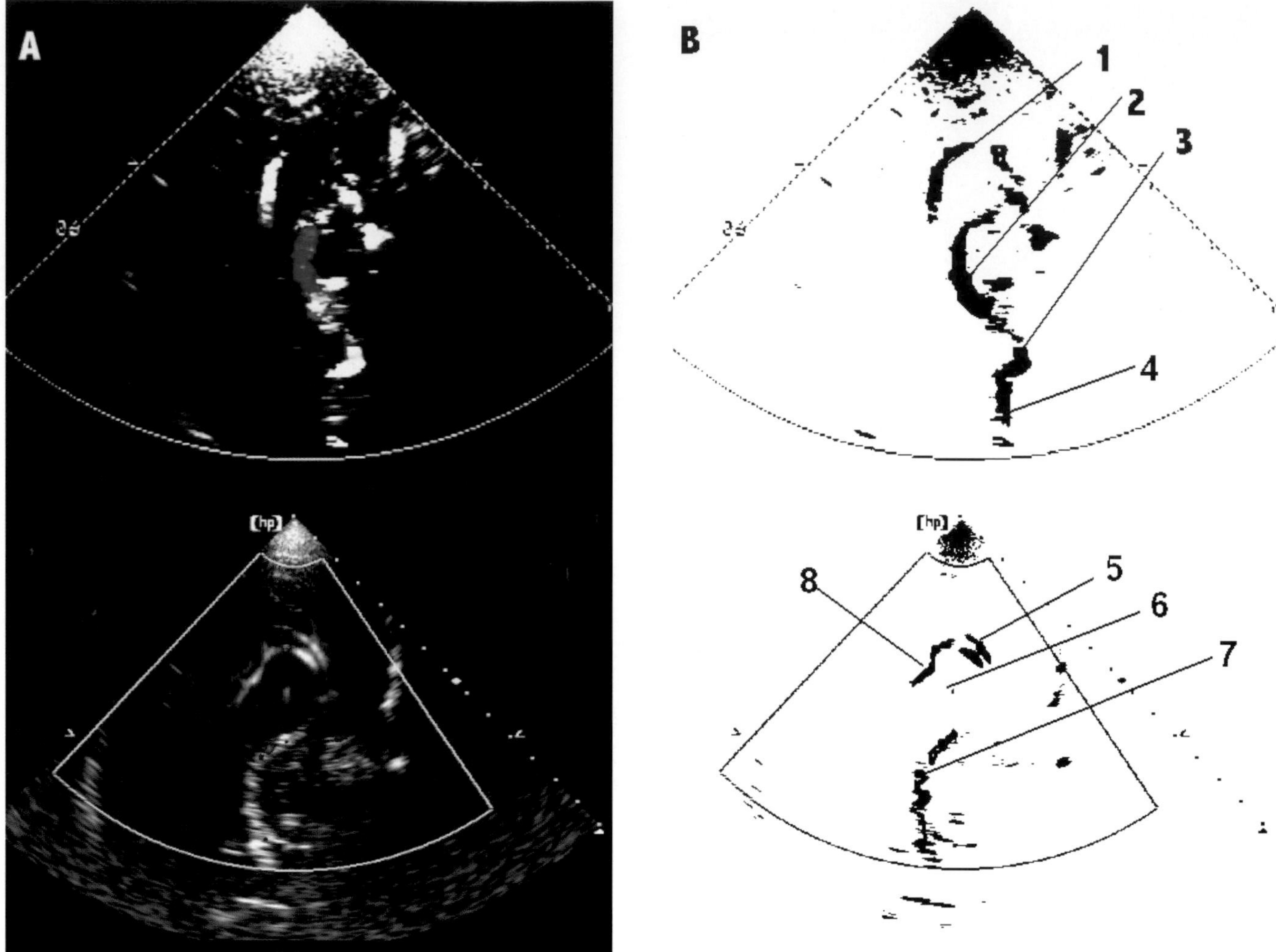

FIGURE 20-5. Paramedian frontal bone window after echo-contrast enhancement. **A.** Frequency coded. **B.** Power mode. *1.* Pericallosal artery. *2.* Internal cerebral vein. *3.* Great cerebral vein of Galen. *4.* Straight sinus. *5.* Callosomarginal artery. *6.* Splenium of the callosal body. *7.* Choreoid plexus of the third ventricle. *8.* Pericallosal artery.

vessel patency. Second, transcranial sonography, especially when contrast enhanced, can be used to select acutely ill patients for new stroke treatments according to their vascular status.

ECEAs improve the imaging of intracranial collateral flow conditions.[38] This applies especially to the posterior communicating artery, because the insonation angle is usually unfavorable. They also have advantages when examining the intracranial vertebrobasilar system. The insonation depth of the basilar artery is significantly increased.[39,40] They increase the quality of vessel depiction and, hence, increase diagnostic confidence so that further diagnostic tests, such as angiography, are no longer necessary for some patients.

An additional field of interest is the intracranial venous system. In this area, promising results have been reported in patients with acute cerebral venous thrombosis.[41,42] Although the deep intracranial veins can frequently be examined without echo-contrast enhancement, ECEAs facilitate the depiction of the large posterior fossa sinuses.[43]

The standard approach of transcranial ultrasound is insonation through the temporal bone and the foramen magnum, because at these acoustic windows the ultrasound attenuation is relatively low. With the aid of ECEAs, new acoustic bone windows can be used to provide additional examination planes. The lateral frontal bone window allows insonation of the circle of Willis in a frontal axial plane. Midline structures such as the A2 segment of the anterior cerebral artery, pericallosal artery, internal cerebral veins, and the straight sinus are imaged in a frontal sagittal plane using the paramedian frontal bone window[44] (Figure 20-5).

ECEAs can also be used for measurement of the cerebral transit time. The method is based on a comparison of signal intensity–time curves in the arterial and venous systems after administration of a contrast bolus. The time latency between the curves represents the cerebral transit time. The extracranial internal carotid artery, jugular vein, posterior cerebral artery's P2 segment, and great cerebral vein of Galen give reliable intensity-time curves.[45,46] In one study, patients with vascular dementia displayed significantly increased transit times compared to both healthy controls and patients with Alzheimer's-type dementia.[45]

For most clinical applications, a bolus intravenous injection of an ECEA is sufficient. The bolus injection is easy to perform and allows satisfactory enhancement for approximately 10–15 minutes. Continuous intravenous administration by a pump system reduces the blooming artifact and can increase the diagnostically useful time to 20–25 minutes. In principle, the clinical applications of ECEAs work with conventional continuous or pulsed wave Doppler systems as well, but the full range of improvements can only be appreciated with color-coded duplex sonography systems.

New Imaging Techniques Based on Echo-Contrast–Enhancing Agents

The established clinical applications of ECEAs use signal enhancement in the linear power range. In the nonlinear power range, microbubbles exhibit behaviors that are unique for gas bubbles: resonance and SAE. Brain tissue resonance is extremely low when compared to bubble resonance, so that using the nonlinear properties of microbubbles for imaging purposes results in a marked increase in the signal to noise ratio.[47] Bubble resonance as well as SAE can be used for detection of blood flow within brain tissue. Current research efforts have concentrated on the development of a qualitative and noninvasive sonographic measurement of brain tissue perfusion.

In *second harmonic imaging*, the ultrasound system emits a fundamental frequency in the range of 1.6–1.8 MHz and receives the first harmonic frequency that is the double of the fundamental.[47] This technique allows detection of flow even in small or slowly perfused vessels. Results of a prospective study evaluating the vertebrobasilar system indicate that cerebellar arteries and the vertebral venous plexus can be displayed.[48]

Resonating microbubbles not only emit first-order harmonic frequencies but also higher-order harmonic and subharmonic frequencies. To increase the backscattered microbubble signal intensity, *wide-band harmonic imaging* uses the full range of the bubble resonance phenomenon (Figure 20-6). This is important not only because the signal intensity of the harmonic emissions is much lower than that of the fundamental frequency, but also because the harmonic backscattered signal is subject to a higher signal attenuation by the skull due to its higher frequency content compared to the fundamental.

SAE occurs in a higher ultrasound intensity range. The fundamental ultrasound pulse induces a microbubble rupture. Bursting microbubbles emit a short ultrasound

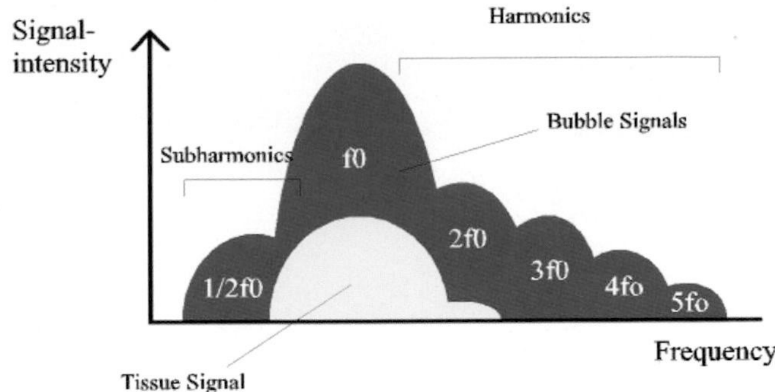

FIGURE 20-6. Schematic drawing of the microbubble resonance phenomenon. Higher harmonics are integer multiples of f0 (fundamental emission frequency); subharmonics are even fractions of f0. Note the increase of the signal to noise ratio for the higher harmonic frequencies.

pulse that can be detected with modern ultrasound systems (Figure 20-7). In the time interval between fundamental pulse traces, some microbubbles coalesce to form larger microbubbles. If a second fundamental ultrasound trace hits these microbubbles, they will emit ultrasound signals at different frequencies and intensities compared to the first fundamental trace. The backscattered signals no longer hold information on flow velocity or direction but indicate the presence of microbubbles.

All ECEA-based imaging techniques have common problems. The first is how to separate the fundamental frequency from the microbubble signals.[49] A relatively ineffective way to achieve this is the filter technique (Figure 20-8). It is important to note that ultrasound systems do not emit a single fundamental frequency; rather, they emit a band of frequencies centered around the fundamental, or center frequency. The more effectively a frequency filter removes fundamental frequencies, the more microbubble signals are filtered out due to overlap. A smaller filter does not remove as much of microbubble signals but decreases the signal to noise ratio by allowing parts of the fundamental frequencies to slip through. Increasing the sensitivity of the ultrasound system can be achieved by transmitting narrow band signals that are tightly centered around the fundamental, which in return deteriorates image resolution. System optimization consists of finding the best balance between these two performance aspects.

A new method is the *pulse inversion technique*. In this technique, after emitting an ultrasound train of pulses with the fundamental frequency, the ultrasound system emits a second train of pulses with a well-timed time delay from the first train. The second train also contains waves of the fundamental frequency but with a 180-degree phase shift. The second train is timed, so that it overlaps with the backscattered signals. The second phase-shifted train of ultrasound waves will add up to zero with the backscattered fundamental frequency con-

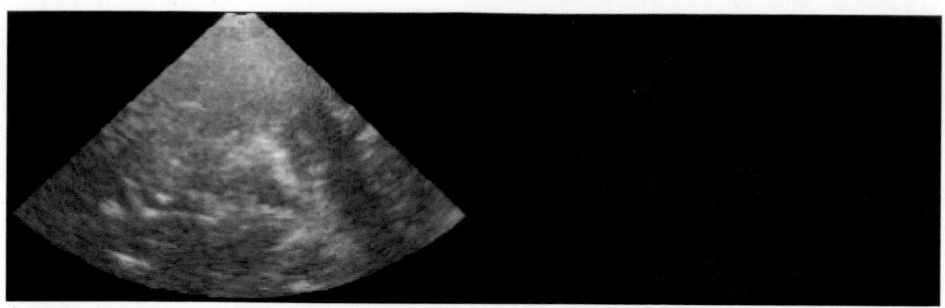

A1

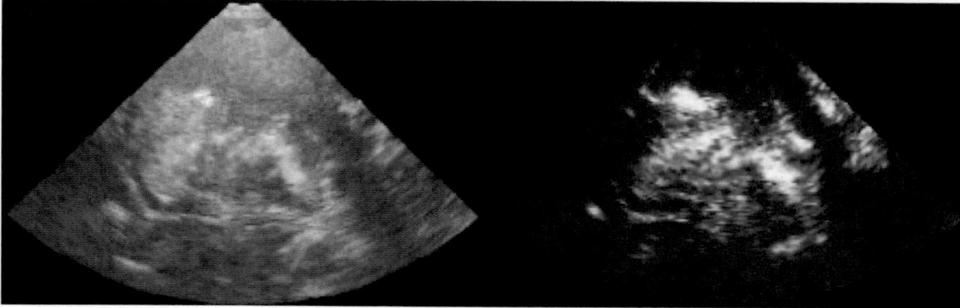

A2

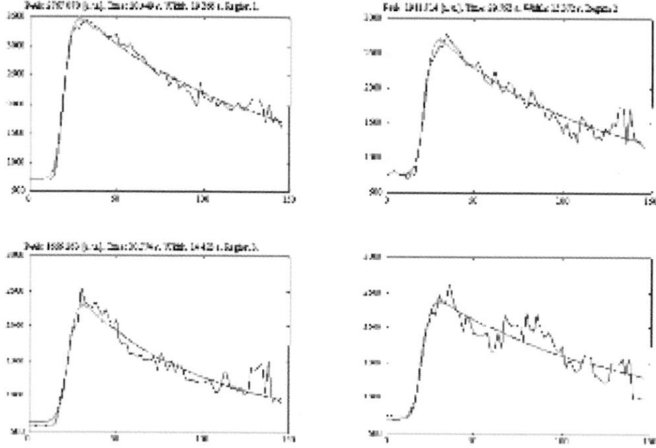

B

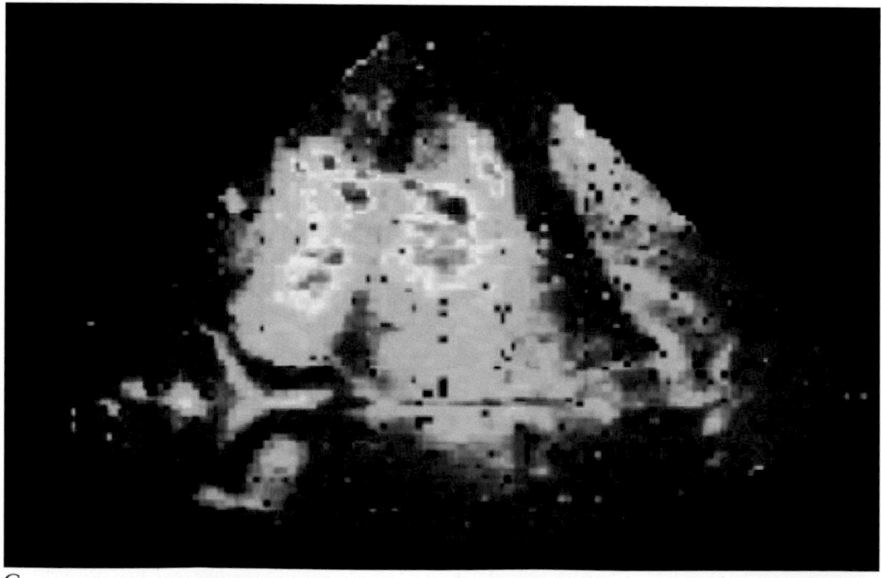

C

FIGURE 20-7. Brain tissue perfusion measurement with stimulated acoustic emission (SAE). **A1.** Gray scale tissue harmonic imaging (*left*) and SAE (*right*) before contrast agent application. **A2.** Gray scale tissue harmonic imaging (*left*) and SAE (*right*) in the phase of maximum-intensity increase after administration of a contrast agent bolus. Note the missing signal in the anterior horns of the lateral ventricle. **B.** Time-intensity curves in regions of interest in the posterior thalamus (*upper left*), the anterior thalamus (*upper right*), the lentiform nucleus (*lower left*), and the hemispheric white substance (*lower right*). **C.** Parameter map coding the peak intensity in the ultrasound plane in 1-mm × 1-mm pixels. (Courtesy of Dr. Thomas Postert, Ruhr University, Dept. of Neurology, St. Josef Hospital, Bochum, Germany.)

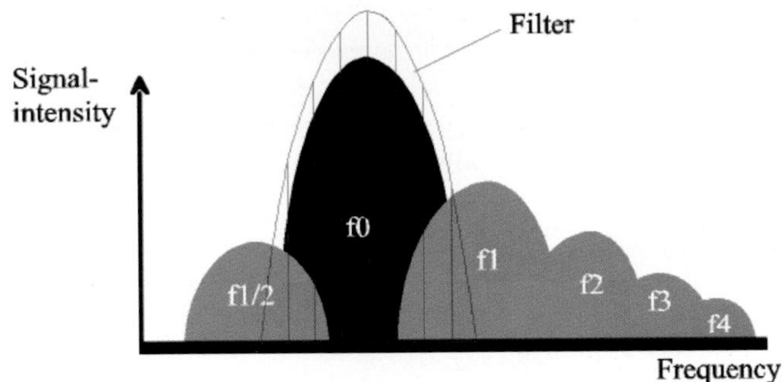

FIGURE 20-8. Separation of the harmonic frequencies from the fundamental by a filter technique. The overlap of frequency bands causes problems in separation. (f0 = fundamental emission frequency.)

tent, allowing microbubble signals to reach the transducer (Figure 20-9). The main advantage of the pulse inversion technique is that it can function over the entire bandwidth of the received echo signals; therefore, it achieves a better image resolution.[50] *Power modulation* is an alternative development (Figure 20-10).

Multipulse release imaging is a novel approach that uses the rupture of echo-contrast agents.[49] It is based on the combination of broadband imaging pulses and a separate destruction burst. Whereas the imaging pulses are used to survey the contrast agent before and after bubble destruction, the destruction pulse induces SAE. The presence of the contrast agent is detected by subtracting the signal response from the imaging pulses.

A problem common to the new ECEA-related ultrasound techniques is the transient response (Figure 20-11). The latter was first observed in echocardiography[51] and is related to the frame rate of the system. It originates from microbubble destruction by

FIGURE 20-9. Schematic drawing summarizing the principles of the pulse inversion technique.

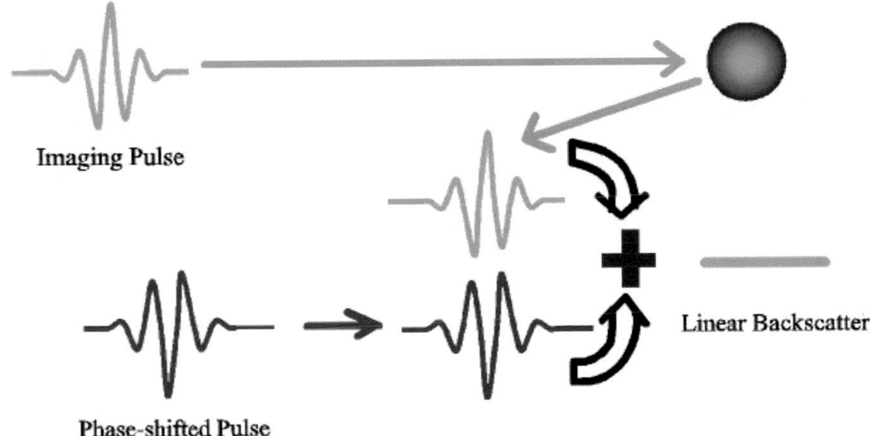

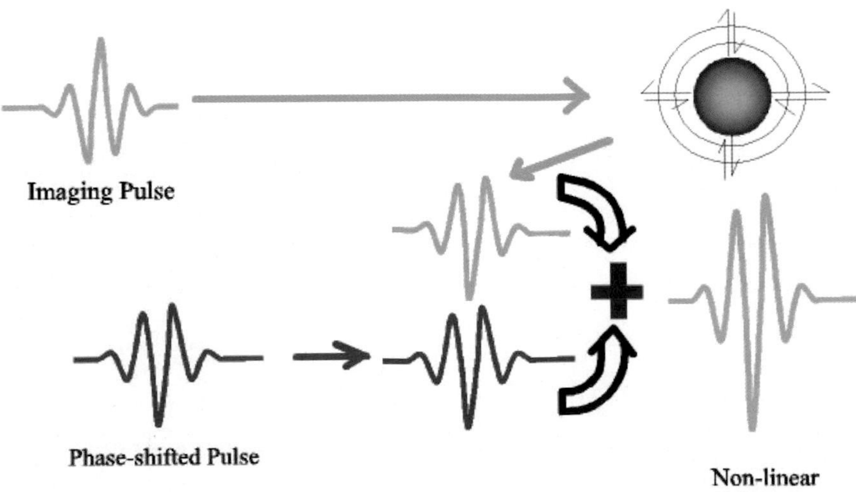

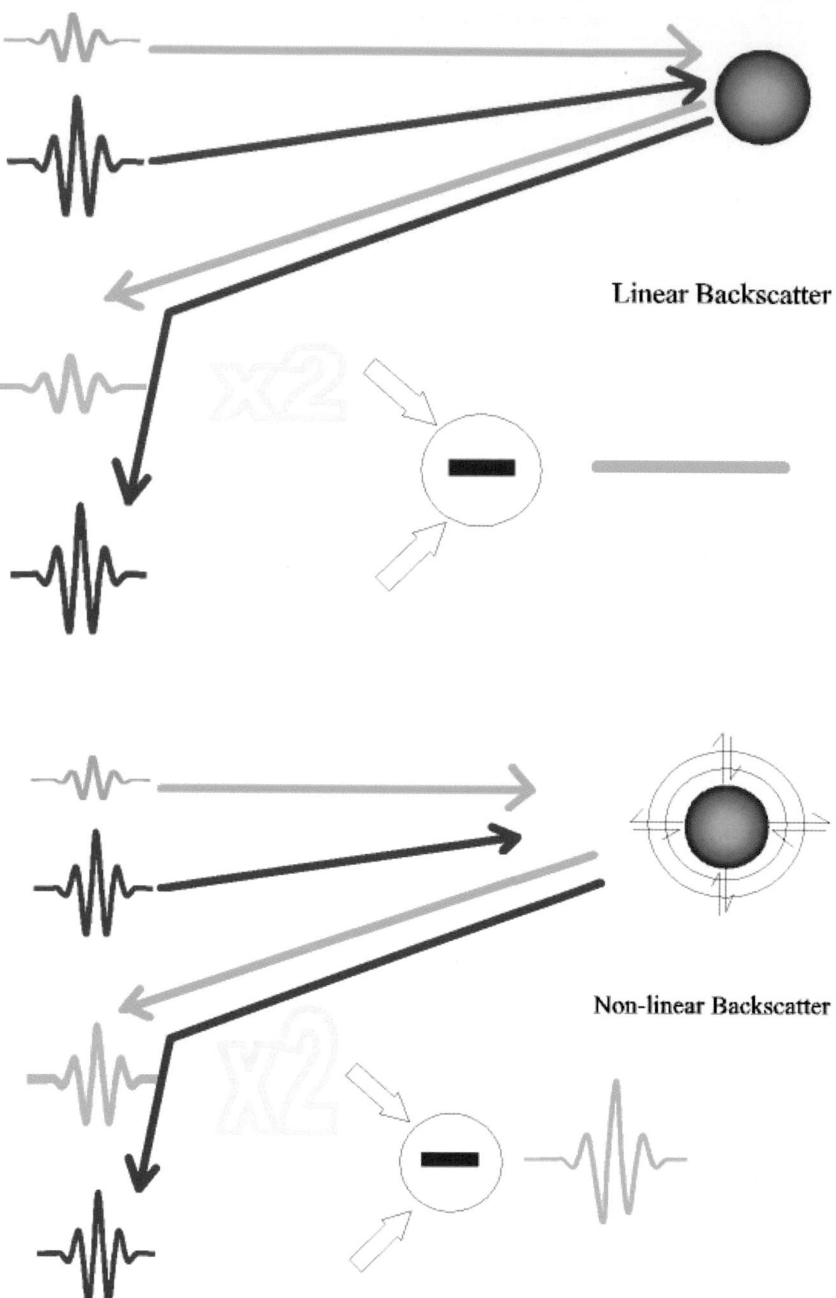

FIGURE 20-10. Schematic drawing of the principles of the power modulation technique. In the nonlinear energy range, the proportionality between power and emitted and received signals becomes lost. Therefore, if the power ratio of two emitted signals is 1 to 2, this ratio is lost in the received signals if backscatter is nonlinear.

the imaging process itself. For the current clinical applications, this effect is marginal. However, for imaging of blood flow in capillaries, this effect can be substantial. To increase the effective microbubble concentration, triggering of the ultrasound system is necessary.

Measurement of Brain Tissue Perfusion

Using a conventional ultrasound system setup, no changes in either gray scale imaging or color mode are noticeable in the brain parenchyma after injection of an echo-contrast bolus. The reasons are low concentration and slow movement of microbubbles in the cerebral microcirculation and signal attenuation by the skull bone that makes measurements in the brain much more demanding than in the heart. Backscattered ultrasound signals from microbubbles in arterioles and capillaries have such a low intensity that they are lost in the system's "noise." The solution for ultrasound brain tissue perfusion measurements is to increase the signal to noise ratio. This can be achieved by using the nonlinear properties of microbubbles in the form of either harmonic imaging or SAE. Furthermore, bubble destruction during the imaging process has to be decreased by reduction of the frame rate of the ultrasound system using a suit-

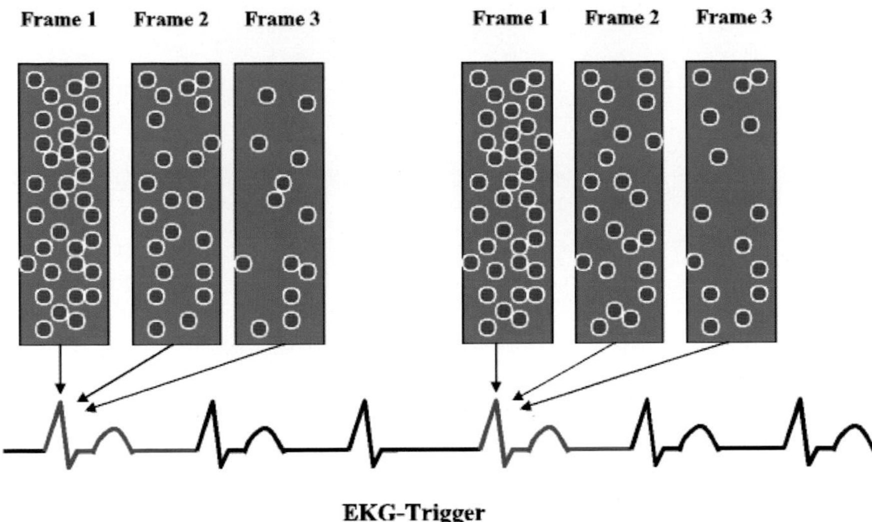

FIGURE 20-11. Transient response. The transient response is caused by the destruction of microbubbles during the imaging process. The effect can be diminished by triggering the pulse emission. (EKG = electrocardiogram.)

able trigger. The resulting techniques are transient response harmonic or transient response SAE imaging. Currently, real-time techniques are in development.

After intravenous injection of an echo-contrast bolus, the bolus is followed, and wash-in and wash-out curves are calculated based on the signal intensity over time in a specific region of interest (Figure 20-12). Based on Fick's dilution theory, attempts are made to quantify these effects, similar to perfusion magnetic resonance imaging or CT. Based on the intensity-time curves, it is possible to calculate parameter images (i.e., peak intensity, time to peak).[52]

Recent studies have shown the feasibility of ultrasound perfusion imaging of the brain in healthy volunteers and stroke patients.[52–57] The results must be regarded as preliminary. An electrocardiogram-triggered gray scale transient response harmonic image is often generated (Figure 20-13). Limitations of the method are now better understood. Imaging results are dependent on the ECEA used.[53] Relatively stable agents, such as Optison (Mallinckrodt Inc., St. Louis, Missouri), give better results than fragile agents such as Levovist. A severe drawback for the quantification of results is the absence of a linear dose-intensity relationship.[56] This means that doubling the concentration or volume of the bolus does not result in a twofold signal increase. In addition, the observed signal increase in brain parenchyma decreases with the insonation depth.[56] These limitations may prevent an exact quantification of brain perfusion with ultrasonic techniques.

Experience with the new *negative bolus contrast* method is limited.[58] In this method, the ECEA is administered via a drip pump at a constant infusion rate. The bubbles in the insonation plane are then destroyed by an intense ultrasound pulse. After a time delay, the intensity

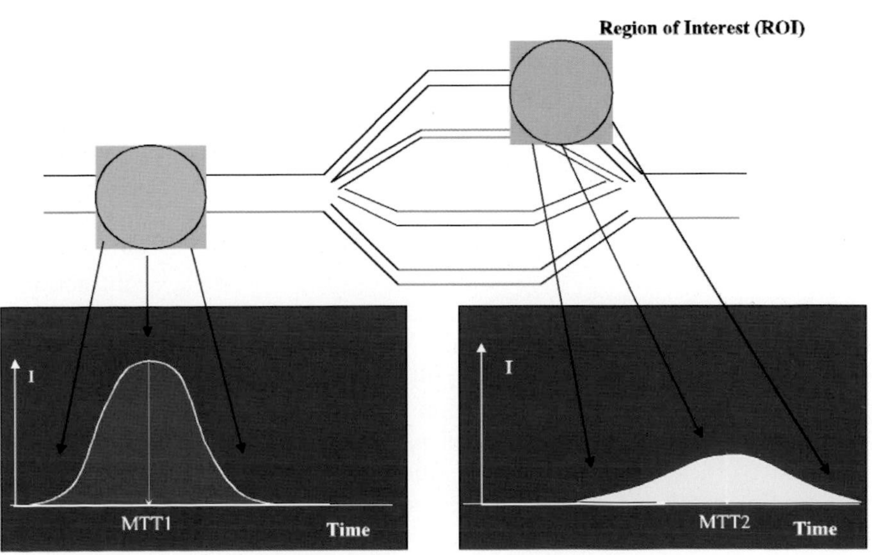

FIGURE 20-12. Measurement of brain tissue perfusion by tracking an echo-contrast agent bolus. With knowledge of the input function, regional cerebral blood flow (rCBF) can be calculated: $rCBF \approx AUC_2/[2AUC_1(MTT_2 - MTT_1)]$. (AUC = area under the curve; MTT = mean transit time.)

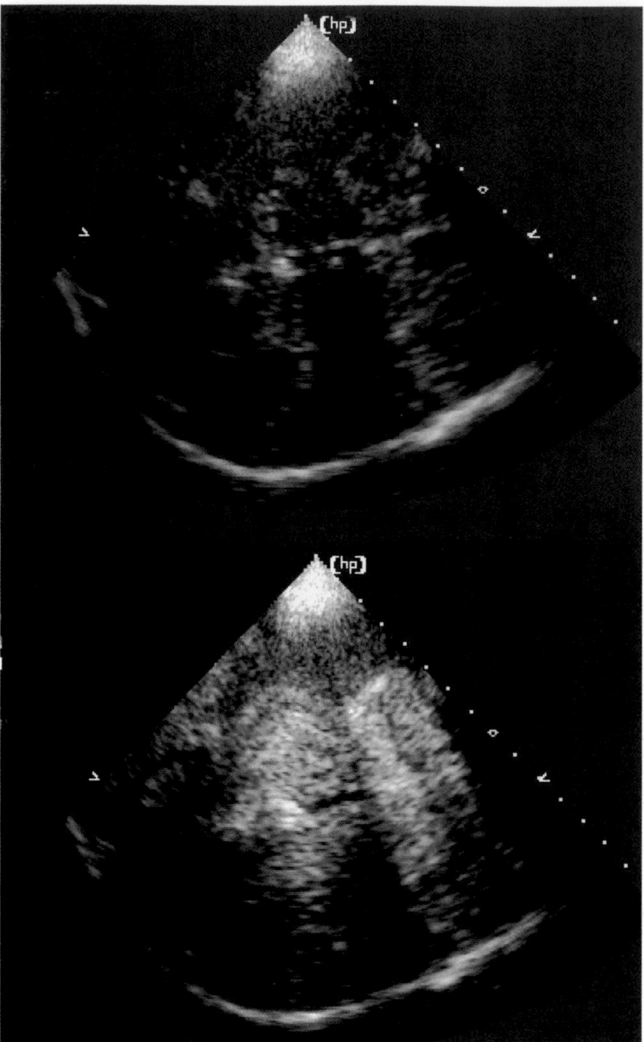

FIGURE 20-13. Gray scale harmonic imaging of the brain tissue perfusion. The upper image is an axial plane through the diencephalon before a contrast agent bolus (Optison [Mallinckrodt Inc., St. Louis, Missouri]), the echo-rich double contour in the middle is a cross section through the third ventricle. Twelve heart cycles after bolus application, a maximum increase in echogenicity of the parenchyma can be demonstrated (*bottom*). Note that the third ventricle does not show any enhancement. There is a clear insonation depth dependence, with a decrease of the effect noticeable in the lower half of the image.

of the backscattered microbubble signals is measured by insonation with a second ultrasound pulse. Depending on the time delay between the two pulses, more or fewer microbubbles can refill the insonation plane. By varying the time delay between the two ultrasound pulses, the hemodynamics of the refill corresponding to the negative bolus produced by the first of the two ultrasound pulses can be measured (Figure 20-14).

Power Doppler

Power Doppler or angio mode techniques have been implemented in most of the high-end duplex sonography systems. Power Doppler does not display the frequency content of a signal but displays power closely related to the signal amplitude and energy (Figures 20-15 and 20-16).[59] All information on flow direction is lost. It is not subject to aliasing phenomena that occur when the pulse repetition frequency is exceeded in frequency-coded color mode. In practice, this hampers the diagnosis of stenoses. Therefore, power mode is not used as a first-line imaging mode. Although it has a superior signal to noise ratio and an increased low-flow detection capacity than frequency mode, power mode is influenced much more by movement artifacts.[49,60]

The underlying physics stipulates that unless insonation at 90 degrees is attempted, the power mode is independent of the insonation angle. Power Doppler is only influenced by the density of reflectors (erythrocytes or echo-contrast agents) within a vessel. Due to its higher sensitivity to low flow, it has an advantage in the visualization of flow in arterial stenoses, in the intracranial venous system, and in aneurysms.[61–64] Power Doppler facilitates the visualization of small arterial branches, such as the posterior communicating artery, M3 segment of the MCA, P2 branch of the posterior cerebral artery, and A2 segment of the anterior cerebral artery.[61]

B-Flow Imaging

An integral part of the *B-flow technique* is coded excitation for the visualization of blood flow.[65] Coded excitation works on the principle of key and lock. All emitted and backscattered ultrasound signals contain an identifying sequence. Only when this sequence or pulse signature is recognized by the system are signals allowed further in the imaging process. The signal to noise ratio is thereby increased. A second component of B-flow imaging is the coded emission of two pulses along one beam line. Received pulses contain information regarding echoes reflected by erythrocytes and tissue. Subtraction of the received pulses yields zero in instances of stationary reflectors. However, depending on the blood flow velocity and the number of erythrocytes, more or fewer reflectors enter the insonation plane. Therefore, subtraction of received pulses along a beam line gives a result other than zero if moving reflectors are insonated. This technique allows coding of flow direction.[66]

B-flow imaging is based on signal amplitude and is less affected by the insonation angle than the frequency-coded modes. An advantage of this technique is the simultaneous generation of the B-mode image and of flow information, avoiding artifacts caused by sequential superimposition of the tissue and blood flow signals.

spherosome-based ultrasound contrast agent (BY963). A transcranial Doppler sonography study. J Neuroimaging 1998;8:83–87.

16. Seidel G, Greis C, Sonne J, Kaps M. Harmonic grey scale imaging of the human brain. J Neuroimaging 1999;9:171–174.

17. Schlief R, Schürmann R, Balzer T, et al. Saccharide Based Contrast Agents. In N Nanda, R Schlief (eds), Advances in Echo Imaging Using Contrast Enhancement. Amsterdam: Kluwer Academic Publishers, 1993;71–96.

18. Gahn G, Ackerman, RH, Candia, MR, et al. Dodecafluoropentane ultrasonic contrast enhancement in carotid diagnosis: preliminary results. J Ultrasound Med 1999;18:101–108.

19. Sitzer M, Fürst G, Siebler M, Steinmetz H. Usefulness of an intravenous contrast medium in the characterization of high-grade internal carotid stenosis with color Doppler-assisted duplex imaging. Stroke 1994;25:385–389.

20. Fürst G, Sitzer M, Hofer M, et al. Kontrastmittelverstärkte farbkodierte Duplexsonographie hochgradiger Karotisstenosen. Ultraschall Med 1995;16: 140–144.

21. Sitzer M, Rose G, Steinmetz H, et al. Characteristics and clinical value of an intravenous echo-enhancement agent in evaluation of high-grade internal carotid stenosis. J Neuroimaging 1997;7[suppl 1]:S22–S25.

22. Droste DW, Jurgens R, Nabavi DG, et al. Echo contrast-enhanced ultrasound of extracranial internal carotid artery high-grade stenosis and occlusion. Stroke 1999;30:2302–2306.

23. Hetzel A, Eckenweber B, Trummer B, et al. Colour-coded duplex sonography of preocclusive carotid stenoses. Eur J Ultrasound 1998;8:181–191.

24. Nabavi DG, Droste DW, Schulte-Altedorneburg G, et al. Klinische bedeutung der echokontrastverstärkung in der neurovaskulären diagnostik. Fortschr Neurol Psychiat 1998;66:466–473.

25. Forsberg F, Liu JB, Burns PN, et al. Artifacts in ultrasonic contrast agent studies. J Ultrasound Med 1994;13:357–365.

26. Postert T, Braun B, Federlein J, et al. Diagnosis and monitoring of middle cerebral artery occlusion with contrast-enhanced transcranial color-coded realtime sonography in patients with inadequate acoustic bone windows. Ultrasound Med Biol 1998;24:333–340.

27. Nabavi DG, Droste DW, Kemeny V, et al. Potential and limitations of echocontrast-enhanced ultrasonography in acute stroke patients: a pilot study. Stroke 1998;29:949–954.

28. Nabavi DG, Droste DW, Schulte-Altedorneburg G, et al. Diagnostic benefit of echocontrast enhancement for the insufficient transtemporal bone window. J Neuroimaging 1999; 9:102–107.

29. Goertler M, Kross R, Baeumer M, et al. Diagnostic impact and prognostic relevance of early contrast-enhanced transcranial color-coded duplex sonography in acute stroke. Stroke 1998;29:955–962.

30. Gerriets T, Seidel G, Fiss I, et al. Contrast-enhanced transcranial color-coded duplex sonography: efficiency and validity. Neurology 1999;52:1133–1137.

31. Gahn G, Gerber J, Hallmeyer S, et al. Noninvasive assessment of the circle of Willis in cerebral ischemia: the potential of CT angiography and contrast-enhanced transcranial color-coded duplex sonography. Cerebrovasc Dis 1999;9:290–294.

32. Gahn G, Gerber J, Hallmeyer S, et al. Contrast-enhanced transcranial color-coded duplex sonography in stroke patients with limited bone windows. AJNR Am J Neuroradiol 2000;21:509–514.

33. National Institute of Neurological Disorders and Stroke rt-PA Study Group. Tissue plasminogen activator for acute ischemic stroke. N Engl J Med 1995;333:1581–1587.

34. Hacke W, Kaste M, Fieschi C, et al. Intravenous thrombolysis with recombinant tissue plasminogen activator for acute hemispheric stroke. The European Cooperative Acute Stroke Study (ECASS). JAMA 1995;274:1017–1025.

35. Hacke W, Kaste M, Fieschi C, et al. Randomised double-blind placebo-controlled trial of thrombolytic therapy with intravenous alteplase in acute ischemic stroke (ECASSII). Second European-Australasian Acute Stroke Study Investigators. Lancet 1998;352:1245–1251.

36. Furlan A, Higashida R, Wechsler L, et al. Intra-arterial prourokinase for acute ischemic stroke. The PROACT II study: a randomized controlled trial. Prolyse in acute cerebral thromboembolism. JAMA 1999;282:2003–2011.

37. Gerriets T, Postert T, Goertler M, et al. DIAS I: Duplex-sonographic assessment of the cerebrovascular status in acute stroke. A useful tool for future stroke trials. Stroke 2000;31:2342–2345.

38. Droste DW, Jurgens R, Weber S, et al. Benefit of echocontrast-enhanced transcranial color-coded duplex ultrasound in the assessment of intracranial collateral pathways. Stroke 2000;31:920–923.

39. Becker G, Lindner A, Bogdahn U. Imaging of the vertebrobasilar system by transcranial color-coded real-time sonography. J Ultrasound Med 1993;12:395–401.

40. Droste DW, Nabavi DG, Kemeny V, et al. Echo contrast enhanced transcranial colour-coded duplex offers improved visualization of the vertebrobasilar system. Acta Neurol Scand 1998;98:193–199.

41. Stolz E, Kaps M, Dorndorf W. Transcranial color-coded duplex sonography of intracranial veins and sinuses in adults. Reference data from 130 volunteers. Stroke 1999;30:1070–1075.

42. Baumgartner RW, Gönner F, Arnold M, Müri RM. Transtemporal power- and frequency-based color-coded duplex sonography of cerebral veins and sinuses. AJNR Am J Neuroradiol 1997;18:1771–1781.

43. Stolz E, Kaps M, Dorndorf W. Assessment of intracranial venous hemodynamics in normals and patients with cerebral venous thrombosis. Stroke 1999;30:70–75.

44. Stolz E, Kaps M, Dorndorf W. Frontal bone windows for transcranial color-coded duplex sonography. Stroke 1999;30:814–820.

45. Puls I, Hauck K, Demuth K, et al. Diagnostic impact of cerebral transit time in the identification of microangiopathy in dementia: a transcranial ultrasound study. Stroke 1999;30:2291–2295.

46. Hoffmann O, Weih M, Schreiber S, et al. Measurement of cerebral circulation time by contrast-enhanced Doppler sonography. Cerebrovasc Dis 2000;10:142–146.

47. Burns PN. Harmonic imaging with ultrasound contrast agents. Clin Radiol 1996;51[suppl 1]:50–55.

48. Seidel G, Kaps M. Harmonic imaging of the vertebrobasilar system. Stroke 1997;28:1610–1613.

49. Frinking PJA, Bouakaz A, Kirkhorn J. Ultrasound contrast imaging: current and new potential methods. Ultrasound Med Biol 2000;26:965–975.

50. Burns PN, Simpson DH, Averkiou MA. Nonlinear imaging. Ultrasound Med Biol 2000;26[suppl 1]:S19–S22.

51. Porter TR. Transient response during contrast echocardiography. Adv Card Echo Contrast 1997;5:47–55.

52. Wiesmann M, Seidel G. Ultrasound perfusion imaging of the human brain. Stroke 2000;31:2421–2425.

53. Seidel G, Algermissen C, Katzer CA, Kaps M. Visualization of brain perfusion with harmonic gray scale and power Doppler technology: an animal pilot study. Stroke 2000;31:1728–1734.

54. Postert T, Braun B, Meves S, et al. Contrast-enhanced transcranial color-coded sonography in acute hemispheric brain infarction. Stroke 1999;30:1819–1826.

55. Postert T, Hoppe P, Federlein J, et al. Ultrasonic assessment of brain perfusion. Stroke 2000;31:1460–1462.

56. Seidel G, Algermissen C, Claassen L, et al. Harmonic imaging of the human brain. Visualization of brain perfusion with ultrasound. Stroke 2000;31:151–154.

57. Postert T, Federlein J, Weber S, et al. Second harmonic imaging in acute middle cerebral artery infarction. Preliminary results. Stroke 1999;30:1702–1706.

58. Wei K, Jayaweera AR, Firoozan S, et al. Quantification of myocardial blood flow with ultrasound-induced destruction of microbubbles administered as a constant venous infusion. Circulation 1998;97:473–483.

59. Haerten R. Power-Doppler-Verfahren. In U Bogdahn, G Becker, F Schlachetzki (eds), Echosignalverstärker und Transkranielle Farbduplex-Sonographie. Berlin: Blackwell, 1998;93–99.

60. Rubin JM, Adler RS. Power Doppler expands standard color capability. Diagn Imaging 1993;15(12):66–69.

61. Postert T, Meves S, Bornke C, et al. Power Doppler compared to color-coded duplex sonography in the assessment of the basal cerebral circulation. J Neuroimaging 1997;7:221–226.

62. Griewing B, Motsch L, Piek J, et al. Transcranial power mode Doppler duplex sonography of intracranial aneurysms. J Neuroimaging 1998;8:155–158.

63. Griewing B, Schminke U, Motsch L, et al. Transcranial duplex sonography of middle cerebral artery stenosis: a comparison of colour-coding techniques—frequency—or power-based Doppler and contrast enhancement. Neuroradiology 1998;40:490–495.

64. Baumgartner RW, Nirkko AC, Müri RM, Gönner F. Transoccipital power-based color-coded duplex sonography of cerebral sinuses and veins. Stroke 1997;28:1319–1323.

65. O'Donell M. Codex excitation systems for improving the penetration of real-time phased array imaging systems. EEE Trans Ultrason Ferroelectr Freq Control 1992;39:341–351.

66. Weskott HP. B-Flow—eine neue Methode zur Bluflussdetektion. Ultraschall Med 2000;21:59–65.

67. Tranquart F, Grenier N, Eder V, Pourcelot L. Clinical use of ultrasound tissue harmonic imaging. Ultrasound Med Biol 1999;25:889–894.

68. Puls I, Berg D, Mäurer M, et al. Transcranial sonography of the brain parenchyma: comparison of B-mode imaging and tissue harmonic imaging. Ultrasound Med Biol 2000;26:189–194.

69. Stolz E, Gerriets T, Fiss I, et al. Correlation of transcranial color-coded duplex sonography and CCT measurements for determining third ventricular midline shift in space occupying stroke. AJNR Am J Neuroradiol 1999;20:1567–1571.

70. Gerriets T, Stolz E, Modrau B, et al. Sonographic midline shift in hemispheric infarctions. Neurology 1999;52:45–49.

71. Nelson TR, Pretorius D. Three-dimensional ultrasound imaging. Ultrasound Med Biol 1998;24:1243–1270.

72. Palombo C, Kozakova M, Morizzo C, et al. Ultrafast three-dimensional ultrasound. Application to carotid artery imaging. Stroke 1998;29:1631–1637.

73. Schminke U, Motsch L, Hilker L, Kessler C. Three-dimensional ultrasound observation of carotid artery plaque ulceration. Stroke 2000;31:1651–1655.

CHAPTER 21

New Techniques in Computed Tomography, Magnetic Resonance Imaging, and Optical Imaging in Cerebrovascular Disease

Walter J. Koroshetz

A variety of imaging technologies enables the identification of cerebral ischemia and ischemic brain injury. Each has its own set of advantages and disadvantages as applied to patients with cerebrovascular disease. Over the past decade, the introduction of new imaging technology into the clinical arena has been impressive, and there is no sign that this trend toward more detailed imaging of brain ischemia and ischemic injury will slow down. The challenge is to understand the limitations of each imaging technique and to develop methods that overcome or minimize them. In addition, completely new imaging technology may fill important gaps that existing methods cannot. Two primary scenarios rule on the demand side: The first is the application of imaging technology to guide acute therapy in the patient with new-onset brain ischemia, and the second is the study of brain blood flow and metabolism as they relate to brain function, cerebrovascular reserve, the effects of vasoactive drugs, and interventional procedures. Advances in technology are driven by the needs of both neuroscience research and clinical practice. Characteristics of imaging technology that are highly regarded in clinical practice include accessibility, cost, ease, rapidity of image interpretation, and usefulness for a large segment of patients with cerebrovascular disease. Research questions vary depending on the line of biological investigation but often stress quantification and spatial or temporal resolution.

It is not possible to predict with accuracy all the techniques that will be developed to fill a void in clinical or research imaging of cerebrovascular disease. A number of techniques, however, have already demonstrated promise and are reviewed in this chapter.

FUTURE ADVANCES IN MAGNETIC RESONANCE IMAGING IN CEREBROVASCULAR DISEASE

Qualitative Perfusion Imaging

Currently, bolus-tracking perfusion magnetic resonance imaging (MRI) enables the physician or researcher to identify regions of brain with abnormal cerebral perfusion in stroke patients. The speed of echo-planar MRI allows multislice tracking of an intravenously delivered bolus of gadolinium as it passes through the brain vessels and parenchyma. The kinetics of this first-pass fall in signal intensity due to the magnetic susceptibility effects of the gadolinium can be analyzed to provide maps of relative cerebral blood flow (rCBF), increased relative mean transit time (rMTT), or decreased relative cerebral blood volume (rCBV). However, with bolus-tracking perfusion MRI, the degree of the perfusion abnormality can only be expressed as relative to other brain regions. Lack of quantification is one of the major limitations of the currently used perfusion techniques. Without the ability to quantify the change in flow, it is difficult to judge the physiologic significance of the perfusion abnormality. Positron emission tomography (PET) and xenon computed tomography (CT) have the advantage that flow can be quantified. Quantitative CBF thresholds have been established for tissue that will die and thresholds for tissue that is ischemic but salvageable (penumbra).[1] PET has the ability to detect the metabolic consequence of the decreased flow (increased oxygen extraction fraction, decreased glucose metabolism, decreased oxygen metabolism). PET thereby can determine whether the CBF decrease actually causes tissue ischemia. In the acute stroke patient, decreased apparent diffusion coefficient (ADC) on MRI provides evidence of ischemic injury. This diffusion-weighted MRI (DWI) abnormality, however, comes with a variable delay after the onset of ischemia. The fate of regions with normal blood volume, normal ADC but increased MTT, and decreased CBF are difficult to predict. In patients with this mismatch—rMTT lesion greater than DWI lesion—the size of the perfusion abnormality usually exceeds the size of the final infarct but by an unpredictable amount (Figure 21-1). The significance of finding decreased rCBF or increased rMTT outside of the acute stroke scenario is even more difficult to know with certainty.[2]

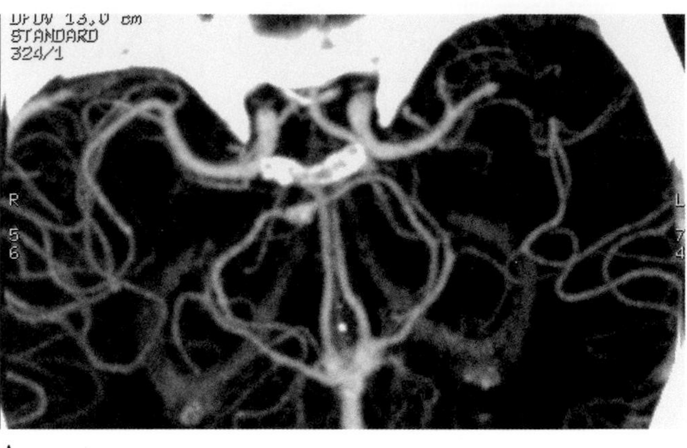

A

FIGURE 21-1. This patient presented with aphasia and right hemiparesis after awakening. The initial computed tomographic contrast study demonstrated distal occlusion of middle cerebral artery as seen in (**A**). (*continued*)

Maps of the Probability of Infarction

One strategy used to circumvent the lack of specificity inherent in relative perfusion imaging has been to empirically examine the acute images and compare them region by region with the final infarct. The degree of the relative perfusion abnormality in a specific clinical setting is used to help determine the most likely outcome of the tissue. Based on the MR signature provided by the various image sequences, the tissue is ascribed a specific probability of dying or living.[3] We examine the probability of tissue death by a reiterative process of analyzing pixel by pixel data from the rCBF, rCBV, rMTT, and DWI images from multiple patients to derive a computer model that predicts eventual tissue fate (Figure 21-2).[4] The model provides a powerful statistical tool with which to evaluate therapies for their ability to alter the expected distribution of the infarct. However, this is a purely empiric method, and its applicability is likely limited to the acute stroke scenario in which the model was developed. Such models may give different results depending on the interval between symptom onset and the image acquisition. For instance, at 24 hours from onset, the DWI abnormality is a much better predictor of infarct size than the rMTT abnormality, but DWI grossly underestimates infarct size 30 minutes from onset; in this time frame, perfusion maps may more accurately predict final infarct. A second general method is to examine the perfusion data for specific abnormalities that occur early on and are predictive of infarction. The decrease in rCBV is one such transition, which is highly predictive of infarct. Another method uses the noise in the perfusion data to establish patterns, which are highly correlated with infarction. In normally perfused brain tissue, there is heterogeneity to the kinetics of flow through the small vessels. In ischemic tissue, the flow becomes more homogeneous. A function related to the degree of lost flow heterogeneity was found to predict regions in the zone of abnormal perfusion most likely to be included in the final infarct (Figure 21-3).[5]

Absolute quantification of CBF with bolus-tracking perfusion MRI is difficult. One reason is that the amount of blood entering the tissue to be imaged is not known. This is estimated by measuring an arterial input function (AIF) taken from the gadolinium signal change originating from pixels associated with a feeding artery. However, this vascular signal intensity is not directly proportional to the concentration of gadolinium. The flow velocity, the size of the vessel, and the orientation of the vessel with respect to the magnetic field affect the signal intensity. In patients with multiple stenotic or occlusive lesions, the AIF for one vascular territory may not be the exact AIF for all the other brain regions. Current techniques are also overly sensitive to delay in arrival of blood to the microvascular bed and dispersion of the input function due to vascular stenosis or multiple pathways of blood flow to the tissue. What would be most desirable is an AIF for each pixel imaged. The use of an AIF over a single large feeding artery is often not optimal. Without a quantitative measurement of the AIF, it is not possible to quantify the parenchymal flow. Improvement is still possible. Compensation for the nonlinearity in the AIF may improve perfusion mapping in the future.[6] Using contrast agents with higher magnetic susceptibility effects may help the currently used qualitative perfusion measurements in the future. This will allow greater signal intensity and a more rapid injection of the bolus (less volume injected at the same rate), which will result in a tighter AIF.

Arterial Spin Labeling

One MR technique promises to overcome the problem of lack of quantification of CBF. Called *arterial spin*

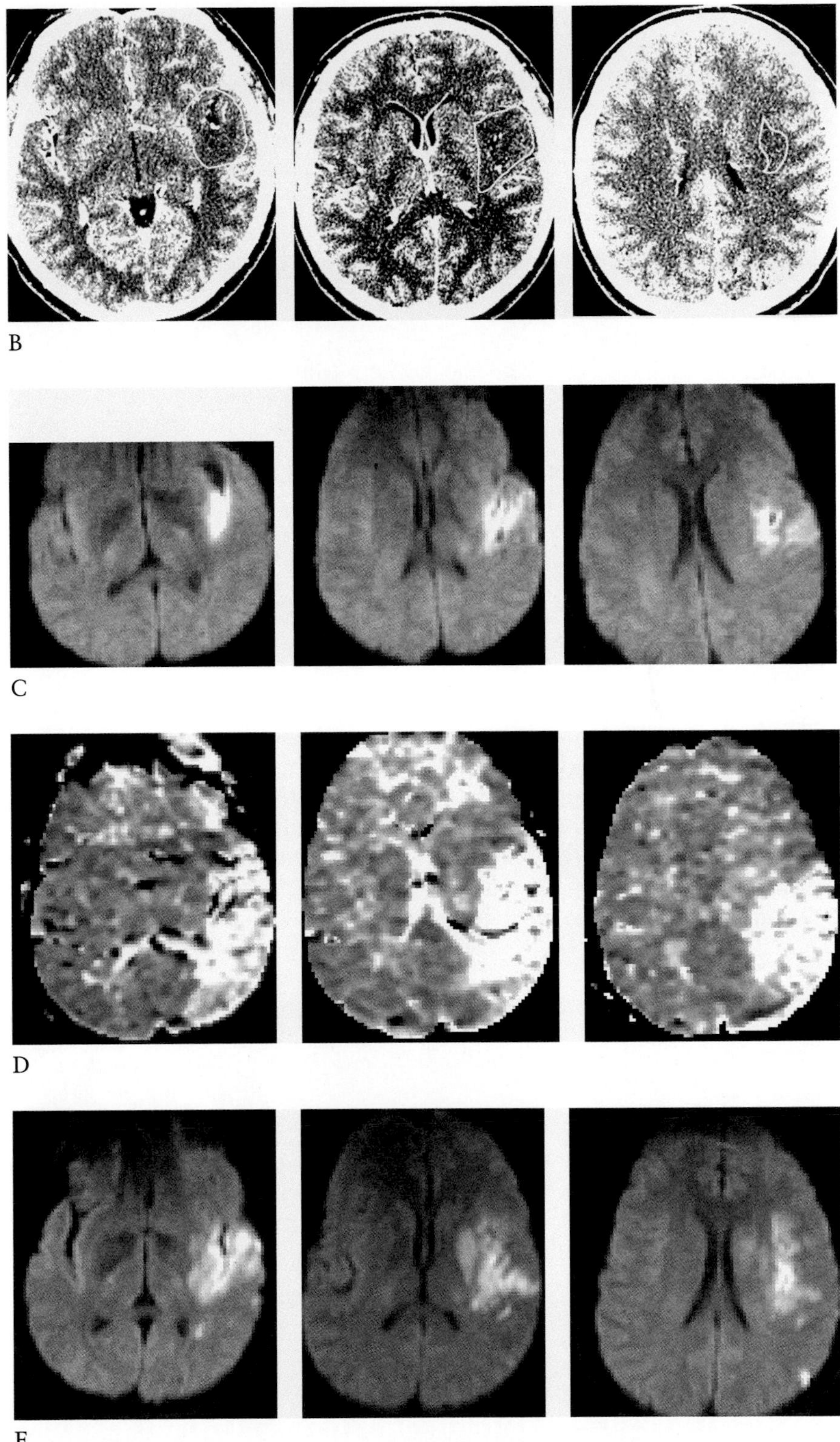

FIGURE 21-1. *Continued.* Unprocessed contrast-enhanced images (whole-brain perfused blood volume images) demonstrate low density in the perisylvian and superior division (**B**). Diffusion-weighted magnetic resonance imaging (MRI) performed 15 minutes later shows similar distribution of abnormality (**C**), as did the computed tomographic images. The relative mean transit time maps from perfusion MRI (**D**) show a much wider territory of abnormal perfusion. However, the relative mean transit time does not specifically define the final infarct. The final infarct seen on the diffusion-weighted MRI 5 days later (**E**) shows enlargement of the infarct, but most of the territory that is abnormal on the initial relative mean transit time maps remains unscathed.

labeling (ASL), this technique uses electromagnetically labeled arterial water as a diffusible tracer. It comes close to providing a separate AIF for each imaged pixel without the contamination due to delay or dispersion that occurs with the bolus-tracking technique. ASL thereby enables quantitative MR measurements of brain blood flow.[7] CBF measurements using ASL have been validated using quantitative H_2 oxygen-15 PET.[8] ASL is not routinely used at present, because it has a much-decreased signal to noise ratio as compared to bolus tracking. Therefore, longer imaging time is required for multislice studies. Consequently, it is

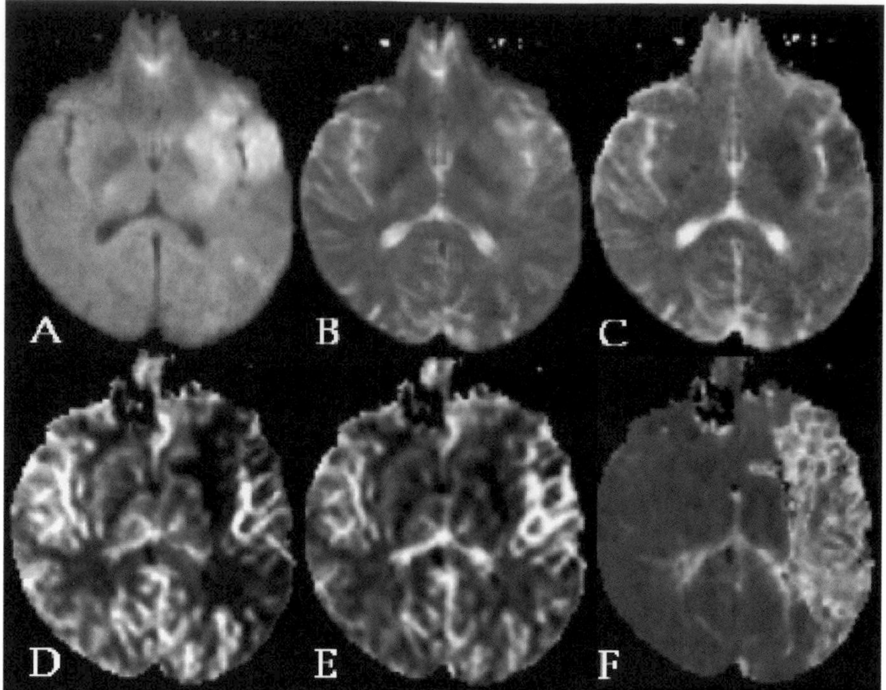

FIGURE 21-2. Magnetic resonance study at 7 hours after onset in a patient presenting with symptoms of right-sided homonymous hemianopia, aphasia, and hemiparesis. Shown are the initial diffusion-weighted magnetic resonance image (**A**), T2 echo-planar image (**B**), apparent diffusion coefficient (**C**), cerebral blood flow (**D**), cerebral blood volume (**E**), and mean transit time maps (**F**). Relative cerebral blood flow and relative mean transit time are abnormal throughout the left middle cerebral artery territory. The diffusion-weighted magnetic resonance image shows injury only in the perisylvian region.

also more sensitive to patient motion. Methodologic advances and higher field strength magnets may make it the preferred method of perfusion MRI in the future.[9] The ASL technique can also be combined with an intravascular contrast agent to enable the simultaneous measurement of both CBV and CBF.[10] A different application of this ability to label inflowing water is also of potential interest. The water flowing through a specific vessel (e.g., one carotid artery) can be electromagnetically tagged and then followed as it passes through the brain vessels and parenchyma. This allows characterization of the vascular territory of a single vessel, providing information similar to the delayed phase of direct cerebral angiography.[11]

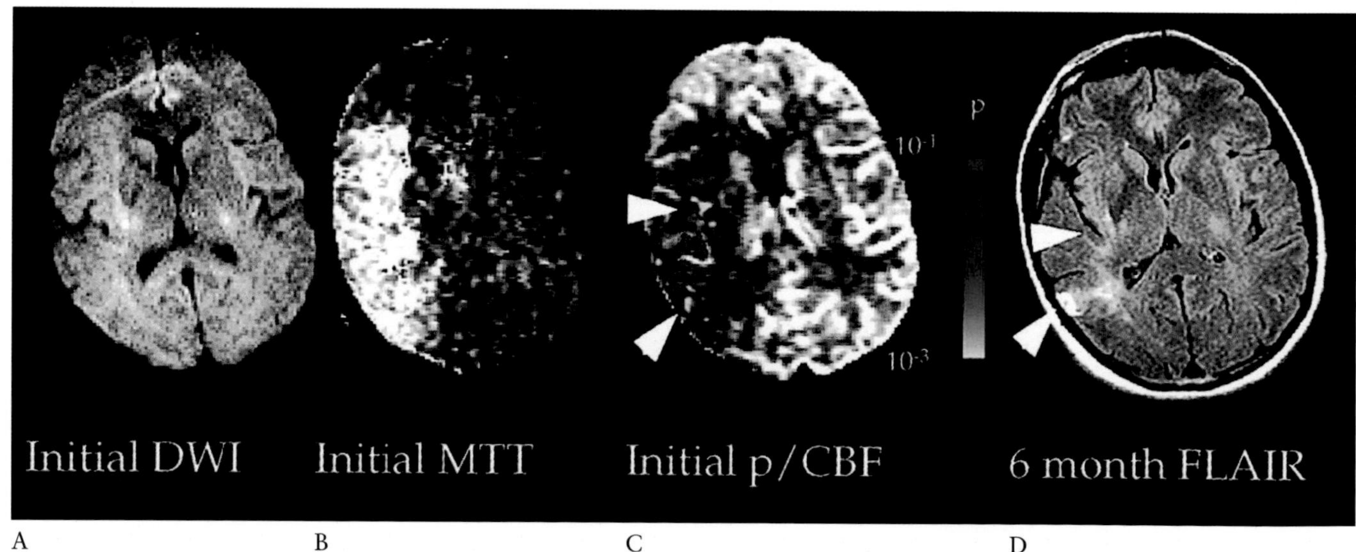

FIGURE 21-3. Map of flow heterogeneity in a patient presenting with right middle cerebral stroke syndrome. The diffusion-weighted magnetic resonance image (DWI) (**A**) is still normal, but the mean transit time (MTT) (**B**) and cerebral blood flow (CBF) (**C**) maps show abnormal perfusion (p) throughout the right middle cerebral territory. Infarction as seen on the 6-month follow-up study developed in those regions with reduced flow heterogeneity (color overlay of the p function of flow heterogeneity on the CBF map). **D.** Six-month fluid-attenuated inversion recovery (FLAIR). (Courtesy of Dr. Leif Ostergaard.)

Blood Oxygen Level–Dependent Technique in Cerebrovascular Disease

Blood oxygen level–dependent (BOLD) imaging has revolutionized the study of topographic brain activation. A change in regional magnetic susceptibility occurs, which may be due to change in the concentration of deoxyhemoglobin or a change in CBV, and is linked to physiologic brain activation. The signal difference is quite small so that the technique is most suited to activation paradigms that allow subtraction of the resting state images. In patients with cerebrovascular disease, the technique has importance in allowing the study of reallocation of neurologic functions to other brain regions during recovery from stroke-related deficits. The region of brain that is activated during performance of a specific neurologic task can be followed as performance on the task improves in the months after stroke. It also offers the potential to study cerebrovascular reserve in response to hypercapnia, acetazolamide,[12] or the effects of vasoactive drugs.[13] Recently, the technique has been used to detect spreading perfusion changes associated with spreading migraine aura.[14] Resting state BOLD maps in patients with ischemic stroke currently suffer from very low signal intensity, but the technique may yet have value in detecting clinically significant alterations in blood volume.[15]

Diffusion Tensor Imaging

Diffusion imaging is sensitive to the changes in the ease with which water can diffuse in the brain tissue. Its value in acute stroke comes from the drop in the ADC of water. This occurs when water shifts from the extracellular to the intracellular space as a consequence of energy failure. The technique is also sensitive enough to distinguish the ease with which water can diffuse in different directions. This component, related to differential diffusion of water in different directions, is called *anisotropy*. Anisotropy is most conspicuous in the white matter, whereas water is more likely to diffuse along the path of the axons/myelin than perpendicular to this path. Computational methods have been brought to use this feature of DWI to identify and map fiber tracts in the brain.[16] Diffusion tensor images are composed of vectors indicating the direction of the white matter fibers. This technique may finally allow tract finding in human white matter. It will be important in the identification of the consequences of Wallerian degeneration[17] and the disconnection of gray matter circuits that occurs after white matter injury. In addition, changes in anisotropy occur in an early stage of white matter ischemia, likely due to the disruption of normal bundling of fiber tracts with interspersed layers of extracellular water.[18] This change in anisotropy in ischemic white matter may be more sensitive than the commonly used technique of isotropic DWI.[19]

Magnetic Resonance Spectroscopy

Nuclear MR spectroscopy can provide information on the relative concentrations of brain chemicals. Above all others, this method has the greatest potential to help unravel the biochemical events that occur in ischemic brain. It relies on the electromagnetic excitation of atoms with unpaired electrons in their outer shell. Hydrogen, because it has only one electron, absorbs energy, and the frequency at which this excitation occurs depends on the local magnetic field in which the hydrogen-1 (^{1}H) is located. The strength of the local magnetic field around the hydrogen atoms varies for different molecules. This dependence of the resonance frequency for excitation or chemical shift allows the separation of the hydrogen spectra into peaks, each of which is due to a specific molecule. The height of any single peak is proportional to the number of hydrogen atoms giving rise to the peak. Peak height (or area under the peak) is, therefore, related to the concentration of the chemical species in the brain region from which the spectra are obtained. To obtain sufficient signal, the spectra are obtained from voxels of brain tissue. The investigator can set the size and brain location of the voxel. The signal from water must be suppressed or else it dwarfs all the other neurochemicals. The primary technical problem is the difficulty in separating the myriad of peaks related to all the different molecules in brain. This is a function of the multiple chemicals present, the low signal strength, and the difficulty in establishing a homogeneous magnetic field throughout the voxel of tissue to be measured. As a result, currently available spectra from brain show broadening of the spectral peaks arising from different chemicals. Line width broadening leads to overlap of the spectra and results in the inability to resolve many of the different chemical peaks.

^{1}H nuclear MR spectroscopy has been used to study a number of brain disorders, including stroke.[20] Its usefulness now relies primarily on its ability to resolve the spectral peaks—and therefore on the ability to measure relative concentrations—of only a handful of chemicals. These more easily measured chemicals include (1) *N*-acetyl aspartate, a neuronal marker that decreases in cerebral ischemia and other conditions associated with neuronal or axonal loss; (2) choline, which is present in lipid and is increased in gliosis; (3) creatine, which is relatively constant throughout the various neural cells; (4) lactate, which is generated through anaerobic metabolism by neural and inflammatory cells (it is a known marker of brain ischemia); and (5) lipid. The hydrogen spectra from brain, however, contain peaks from many more biochemicals. With improved techniques and higher field strength magnets, the spectra related to other biochemicals that are important in stroke might be resolved. The technique promises to become more important in stroke research in the future.

A variety of other atoms are amenable to MR spectroscopy. Phosphorus-31 (^{31}P) spectroscopy has been proved valuable in a variety of clinical and neuroscientific contexts. ^{31}P spectroscopy allows resolution of peaks due to adenosine triphosphate (ATP) and inorganic phosphorus. The technique, therefore, allows detection of a fall in the ratio of brain ATP/brain inorganic phosphorus as occurs with energy failure in the setting of ischemia. Together with ^{1}H lactate spectroscopy, ^{31}P spectroscopy provides information on the metabolic consequences of a change in blood flow. This is needed to differentiate physiologically acceptable decreases in CBF from those that are associated with impaired metabolism (i.e., tissue ischemia). As PET defines ischemia by decreased CBF associated with increased oxygen extraction fraction, tissue ischemia by MR spectroscopy could be defined as a decrease in CBF associated with inadequate levels of ATP and a shift to glycolytic metabolism-elevating lactate. Carbon-13 (^{13}C) MR spectroscopy may also enable more detailed examination of brain metabolism. Administration of ^{13}C-labeled glucose can be followed by MR spectroscopy measurements of the concentrations of tricarboxylic acid cycle metabolites on the pathway to ATP synthesis.[21] The use of MR spectroscopy to dissect abnormalities in brain metabolism is in its infancy.

Technical advances, together with the application of advanced MR spectroscopy techniques to the study of brain ischemia, should open a new field of in vivo imaging of brain metabolism. As discussed, concerns for adequate signal strength necessitate measurement in fairly large voxels of brain tissue. Because of the regional heterogeneity that occurs in the brain of stroke patients, single-voxel imaging offers limited information. Interpretation is always impaired by the concern that the measurements are determined by voxel location (e.g., core vs. periphery of infarct, volume averaging with normal brain). The MR spectroscopy signal, however, is amplified at higher magnetic field strengths. With 1.5T- and high field strength magnets, it is possible to obtain signal from multiple smaller voxels[22] and actually construct a brain image based on the concentration of a specific brain chemical. This technique, called *chemical shift imaging*, may be exceedingly valuable for the study of stroke. High field strength—3T- or 7T-magnets—are now being used to improve the signal to noise ratio. New methods of providing a homogeneous magnetic field throughout the brain are also being developed to further this technology.[23] Multislice maps of brain lactate/creatine or *N*-acetyl aspartate/creatine ratios[24] or ATP[25] may soon allow study of the metabolic consequences of a drop in CBF or increased MTT in stroke patients. Combining metabolic chemical shift imaging, quantitative perfusion imaging, DWI, and anatomic imaging, MR should rival PET as the most powerful investigational method to study brain ischemia in humans.

BOLUS-TRACKING COMPUTED TOMOGRAPHY PERFUSION IMAGING

Much like perfusion MRI, the helical CT x-ray scanners are now fast enough to follow the first pass of an intravenous bolus of CT dye through the brain parenchyma. The same algorithms underlying bolus-tracking perfusion MRI can be modified to compute CBF, CBV, and MTT after an intravenous bolus of CT contrast. In addition, as opposed to the situation with MR contrast, the change in signal intensity (Hounsfield units) in the large artery chosen for the AIF is directly proportional to the concentration of CT contrast. Therefore, unlike bolus-tracking perfusion MRI, CT perfusion imaging enables better quantitative measurement of CBF, MTT, and CBV.[26,27] Values of perfusion parameters using the bolus-tracking CT perfusion technique have been validated against other means of measuring quantitative blood flow.[28]

The major disadvantage of CT perfusion imaging, as opposed to MR, is the current limitation to a single slice of brain. The most advanced helical CT scanner on the market currently has four detectors separated by 0.5 cm. This allows imaging the first pass of an intravenous bolus of contrast through the brain with repetitive scanning but only in a 2-cm slab. Echo-planar MRI is fast enough to repetitively image the passage of gadolinium on multiple slices covering the whole brain. Recent studies have demonstrated that thresholds of CBF and CBV measured by single-slice CT perfusion predict which brain regions in the slice will be included in the final infarct.[29,30] Although it provides quantitative data that are useful for investigative questions, the clinical significance of the study may vary with slice placement. Quantitation is also dependent on selection of the AIF from a large artery directly supplying the tissue in question. Values may vary with the artery selected, and obtaining an accurate input function from a given artery may not always be possible. Correlations with established quantitative CBF techniques such as xenon CT or PET have provided only limited data thus far. This technique will become exceedingly powerful in the future if new-generation helical CT scanners incorporate enough spread between the detectors to allow more complete sampling of the entire brain and improvement in the accuracy of the AIF.

Less important negative aspects of the CT perfusion technique include x-ray exposure and the potential renal toxicity of the x-ray contrast. The major advantage of CT perfusion imaging stems from its ease of performance and ability to quantify blood flow. Most emergency services are organized to perform CT scanning for diagnostic imaging in critically ill patients. The perfusion study, coming immediately after a standard CT scan for acute stroke, adds only an additional 5 minutes. Most likely, CT measurement of CBF/CBV will be performed as part of the anatomic contrast study of the cerebral vasculature (CT angiography combined with whole-brain blood volume imaging; see the section Whole-Brain Blood Volume Imaging). Currently, quantitative CT perfusion imaging requires a separate bolus injection in addition to that needed for CT angiography.

Whole-Brain Blood Volume Imaging

In performing CT angiography, a number of groups noticed that if the imaging sequence is continued above the circle of Willis and through the entire brain, there is obvious heterogeneity in the parenchymal contrast enhancement.[31] Brain tissue in the region of the suspected infarction appears darker than the surrounding normal tissue. Brain tissue with vessels that can no longer be filled with blood accumulates less intravascular contrast and appears less bright on CT. These regions have reduced blood volume. Though not quantitative, these simple whole-brain images of "perfused blood volume" demonstrate a decrease in contrast enhancement after bolus injection in brain regions with high probability of infarction. MR-based CBV studies have shown the value of abnormal CBV in predicting eventual infarction. This transition to abnormal blood volume may have an important biologic basis and consequences. Occlusion of the microvasculature due to platelet, fibrin, or inflammatory processes would be expected to lead to severe reduction in tissue blood volume and result in permanent infarction if the microvascular plugging precludes tissue reperfusion (i.e., no-reflow phenomenon).

The imaging of brain parenchyma immediately after bolus contrast injection for CT angiography has proved valuable in the acute stroke setting. It is easy to obtain, as it only requires bolus injection of CT contrast and triggering the scanner to begin imaging, when the bolus is expected to reach the cerebral vessels. In most institutions, whole-brain CT perfusion is done by continuing the CT angiography imaging sequence to include axial images of the whole brain. Interpretation does not require post-processing, although it is beneficial to set the window and level settings to allow a high contrast (W30, L30) when viewing the images for regions of hypodensity. In our experience, the whole-brain perfused blood volume images (WBPBVI) have been found to (1) increase the sensitivity of detecting abnormalities related to stroke on CT,[32] (2) increase the clinician's ability to predict the clinical stroke subtype and the brain territory affected,[32] and (3) predict with high specificity that regions abnormal on WBPBVI go on to infarction.[33] In our study of patients undergoing successful recanalization of the middle cerebral artery, we found that the eventual stroke volume size was equal to size of the initial WBPBVI abnormality. In contrast, in patients in whom the recanalization attempts were unsuccessful, the final infarct size was much larger than the initial WBPBVI abnormality. These data indicate that brain regions with CBV that are decreased to the point that there is hypodensity on the CT perfusion images are likely to progress to infarction, even if the middle cerebral artery reopens. In fact, our studies of WBPBVI followed by MRI (Figure 21-4) demonstrate that the regional hypodensity on the CT perfusion highly correlates with the regional hyperdensity on the subsequent DWI.[34] This relationship is expected based on the MR experience, indicating that regions with decreased rCBV usually are abnormal on DWI.

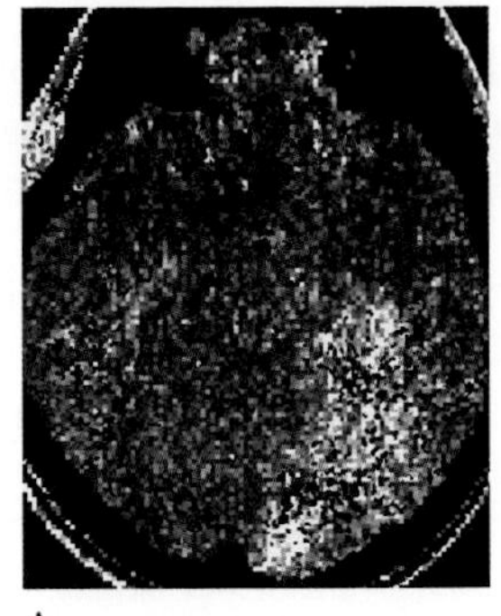

A

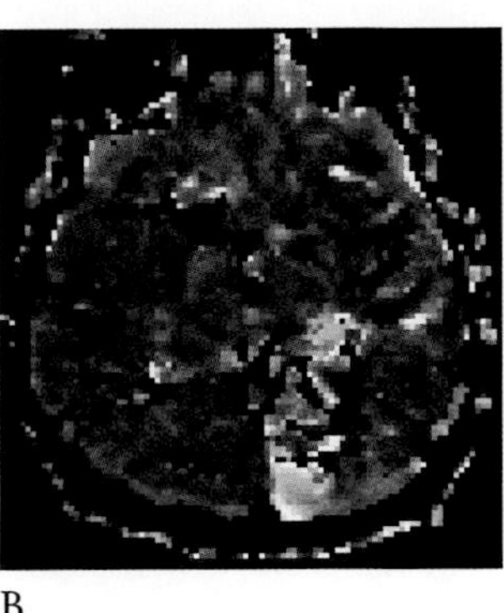

B

FIGURE 21-4. Mean transit time maps in a patient with an acute left posterior cerebral artery stroke. **A.** Computed tomography bolus-tracking technique. **B.** Magnetic resonance. (Courtesy of Dr. Michael Lev.)

This easy and inexpensive technique is available to any program using a helical CT scanner. It has the potential to revolutionize stroke imaging. CT scan is currently the standard first imaging technique for the patient with a stroke-like syndrome. It is fast and easily accessible in any primary stroke center. The addition of an intravenous bolus of CT contrast enables both assessment of the vascular lesion by CTA and identification of regions with abnormal perfused blood volume. CT, once considered to be normal in the acute ischemic stroke patient, now can be used to issue a complete diagnostic workup in a matter of minutes.

TRANSCRANIAL OPTICAL IMAGING OF BRAIN ISCHEMIA

In the coming decades, the imaging techniques discussed previously will give more detailed information about brain ischemia and its metabolic and structural consequences. However, each provides a "snapshot" of brain pathology and is limited by the relative difficulty of performing serial studies. CT and MR are poorly suited as "monitors" of brain ischemia. A method to continuously monitor cerebral perfusion and metabolism would be tremendously valuable in guiding therapy and detecting important changes. Diffuse optical tomography (DOT) is a method under development that may fill this gap.

Biologic tissue is relatively transparent to light in the near-infrared range between 700 to 1,000 nm. This is due to the fact that water absorption and hemoglobin absorption are relatively small within this wavelength region. This near-infrared wavelength range represents an "optical window" for the noninvasive assessment of brain tissue.[35] Oxyhemoglobin, deoxyhemoglobin, and an exogenous agent, indocyanine green, absorb at different wavelengths in the near-infrared range. Near-infrared spectroscopy is currently in clinical use, using devices with single source and detector, acting as a global brain partial pressure of oxygen monitor. These devices are poorly suited for stroke patients in whom the abnormalities are regional, not global. DOT uses multiple sender-receiver pairs to obtain spatial information regarding the absorption of light by oxyhemoglobin and deoxyhemoglobin cytochromes. The hope is that DOT will offer images of regional oxyhemoglobin to deoxyhemoglobin ratio and blood volume. Changes in brain hemoglobin concentration and oxygen saturation can now be detected with DOT in response to brain activation. The basis for this effect is likely similar to that discussed in the section Blood Oxygen Level–Dependent Technique in Cerebrovascular Disease. Blood flow and volume may be estimated by tracking an intravenous bolus of indocyanine green through the brain. Although signals related to brain activation can be obtained with transcranial near-infrared spectroscopy spatial localization of the signal, differentiation of scalp from brain signal and validation of the technique in patients with brain ischemia are yet needed to show value in clinical stroke. The technique is especially well suited to the study of infants and children because the skull is less of an impediment and the brain is smaller. Other techniques, such as CT and MRI, are difficult in young patients because of the need for immobilization.

DOT can noninvasively detect the changes in hemoglobin absorption that accompany brain activity in adult human subjects. Several types of brain activities have been assessed, including motor activity,[36] visual activation,[37] auditory stimulation,[38] and performance of cognitive tasks.[39] In recent years, a more sophisticated system allowing diffuse optical imaging has been developed.

Four properties of optical spectroscopy make it the futuristic device of choice in monitoring stroke patients. First, optical spectroscopy can be used to monitor blood oxygenation and volume as reflected by the relative absorption of oxyhemoglobin and deoxyhemoglobin. Second, optical spectroscopy imaging can detect regions of intracerebral hemorrhage as reflected by a change in the reflectance of the brain tissue and major increase in hemoglobin concentration. Third, optical spectroscopy can be extended to obtain tomographic images that reveal spatial variations in the cortical blood oxygenation and tissue perfusion and brain hemorrhage. Fourth, optical imaging can be used to map CBF by analyzing the kinetics of the first pass of an intravenous bolus of indocyanine green.[40] Indocyanine green is an intravascular dye commonly used to compute cardiac output in patients.

CONCLUSION

Advances in brain imaging have completely redefined how we diagnose and manage acute stroke patients. Some techniques are expensive and exquisitely detailed, others inexpensive and widely available. It is now possible to measure the changes in brain perfusion and to determine whether treatment can prevent brain tissue from dying or reverse the level of ischemia. The brain of the patient with cerebrovascular disease no longer needs to be treated as a black box. The technology to measure cerebral perfusion and early phases of ischemic injury has advanced far faster than our knowledge of its clinical usefulness. However, with the dispersion of the technology into stroke centers around the world, the clinical/imaging correlation information should begin to accumulate. Besides the challenge of developing new technology, we must also meet the challenge to assess existing technology for its ability to decrease patient mortality and morbidity, improve eventual functional disability, and limit overall stroke-related medical costs.

REFERENCES

1. Baron JC. Perfusion thresholds in human cerebral ischemia: historical perspective and therapeutic implications. Cerebrovasc Dis 2001;11:[Suppl 1]:2–8.

2. Lythgoe DJ, Ostergaard L, William SC, et al. Quantitative perfusion imaging in carotid artery stenosis using dynamic susceptibility contrast-enhanced magnetic resonance imaging. Magn Reson Imaging 2000; 18(1):1–11.

3. Jacobs MA, Zhang ZG, Knight RA, et al. A model for multiparametric MRI tissue characterization in experimental cerebral ischemia with histological validation in rat: part 1. Stroke 2001;32(4):943–949.

4. Wu O, Koroshetz WJ, Ostergaard L, et al. Predictive models of tissue outcome in acute human cerebral ischemia based on combined diffusion- and perfusion-weighted imaging. Stroke 2001;32:933–942.

5. Ostergaard L, Sorensen AG, Chesler DA, et al. Combined diffusion-weighted and perfusion-weighted heterogeneity magnetic resonance imaging. Stroke 2000;31:1097.

6. Ellinger R, Kremser C, Schocke MF, et al. The impact of peak saturation of the arterial input function on quantitative evaluation of dynamic susceptibility

contrast-enhanced MR studies. J Comp Assist Tomogr 2000;24(6):942–948.

7. Chalela JA, Alsop DC, Gonzalez-Atavales JB, et al. Magnetic resonance perfusion imaging in acute ischemic stroke using continuous arterial spin labeling Stroke 2000;31(3):680–687.

8. Ye FQ, Berman KF, Ellmore T, et al. $H_2{}^{15}O$ PET validation of steady-state arterial spin tagging cerebral blood flow measurements in humans. Magn Reson Med 2000;44(3):450–456.

9. Franke C, van Dorsten FA, Olah L. Arterial spin tagging perfusion imaging of rat brain: dependency on magnetic field strength. Magn Reson Imaging 2000;18(9):1109–1113.

10. Zaharchuk G, Bogdanov AA Jr, Marota JJ, et al. Continuous assessment of perfusion by tagging including volume and water extraction (CAPTIVE): a steady-state contrast agent technique for measuring blood flow, relative blood volume fraction, and the water extraction fraction. Magn Reson Med 1998; 40(5):666–678.

11. Zaharchuk G, Ledden PJ, Kwong KK, et al. Multislice perfusion and perfusion territory imaging in humans with separate label and image coils. Magn Reson Med 1999;41(6):1093–1098.

12. Kastrup A, Kruger G, Neumann-Haefelin T, Moseley ME. Assessment of cerebrovascular reactivity with functional magnetic resonance imaging: comparison of CO_2 and breath holding. Magn Reson Imaging 2001;19(1):13–20.

13. Mandeville G, Jenkins BG, Kosofsky BE, et al. Regional sensitivity and coupling of BOLD and CBV changes during stimulation of rat brain. Magn Reson Med 2001;45(3):443–447.

14. Hadjikhani N, Sanchez del Rio M, Wu O, et al. Mechanisms of migraine aura revealed by functional MRI in human visual cortex. Proc Natl Acad Sci U S A 2001;98(8):4687–4692.

15. Kavec M, Grohn OH, Kettunen MI, et al. Use of spin echo T(2) in assessment of cerebral misery perfusion at 1.5 T. MAGMA 2001;12(1):32–39.

16. Le Bihan D, Mangin JF, Poupon C, et al. Diffusion tensor imaging: concepts and applications. J Magn Reson Imaging 2001;13(4):534–546.

17. Werring DJ, Toosy AT, Clark CA, et al. Diffusion tensor imaging can detect and quantify corticospinal tract degeneration after stroke. J Neurol Neurosurg Psychiatry 2000;69(2):269–272.

18. Sorensen AG, Wu O, Copen WA, et al. Human acute cerebral ischemia: detection of changes in water diffusion anisotropy by using MR imaging. Radiology 1999;212:785–792.

19. Mukherjee P, Bahn MM, McKinstry RC, et al. Differences between gray matter and white matter water diffusion in stroke: diffusion-tensor MR imaging in 12 patients. Radiology 2000;215(1):211–220.

20. Wardlaw JM, Marshall I, Wild J, et al. Studies of acute ischemic stroke with proton magnetic resonance spectroscopy: relation between time from onset, neurological deficit, metabolite abnormalities in the infarct, blood flow, and clinical outcome. Stroke 1998; 29(8):1618–1624.

21. Chen W, Zhu XH, Gruetter R, et al. Study of tricarboxylic acid cycle flux changes in human visual cortex during Hemifield visual stimulation using ^1H-^{13}C MRS and fMRI. Magn Reson Med 2001;45(3):349–355.

22. Hanson LG, Adalsteinsson E, Pfefferbaum A, Spielman DM. Optimal voxel size for measuring global gray and white matter proton metabolite concentrations using chemical shift imaging. Magn Reson Med 2000;44(1):10–18.

23. Spielman DM, Adalsteinsson E, Lim KO. Quantitative assessment of improved homogeneity using higher-order shims for spectroscopic imaging of the brain. Magn Reson Med 1998;40(3):376–382.

24. Guimaraes AR, Baker JR, Jenkins BG, et al. Echoplanar chemical shift imaging. Magn Reson Med 1999;41(5):877–882.

25. Zakian KL, Koutcher JA, Ballon D. A dual-tuned resonator for proton-decoupled phosphorus-31 chemical shift imaging of the brain. Magn Reson Med 1999;41(4):809–815.

26. Cenic A, Nabavi DG, Craen RA, et al. Dynamic CT measurement of cerebral blood flow: a validation study. AJNR Am J Neuroradiol 1999;20:63–73.

27. Nabavi DG, Cenic A, Craen RA, et al. CT assessment of cerebral perfusion: experimental validation and initial clinical experience. Radiology 1999; 213:141–149.

28. Wintermark M, Thiran JP, Maeder P, et al. Simultaneous measurement of regional cerebral blood flow by perfusion CT and stable xenon CT: a validation study. AJNR Am J Neuroradiol 2001;22(5):905–914.

29. Koenig M, Kraus M, Theek C, et al. Quantitative assessment of the ischemic brain by means of perfusion-related parameters derived from perfusion CT. Stroke 2001;32(2):431–437.

30. Mayer TE, Hamann GF, Baranczyk J, et al. Dynamic CT perfusion imaging of acute stroke. Am J Neuroradiol 2000;21(8):1441–1449.

31. Hunter GJ, Hamberg LM, Ponzo JA, et al. Assessment of cerebral perfusion and arterial anatomy in hyperacute stroke with three-dimensional functional CT: early clinical results. AJNR Am J Neuroradiol 1998;19:29–37.

32. Ezeddine M, Lev MH, McDonald C, et al. Impact of Contrast CT Angiography and Whole Brain Contrast CT Perfusion Study on the Accuracy of Cerebrovascular Diagnosis in Patients Presenting with a Major Strokelike Syndrome. 26th International Confer-

ence on Stroke and Cerebral Circulation, Ft. Lauderdale, Florida, 2001.

33. Lev MH, Segal AZ, Farkas J, et al. Utility of perfusion-weighted CT imaging in acute middle cerebral artery stroke treated with intra-arterial thrombolysis: prediction of final infarct volume and clinical outcome. Stroke 2001;32:2021–2028.

34. Lev MH, Berzin TM, Symons S, et al. CT perfusion imaging versus MR diffusion weighted imaging: acute stroke detection and prediction of final infarct size. Proceedings of the 39th Annual Meeting of the American Society of Neuroradiology, Boston, Massachusetts, 2001.

35. Jobsis FF. Noninvasive infrared monitoring of cerebral and myocardial oxygen sufficiency and circulatory parameters. Science 1977;198:1264–1267.

36. Maki A, Yamashita Y, Ito Y, et al. Spatial and temporal analysis of human motor activity using noninvasive NIR tomography. Med Phys 1995;22:1997–2005.

37. Villringer A, Planck J, Hock C, et al. Near infrared spectroscopy (NIRS): a new tool to study hemodynamically changes during activation of brain function in human adults. Neurosci Lett 1993;154:101–104.

38. Hoshi Y, Tamura M. Dynamic multichannel near-infrared optical imaging of human brain activity. J Appl Physiol 1993;75:1842–1846.

39. Chance B, Kang K, He L, et al. Highly sensitive object location in tissue models with linear in-phase and anti-phase multi-element optical arrays in one and two dimensions. Proc Natl Acad Sci U S A 1993;90:3423–3427.

40. Kusaka T, Isobe K, Nagano K, et al. Estimation of regional cerebral blood flow distribution in infants by near-infrared topography using indocyanine green. Neuroimage 2001;13(5):944–952.

Index

Note: Numbers followed by *f* indicate figures; numbers followed by *t* indicate tables.